FIRST AID FOR THE® USMLE Step 3

Fourth Edition

TAO LE, MD, MHS
Associate Clinical Professor of Medicine and Pediatrics
Chief, Section of Allergy and Immunology
Department of Medicine
University of Louisville

VIKAS BHUSHAN, MD
Diagnostic Radiologist

JAMES S. YEH, MD, MPH
Attending Physician
Research Fellow
Department of Medicine
Brigham and Women's Hospital
Harvard Medical School

KACHIU CECILIA LEE, MD, MPH
Clinical and Research Fellow
Wellman Center for Photomedicine
Department of Dermatology
Massachusetts General Hospital
Harvard Medical School

New York   Chicago   San Francisco   Athens   London   Madrid   Mexico City
Milan   New Delhi   Singapore   Sydney   Toronto

First Aid for the® USMLE Step 3, Fourth Edition

Copyright © 2016 by Tao Le and Vikas Bhushan. All rights reserved. Printed in the United States of America. Except as permitted under the United States Copyright Act of 1976, no part of this publication may be reproduced or distributed in any form or by any means, or stored in a data base or retrieval system, without the prior written permission of the publisher.

Previous editions copyright © 2010, 2008, 2005 by Tao Le and Vikas Bhushan.

First Aid for the® is a registered trademark of McGraw-Hill Education. All rights reserved.

1 2 3 4 5 6 7 8 9 0   DOW/DOW   19 18 17 16 15

ISBN 9780071825962
MHID 0071825967
ISSN 1554-1363

NOTICE

Medicine is an ever-changing science. As new research and clinical experience broaden our knowledge, changes in treatment and drug therapy are required. The authors and the publisher of this work have checked with sources believed to be reliable in their efforts to provide information that is complete and generally in accord with the standards accepted at the time of publication. However, in view of the possibility of human error or changes in medical sciences, neither the authors nor the publisher nor any other party who has been involved in the preparation or publication of this work warrants that the information contained herein is in every respect accurate or complete, and they disclaim all responsibility for any errors or omissions or for the results obtained from use of the information contained in this work. Readers are encouraged to confirm the information contained herein with other sources. For example and in particular, readers are advised to check the product information sheet included in the package of each drug they plan to administer to be certain that the information contained in this work is accurate and that changes have not been made in the recommended dose or in the contraindications for administration. This recommendation is of particular importance in connection with new or infrequently used drugs.

This book was set in Electra LT Std by Rainbow Graphics.
The editors were Catherine A. Johnson and Christina M. Thomas.
The production supervisor was Jeffrey Herzich.
Project management was provided by Rainbow Graphics.
The designer was Alan Barnett.
RR Donnelley was printer and binder.

This book is printed on acid-free paper.

International Edition ISBN 978-1-25-925324-9, MHID 1-25-925324-4.
Copyright © 2016. Exclusive rights by McGraw-Hill Education for manufacture and export. This book cannot be re-exported from the country to which it is consigned by McGraw-Hill Education. The International Edition is not available in North America.

McGraw-Hill Education books are available at special quantity discounts to use as pre.miums and sales promotions or for use in corporate training programs. To contact a representative, please visit the Contact Us pages at www.mhprofessional.com.

DEDICATION

To Andrea "Andi" Fellows, who loyally shepherded
countless *First Aid* manuscripts and proofs to publication
for the benefit of students and physicians everywhere.

Contents

AUTHORS

Eike Blohm, MD
Toxicology Fellow, Department of Emergency Medicine
University of Massachusetts

Mirjana Domakonda, MD
Fellow, Division of Child and Adolescent Psychiatry
Department of Psychiatry
New York-Presbyterian Hospital of Columbia and Cornell
    Universities

Julie C. Fu, MD
Fellow, Department of Hematology/Oncology
Tufts Medical Center

Pourya Ghazi , MD
Hospitalist
Optum Medical Partners
Monarch HealthCare

Kate Humphrey, MD
Faculty, Division of Patient Safety and Quality
Pediatric Hospitalist, Division of General Pediatrics
Department of Medicine
Boston Children's Hospital

Joshua M. Liao, MD
General Internal Medicine Fellow
University of Pennsylvania School of Medicine

Rupal D. Mathur, MD
Resident, Department of Medicine
Massachusetts General Hospital
Harvard Medical School

Valentina Rodriguez-Triana, MD, MS
Health Sciences Assistant Clinical Professor
Department of Obstetrics and Gynecology
David Geffen School of Medicine
University of California at Los Angeles

Sonali Saluja, MD, MPH
General Internal Medicine Fellow
Cambridge Health Alliance
Harvard Medical School

Yifan Zheng, MD
Clinical Research Fellow, Division of Thoracic Surgery
Department of Surgery
Brigham and Women's Hospital
Harvard Medical School

IMAGE EDITOR

Mariam Aboian, MD, PhD
Resident, Department of Radiology
University of California, San Francisco

FACULTY REVIEWERS

Aaron Berkowitz, MD, PhD
Associate Neurologist
Department of Neurology
Brigham and Women's Hospital
Instructor in Neurology
Harvard Medical School

Fabienne Bourgeois, MD, MPH
Pediatric Hospitalist, Division of General Pediatrics
Department of Medicine
Boston Children's Hospital

Eddy J. Chen, MD
Instructor of Medicine
Department of Medical Oncology
Dana-Farber Cancer Institute

Emily Grover, MD
Fellow in Medical Simulation and Education
STRATUS Center for Medical Simulation
Department of Emergency Medicine
Brigham and Women's Hospital
Harvard Medical School

Kathleen J. Haley, MD
Associate Physician, Pulmonary and Critical Care Medicine
Brigham and Women's Hospital
Associate Professor of Medicine
Harvard Medical School

Ole-Petter R. Hamnvik, MB, BCh, BAO, MMSc
Associate Director, Fellowship Program
Division of Endocrinology, Diabetes, and Hypertension
Department of Medicine
Brigham and Women's Hospital
Harvard Medical School

Hamed Khalili, MD, MPH
Instructor of Medicine, Division of Gastroenterology
Massachusetts General Hospital
Harvard Medical School

Katherine Lupton, MD
Instructor, Department of Medicine
Cambridge Health Alliance
Harvard Medical School

Richard J. Pels, MD
Director, Internal Medicine Residency Program
Cambridge Health Alliance
Harvard Medical School

Corinne Rhodes, MD
Fellow, Division of General Internal Medicine
Department of Medicine
Massachusetts General Hospital
Harvard Medical School

Brianne Romeroso, MD
Assistant Clinical Professor, Obstetrics and Gynecology
University of California, Los Angeles

Heather F. Sateia, MD
Instructor, Division of General Internal Medicine
Department of Medicine
Johns Hopkins School of Medicine

Joji Suzuki, MD
Director, Division of Addiction Psychiatry
Department of Psychiatry
Brigham and Women's Hospital
Harvard Medical School

Athe Tsibris, MD, MS
Associate Physician, Infectious Diseases
Brigham and Women's Hospital
Assistant Professor of Medicine
Harvard Medical School

Amanda R. Vest, MBBS
Assistant Professor, Division of Cardiology
Department of Medicine
Tufts University School of Medicine

Daniella A. Zipkin, MD
Associate Professor of Medicine
Department of Medicine
Duke University Medical Center

Preface

With *First Aid for the USMLE Step 3*, we continue our commitment to providing residents and international medical graduates with the most useful and up-to-date preparation guides for the USMLE exams. This fourth edition represents a thorough review in many ways and includes the following:

- An updated review of hundreds of high-yield Step 3 topics, presented in a format designed to highlight board-relevant information.
- A renewed emphasis on integrated pathophysiology and on the "next step" in diagnosis and management.
- More high-yield, vignette-style "flash cards" and four-color images designed to enhance study.
- A thoroughly revised exam preparation guide for the USMLE Step 3 with test-taking strategies pertinent to the newly revised exam.
- A high-yield guide to the Computer-based Case Simulations (CCS) that includes invaluable tips and shortcuts.
- One hundred updated minicases with presentations and management strategies similar to those of the actual CCS cases.

We invite you to share your thoughts and ideas to help us improve *First Aid for the USMLE Step 3*. See How to Contribute, p. xiii.

Tao Le
Louisville

Vikas Bhushan
Los Angeles

James S. Yeh
Boston

Kachiu Cecilia Lee
Boston

Acknowledgments

This has been a collaborative project from the start. We gratefully acknowledge the thoughtful comments, corrections, and advice of the residents, international medical graduates, and faculty who have supported the authors in the development of *First Aid for the USMLE Step 3*.

For support and encouragement throughout the process, we are grateful to Thao Pham, Isabel Nogueira, and Louise Petersen.

Thanks to our publisher, McGraw-Hill, for the valuable assistance of their staff. For enthusiasm, support, and commitment to this challenging project, thanks to our editor, Catherine Johnson. We also thank Rainbow Graphics—especially David Hommel, Donna Campbell, and Susan Cooper—for remarkable editorial and production work.

Finally, we want to give very special thanks and acknowledgment to Andrea "Andi" Fellows, who edited this book and has edited every book in the *First Aid for the Boards* series, including *First Aid for the USMLE Step 1*, over the past 20 years. Her wry humor and fanatical attention to detail are evident throughout our pages. The author team has been blessed to have her as a friend and colleague over the years.

Tao Le
Louisville

Vikas Bhushan
Los Angeles

James S. Yeh
Boston

Kachiu Cecilia Lee
Boston

How to Contribute

To help us continue to produce a high-yield review source for the USMLE Step 3 exam, you are invited to submit any suggestions or corrections. We also offer **paid internships** in medical education and publishing ranging from three months to one year (see below for details).

Please send us your suggestions for:

- Study and test-taking strategies for the computerized USMLE Step 3.
- New facts, mnemonics, diagrams, and illustrations.
- CCS-style cases.
- Low-yield topics to remove.

For each entry incorporated into the next edition, you will receive up to a $20 gift certificate as well as personal acknowledgment in the next edition. Diagrams, tables, partial entries, updates, corrections, and study hints are also appreciated, and significant contributions will be compensated at the discretion of the authors. Also let us know about material in this edition that you feel is low yield and should be deleted.

The preferred way to submit entries, suggestions, or corrections is via the First Aid Team's blog at:

www.firstaidteam.com

Please include name, address, school affiliation, phone number, and e-mail address (if different from the address of origin).

NOTE TO CONTRIBUTORS

All entries become property of the authors and are subject to editing and reviewing. Please verify all data and spellings carefully. In the event that similar or duplicate entries are received, only the first entry received will be used. Include a reference to a standard textbook to facilitate verification of the fact. Please follow the style, punctuation, and format of this edition if possible.

INTERNSHIP OPPORTUNITIES

The author team is pleased to offer part-time and full-time paid internships in medical education and publishing to motivated physicians. Internships may range from three months (eg, a summer) up to a full year. Participants will have an opportunity to author, edit, and earn academic credit on a wide variety of projects, including the popular *First Aid* series. Writing/editing experience, familiarity with Microsoft Word, and Internet access are desired. For more information, e-mail a résumé or a short description of your experience along with a cover letter to the authors at firstaidteam@yahoo.com.

Introduction

The USMLE Step 3 is one of the last steps one must take toward becoming a licensed physician. The exam assesses the extent to which one can apply medical knowledge to the unsupervised practice of medicine. For international medical graduates (IMGs) who are applying for residency training in the United States, it also represents an opportunity to strengthen the residency application. The Step 3 exam focuses on the initial and **long-term** management of **common** clinical problems in **outpatient** settings. The content and format of the test were revised beginning with the November 2014 testing schedule.

In this section, we will provide an overview of the newly revised Step 3 exam and will offer you proven approaches toward conquering it. For a detailed description of Step 3, visit **www.usmle.org** or refer to the two booklets provided on the USMLE Web site: *USMLE Step 3 Content Description and General Information* and *USMLE Step 3 Sample Test Questions*.

USMLE Step 3

HOW IS STEP 3 STRUCTURED?

The Step 3 exam is administered on two separate days that need not be consecutively scheduled. The first day of the exam covers the Foundations of Independent Practice (FIP). The second day emphasizes Advanced Clinical Medicine (ACM).

Foundations of Independent Practice (FIP). Day 1 of testing lasts seven hours and consists of six blocks of 42–43 multiple-choice questions for a total of 256 questions. Test takers are given a maximum of 60 minutes to complete each block. There is a 45-minute break as well as an optional five-minute tutorial. Break time can be extended if a test taker skips the optional tutorial or finishes a test block early. Once you finish a test block, you cannot go back to it.

The content material on day 1 focuses on the basic principles required for the provision of effective health care. This includes basic foundational science (ie, knowledge of the underlying mechanisms of both normal and abnormal physiologic processes); knowledge of the history and physical examination, the diagnostic process, and use of studies in diagnosing diseases; the principles and interpretation of biostatistics, epidemiology, and population health; and the application of social sciences, including interpersonal skills, medical ethics, systems-based practice, and patient safety, to the provision of health care. Also included on day 1 are items that test one's ability to interpret the medical literature and pharmaceutical advertisements.

Advanced Clinical Medicine (ACM). Day 2 lasts approximately nine hours and consists of six blocks of 33 multiple-choice questions for a total of 198 questions. Test takers are given 45 minutes to complete each block. There is an optional five-minute tutorial. Day 2 also includes a Computer-based Clinical Simulation (CCS) component in which 13 case simulations are presented. Each case is allotted 10–20 minutes. There is also an optional seven-minute CCS tutorial and a 45-minute break. As on day 1, test takers can add

KEY FACT

Step 3 is not a retread of Step 2.

How to Contribute

To help us continue to produce a high-yield review source for the USMLE Step 3 exam, you are invited to submit any suggestions or corrections. We also offer **paid internships** in medical education and publishing ranging from three months to one year (see below for details).

Please send us your suggestions for:

- Study and test-taking strategies for the computerized USMLE Step 3.
- New facts, mnemonics, diagrams, and illustrations.
- CCS-style cases.
- Low-yield topics to remove.

For each entry incorporated into the next edition, you will receive up to a $20 gift certificate as well as personal acknowledgment in the next edition. Diagrams, tables, partial entries, updates, corrections, and study hints are also appreciated, and significant contributions will be compensated at the discretion of the authors. Also let us know about material in this edition that you feel is low yield and should be deleted.

The preferred way to submit entries, suggestions, or corrections is via the First Aid Team's blog at:

www.firstaidteam.com

Please include name, address, school affiliation, phone number, and e-mail address (if different from the address of origin).

NOTE TO CONTRIBUTORS

All entries become property of the authors and are subject to editing and reviewing. Please verify all data and spellings carefully. In the event that similar or duplicate entries are received, only the first entry received will be used. Include a reference to a standard textbook to facilitate verification of the fact. Please follow the style, punctuation, and format of this edition if possible.

INTERNSHIP OPPORTUNITIES

The author team is pleased to offer part-time and full-time paid internships in medical education and publishing to motivated physicians. Internships may range from three months (eg, a summer) up to a full year. Participants will have an opportunity to author, edit, and earn academic credit on a wide variety of projects, including the popular *First Aid* series. Writing/editing experience, familiarity with Microsoft Word, and Internet access are desired. For more information, e-mail a résumé or a short description of your experience along with a cover letter to the authors at firstaidteam@yahoo.com.

GUIDE TO THE USMLE STEP 3

Introduction

The USMLE Step 3 is one of the last steps one must take toward becoming a licensed physician. The exam assesses the extent to which one can apply medical knowledge to the unsupervised practice of medicine. For international medical graduates (IMGs) who are applying for residency training in the United States, it also represents an opportunity to strengthen the residency application. The Step 3 exam focuses on the initial and **long-term** management of **common** clinical problems in **outpatient** settings. The content and format of the test were revised beginning with the November 2014 testing schedule.

In this section, we will provide an overview of the newly revised Step 3 exam and will offer you proven approaches toward conquering it. For a detailed description of Step 3, visit **www.usmle.org** or refer to the two booklets provided on the USMLE Web site: *USMLE Step 3 Content Description and General Information* and *USMLE Step 3 Sample Test Questions*.

KEY FACT

Step 3 is not a retread of Step 2.

USMLE Step 3

HOW IS STEP 3 STRUCTURED?

The Step 3 exam is administered on two separate days that need not be consecutively scheduled. The first day of the exam covers the Foundations of Independent Practice (FIP). The second day emphasizes Advanced Clinical Medicine (ACM).

Foundations of Independent Practice (FIP). Day 1 of testing lasts seven hours and consists of six blocks of 42–43 multiple-choice questions for a total of 256 questions. Test takers are given a maximum of 60 minutes to complete each block. There is a 45-minute break as well as an optional five-minute tutorial. Break time can be extended if a test taker skips the optional tutorial or finishes a test block early. Once you finish a test block, you cannot go back to it.

The content material on day 1 focuses on the basic principles required for the provision of effective health care. This includes basic foundational science (ie, knowledge of the underlying mechanisms of both normal and abnormal physiologic processes); knowledge of the history and physical examination, the diagnostic process, and use of studies in diagnosing diseases; the principles and interpretation of biostatistics, epidemiology, and population health; and the application of social sciences, including interpersonal skills, medical ethics, systems-based practice, and patient safety, to the provision of health care. Also included on day 1 are items that test one's ability to interpret the medical literature and pharmaceutical advertisements.

Advanced Clinical Medicine (ACM). Day 2 lasts approximately nine hours and consists of six blocks of 33 multiple-choice questions for a total of 198 questions. Test takers are given 45 minutes to complete each block. There is an optional five-minute tutorial. Day 2 also includes a Computer-based Clinical Simulation (CCS) component in which 13 case simulations are presented. Each case is allotted 10–20 minutes. There is also an optional seven-minute CCS tutorial and a 45-minute break. As on day 1, test takers can add time to the break by completing a test block early or by skipping the optional tutorial. At the end of the day, there is an optional survey.

Day 2 of the exam focuses on the test taker's ability to apply medical knowledge in the context of patient management and the evolving manifestations of disease over time. The test focuses on knowledge of medical decision making, diagnosis and management, and disease prognosis and outcome. Additional emphasis is placed on screening and health maintenance management. Also included are multiple-choice questions and computer-based case simulations. Tables 1-1 and 1-2 graphically depict the areas of concentration of the revised Step 3 exam.

WHAT TYPES OF QUESTIONS ARE ASKED?

Virtually all questions on Step 3 are case based. A substantial amount of extraneous information may be given, or a clinical scenario may be followed by a question that one could answer without actually reading the case. It is your job to determine which information is superfluous and which is pertinent to the case at hand. There are three question formats:

TABLE 1-1.   Step 3 Content Areas Tested

CATEGORY	PERCENT OF OVERALL CONTENT
General Principles of Foundational Science[a]	1–3%
Biostatistics and Epidemiology/Population Health and Interpretation of the Medical Literature Social Science	14–18%

Individual Organ Systems[b]
   Immune System
   Blood and Lymphoreticular System
   Behavioral Health
   Nervous System and Special Senses
   Skin and Subcutaneous Tissue
   Musculoskeletal System
   Cardiovascular System
   Respiratory System
   Gastrointestinal System
   Renal and Urinary System
   Pregnancy, Childbirth, and the Puerperium
   Female Reproductive System and Breast
   Male Reproductive System
   Endocrine System
   Multisystem Processes and Disorders
	80–85%

[a] This category includes test items covering underlying physiologic mechanisms that are normal and not limited to specific organ systems.

[b] This category includes test items covering both normal and abnormal physiologic processes that affect specific organ systems.

TABLE 1-2.   Step 3 Competencies Tested[a]

COMPETENCY	DAY 1: FIP	DAY 2: ACM
Medical Knowledge/Scientific Concepts	18–22%	—
Patient Care: Diagnosis	40–45%	—
▪ History/Physical Exam		
▪ Laboratory/Diagnostic Studies		
▪ Diagnosis		
▪ Prognosis/Outcome	—	20–25%
Patient Care: Management	—	75–80%
▪ Health Maintenance/Disease Prevention		
▪ Pharmacotherapy		
▪ Clinical Interventions		
▪ Mixed Management		
▪ Surveillance for Disease Recurrence		
Communication and Professionalism	8–12%	—
Systems-based Practice/Patient Safety and Practice-based Learning	22–27%	—

[a] The competencies listed in rows 2–4 (Patient Care: Diagnosis and Management) are also tested on the CCS.

- **Single items.** This is the **most frequent** question type. It consists of the traditional single-best-answer question with 4–5 choices.
- **Multiple-item sets.** This consists of a clinical vignette followed by 2–3 questions regarding that case. These questions can be answered **independently.** Again, there is only one best answer.
- **Cases.** This is a clinical vignette followed by 2–5 questions. You actually receive additional information as you answer questions, so it is important that you answer questions sequentially without skipping. As a result, once you proceed to the next question in the case, you cannot change the answer to the previous question.

Questions are organized by clinical **setting** and include an outpatient office/community health center, an inpatient hospital, and an emergency department. The clinical care situations you will encounter in these settings include:

- **Initial workup:** This is characterized by the initial assessment and management of clinical issues among patients typically seen in an outpatient setting.
- **Continued care:** This physician-patient encounter typically occurs in an ambulatory context but may also take place in an inpatient setting. The encounter focuses on the management of previously diagnosed conditions and issues surrounding health maintenance. Encounters are characterized by the evaluation and management of acute exacerbations or complications of chronic and progressive medical illnesses.
- **Urgent intervention:** This encounter tests the prompt recognition and management of life-threatening emergencies, typically in emergency departments or in the context of hospitalized patients.

KEY FACT

For long vignettes, read the question stem first, and then read the case.

KEY FACT

Remember that Step 3 tends to focus on outpatient continuing-management scenarios.

When approaching vignette questions, you should keep a few things in mind:

- Be sure to note the age and race of the patient in each clinical scenario. When ethnicity is given, it is often relevant. Know these associations well (see high-yield facts), especially for more common diagnoses.
- Be able to recognize key facts that distinguish major diagnoses.
- Questions often describe clinical findings rather than naming eponyms (eg, they cite "audible hip click" instead of "positive Ortolani's sign").

HOW ARE THE SCORES REPORTED?

Like the Step 1 and 2 score reports, your Step 3 report includes your pass/fail status, a score with a three-digit scale, and a graphical performance profile organized by discipline and disease process. A minimum score of **190** is required for passing. According to the USMLE, the mean score for first-time test takers from accredited US medical schools ranges from 215 to 235 with a standard deviation of approximately 20.

According to recent data from the USMLE Web site, approximately **95%** of graduates from US and Canadian medical schools passed Step 3 on their first try, whereas 80–85% of IMGs passed on their first attempt. Detailed, year-to-year performance information can be found at www.usmle.org/performance-data/.

HOW DO I REGISTER TO TAKE THE EXAM?

The process of registering for the Step 3 exam varies depending on whether you are a US or a Canadian-based medical student, an allopathic or osteopathic student, or a student living outside the United States or Canada. For US and Canadian medical students, application is made through the Web site of the Federation of State Medical Boards (FSMB), **www.fsmb.org**. The registration fee varies and was $815 in 2015. Note again that **the two days of the exam do not need to be scheduled consecutively.**

Your scheduling permit is sent via e-mail to the e-mail address provided on the application materials. Once you have received your scheduling permit, it is your responsibility to print it and decide when and where you would like to take the exam. For a list of Prometric locations nearest you, visit **www.prometric.com**. Call Prometric's toll-free number or visit www.prometric.com to arrange a time to take the exam.

The electronic scheduling permit you receive will contain the following important information:

- Your USMLE identification number.
- The eligibility period in which you may take the exam.
- Your "scheduling number," which you will need to make your exam appointment with Prometric.
- Your Candidate Identification Number, or CIN, which you must enter at your Prometric workstation in order to access the exam.

Prometric has no access to these codes or your scheduling permit and will not be able to supply them for you. You will not be allowed to take Step 3 unless you present your permit, printed ahead of time, along with an unexpired, government-issued photo identification that contains your signature (eg, a driver's license or passport). Make sure the name on your photo ID exactly matches the name that appears on your scheduling permit.

KEY FACT

As part of its multiple-choice questions, the exam tests your ability to understand and interpret medical journal abstracts and pharmaceutical advertisements.

KEY FACT

Check the "FAQ" and "Scores" tabs of the USMLE Web site for the latest score information.

KEY FACT

The exam is scheduled on a "first-come, first-served" basis, so contact Prometric as soon as you receive your scheduling permit!

WHAT IF I NEED TO RESCHEDULE THE EXAM?

You can change your date and/or center within your three-month eligibility period at no charge by contacting Prometric. If space is available, you may reschedule up to five days before your test date. If you reschedule within five days of your test date, Prometric will charge a rescheduling fee. If you need to reschedule outside your initial three-month period, you can apply for a single three-month extension (eg, April/May/June can be extended through July/August/September) after your eligibility period has begun (go to **www.nbme.org** for more information). For other rescheduling needs, you must submit a new application along with another application fee.

WHAT ABOUT TIME?

Time is of special interest on the exam. As you take the exam, the computer will keep track of how much time has elapsed. However, the computer will show you only how much time remains in a given test block (unless you look at the full clock by using the **Alt-T** command). Therefore, it is up to you to determine if you are pacing yourself properly. Note that on both days of the exam, you have approximately **75 seconds** per multiple-choice question. If you feel that you can't answer a question within a reasonable period of time, take an educated guess and move on, as there are **no penalties** for wrong answers.

It should be noted that 45 minutes is allowed for break time. However, you can elect not to use all of your break time, or you can gain extra break time either by skipping the tutorial or by finishing a block ahead of the allotted time. **The computer will not warn you** if you have used more than your allotted break time.

KEY FACT

Never, ever leave a question blank! You can always mark it and come back later.

IF I LEAVE DURING THE EXAM, WHAT HAPPENS TO MY SCORE?

You are considered to have started the exam once you have entered your CIN onto the computer screen. In order to receive an official score, however, you must finish the entire exam. This means that you must start an exam block and either finish it or run out of time. If you do **not** complete all the blocks, your USMLE score transcript will document your exam as an incomplete attempt, and no actual score will be reported.

The exam ends when all blocks have been completed or time has elapsed. As you leave the testing center, you will receive a written test-completion notice to document your completion of the exam.

HOW LONG WILL I HAVE TO WAIT BEFORE I GET MY SCORES?

The USMLE typically reports scores 3–4 weeks after the examinee's test date. During peak periods, however, it may take **up to eight weeks** for scores to be made available. Official information concerning the time required for score reporting is posted on the USMLE Web site.

USMLE/NBME Resources

We strongly encourage you to use and study the free materials provided by the testing agencies as well as those found on the USMLE Web site at www.usmle.org/practice-materials/index.html. These include:

USMLE Step 3 Content Description and General Information
 USMLE Step 3 Sample Test Questions
 Tutorial and Practice Test Items for Multiple-Choice Questions
 Primum Computer-based Case Simulations (CCS)

In addition, computer-based practice tests are available for a fee through the NBME for those who seek to become familiar with the Prometric test center environment.

Testing Agencies

National Board of Medical Examiners (NBME)
Department of Licensing Examination Services
3750 Market Street
Philadelphia, PA 19104-3102
215-590-9500
Fax: 215-590-9457
www.nbme.org

Educational Commission for Foreign Medical Graduates (ECFMG)
3624 Market Street
Philadelphia, PA 19104-2685
215-386-5900
Fax: 215-386-9196
www.ecfmg.org

Federation of State Medical Boards (FSMB)
400 Fuller Wiser Road, Suite 300
Euless, TX 76039
817-868-4000
Fax: 817-868-4041
www.fsmb.org

USMLE Secretariat
3750 Market Street
Philadelphia, PA 19104-3102
215-590-9700
Fax: 215-590-9460
www.usmle.org

NOTES

GUIDE TO THE CCS

Introduction

The Primum CCS is a computerized patient simulation that is administered on the second day of the Step 3 exam. You will be given nine cases over four hours and will have up to 25 minutes to complete each case. As with the rest of the Step 3 exam, the CCS aims to test your ability to properly diagnose and manage common conditions in a variety of patient settings. Many of the conditions tested are obvious or easily diagnosed.

Clinical problems presented on the CCS may be acute or chronic and may range from mild to life-threatening. Cases may last anywhere from a few minutes to a few months in **simulated time**, but you will be allotted only 25 minutes of real time to complete each. Regardless of the setting (eg, office, ED, ICU), you will serve as the patient's primary physician and will assume complete responsibility for his or her care.

What Is the CCS Like?

OVERVIEW

If you wish to excel on the CCS, there is no substitute for downloading and trying out the sample cases from the USMLE Web site (www.usmle.org/practice-materials/index.html). Devoting at least a few hours to these cases and familiarizing yourself with the CCS interface will improve your performance on the exam regardless of your level of computer expertise.

For each case, you will be presented with a chief complaint, vital signs, and a history of present illness (HPI). You will then initiate patient management, continue care, and advance the case by taking one of the following four actions represented on the computer screen:

1. Get Interval History or Physical Exam. You can obtain either a focused or a full physical exam. You can also obtain an interval history to see how a patient is doing. Getting an interval history or performing a physical exam will automatically advance the clock in simulated time.

Quick tips and shortcuts:

- If the patient's vital signs are unstable, remember that you may have to write some orders (eg, IV fluids, oxygen, type and cross-match) before performing the physical exam.
- Remember to keep the physical exam **focused.** Conducting a full physical exam may be wasteful and may cost you valuable simulated time. You can always perform additional exam components as they become necessary.

2. Write Order or Review Chart. You can manage the patient by typing orders. For example, you can order tests, monitoring, treatments, procedures, consultations, and counseling. The order sheet on the CCS is formatted as free-text entry, so you can type whatever you choose; the computer has a 12,000-term vocabulary that can accommodate approximately 2500 orders or actions.

When you order a medication, you will also need to specify the **route** and **frequency** of administration. If a patient comes into a case with preexisting

KEY FACT

Cases can, and frequently do, end in < 25 minutes.

KEY FACT

You will see few diagnostic "zebras" on the CCS. The focus here is on management, management, management!

KEY FACT

Orders on the CCS require free-text entry. There are no multiple-choice options here!

medications, these meds will appear on the order sheet with an order time of "Day 1 @00:00." The medications will continue to be administered unless you decide to cancel them. Unlike the interval history or physical exam, you must **manually** advance simulated time to see the results of your orders.

Quick tips and shortcuts:

- As long as the computer can recognize the **first three characters** of your order, it can provide a list of orders from which to choose.
- When inputting an order, simply type the name of the test, therapy, or procedure you wish to obtain. Don't type verbs such as "get," "administer," or "do."
- Do the sample cases to get a sense of the types of abbreviations that the computer will recognize (eg, CBC, CXR, ECG).
- Familiarize yourself with the routes of administration and dosing frequencies of common medications. You do **not** need to know dosages or drip rates.
- Never assume that other health care staff or consultants will write orders for you. On the contrary, you are responsible for writing all orders, including routine actions such as IV fluids, oxygen, monitoring, and diabetic diet. If a patient is preop, don't forget NPO, type and cross-match, and antibiotics.
- You can always change your mind about an order and cancel it as long as the clock has not advanced.
- Review any preexisting medications on the order sheet. Sometimes the patient's problem may be due to a preexisting medication **side effect** or a drug interaction!

3. Obtain Results or See Patient Later. To determine how a given case evolves after you have entered your orders, you must advance the clock. You can specify a time to see the patient either in the future or when the next results become available. Upon advancing the clock, you may receive messages from the patient, family, or health care staff updating you on the patient's status before the specified time or results are made available. If you stop a clock advance to a future time (eg, a follow-up appointment) to review results from previous orders, that future event will be canceled.

Quick tips and shortcuts:

- Before advancing the clock, ask yourself whether the patient will be okay during that time period. Also ask yourself whether the patient is in the appropriate location or whether he or she should be transferred to another setting.
- If you receive an update while the clock is advancing, be sure to review your current management, especially if the patient's condition is worsening.

4. Change Location. In the simulated exam, you will have an outpatient office with admitting privileges to a 400-bed tertiary-care facility. As in real life, the patient will typically present to you in either an office or an ED. Once you've done all you can for the patient, you can elect to transfer him or her to another setting, such as the ward or the ICU, for appropriate care. Note that in the context of the CCS, "ICU" is a blanket term that encompasses all types of intensive care units, including medical, surgical, pediatric, obstetrics, and neonatal. Where appropriate, the patient may be discharged home with follow-up.

KEY FACT

Wherever the patient goes, you go!

KEY FACT

The final diagnosis and reasons for consultation do not count toward your score!

<u>Q</u>uick tips and shortcuts:

- Always ask yourself if the patient is in the right setting to receive optimal management.
- Remember that you will remain the patient's **primary physician** regardless of where he or she goes.
- When changing locations (and especially when discharging the patient), remember to discontinue orders that are no longer needed.
- Remember that patients who are discharged home will require a follow-up appointment.
- Before discharging a patient, think about whether he or she needs any health maintenance or counseling.

FINISHING THE CASE

On the CCS, each case ends when you have used up your allotted 25 minutes. If the measurement objectives for the case have already been met before this 25-minute period has elapsed, the computer may ask you to exit early. Toward the end, you will be given a warning that the case is about to conclude. You will then be given an opportunity to cancel existing orders as well as to write new short-term orders. You will be asked for a final diagnosis before exiting.

How Is the CCS Graded?

Your grade will be determined by a scoring algorithm that is based on generally accepted practices of care. This algorithm allows for wide variation and recognizes that there may be more than one appropriate way to approach a case. In general, you will **gain** points for appropriate management actions and will **lose** points for actions that are not indicated or are potentially harmful to your patient. These actions are **weighted** such that key actions (eg, ordering an emergent needle thoracostomy for a patient with tension pneumothorax) will earn you a comparatively greater number of points, whereas highly inappropriate actions (eg, ordering a liver biopsy for a patient with an ear infection) will cost you relatively more points.

Note, however, that even if your management actions are correct, you may not be given full credit for them if you perform them **out of sequence** or following an **inappropriate delay** in simulated time. **Unnecessary or excessive orders**—even if they pose no risk to the patient—will cost you points as well. The bottom line is that the CCS tends to reward thorough but efficient medicine.

High-Yield Strategies for the CCS

As mentioned earlier, it is essential that you practice the sample CCS cases before taking the actual exam. Make sure you do both outpatient and inpatient cases. Try different abbreviations to get a feel for the vocabulary you should use when you write orders. You can also apply different approaches toward the same case to see how the computer reacts.

Read through the 100 cases in **Chapter 19, High-Yield CCS Cases.** They will show you how clinical conditions can present and play out in the CCS. Remember that the computer wants you to do the **right things** at the **right** times while incurring **minimal waste and risk** to the patient. When taking the exam, also bear the following in mind:

- **Read the HPI carefully.** Use the HPI to develop a short differential that will direct your physical exam and initial management. Often the diagnosis will become apparent to you before you begin the physical exam. Jot down pertinent positives and negatives so that you don't have to come back and review the chart. Keep in mind any drug allergies that the patient might have.

- **Remember that unstable patients need immediate management.** If a patient's vital signs are unstable, you may want to take some basic management measures, such as administering IV fluids and oxygen, before starting the physical exam. With unstable patients, your goal should be to order tests that will help identify and manage the patient's underlying condition while incurring minimal delay.

- **Consultants are rarely helpful.** Although you will earn some points for calling a consultant for an indicated procedure (eg, a surgeon for an appendectomy), consultants will generally offer little in the way of diagnostic or management assistance.

- **Don't forget health maintenance, education, and counseling.** After treating tension pneumothorax, counsel the patient about smoking cessation if the HPI mentions that he or she is an active smoker.

- **Don't treat the patient alone.** The computer will not permit you to treat a patient's family or sexual partner, but it will allow you to provide education or counseling. If a female patient is of childbearing age, check a pregnancy test before starting a potentially teratogenic treatment.

- **Some patients will worsen despite good care, while others will improve despite poor management.** If a case is not going your way, reassess your approach to make sure you're not missing anything. If you're confident about your diagnosis and management strategy, stop second-guessing it. Sometimes the CCS tests your ability to handle difficult clinical situations.

KEY FACT

A patient whose condition is worsening may reflect the testing goals of the case rather than an error on your part.

NOTES

CHAPTER 2

AMBULATORY MEDICINE

Ophthalmology

GLAUCOMA

A form of optic neuropathy that is caused by ↑ intraocular pressure (defined as > 20 mm Hg) and results in loss of vision if left untreated. Table 2-1 contrasts open-angle with closed-angle glaucoma.

DIABETIC RETINOPATHY

- Asymptomatic, gradual vision loss in patients with diabetes. The leading cause of blindness in the United States. Divided into nonproliferative and proliferative forms.
- **Sx/Exam: Funduscopic findings** include neovascularization, microaneurysms, flame hemorrhages, and macular edema.
- **Tx:** Proliferative retinopathy may be treated, and progression slowed, with laser photocoagulation surgery or vitrectomy.
- **Prevention:**
  - Patients with diabetes should have a comprehensive ophthalmologic exam at least annually to screen for signs of retinopathy.
  - Progression can be slowed with tight glucose and BP control.

TABLE 2-1. Open-Angle vs Closed-Angle Glaucoma

	OPEN-ANGLE GLAUCOMA	CLOSED-ANGLE GLAUCOMA
Etiology/risk factors	Drainage canals are blocked; the angle between the iris and cornea is open. Most common.	The angle between the iris and cornea (anterior chamber angle) is closed, impairing drainage. Risk factors include African American ethnicity, a ⊕ family history, female gender, and age > 40–50.
Symptoms	Chronic; gradual loss of peripheral vision.	Acute; presents with eye pain, headache, nausea, conjunctival injection, halos around lights, and fixed, dilated pupils.
Diagnosis	High intraocular pressures and an abnormal cup-to-disk ratio (> 50%) (see Figure 2-1).	High intraocular pressures (≥ 30 mm Hg; normal 8–21 mm Hg).
Treatment	Nonselective topical β-blockers (eg, timolol, levobunolol). Topical adrenergic agonists (eg, epinephrine). Topical cholinergic agonists (eg, pilocarpine, carbachol). Topical carbonic anhydrase inhibitors (eg, dorzolamide, brinzolamide).	**Contact an ophthalmologist immediately!** **Pupillary constriction:** Topical pilocarpine. **↓ intraocular pressure:** Timolol, acetazolamide. Laser iridotomy. **Systemic:** Acetazolamide, mannitol.

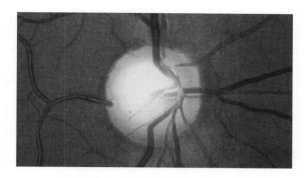

FIGURE 2-1. **Open-angle glaucoma.** Note the change in the cup-to-disk ratio. (Reproduced with permission from USMLE-Rx.com.)

HERPES ZOSTER OPHTHALMICUS

■ Infection of the V1 branch of CN V (the ophthalmic division of the trigeminal nerve; see Figure 2-2). Particularly common in immunocompromised states such as HIV infection.

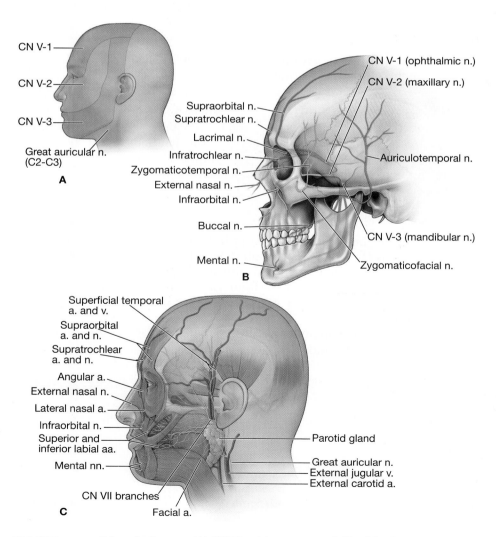

FIGURE 2-2. **Trigeminal nerve.** (A) CN V and its cutaneous fields of the face. (B) Branches of CN V in the face. (C) Vasculature of the face. (Reproduced with permission from Morton DA et al. *The Big Picture: Gross Anatomy.* New York: McGraw-Hill, 2011, Fig. 20-1A and B.)

Q

A 42-year-old woman presents with headache, nausea, vomiting, and a red eye that has progressively worsened since this morning. She also notes vision changes. Exam reveals conjunctival injection; a moderately fixed, dilated pupil; and no focal weaknesses in the extremities. What should you do next?

- **Sx/Exam:** Presents with fever, headache, malaise, periorbital burning/itching, conjunctivitis, keratitis, ↑ intraocular pressure, optic neuropathy, and cranial nerve palsies. Vesicles are purulent and progress to crusting.
- **Tx:**
  - IV acyclovir/valacyclovir/famciclovir within 72 hours after the appearance of the rash ↓ the incidence of complications.
  - **Refer immediately to an ophthalmologist.**

Ear, Nose, and Throat (ENT)

INFLUENZA

An acute respiratory illness caused by influenza A or B. Occurs primarily during the winter.

SYMPTOMS/EXAM

Generally presents following an incubation period of 1–2 days with acute-onset upper and lower respiratory tract symptoms, myalgias, fevers, and weakness.

DIAGNOSIS

Rapid antigen tests have a sensitivity of only 40–60%. Diagnosis may be established through PCR testing or viral culture.

TREATMENT

- The antiviral drugs zanamivir and oseltamivir can be used prophylactically or to treat existing infection in at-risk individuals; most effective when given within 48 hours of exposure or at symptom onset.
- Most influenza strains have become resistant to amantadine and rimantadine.

COMPLICATIONS

- Pneumonia is the 1° complication of influenza. Risk factors include diabetes mellitus (DM) and cardiopulmonary disease. Patients > 50 years of age and nursing home residents are also at risk.
- 2° bacterial pneumonia, often from *Streptococcus pneumoniae*, is an important complication and is responsible for one-quarter of influenza-related deaths.
- Other complications include myositis, rhabdomyolysis, CNS involvement, myocarditis, and pericarditis.

HEARING LOSS

Common in the elderly. Table 2-2 contrasts conductive with sensorineural hearing loss.

ALLERGIC RHINITIS

Affects up to 20% of the adult population. Patients may also have asthma and atopic dermatitis.

KEY FACT

Otosclerosis is the most common cause of conductive hearing loss in young adults.

Use tonometry to check intraocular pressures. A pressure of ≥ 30 mm Hg confirms the diagnosis of closed-angle glaucoma. Refer to ophthalmology. Initial treatments include timolol, acetazolamide, and topical pilocarpine.

TABLE 2-2.   Conductive vs Sensorineural Hearing Loss

	CONDUCTIVE	SENSORINEURAL
Location of damage	Outer and middle ear.	Inner ear.
Diagnosis	**Weber test:** A vibrating tuning fork in the middle of the patient's forehead will sound louder in the **affected** ear. **Rinne test:** Place a vibrating tuning fork against the patient's mastoid bone and replace immediately near the external meatus once it is no longer audible; bone conduction will be audible longer than air conduction.	**Weber test:** A vibrating tuning fork in the middle of the patient's forehead will sound louder in the **normal** ear. **Rinne test:** Same maneuver; air conduction will be audible longer than bone conduction.
Examples	Cerumen impaction Foreign bodies Otitis externa Tumor/mass Otosclerosis (progressive fixation of stapes)	Otitis media Barotrauma Perforation of the tympanic membrane Presbycusis (age related) Drug induced (eg, aspirin, aminoglycosides)

SYMPTOMS/EXAM

- Presents with congestion, rhinorrhea, sneezing, eye irritation, and postnasal drip.
- Identify exposure to environmental allergens such as pollens, animal dander, dust mites, and mold spores. May be seasonal.
- Exam reveals edematous, pale mucosa; cobblestoning in the pharynx; scleral injection; and blue, boggy turbinates.

DIAGNOSIS

- Diagnosed by clinical exam.
- Skin prick testing to a standard panel of antigens can be performed, or blood testing can be conducted to look for specific IgE antibodies via radioallergosorbent testing (RAST).

TREATMENT

- **Allergen avoidance:** Use dust mite–proof covers on bedding and remove carpeting. Keep the home dry and avoid pets.
- **Drugs:**
  - **Antihistamines (diphenhydramine, fexofenadine):** Block the effects of histamine released by mast cells. Selective antihistamines such as fexofenadine may cause less drowsiness than nonselective agents such as diphenhydramine.
  - **Intranasal corticosteroids:** Anti-inflammatory properties yield excellent symptom control.
  - **Sympathomimetics (pseudoephedrine):** α-adrenergic agonist effects result in vasoconstriction.
  - **Intranasal anticholinergics (ipratropium):** ↓ mucous membrane secretions.
  - **Immunotherapy ("allergy shots"):** Slow to take effect, but useful for difficult-to-control symptoms.

Q   1

A 71-year-old man with a history of well-controlled asthma presents in November for his annual checkup. He has no complaints, and his physical exam is unremarkable. He received the pneumococcal vaccine 3 years ago. What should he be given before the completion of his visit?

Q   2

A 68-year-old woman is brought to your office because her son is concerned that she is losing her memory. He describes several instances in which she forgot what he had just told her, adding that she was recently unaware that he was calling to her at a crowded park. She spends most of her time at home watching television. What is the diagnosis?

EPISTAXIS

Bleeding from the nose or nasopharynx. **Roughly 90% of cases are anterior nasal septum bleeds at Kiesselbach's plexus** (see Figure 2-3). The most common etiology is local trauma 2° to digital manipulation. Other causes include dryness of the nasal mucosa, nasal septal deviation, use of antiplatelet medications, bone abnormalities in the nares, rhinitis, and bleeding diatheses.

Symptoms/Exam
- **Posterior bleeds:** More brisk and less common; blood is swallowed and may not be seen.
- **Anterior bleeds:** Usually less severe; bleeding is visible as it exits the nares.

Treatment
- Treat with prolonged and sustained direct pressure and topical nasal vasoconstrictors (phenylephrine or oxymetazoline).
- If bleeding does not stop, cauterize with silver nitrate or insert nasal packing (with antibiotics to prevent toxic shock syndrome, covering for *S aureus*).
- If severe, type and screen, obtain IV access, and consult an ENT surgeon.

Dermatology

"DERM TERMS"

Table 2-3 gives examples of common dermatologic lesions.

ATOPIC DERMATITIS (ECZEMA)

Pruritic, lichenified eruptions that are classically found in the antecubital fossa but may also appear on the neck, face, wrists, and upper trunk. Has a chronic course with remissions.

- Characterized by an early age of onset (often in childhood).
- Associated with a ⊕ family history and a personal history of atopy.
- Patients tend to have ↑ serum IgE and repeated skin infections.

KEY FACT

Leukoplakia consists of white patches/plaques on the oral mucosa (see Figure 2-4) that cannot be removed by rubbing mucosal surface (vs *Candida*). Chewing tobacco is a risk factor.

1 **A**

Annual influenza vaccination is recommended for all patients > 6 months of age who lack contraindications.

2 **A**

Presbycusis, or age-related hearing loss. Hearing loss in the elderly must be evaluated. Patients may have difficulty distinguishing voices in a crowd, which is often misinterpreted as memory loss. Patients may become socially isolated.

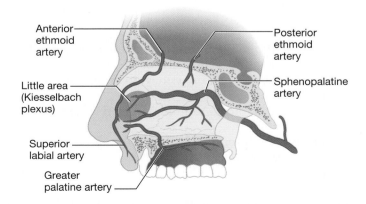

FIGURE 2-3. Blood supply to the nasal cavity. The most common site of hemorrhage is from Kiesselbach's plexus. The most common site of posterior hemorrhage is from the sphenopalatine artery. (Reproduced with permission from Tintinalli JE et al. *Tintinalli's Emergency Medicine: A Comprehensive Study Guide,* 7th ed. New York: McGraw-Hill, 2011, Fig. 239-1.)

TABLE 2-3.   Types of Dermatologic Lesions

TYPE	DESCRIPTION	EXAMPLES
Macule	Flat, circumscribed, < 0.5 cm in diameter.	Lentigo, café-au-lait spot, nevi (Image A).
Patch	Flat, > 0.5 cm in diameter.	Café-au-lait spot, vitiligo (Image B).
Papule	Elevated, palpable, < 0.5 cm in diameter.	Elevated nevi, molluscum contagiosum (Image C).
Plaque	Elevated, palpable, > 0.5 cm in diameter.	Psoriasis (Image D), lichen simplex chronicus, oral leukoplakia.
Nodule	Circumscribed, elevated, solid, 0.5–2.0 cm in diameter; located in the epidermis or deeper.	Rheumatoid nodules, xanthomas (Image E).
Tumor	Large, circumscribed, solid; located deep in tissue.	Neoplasms (Image F).

TABLE 2-3. Types of Dermatologic Lesions *(continued)*

TYPE	DESCRIPTION	EXAMPLES
Vesicle	Circumscribed, elevated, fluid filled, < 0.5 cm in diameter.	Herpes lesions (Image G), varicella-zoster lesions.
Bullae	Circumscribed, elevated, fluid filled, > 0.5 cm in diameter.	Coma blisters, pemphigus (Image H), epidermolysis bullosa.
Pustule	Circumscribed, elevated, purulent.	Folliculitis, acne, pyoderma (Image I).

Images A and C reproduced with permission from Longo DL et al. *Harrison's Principles of Internal Medicine,* 18th ed. New York: McGraw-Hill, 2012, Figs. 51-2 and 183-1. Images B, F, H, and I reproduced with permission from Goldsmith LA et al. *Fitzpatrick's Dermatology in General Medicine,* 8th ed. New York: McGraw-Hill, 2012, Figs. 74-4, 129-1, 200-32, and 5-15. Image D reproduced with permission from McKean SC et al. *Principles and Practice of Hospital Medicine.* New York: McGraw-Hill, 2012, Fig. 143-4. Images E and G reproduced with permission from Wolff K et al. *Fitzpatrick's Color Atlas and Synopsis of Clinical Dermatology,*7th ed. New York: McGraw-Hill, 2013, Figs. 15-14 and 27-31.

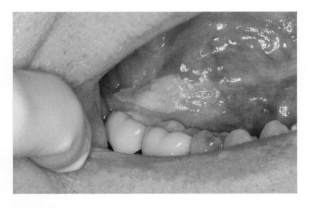

FIGURE 2-4. **Oral leukoplakia.** White plaques are seen on the lateral tongue. (Reproduced with permission from Goldsmith LA et al. *Fitzpatrick's Dermatology in General Medicine,* 8th ed. New York: McGraw-Hill, 2012, Fig. 76-9.)

SYMPTOMS/EXAM

- Presents with severe pruritus, with distribution generally in the face, neck, upper trunk, and bends of the elbows and knees. The skin is dry, leathery, and lichenified (see Figure 2-5).
- The condition usually worsens in the winter and in low-humidity environments.

DIFFERENTIAL

Seborrheic dermatitis, contact dermatitis, impetigo.

DIAGNOSIS

Diagnosis is clinical.

TREATMENT

Keep skin moisturized. **Topical steroid creams should be used sparingly** and should be tapered once flares resolve. The first-line steroid-sparing agent is tacrolimus ointment.

CONTACT DERMATITIS

Caused by exposure to allergens in the environment; may lead to acute, subacute, or chronic eczematous inflammation.

- **Irritant contact dermatitis:** Non-immune-mediated irritation caused by a substance; usually presents as burning, pruritus, and pain from dry, cracked skin. Has no clearly demarcated borders.
- **Allergic contact dermatitis:** Type IV hypersensitivity; usually occurs as pruritus from vesicles and bullae in a demarcated rash.

SYMPTOMS

Patients complain of itching, burning, and an intensely pruritic rash.

EXAM

- **Acute:** Presents with papular erythematous lesions and sometimes with vesicles, weeping erosions where vesicles have ruptured, crusting, and excoriations. The pattern of lesions often reflects the mechanism of exposure (eg, a line of vesicles or lesions under a watchband; see Figure 2-6).
- **Chronic:** Characterized by hyperkeratosis and lichenification.

DIAGNOSIS

- A clinical diagnosis that is made in the setting of a possible exposure.
- Patch testing can be used to elicit the reaction with the agent that caused the dermatitis.
- Consider the occupation and hobbies of the individual and the exposure area of the body to determine if they suggest a diagnosis.

TREATMENT

- Avoid causative agents.
- Cold compresses and oatmeal baths help soothe the area.
- Administer topical steroids. A short course of oral steroids may be needed if a large region of the body is involved.

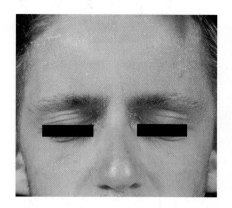

FIGURE 2-5. **Atopic dermatitis.** Erythematous plaques with scaling are seen in an adolescent with atopic dermatitis. (Reproduced with permission from Wolff K et al. *Fitzpatrick's Dermatology in General Medicine,* 7th ed. New York: McGraw-Hill, 2008, Fig. 14-6.)

KEY FACT

Common causes of contact dermatitis include nickel (earrings, watches, necklaces) and poison ivy.

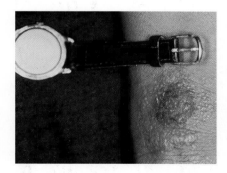

FIGURE 2-6. **Contact dermatitis.** The erythematous, edematous base of the eruption corresponds to the posterior surface of the watch. (Used with permission of the Department of Dermatology, Wilford Hall USAF Medical Center and Brooke Army Medical Center, San Antonio, TX, as published in Knoop KJ et al. *The Atlas of Emergency Medicine,* 2nd ed. New York: McGraw-Hill, 2010, Fig. 13-50.)

Q

A 24-year-old medical student develops a rash when he puts on a pair of latex examination gloves. What is the mechanism leading to this rash?

KEY FACT

Psoriatic arthritis characteristically involves the DIP joints.

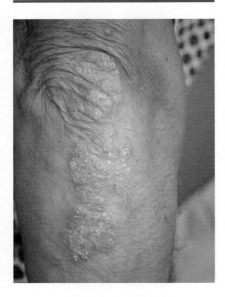

FIGURE 2-7.   Psoriasis. Note the well-demarcated, erythematous plaque with micaceous silvery scale of the elbow. (Reproduced with permission from USMLE-Rx.com.)

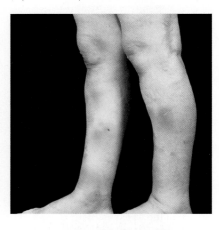

FIGURE 2-8.   Erythema nodosum. Note the bilateral erythematous nodules localized over the shins. (Reproduced with permission from Goldsmith LA et al. *Fitzpatrick's Dermatology in General Medicine,* 8th ed. New York: McGraw-Hill, 2012, Fig. 70-2.)

Allergic contact dermatitis is a result of delayed contact (type IV) hypersensitivity caused by allergen-primed memory T lymphocytes (vs irritant contact dermatitis, which results from cytokines released following irritant contact).

PSORIASIS

An immune-mediated skin disease characterized by pink plaques with silvery scale and sharply defined margins. The condition is often chronic with a probable genetic predisposition.

SYMPTOMS/EXAM

Presents with well-demarcated, silvery, scaly plaques on the knees, elbows, gluteal cleft, and scalp (see Figure 2-7). **Nails may show pitting** and onycholysis.

TREATMENT

- **Limited disease:** Topical steroids, topical vitamin D analogs, topical retinoids.
- **Generalized disease (involving > 30% of the body):** UVB light exposure; PUVA (psoralen and UVA) if UVB is not effective. Methotrexate, acitretin, and anti-TNF agents may also be used for severe cases.

ERYTHEMA NODOSUM

An inflammatory condition that is characterized by tender red or violet nodules. More common in women than in men. Although often idiopathic, it may also be 2° to sarcoidosis, IBD, and **infections (streptococcal infection, coccidioidomycosis, TB).**

SYMPTOMS/EXAM

- Lesions are painful and may be preceded by fever, malaise, and arthralgias. Recent URI or diarrheal illness may suggest a cause.
- Exam reveals deep-seated, poorly demarcated, painful red nodules without ulceration on the shins (see Figure 2-8).

DIFFERENTIAL

Cellulitis, trauma, thrombophlebitis.

TREATMENT

- Treat the underlying disease. The condition is usually self-limited, but NSAIDs are helpful for pain.
- In more persistent cases, potassium iodide drops and systemic corticosteroids may be of benefit.

ROSACEA

Most commonly affects people with fair skin, those with light hair and eyes, and those who have frequent flushing.

SYMPTOMS/EXAM

- Presents with erythema and with inflammatory papules that mimic acne and appear on the cheeks, forehead, nose, and chin.
- Open and closed comedones (whiteheads and blackheads) are **not** present.
- **Recurrent flushing may be elicited by spicy foods, alcohol, or emotional reactions.**

- Rhinophyma (an enlarged nose with an irregular texture) occurs late in the course of the disease and results from sebaceous gland hyperplasia (see Figure 2-9).
- Patients may have ocular symptoms such as blepharitis, conjunctival injection, and lid margin telangiectasias.

DIFFERENTIAL

The absence of comedones in rosacea and the patient's age help distinguish the condition from acne vulgaris.

TREATMENT

- **Initial therapy:** The goal is to control rather than cure the chronic disease. Use mild cleansers, azelaic acid, and/or metronidazole topical gel +/– oral antibiotics as initial therapy.
- **Persistent symptoms:** Treat with oral antibiotics (doxycycline, minocycline) and tretinoin cream.
- **Maintenance therapy:**
  - Topical metronidazole may be used once daily.
  - Clonidine or α-blockers may be effective in the management of flushing, and patients should avoid triggers.
  - Consider referral for surgical evaluation if rhinophyma is present and is not responding to treatment.
  - Any patient with ocular symptoms (eg, grittiness, dryness) should be started on oral or topical local antibiotics and ocular lubricants.

ERYTHEMA MULTIFORME (EM)

An acute inflammatory disease that is sometimes recurrent (type IV hypersensitivity). The most common etiologic factors are HSV and *Mycoplasma pneumoniae*. May also be caused by medications such as sulfa drugs. Many cases are idiopathic and recurrent.

SYMPTOMS/EXAM

- May be preceded by malaise and fever or by itching and burning at the site where the eruptions will occur.
- Presents with sudden onset of rapidly progressive, symmetrical lesions.
- Targetoid papules are typically located on the back of the hands and on the palms, soles, and limbs (see Figure 2-10). However, they can be found anywhere (see Figure 2-11). Lesions recur in crops for 2–3 weeks.

DIAGNOSIS

Typically a clinical diagnosis.

TREATMENT

- Mild cases can be treated symptomatically with histamine blockers for pruritus.
- If many targetoid lesions are present, patients usually respond to prednisone for 1–3 weeks.
- Azathioprine has been helpful in cases that are unresponsive to other treatments.
- When HSV causes recurrent EM, maintenance acyclovir or valacyclovir can ↓ recurrences of both.

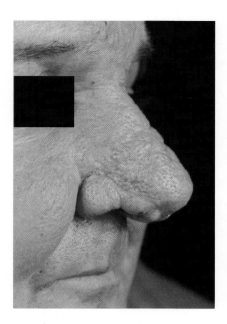

FIGURE 2-9. Rhinophyma. (Reproduced with permission from Wolff K et al. *Fitzpatrick's Color Atlas & Synopsis of Clinical Dermatology*, 5th ed. New York: McGraw-Hill, 2005: 11.)

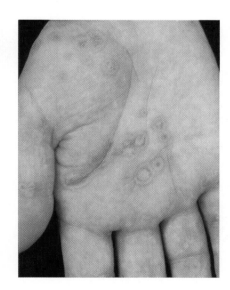

FIGURE 2-10. Erythema multiforme. Note the typical targetoid lesions on the palm. (Reproduced with permission from Goldsmith LA et al. *Fitzpatrick's Dermatology in General Medicine*, 8th ed. New York: McGraw-Hill, 2012, Fig. 39-3.)

Q

A 26-year-old man presents with targetoid papules that appeared on his palms 2 days ago. He states that he was recently prescribed a new antiseizure medication for his epilepsy. He denies any other symptoms, and exam reveals no other lesions. What is the diagnosis?

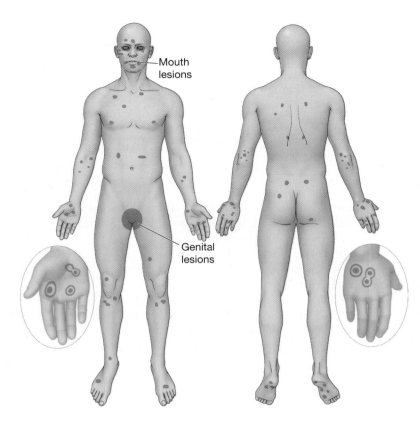

Mouth
lesions

Genital
lesions

FIGURE 2-11. **Distribution of erythema multiforme.** (Reproduced with permission from Wolff K et al. *Fitzpatrick's Color Atlas and Synopsis of Clinical Dermatology*, 7th ed. New York: McGraw-Hill, 2013, Fig. 14-18.)

PEMPHIGUS VULGARIS

An autoimmune disease in which blisters are formed as a result of **autoantibodies targeting desmoglein 3 and 1 in the desmosomal complex** in skin cells. Pemphigus vulgaris is the most common subtype of pemphigus.

SYMPTOMS/EXAM

- Presents with **flaccid bullae** and with **erosions** where bullae have been unroofed (see Figure 2-12). Oral lesions usually precede skin lesions.
- If it is not treated early, the disease usually generalizes and can affect the esophagus.
- Nikolsky's sign is elicited when gentle lateral traction on the skin separates the epidermis from underlying tissue.

DIAGNOSIS

Skin biopsy.

TREATMENT

Corticosteroids and immunosuppressive agents.

BULLOUS PEMPHIGOID

An autoimmune disease characterized by **antibodies against basement membrane proteins that lead to subepidermal bullae.** More common than pemphigus vulgaris, and typically occurs in those > 60 years of age (the median age at onset is 80 years).

KEY FACT

Pemphigus vulgaris presents with flaccid bullae, whereas bullous pemphigoid is characterized by tense bullae.

A

Erythema multiforme (EM) 2° to the new antiseizure medication. EM differs from Stevens-Johnson syndrome/toxic epidermal necrolysis in that lesions are generally localized to the extremities (vs spreading from the face and trunk), and the disease course is usually less severe.

SYMPTOMS/EXAM

Presents as large, tense bullae with few other symptoms (see Figure 2-13).

DIFFERENTIAL

Pemphigus vulgaris, dermatitis herpetiformis.

DIAGNOSIS

Diagnosis is made with skin biopsy, with confirmation via immuno- and histo-pathology.

TREATMENT

Topical steroids.

ACNE VULGARIS (COMMON ACNE)

Results from ↑ pilosebaceous gland activity, *Propionibacterium acnes,* and plugging of follicles.

SYMPTOMS/EXAM

Characterized by a variety of lesions, including closed comedones (whiteheads), open comedones (blackheads), inflammatory papules, nodules, and scars. Lesions are typically seen over the face, back, and chest.

DIFFERENTIAL

Rosacea, folliculitis.

DIAGNOSIS

Diagnosis is clinical.

TREATMENT

- Begin with topical benzoyl peroxide, topical retinoids, or topical antibiotics such as erythromycin.
- A 2° line of treatment includes addition of oral antibiotics such as minocycline or doxycycline.
- Isotretinoin (Accutane) can be used but is teratogenic and should thus be prescribed with caution in women of childbearing age. Concomitant contraception and pregnancy tests are necessary.

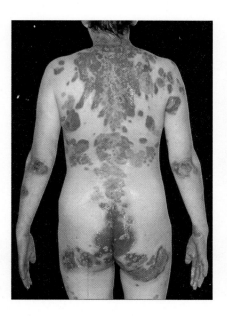

FIGURE 2-12.   Pemphigus vulgaris. Note the extensive erosions due to blistering and the intact, flaccid blisters at the lower border of the eroded lesions. (Reproduced with permission from Goldsmith LA et al. *Fitzpatrick's Dermatology in General Medicine,* 8th ed. New York: McGraw-Hill, 2012, Fig. 54-3.)

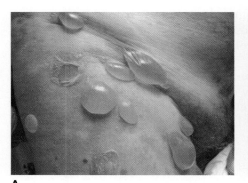

A

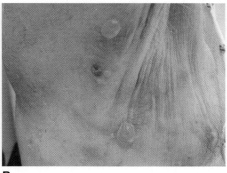

B

FIGURE 2-13.   Bullous pemphigoid. (A) Large, tense bullae and erythematous patches are seen on the thighs and lower legs. **(B)** Urticarial plaques with overlying tense vesicles and bullae are seen in the axilla. (Reproduced with permission from Goldsmith LA et al. *Fitzpatrick's Dermatology in General Medicine,* 8th ed. New York: McGraw-Hill, 2012, Fig. 56-3.)

HERPES ZOSTER (SHINGLES)

Caused by reactivated varicella-zoster virus (VZV), which remains dormant in the **dorsal roots** of nerves. Risk factors include ↑ age and immunosuppression. After the eruption, patients can develop postherpetic neuralgia, a painful disorder.

SYMPTOMS/EXAM

Presents with the cutaneous finding of **painful vesicles evolving into crusted lesions in a dermatomal distribution.** Lesions are typically preceded by paresthesias in the area of distribution.

DIFFERENTIAL

Contact dermatitis.

DIAGNOSIS

Diagnosis is largely clinical. PCR or culture can be confirmatory.

TREATMENT

- Pain management.
- If initiated within 72 hours of rash onset, antiviral treatment with acyclovir, valacyclovir, or famciclovir can ↓ the duration of illness and may also ↓ the occurrence of postherpetic neuralgia. Use of glucocorticoids is controversial and is generally not recommended.
- Patients are infectious until crusts have formed over the vesicles. Keep the area covered to prevent the spread of virus to immunocompromised patients.
- Vaccination is recommended for people ≥ 60 years of age and helps ↓ the risk of both shingles and postherpetic neuralgia.

DERMATOPHYTOSES

Dermatophytes attach to and proliferate on the superficial layers of the epidermis, nails, and hair. Examples are given in Table 2-4.

BASAL CELL CARCINOMA

- The most common skin cancer. Slow growing and rarely metastasizes. Caused by excessive sun exposure.
- **Sx/Exam:** Pearly papules with central depression that may be ulcerated. Most commonly found on sun-exposed areas.
- **Dx:** Skin biopsy shows palisading cells with retraction.
- **Tx:**
  - Curettage, cryosurgery, radiation, or excision by surgery depending on the size, location, and histology of the tumor as well as on prior treatment and cosmetic considerations.
  - Mohs' micrographic surgery for lesions on areas of the face that are difficult to reconstruct.

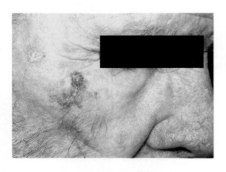

FIGURE 2-14. **Actinic keratosis.**
(Reproduced with permission from Wolff K et al. *Fitzpatrick's Color Atlas and Synopsis of Clinical Dermatology,* 7th ed. New York: McGraw-Hill, 2013, Fig. 10-28.)

SQUAMOUS CELL CARCINOMA

- The second most common skin cancer. Actinic keratoses are premalignant precursors (see Figure 2-14).

TABLE 2-4. **Common Dermatophytoses**

Condition	Description	Example
Tinea capitis	Erythema and scaling of the scalp with thickened, broken-off hairs and scalp kerion (Image A). Etiology: *Trichophyton tonsurans, Microsporum canis.* Treatment: Griseofulvin, itraconazole.	
Tinea corporis	Annular plaques with a thin scale and central clearing (Image B). Etiology: *Trichophyton mentagrophytes, M canis.* Treatment: Griseofulvin, itraconazole, clotrimazole cream.	
Tinea pedis	Red, scaly soles with maceration and fissuring between the toes +/− blisters (Image C). Etiology: *Trichophyton rubrum.* Treatment: Griseofulvin, terbinafine, itraconazole, antifungal powders.	
Onychomycosis	Hyperkeratosis and yellowing of the nail plate; scaling (Image D). Etiology: *T rubrum, T mentagrophytes.* Treatment: Terbinafine.	
Tinea versicolor	Hypopigmented macules in areas of sun-induced pigmentation; reddish-brown appearance in winter (Image E). Etiology: *Malassezia globosa, Malassezia furfur.* Treatment: Itraconazole, topical selenium sulfide/ketoconazole.	

Image A courtesy of the Centers for Disease Control and Prevention, Atlanta, GA. Image B reproduced with permission from Stern SD et al. *Symptom to Diagnosis: An Evidence-Based Guide,* 2nd ed. New York: McGraw-Hill, 2010, Fig. 24-11. Images C–E reproduced with permission from Wolff K et al. *Fitzpatrick's Color Atlas and Synopsis of Clinical Dermatology,* 7th ed. New York: McGraw-Hill, 2013, Figs. 26-29, 26-32, and 26-19.

Q

A 71-year-old man complains of a lesion on his right flank that was preceded by tingling in the same area 1 day ago. Exam reveals a 4-inch band of painful vesicles with 2° crusting and a clear midline border. What test do you send to confirm your clinical diagnosis?

- Risk factors include a history of actinic keratosis, immunosuppression, smoking, arsenic exposure, and exposure to industrial carcinogens.
- **Sx/Exam:**
  - **Actinic keratosis:** Presents as gritty or scaly plaques occurring in areas of sun exposure.
  - **Squamous cell carcinoma:** Pink plaques with scale or erosion; may spread to regional lymph nodes.
- **Dx:** Skin biopsy shows irregular masses of anaplastic epidermal cells proliferating down to the dermis.
- **Tx:**
  - Surgical excision for larger lesions; actinic keratoses may be treated with topical chemotherapeutics or liquid nitrogen.
  - Mohs' micrographic surgery for lesions on areas of the face that are difficult to reconstruct.

MELANOMA

- Malignant proliferation of melanocytes.
- Risk factors include sun exposure, fair skin, a ⊕ family history, a large number of nevi, and dysplastic nevi.
- **Sx/Exam:** Look for nevi with an irregular appearance (**ABCDE = A**symmetry, **B**order irregularity, **C**olor irregularity, **D**iameter > 6 mm, **E**volution).
- **Dx:** Skin biopsy (melanocytes with cellular atypia); imaging may be warranted for metastatic evaluation.
- **Tx:** Surgical excision; adjuvant therapy for patients with advanced disease.

Genitourinary Disorders

ERECTILE DYSFUNCTION (ED)

Inability to achieve or maintain an erection sufficient for penetration and ejaculation. Affects 30 million men. Associated with age; some degree of ED is seen in 40% of 40-year-olds and 70% of 70-year-olds. Etiologies are as follows:

- **Psychological:**
  - Symptoms often have a sudden onset.
  - Patients are unable to sustain or sometimes even obtain an erection.
  - Patients have **normal nocturnal penile tumescence** (those with organic causes do not).
- **Organic:**
  - **Endocrine:** DM, hypothyroidism or thyrotoxicosis, pituitary or gonadal disorders, ↑ prolactin.
  - **Vascular:** Atherosclerosis, vascular steal.
  - **Neurologic:** Stroke, DM, MS, spinal surgery, neuropathy.
  - **Exogenous:** β-blockers, SSRIs, α-blockers, clonidine, CNS depressants, anticholinergics, chronic opioids, TCAs.

EXAM

- Look for exam findings suggesting an organic cause—eg, small testes, evidence of Peyronie's disease, perineal sensation/cremaster reflex, or evidence of peripheral neuropathy/vasculopathy.
- Assess peripheral pulses; look for skin atrophy, hair loss, and low skin temperature.

Although a clinical exam is typically sufficient for the diagnosis of herpes zoster, a PCR of fluid from the lesion can be confirmatory. NSAIDs may be useful for pain control, and antiviral therapy may speed resolution and ↓ the likelihood of postherpetic neuralgia.

DIAGNOSIS

Assess testosterone; if there is concern about 2° causes, check TSH, prolactin, and glucose (to assess for diabetes).

TREATMENT

- Treat underlying disease.
- PDE-5a inhibitors (sildenafil, tadalafil, vardenafil) inhibit cGMP-specific phosphodiesterase type 5a, thereby improving relaxation of smooth muscle in the corpora cavernosa. Side effects include flushing, headache, and ↓ BP. Patients cannot be on nitrates or α-blockers.
- Injectable therapies such as alprostadil may also be used.
- For those who fail medical therapy, an external penile pump or an inflatable penile prosthesis can be tried.
- Testosterone for hypogonadism; behavioral treatment for depression and anxiety. A PDE-5a inhibitor may be effective for patients with psychogenic causes.
- Vascular surgery if indicated.

BENIGN PROSTATIC HYPERPLASIA (BPH)

Hyperplasia of the prostate that leads to bladder outlet obstruction. Incidence ↑ with age. Common in patients > 45 years of age. In those < 45 years of age with urinary retention, consider an alternative diagnosis such as urethral stricture or a neuropathic etiology.

SYMPTOMS/EXAM

- Patients complain of frequency, urgency, nocturia, ↓ force and size of the urinary stream, and incomplete emptying leading to overflow incontinence.
- Exam reveals a firm, rubbery, smooth prostatic surface (vs rock-hard areas that suggest prostate cancer).

DIAGNOSIS

- Diagnosed by history and exam. Check a UA for infection or hematuria, both of which should prompt further evaluation.
- PSA is ↑ in up to 50% of patients but is not diagnostically useful.

TREATMENT

- α-blockers (terazosin), 5α-reductase inhibitors (finasteride).
- Avoid anticholinergics, antihistamines, or narcotics.
- If the condition is refractory to medications, consider surgical options such as transurethral resection of the prostate (TURP). An open procedure is appropriate if gland size is > 75 g. In general, indications for TURP include recurrent UTIs, bladder stones, hematuria, episodes of acute urinary retention, and renal failure 2° to obstruction.

TESTICULAR MASSES/GROIN PAIN IN MEN

Epididymitis/Orchitis

- **Epididymitis** is defined as an acute infection that results in posterior and superior testicular tenderness. It is the most common cause of scrotal pain in adults. **Orchitis** is associated with diffuse testicular pain.
  - In men > 35 years of age, *E coli* is the most common cause.
  - In men < 35 years of age, *Chlamydia* is most common.

Q 1

A patient presents for evaluation of a pigmented skin lesion. Biopsy reveals melanocytes with marked atypia characteristic of melanoma. What feature is the most important prognostic factor?

Q 2

A 74-year-old man presents with inability to maintain an erection. Although the problem started several years ago, he states that he ignored it because he thought it was a normal part of aging. How should the patient be counseled?

Q 3

A 70-year-old man is prescribed terazosin for his BPH. How does the drug treat this condition, and what other medical condition does its mechanism of action address?

- **Dx:** CBC, UA and urine culture, Gram stain for gonococcal infection and trichomoniasis, nucleic acid amplification tests for *Neisseria gonorrhoeae* and *Chlamydia trachomatis*, Doppler ultrasound (shows ↑ blood flow).
- **Tx:** Antibiotics and supportive therapy (analgesics, ice packs, scrotal support and elevation).

Testicular Torsion

- A urologic emergency that requires immediate intervention owing to the potential for resulting infertility.
- **Sx/Exam:** The affected testicle sits higher and is painful.
- **Dx:** CBC, UA and urine culture, Gram stain, nucleic acid amplification tests, Doppler ultrasound (shows ↓ blood flow).
- **Tx:** Manual detorsion or surgical intervention.

Health Care Maintenance

CANCER SCREENING

Table 2-5 outlines recommended guidelines for the screening of common forms of cancer.

OTHER ROUTINE SCREENING

- **Hypertension:** BP screening should be done every 2 years in normotensive adults and every year for those with a systolic BP of 120–139 or a diastolic BP of 80–90. For young patients (age < 50) with an ↑ BP, look for 2° causes of hypertension, such as chronic kidney disease, pheochromocytoma, thyroid/parathyroid disease, sleep apnea, renovascular disease, Cushing's syndrome, coarctation of the aorta, and 1° hyperaldosteronism.
- **Hyperlipidemia:** The US Preventive Services Task Force (USPSTF) strongly recommends screening men ≥ 35 years of age and women ≥ 45 years of age (20–45 years of age in the setting of CAD risk factors) for lipid disorders. Treatment measures are outlined in Table 2-6. Risk factors that modify LDL goals include:
    - Cigarette smoking
    - Hypertension (BP ≥ 140/90 or on antihypertensive medication)
    - Diabetes
    - Age (men ≥ 45 years; women ≥ 55 years) and male gender
    - Obesity
- **Diabetes:** The ADA recommends testing for diabetes or prediabetes in all adults with a BMI ≥ 25 kg/m² and 1 or more additional risk factors for diabetes (see below). For those without risk factors, testing should begin at age 45. A fasting plasma glucose, a 2-hour oral glucose tolerance test, or an HbA_{1c} (≥ 6.5%) is appropriate. Additional risk factors for diabetes are as follows:
    - A family history of DM in a first-degree relative
    - Habitual physical inactivity
    - Belonging to a high-risk ethnic or racial group (eg, African American, Hispanic, Native American, Asian American, Pacific Islander)
    - A history of delivering a baby weighing > 4.1 kg (9 lbs) or of gestational diabetes

---

1 **A**

Depth of invasion of the melanoma.

2 **A**

Although ED is associated with age, it is still considered abnormal, and patients presenting with complaints of ED should be adequately evaluated for all potential causes.

3 **A**

α_1-blockers such as terazosin act on smooth muscle in the prostate, bladder neck, and urethra. They also act on vascular smooth muscle, causing vasodilation; therefore, they have an effect on hypertension as well.

TABLE 2-5. **Recommended Cancer Screening Guidelines**

TYPE	RECOMMENDATIONS
Cervical cancer	A Pap smear is recommended starting at age 21 until age 75. Patients may be screened every 3 years if they have had a normal Pap. Those > 30 years of age may ↑ the screening interval to 5 years if the Pap is performed with HPV PCR testing.
Breast cancer	Mammography should be conducted every 2 years after age 50 (may begin earlier if there is a ⊕ family history at a young age). The age at which mammographic screening should begin is controversial. The USPSTF recommends biennial screening mammography for women 50–74 years of age. For patients in their 40s, it is recommended that the decision to begin screening be thoroughly discussed with their doctors.
Colon cancer	Hemoccult annually (especially in patients > 50 years of age); flexible sigmoidoscopy (every 3–5 years in those > 50) or colonoscopy (every 10 years in those > 50). If a first-degree relative has colon cancer, begin screening at age 40 or when the patient is 10 years younger than the age at which that relative was diagnosed, whichever comes first.
Prostate cancer	Controversial. Some groups (eg, the USPSTF) recommend no screening; others recommend a yearly rectal exam and PSA beginning at age 45, especially for African Americans, patients with a strong family history, or those with any changes in urinary symptoms.
Lung cancer	Controversial. The USPSTF recommends annual screening for lung cancer with a low-dose CT scan at 55–80 years of age if the patient has a 30-pack-year smoking history and is currently smoking or quit within the past 15 years.

- Hypertension (BP ≥ 140/90)
- Dyslipidemia
- Polycystic ovarian syndrome
- A history of vascular disease
- **Osteoporosis:** The USPSTF recommends that women ≥ 65 years of age be screened no more than every 2 years. Screening should begin earlier for postmenopausal women who are at ↑ risk for osteoporotic fractures (eg, low weight, low estrogen state, long-term use of oral or injected steroids). DEXA is the screening test of choice.
- **Abdominal aortic aneurysm (AAA):** The USPSTF recommends 1-time screening for AAA in men 65–75 years of age who have smoked at any time. Abdominal ultrasound is the screening test of choice.

TABLE 2-6. **Treatment of Hyperlipidemia**

RISK FACTOR	LDL TREATMENT
CAD history 40–75 years of age with DM 40–75 years of age without CAD with a 10-year risk for MI/stroke > 7.5% > 21 years of age with LDL > 190 mg/dL	Moderate- to high-intensity statin; follow up by measuring lipid panel; no titration to specific LDL cholesterol goal.

Q

A 41-year-old woman with no significant medical history comes to your clinic for her first checkup. She has no children and is in a monogamous relationship. Her mother had type 2 DM. Her physical exam is within normal limits. Which screening tests might you recommend?

IMMUNIZATIONS

Table 2-7 lists indications for adult immunizations.

TABLE 2-7.   **Indications for Immunization in Adults**

IMMUNIZATION	INDICATION/RECOMMENDATION
Tetanus	Give 1° series in childhood followed by boosters every 10 years (see Chapter 4).
Hepatitis B	Administer to all infants and to patients at ↑ risk (eg, IV drug users, health care providers, those with chronic liver disease).
Pneumococcal	Give to those ≥ 65 years of age or to any patient at ↑ risk (eg, patients with splenectomy, COPD, or diabetes; alcoholics; or immunocompromised patients such as those on chemotherapy, posttransplant, or HIV ⊕).
Influenza	Give annually to all patients > 6 months of age.
Hepatitis A	Give to those traveling to endemic areas, those with chronic liver disease (HBV or HCV), and IV drug abusers.
Zoster	Recommended for all patients ≥ 60 years of age who have no contraindications, including those who report a previous episode of zoster or who have chronic medical conditions.
Smallpox	Currently recommended only for those working in laboratories in which they are exposed to the virus.
Meningococcal	Not recommended for routine use. Used in outbreaks. The CDC recommends that all children 11–12 years of age be vaccinated and that a booster dose be given at age 16.

A

A Pap smear; hypertension screening; and a fasting glucose test, a 2-hour glucose tolerance test, or an HbA$_{1c}$. Given the patient's age, a screening mammogram is controversial. It is important to discuss the risks, benefits, and alternatives of screening before proceeding.

CARDIOVASCULAR

KEY FACT

Major risk factors for ischemic heart disease:
- Age > 65
- Male gender
- Family history
- Hypertension
- Smoking
- Hyperlipidemia
- Diabetes mellitus

KEY FACT

Unstable angina is any new angina in previously asymptomatic patients, or accelerating or new rest angina in patients with prior stable angina.

KEY FACT

Certain patients—including diabetics, women, and the elderly—can present with ischemic disease with highly atypical symptoms. Diabetes is considered a CAD risk equivalent.

Ischemic Heart Disease

The 1° cause of ischemic heart disease is atherosclerotic occlusion of the coronary arteries. **Major risk factors** include age, family history (particularly of early CAD in a first-degree relative, as defined by significant disease in male relatives before age 55 or in female relatives before age 65), smoking, diabetes, hypertension, and hyperlipidemia.

SYMPTOMS

- **May be asymptomatic** or present as follows:
  - **Stable angina:** Substernal chest tightness/pain or shortness of breath with a consistent amount of exertion; relief is obtained with rest or nitroglycerin. Reflects a stable, flow-limiting plaque.
  - **Unstable angina or MI (acute coronary syndrome):** Chest tightness/pain and/or shortness of breath, typically at rest, with a duration of > 20 minutes (in patients with known stable angina, unstable angina may present with acceleration or worsening of prior anginal symptoms). Pain tends not to improve markedly with nitroglycerin or recurs soon after its use. Reflects plaque rupture with formation of a clot in the lumen of the blood vessel.
- Not all patients present with typical anginal symptoms. Ask about other symptoms that are considered "anginal equivalents," such as dyspnea.

EXAM

- Exam may be normal when patients are asymptomatic. During episodes of angina, a left ventricular S4 or a mitral regurgitation murmur may occasionally be heard.
- Look for signs of heart failure (eg, ↑ JVP, inspiratory crackles, hepatomegaly, lower extremity edema) that could be due to prior MI and may be causing left ventricular dysfunction.
- Look for vascular disease elsewhere—eg, carotid, abdominal, and femoral bruits; asymmetric or diminished pulses; and lower extremity ischemic ulcers.

DIFFERENTIAL

Consider pericarditis, pulmonary embolism, pneumothorax, aortic dissection, peptic ulcer, esophageal disease (including diffuse esophageal spasm), GERD, and musculoskeletal causes. Chest pain from anxiety should be a diagnosis of exclusion.

DIAGNOSIS

- **Initial workup:** Look for elevated cardiac biomarkers (troponin, CK, CK-MB) +/– ECG changes (ST-segment elevation/depression/Q waves) in the distribution of the coronary arteries (see Table 3-1, Table 3-2, and Figure 3-1); check a CXR for other causes of chest pain. Non-ST-segment-elevation MI (NSTEMI) can be distinguished from unstable angina by the presence of elevated cardiac biomarkers.
- **Stress testing:** Exercise, dobutamine, or vasodilator stress; ECG, echocardiography, or radionuclide imaging to assess perfusion (see the discussion of advanced cardiac evaluation below).
- **Cardiac catheterization:** Defines anatomy and the location and severity of lesions. ST-segment-elevation MI (STEMI) is a high-risk MI that requires emergency catheterization for reperfusion.

TABLE 3-1.   Arterial Supply of the Heart in Right-Dominant Coronary Circulation

LEFT ANTERIOR DESCENDING (LAD) ARTERY	LEFT CIRCUMFLEX ARTERY	RIGHT CORONARY ARTERY/ POSTERIOR DESCENDING ARTERY (RCA/PDA)
Apex	Lateral wall of LV	Lateral wall of right ventricle (RV)
Anterior wall of left ventricle (LV)	Posterior wall of LV (20%)	Posterior wall of LV (80%)
Anterior two-thirds of interventricular septum (IVS)	Posterior one-third of IVS (20%)	Posterior one-third of IVS (80%)
		SA node
		AV node

TREATMENT

- **Acute coronary syndrome:**
    - Initial treatment includes anticoagulation (LMWH, unfractionated heparin), aspirin, nitroglycerin, O_2, and a β-blocker in hemodynamically stable patients. Antiplatelet agents (clopidogrel, prasugrel, ticagrelor) are often used as well if a percutaneous stent is placed. Glycoprotein IIb/IIIa antagonists (abciximab, eptifibatide, tirofiban) or bivalirudin may be used in the catheterization laboratory when angioplasty is pursued.
    - STEMIs or NSTEMIs with high-risk features should be managed by percutaneous coronary intervention. If possible, an ACEI should be started before discharge.
- **Angina:** β-blockers ↓ HR, ↑ myocardial perfusion time, and ↓ cardiac workload, which ↓ exertional angina. If symptoms arise on a β-blocker, a long-acting nitrate or calcium channel blocker (CCB) can be added. Ranolazine can be added for refractory angina.

PREVENTION

2° prevention measures include:

- **Risk factor modification (to slow progression):** Control diabetes, ↓ BP, ↓ cholesterol (**specifically LDL**), and encourage smoking cessation.
- **Prevention of MI: Aspirin;** clopidogrel can be given to aspirin-sensitive patients.
- **Drugs that improve mortality after MI:** Aspirin, β-blockers, ACEIs (or ARBs in ACEI-intolerant patients), HMG-CoA reductase inhibitors (statins), and spironolactone in high-risk subgroups. Antiplatelet agents are used following coronary stent placement, usually for a minimum of 12 months.

TABLE 3-2.   ECG Findings with MI in Right-Dominant Coronary Circulation

AREA OF INFARCT	CORONARY ARTERY INVOLVED	LEADS WITH ST CHANGES
Inferior wall (RV)	RCA/PDA	II, III, aVF
Septum	LAD	V2, V3
Lateral wall (LV)	Left circumflex	I, aVL, V5, V6

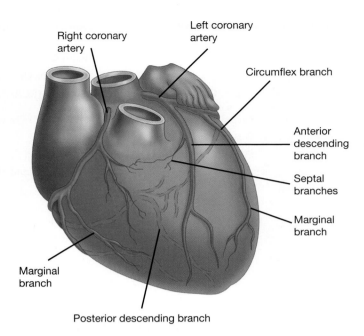

FIGURE 3-1.   Coronary artery anatomy. (Reproduced with permission from Le T, Krause K. *First Aid for the Basic Sciences: Organ Systems,* 2nd ed. New York: McGraw-Hill, 2011, Fig. 1-9.)

KEY FACT

Any condition that causes delayed left ventricular emptying (eg, aortic stenosis, LBBB) can be associated with paradoxical splitting. Delayed emptying leads to delayed A2, with P2 heard before A2. On inspiration, A2 and P2 move closer together, eliminating a split S2.

KEY FACT

VSDs produce holosystolic murmurs that radiate throughout the precordium, often with a thrill. They are the most common cardiac malformation at birth.

Valvular Disease

Table 3-3 describes the clinical characteristics and treatment of common valvular lesions.

Congestive Heart Failure

Defined as inability of the heart to pump adequate blood to meet the demands of the body. Can be categorized in different ways. One categorization scheme includes:

- Systolic heart failure (aka "heart failure with reduced EF")
- Diastolic heart failure (aka "heart failure with preserved EF")
- Heart failure related to valvular disease
- Heart failure related to arrhythmias

SYSTOLIC HEART FAILURE

Weakened pumping function of the heart. Common causes include **ischemic heart disease, long-standing hypertension,** toxins (eg, alcohol), and viral or idiopathic cardiomyopathy in younger patients.

SYMPTOMS

- Patients present with poor exercise tolerance, exertional dyspnea, and easy fatigability.
- Volume-overloaded patients may present with **orthopnea,** paroxysmal nocturnal dyspnea, poor appetite, RUQ pain, and ankle swelling.

TABLE 3-3.   **Presentation and Treatment of Select Valvular Lesions**

LESION	SYMPTOMS	EXAM	TREATMENT	COMMENTS
Mitral stenosis	Symptoms of heart failure; hemoptysis; atrial fibrillation (AF).	Diastolic murmur best heard at the apex; opening snap; usually does not radiate.	HR control, balloon valvuloplasty, valve replacement.	Usually caused by **rheumatic fever.**
Mitral regurgitation	Has a long asymptomatic period; when severe or acute, presents with symptoms of heart failure.	**Blowing** systolic murmur at the apex, **radiating to the axilla.** The posterior leaflet may lead to a murmur along the sternal border.	If acute, surgery is always required. For chronic mitral regurgitation, repair or replace the valve when symptomatic or if the ejection fraction (EF) is < 60%. Surgery is indicated in some patients with an EF > 60% (new AF, pulmonary hypertension).	Long-standing regurgitation dilates the atrium, increasing the chance of AF.
Mitral valve prolapse	Asymptomatic.	Midsystolic click; also murmur if mitral regurgitation is present.	Endocarditis prophylaxis is not required.	Questionable association with palpitations and panic attacks. The most common cause of mitral regurgitation.
Aortic stenosis	Chest pain, syncope, heart failure, shortness of breath.	Harsh systolic crescendo-decrescendo murmur radiating to the carotids along the right sternal border. **A small and slow carotid upstroke** (parvus et tardus), a late-peaking murmur, and loss of clear S2 can be seen with severe stenosis.	**Avoid overdiuresis; avoid vasodilators** such as nitrates and ACEIs given fixed obstruction. Surgery or balloon valvuloplasty for all symptomatic patients.	Once symptoms appear, mortality is 50% at 3 years.
Aortic regurgitation	Usually asymptomatic until advanced; then presents with symptoms of heart failure.	**Wide pulse pressure;** soft, high-pitched diastolic murmur along the left sternal border. Radiates toward the apex.	**Afterload reduction** with ACEIs, hydralazine; valve replacement if symptomatic or in the setting of a ↓ EF.	Many cases are associated with aortic root disease, dissection, syphilis, ankylosing spondylitis, and Marfan's syndrome.

EXAM

Exam often reveals inspiratory crackles (may be absent in chronic heart failure), a diffuse PMI that is displaced to the left (reflects cardiomegaly), an **S3 gallop,** ↑ JVP, and lower extremity edema. Cool extremities and/or confusion may suggest low cardiac output.

DIFFERENTIAL

Deconditioning, lung disease (eg, COPD, chronic thromboembolic pulmonary hypertension, 1° pulmonary hypertension), other categories of heart fail-

A 58-year-old man with long-standing hypertension is admitted to the hospital with dyspnea on exertion and bibasilar crackles, and you suspect CHF as the cause. Which imaging modality would you order to confirm your diagnosis?

ure (eg, diastolic dysfunction), other causes of edema (eg, cirrhosis, vascular incompetence, low albumin, nephrotic syndrome).

DIAGNOSIS

- The history and exam are suggestive, but determination of the EF via an imaging study (eg, **echocardiography,** radionuclide imaging, cardiac MRI) confirms the diagnosis.
- **Look for the cause of the low EF:**
  - Perform a stress test or cardiac catheterization to look for CAD; evaluate for thyroid and renal disease.
  - Look for a history of alcohol use or exposure to offending cardiotoxic medications such as **doxorubicin.**
  - Dilated cardiomyopathy can be seen in postpartum females.
  - A myocardial biopsy may be performed in selected cases to evaluate for infiltrative disease or other rare causes of heart failure when other evaluations are inconclusive.

TREATMENT

- Treatment is based on optimizing cardiac output via the following mechanisms:
  - ↓ preload (reducing cardiac filling pressures).
  - ↓ wall stress and optimization of cardiac contractility.
  - ↓ afterload (making it easier for the heart to pump systemically).
- **Maintenance medications** include:
  - **Preload reduction:** Diuretics (furosemide, torsemide).
  - **↓ wall stress:** β-blockers (metoprolol, bisoprolol, carvedilol).
  - **Optimization of contractility:** Digoxin (may lower the frequency of hospitalizations and improve symptoms but does not ↓ mortality).
  - **Afterload reduction:** Renin-angiotensin-aldosterone antagonists (ACEIs/ARBs; spironolactone if potassium and creatinine are not ↑ and the patient is on optimal dosages of β-blockers and ACEIs/ARBs). Hydralazine and nitrates may be useful additions to ACEIs/ARBs in African American patients or an alternative to ACEIs/ARBs in patients with kidney disease/hyperkalemia. Spironolactone improves mortality in symptomatic systolic heart failure.
- **Exacerbations:** Give **loop diuretics** such as furosemide when the patient is volume overloaded. These are generally given first in IV form and then transitioned to oral form once the patient is closer to euvolemia. β-blockers and afterload reduction agents can be initiated once the patient is euvolemic.
- **Implantable cardiac defibrillators (ICDs)** are associated with ↓ mortality from ventricular tachycardia and ventricular fibrillation (VT/VF) in heart failure patients who are symptomatic and have a ↓ EF (< 35%). **Cardiac resynchronization therapy (CRT)** is sometimes indicated in heart failure patients with both a ↓ EF and intraventricular conduction delay (QRS > 120 msec).
- Treat the underlying cause of the systolic heart failure (eg, CAD).

DIASTOLIC HEART FAILURE

During diastole, the heart is **stiff** and does not relax well, resulting in ↑ diastolic filling pressure. However, the EF is often normal, so isolated diastolic heart failure is sometimes referred to as "heart failure with preserved ejection fraction" (HFpEF). **Hypertension with left ventricular hypertrophy** (LVH) is the most common cause; other causes include hypertrophic cardiomyopathy and infiltrative diseases.

KEY FACT

ACEIs, ARBs, and spironolactone all cause hyperkalemia and should be avoided or used cautiously in patients with hyperkalemia and/or renal impairment.

KEY FACT

Don't forget—systolic heart failure is associated with a low EF, whereas diastolic heart failure often has a normal to elevated EF.

KEY FACT

VT leading to VF is a common cause of death in patients with a ↓ EF. Thus, ICD placement is indicated for patients with an EF < 35%, and CRT is indicated for those with a ↓ EF and intraventricular delay.

Transthoracic echocardiography (TTE). TTE provides specific information, such as LVEF and diastolic compliance and relaxation, that can confirm the diagnosis of systolic and diastolic heart failure. It also yields information about specific etiologies or precipitants, such as valvular or wall motion abnormalities.

SYMPTOMS/EXAM

- Signs and symptoms are the same as those of systolic heart failure.
- Exam findings are similar to those of systolic failure. Listen for an **S4** rather than an **S3** (if rhythm is regular) or an irregular rhythm (AF is commonly associated with diastolic dysfunction).

DIAGNOSIS

- Presents with symptoms of heart failure with a preserved EF on echocardiogram.
- Echocardiography often shows ventricular hypertrophy. Biopsy may be needed to establish the underlying diagnosis if infiltrative disease is suspected. Cardiac MRI is becoming an increasingly popular modality for this purpose.

TREATMENT

- Control hypertension.
- Give diuretics to control volume overload and symptoms, but **avoid over-diuresis,** which can ↓ preload and cardiac output.
- Manage arrhythmias (eg, AF) that are frequently associated with diastolic dysfunction.
- Control renal and vascular disease, both of which are thought to be associated with diastolic heart disease.

HEART FAILURE RELATED TO VALVULAR DISEASE

- Right-sided valvular lesions can cause profound edema that is refractory to diuresis.
- Left-sided valvular lesions can produce heart failure.

HEART FAILURE RELATED TO ARRHYTHMIAS

- Often apparent from either patient-reported palpitations or ECG findings.
- Rhythms that can cause symptoms of heart failure include both tachyarrhythmias (eg, rapid **AF**) and bradyarrhythmias. Others present abruptly with palpitations, shortness of breath, or even syncope.

Cardiomyopathy

Table 3-4 outlines the types and clinical presentations of cardiomyopathies as well as their treatment. Echocardiography is useful for the diagnosis of all types of cardiomyopathy.

Pericardial Disease

PERICARDITIS

Inflammation of the pericardial sac. May be acute (< 6 weeks; most common), subacute (6 weeks to 6 months), or chronic (> 6 months). Causes include bacterial or viral infection (especially enterovirus), mediastinal radiation, post-MI (Dressler's syndrome), cancer, rheumatologic diseases (SLE, RA), uremia, TB, and prior cardiac surgery. May also be idiopathic (the most common cause of acute cases).

KEY FACT

Important 2° causes of diastolic heart failure:
- Sarcoidosis
- Amyloidosis
- Hemochromatosis
- Scleroderma
- Fibrosis (radiation, surgery)

KEY FACT

Active ischemia can acutely worsen diastolic dysfunction and cause systolic dysfunction, so treat any coexisting CAD in patients with diastolic heart failure.

Q

A 54-year-old business executive develops chest pain while at work. His vital signs remain stable. The chest pain is partially relieved by nitroglycerin but worsens with cough and deep inspiration. He is brought to the ED, where his ECG reveals diffuse ST-T elevations. His cardiac enzymes are normal. What is the appropriate treatment?

TABLE 3-4.   Types and Features of Cardiomyopathies

TYPE	ASSOCIATED SYMPTOMS AND CONDITIONS	DISTINGUISHING FEATURES	TREATMENT
Dilated	Ischemia, tachycardia, hypertension, alcohol, and Chagas' disease (in South America).	If the offending source or stimulus is removed, alcoholic and tachycardia-induced cardiomyopathies can be almost completely reversible.	ACEIs, ARBs, β-blockers, and spironolactone. Digoxin can improve symptoms but does not improve mortality.
Restrictive	Sarcoid, amyloid, hemochromatosis, cancer, and glycogen storage disease.	Echocardiography shows LVH, whereas ECG frequently shows low voltage. Biopsy is occasionally required to determine the cause.	Directed at the underlying cause and symptom management with diuretics.
Hypertrophic	Genetically inherited in an autosomal dominant pattern; associated with sudden cardiac death.	Echocardiography may reveal a normal EF and an asymmetrically thickened ventricle.	Avoid inotropes, vasodilators, and excessive diuresis.

KEY FACT

Chronic constrictive pericarditis often presents with ascites, hepatomegaly, and distended neck veins. A common cause in North America is prior pericardiotomy (from cardiac surgery). TB is a cause that is uncommon in North America.

SYMPTOMS/EXAM

- Presents with **chest pain** that is often improved with sitting up or leaning forward. The pain may radiate to the back and to the left trapezial ridge.
- If a large effusion is present, the patient may be short of breath.
- Exam may reveal a pericardial friction rub (a leathery sound that can be present in multiple stages of the cardiac cycle).

DIFFERENTIAL

Myocardial ischemia, aortic dissection, pneumonia, pulmonary embolism, pneumothorax.

DIAGNOSIS

- A number of features can distinguish pericarditis from acute MI (see Table 3-5).
- Echocardiography may reveal an associated pericardial effusion.
- Search for an underlying cause—ie, take a history for viral illness, radiation exposure, and malignancy. Check ANA, PPD, blood cultures if febrile, and renal function.

NSAIDs. The patient most likely has pericarditis, which is a clinical diagnosis.

TABLE 3-5.   Pericarditis vs Acute MI

	PERICARDITIS	MI
Clinical	Pain improves with sitting up or leaning forward; sometimes pleuritic.	Pain is not alleviated or exacerbated by position.
ECG	Diffuse ST-segment elevation, often with upward concavity (see Figure 3-2); PR-segment depression; ST-T changes tend to normalize more rapidly than those in MI.	ST-segment elevation is localized to the distribution of coronary arteries, often with downward concavity.

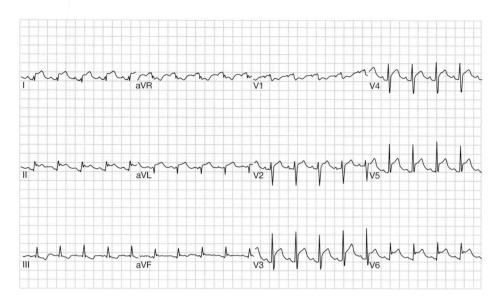

FIGURE 3-2.   Pericarditis. Note diffuse ST-segment elevation.

TREATMENT

- Where possible, treat the underlying disorder (eg, SLE, advanced renal failure).
- For viral or idiopathic pericarditis, give NSAIDs, colchicine, or aspirin. Avoid NSAIDs or steroids in early post-MI pericarditis, as they may interfere with scar formation.

COMPLICATIONS

Patients may develop a clinically significant pericardial effusion and **tamponade** (see below).

PERICARDIAL EFFUSION AND CARDIAC TAMPONADE

Accumulation of fluid (usually chronic) or blood (usually acute and posttraumatic/postsurgical) in the pericardial cavity surrounding the heart.

SYMPTOMS/EXAM

- Symptomatology often depends on the rate of fluid accumulation. If **acute,** patients may present with **shock.** If **chronic,** patients may present with **shortness of breath and heart failure (if gradual, several liters of fluid may accumulate).**
- In patients with pericardial effusions and tamponade physiology, exam classically reveals distant or muffled heart sounds, ↑ JVP, and pulsus paradoxus (a drop of > 10 mm Hg in systolic BP during inspiration).

DIFFERENTIAL

Pneumothorax, acute MI, heart failure.

DIAGNOSIS

Echocardiography is needed to confirm the diagnosis. CXR may reveal an enlarged cardiac silhouette (see Figure 3-3), and ECG may show low voltages and electrical alternans (beat-to-beat variation in R-wave amplitude).

KEY FACT

Pulsus paradoxus occurs in tamponade: inspiration → ↑ venous return to the right side of the heart → ↓ LV filling and output (pericardial fluid creates a fixed volume, so increases in right-sided volume → ↓ left-sided volume).

KEY FACT

Always check a bedside pulsus paradoxus when tamponade is suspected. Echocardiography is the diagnostic procedure of choice.

A 62-year-old man suddenly develops hypotension and shortness of breath 1 day after CABG surgery. Exam reveals JVD and muffled heart sounds, and bedside pulsus paradoxus is present. What are your next diagnostic and therapeutic steps?

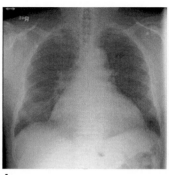
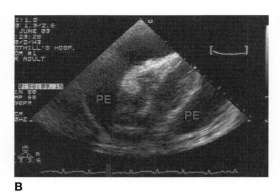

A   **B**

FIGURE 3-3.   **Pericardial effusion and tamponade. (A)** CXR with enlargement of the cardiac silhouette ("water-bottle heart") in a patient with a pericardial effusion. **(B)** Apical 4-chamber transthoracic echocardiogram with a large pericardial effusion (PE) and collapse of the right atrium and right ventricle during diastole in a patient with cardiac tamponade. (Image A reproduced with permission from USMLE-Rx.com. Image B reproduced with permission from Hall JB et al. *Principles of Critical Care,* 3rd ed. New York: McGraw-Hill, 2005, Fig. 28-7A.)

TREATMENT

- Consider emergent pericardiocentesis for patients with post–chest trauma shock as well as for those whose echocardiogram shows evidence of tamponade physiology.
- Also consider a pericardial window for those with recurrent or malignant effusions. While evaluation with echocardiography is being pursued, give IV fluids to maintain preload and systemic BP.

Advanced Cardiac Evaluation

- **Indications for stress testing** include diagnosis of CAD/evaluation of symptoms, preoperative evaluation, risk stratification in patients with known disease, and decision making about the need for revascularization.
- **Contraindications** include severe aortic stenosis, acute coronary syndrome, acute pulmonary embolus, unstable arrhythmias, and decompensated heart failure.
- Testing consists of a stressing modality and an evaluating modality (see Tables 3-6 and 3-7).
- Within available options for pharmacologic stressing modalities, dobuta-

Order an echocardiogram (to look for tamponade physiology) and pursue therapeutic pericardiocentesis or pericardial window.

TABLE 3-6.   **Stressing Modalities in Cardiac Testing**

MODALITY	PROS	CONS
Treadmill	Good for patients who can exercise lightly.	Lower sensitivity in women.
Dobutamine	Good for patients who cannot exercise.	Patients can feel poorly because of β-agonism.
Adenosine or dipyridamole (with nuclear imaging)	Good for patients who cannot exercise.	Can cause bronchospasm; exercise caution in patients with asthma/COPD.

TABLE 3-7. **Evaluating Modalities in Cardiac Testing**

MODALITY	PROS	CONS
ECG	Inexpensive, fast.	Cannot localize the lesion; cannot use with baseline ST-segment abnormalities or left bundle branch block (LBBB); cannot use if the patient is on digoxin.
Echocardiography	Better than ECG in patients with LBBB; cheaper than nuclear imaging.	Quality is provider dependent, which may limit the usefulness of images.
Radionuclide tracer (thallium or technetium)	Localizes ischemia; localizes infarcted tissue.	Expensive. Usefulness can be limited in extensive, multivessel CAD with balanced ischemia in different regions.

mine ↑ cardiac contractility, whereas adenosine and dipyridamole dilate the coronary arteries (the latter ↑ blood flow in healthy arteries but not in already maximally dilated diseased arteries, creating a differential flow that can be detected on nuclear imaging).

Hypertension

A major contributor to cardiovascular disease; more common with increasing age and among African Americans.

SYMPTOMS

Asymptomatic unless severe. If severe without symptoms, it is termed *hypertensive urgency*. If severe with symptoms or evidence of organ damage (dizziness, lightheadedness), it is termed *hypertensive emergency*.

EXAM

- BP > 140/90.
- A displaced PMI or an **S4** suggests LVH.
- Listen for bruits, which indicate peripheral vascular disease.
- Examine fundi, which can show **AV nicking** and "copper-wire" changes to the arterioles. In severe hypertension, look for papilledema and retinal hemorrhages.
- Look for signs suggestive of 2° hypertension.

DIFFERENTIAL

The vast majority of cases are due to essential (1°) hypertension, but in the right clinical settings or in cases of refractory hypertension, consider 2° causes (see Table 3-8).

DIAGNOSIS

- Diagnosed in the setting of a **BP > 140/90** on 3 separate occasions (elevation of either systolic or diastolic BP).
- A systolic BP of 120–139 or a diastolic BP of 80–89 is considered "prehypertension" and predicts the future development of hypertension.

 KEY FACT

Guidelines for goal BP have recently changed for both diabetic and nondiabetic patients.

 Q

A 65-year-old Caucasian man who has a history of diabetes and is currently on metformin has BP readings of 150/90 and 140/95 on multiple office visits. You start him on an ACEI, but he returns for follow-up complaining of a dry cough with a measured BP of 145/92. What is your BP goal for this patient, and what are additional options for treating his hypertension?

TABLE 3-8. Causes of 2° Hypertension

CAUSES	EXAMPLES
Endocrine	Cushing's syndrome, Conn's syndrome (aldosterone-producing tumor), hyperthyroidism, pheochromocytoma.
Renal	Chronic kidney disease (CKD); renal artery stenosis (listen for an abdominal bruit).
Medications	OCPs, NSAIDs.
Other	Fibromuscular dysplasia of the renal arteries and aortic coarctation (in younger patients); obstructive sleep apnea, alcohol.

TREATMENT

- Based on the most recent guidelines, the **goal BP for almost all patients, including those with diabetes or CKD,** is < 140/90. This represents a change from earlier guidelines, which recommended a goal of < 130/80 in diabetics and those with renal insufficiency. (Note: The goal BP recommended in the most recent guidelines has been the subject of controversy.)
- New guidelines also suggest that for patients > 60 years of age without diabetes or CKD, the goal BP should be < 150/90.
- **Interventions** include the following (see also Figure 3-4):
  - **Step 1—lifestyle modification:** Weight loss, exercise, ↓ sodium intake, smoking cessation.

KEY FACT

The goal BP in patients with diabetes or CKD is < 140/90, similar to the general population (previously the goal BP was < 130/80).

Thiazide diuretics, CCBs, ACEIs, and ARBs are all therapeutic options. The BP goal for this patient would be < 140/90. In light of his cough (a potential side effect of ACEIs), you could switch the patient to an ARB.

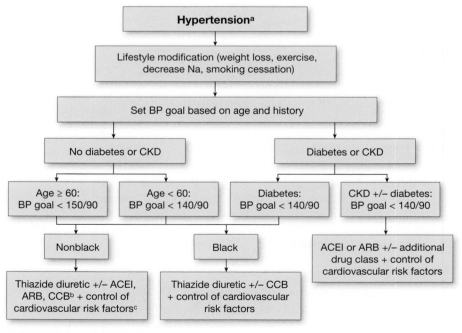

^a BP > 140/90 on 3 separate occasions.
^b Do not use ACEIs and ARBs together.
^c Eg, DM, smoking, hyperlipidemia.

FIGURE 3-4. **Algorithm for the treatment of hypertension.**

- **Step 2—medications: First-line agents** include **thiazide diuretics, CCBs, ACEIs, or ARBs** unless there is a more specific indication for another class of drugs (see Table 3-9). Consider starting 2 drugs initially if systolic BP is > 160.
- Control other cardiovascular risk factors, such as diabetes, smoking, and hypercholesterolemia.

COMPLICATIONS

Long-standing hypertension contributes to renal failure, heart failure (both systolic and diastolic), CAD, peripheral vascular disease, and stroke.

Aortic Dissection

Aortic dissection most commonly occurs in patients with a history of long-standing hypertension, cocaine use, aortic aneurysm, or aortic root disease such as Marfan's syndrome or Takayasu's arteritis.

SYMPTOMS/EXAM

- Presents with sudden onset of severe chest pain that sometimes radiates to the back, often described as a burning, searing, or tearing pain. May also present with neurologic symptoms resulting from occlusion of vessels supplying the brain or spinal cord.
- On exam, evaluate for aortic regurgitation, **asymmetric pulses and blood pressures,** and neurologic findings.

DIFFERENTIAL

MI (aortic dissection can also cause an MI if it extends into a coronary artery), pulmonary embolism, pneumothorax.

TABLE 3-9. Antihypertensive Medications

COMMONLY USED CLASSES	OPTIMAL USE	MAIN SIDE EFFECTS
Thiazide diuretics	First-line agent.	↓ excretion of calcium and uric acid; hyponatremia.
β-blockers	Not recommended as a first-line agent; useful in ↓ EF, **angina,** and **CAD.**	Bradycardia, erectile dysfunction, bronchospasm in asthmatics.
ACEIs	First-line agent; preferred over thiazides or CCBs in patients with CKD with or without diabetes; also useful in patients with ↓ EF and in diabetes with **microalbuminuria.**	**Dry cough,** angioedema, hyperkalemia, acute kidney injury.
ARBs	Same as ACEIs (does not cause cough associated with ACEIs).	Hyperkalemia.
CCBs	First-line agent.	Lower extremity edema.

KEY FACT

The treatment of hypertension in African American patients should begin with thiazide diuretics or CCBs even in those with diabetes.

KEY FACT

Always think about aortic dissection in patients with chest pain!

Q

A 69-year-old hospital administrator presents to the ED with severe, tearing chest pain that radiates to his back. CXR is unrevealing. Given your concern for potential aortic dissection, what is the next diagnostic step?

DIAGNOSIS

- Requires a high index of suspicion.
- CXR has low sensitivity but may show a widened mediastinum or a hazy aortic knob (see Figure 3-5).
- **CT with IV contrast** is diagnostic and shows the extent of dissection.
- Transesophageal echocardiography (TEE) is highly sensitive and specific.
- MRI may also be used, but it is often time consuming and may not be optimal for unstable patients.

TREATMENT

- **Initial medical stabilization:** Aggressive **HR and BP control**, first with β-blockers (typically IV esmolol) and then with IV nitroprusside if needed.
- **Ascending dissection—Stanford type A (involves the ascending aorta):** Emergent surgical repair.
- **Descending dissection—Stanford type B (distal to the left subclavian artery):** Medical management is indicated unless there is intractable pain, progressive dissection in patients with chest pain, or vascular occlusion of the aortic branches (see Figure 3-6).

COMPLICATIONS

Aortic rupture, acute aortic regurgitation, tamponade, MI, neurologic impairment, limb or mesenteric ischemia, renal ischemia.

Peripheral Vascular Disease

Atherosclerotic disease of vessels other than the coronary arteries. Risk factors are similar to those for CAD and include **smoking, diabetes,** hypercholesterolemia, hypertension, and increasing age.

SYMPTOMS

Complaints and presentation depend on the organ affected.

- **Mesenteric ischemia:** Postprandial abdominal pain and food avoidance ("food fear"), bloody diarrhea.
- **Lower extremities:** Claudication, leg ulceration or nonhealing wounds, rest pain.
- **Kidneys:** Usually asymptomatic, but may present with difficult-to-control hypertension.
- **CNS:** Stroke and TIA (see Chapter 13).

EXAM

- **Mesenteric disease:** No specific findings. The patient may be thin because of weight loss from avoidance of food.
- **Abdomen:** Palpate for a pulsatile mass (**abdominal aortic aneurysm**) in the abdominal midline.
- **Lower extremity disease:** Exam reveals ulcers and nonhealing wounds, diminished pulses, ↓ ankle-brachial indices, skin atrophy and loss of hair, and **bruits** over affected vessels (abdominal, femoral, popliteal).
- **Renal artery stenosis:** Listen for a **bruit during systole and diastole** (highly specific).

KEY FACT

Risk factors for aortic aneurysm include age > 60, smoking, hypertension, a family history of aortic aneurysm, and hypercholesterolemia. The risk of rupture is low for aneurysms < 4 cm but ↑ with those ≥ 5 cm.

KEY FACT

Surgery is indicated for rapidly expanding aneurysms (> 0.5 cm/year) as well as for large aneurysms to avert the catastrophe of dissection.

KEY FACT

Peripheral vascular disease is a predictor of CAD.

KEY FACT

Patients with acute vessel occlusion from an embolus or an in situ thrombus present with sudden pain (abdominal or extremity). This represents an emergency.

Chest CT with IV contrast. (TEE is appropriate for patients with a history of allergic reaction to IV contrast.)

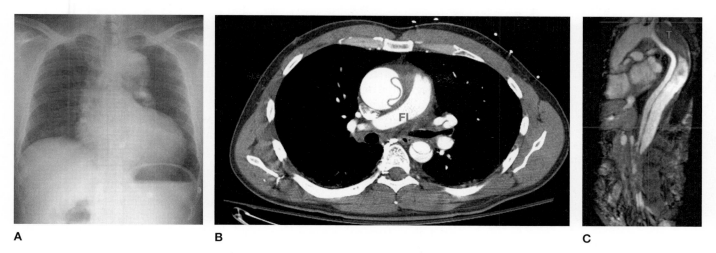

FIGURE 3-5.   Aortic dissection. (A) Frontal CXR showing a widened mediastinum in a patient with an aortic dissection. **(B)** Transaxial contrast-enhanced CT showing a dissection involving the ascending and descending aorta (FL, false lumen). **(C)** Sagittal MRA image showing a dissection involving the descending aorta, with a thrombus (T) in the false lumen. (Images A and C reproduced with permission from USMLE-Rx.com. Image B reproduced with permission from Doherty GM. *Current Diagnosis & Treatment: Surgery,* 13th ed. New York: McGraw-Hill, 2010, Fig. 19-17.)

DIFFERENTIAL

- **Abdominal pain:** Stable symptoms can mimic PUD or biliary colic. If the colon is predominantly involved, episodes of pain and bloody stool can look like infectious colitis.
- **Lower extremities: Spinal stenosis** can produce lower extremity discomfort similar to claudication. Claudication improves with rest (except for severe peripheral arterial disease with rest claudication), but spinal stenosis classically improves with **sitting forward** (lumbar flexion improves spinal stenosis symptoms).

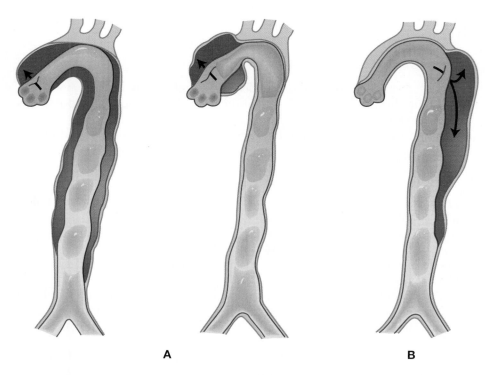

FIGURE 3-6.   Ascending vs descending aortic dissection. (A) Proximal or ascending (type A). **(B)** Distal or descending (type B). (Reproduced with permission from Doherty GM. *Current Diagnosis & Treatment: Surgery,* 13th ed. New York: McGraw-Hill, 2010, Fig. 19-16.)

DIAGNOSIS

- **Mesenteric disease:** A diagnosis of exclusion. Angiography reveals lesions.
- **Lower extremity disease:** Diagnosed via the **ankle-brachial index** (compares BP in the lower and upper extremities) and Doppler ultrasound. Angiography or MRA is used in preparation for revascularization but is generally not used for diagnosis.
- **Renal artery stenosis:** CT angiography, MRA, conventional angiography, or ultrasound with Doppler flow (technically difficult).

TREATMENT

- Control modifiable risk factors, especially smoking.
- **Mesenteric disease:** Treat with surgical revascularization or angioplasty.
- **Lower extremity disease:** Treat with exercise (to improve functional capacity), surgical revascularization, and sometimes angioplasty. Cilostazol is moderately useful (improves pain-free walking distance by 50%), whereas pentoxifylline is of marginal benefit. Antiplatelet therapy (aspirin, clopidogrel) is indicated to prevent cardiovascular events.
- **Renal artery stenosis:** Surgery or angioplasty may be of benefit.

Hypercholesterolemia

One of the principal factors contributing to atherosclerotic vascular disease. ↑ LDL and ↓ HDL are the 1° contributors. Hypercholesterolemia can be idiopathic, genetic, or 2° to other diseases, such as diabetes, nephrotic syndrome, and hypothyroidism.

SYMPTOMS

Generally asymptomatic unless the patient develops ischemia (eg, angina, stroke, claudication) or unless severe hypertriglyceridemia leads to pancreatitis. In certain cases, patients may notice fat deposits (**xanthomas**) in certain body regions.

EXAM

- Look for evidence of atherosclerosis—eg, carotid, subclavian, abdominal and other bruits; diminished or asymmetric pulses; or ischemic foot ulcers or other skin or hair changes.
- Look for xanthomas over the tendons, above the upper eyelid, and on the palms.

DIAGNOSIS

- Diagnosis is based on a lipid panel. A full panel consists of total cholesterol, HDL, LDL, and triglycerides.
- A nonfasting lipid profile can be obtained for ease of testing. Fasting and nonfasting LDL values vary very little. However, triglyceride values ↑ following a meal. If triglyceride values are of concern, fasting levels should be obtained.
- LDL has traditionally not been measured directly but has been **calculated** on the basis of total cholesterol, HDL, and triglycerides (via the Friedewald equation). **High triglycerides** (> 400 mg/dL) make LDL calculation unreliable. However, newer assays can measure LDL directly.
- Look for other contributing conditions. **Check glucose and TSH;** check body weight, and consider nephrotic syndrome.

KEY FACT

The Friedewald equation can be used to calculate LDL cholesterol (in mg/dL):

LDL = Total cholesterol – HDL – (TG/5)

- In patients with a family history of early heart disease, consider novel risk factors such as homocysteine, Lp(a), and CRP. These can be treated with folic acid supplementation, niacin, and statins, respectively.

TREATMENT

Treatment is aimed at preventing pancreatitis when triglycerides are very high (generally >1000 mg/dL) and at preventing atherosclerotic disease (see Table 3-10).

- **LDL:**
  - Traditional treatment has been based on goal LDL (eg, in patients with diabetes or CAD, the goal LDL was < 70 mg/dL; lower-risk patients had higher LDL goals). However, recent guidelines recommend percent reductions in LDL rather than absolute goals (eg, a 50% reduction in LDL in high-intensity treatment and a 30–50% reduction in moderate-intensity treatment) based on patient risk profiles (see Figure 3-7).
  - The mainstay of treatment is diet, exercise, and a statin. LDL control is the 1° cholesterol-related goal in patients with CAD or diabetes.
- **HDL:** Can be modestly ↑ with fibrate or nicotinic acid. Although ↓ HDL has been associated with an ↑ risk of cardiovascular events, using medications to ↑ HDL has not been as promising as hoped.
- **Triglycerides:** If > 500 mg/dL, recommend dietary modification (↓ total fat, ↓ saturated fat, ↓ alcohol) and aerobic exercise, and begin medication (fibrate or nicotinic acid). At lower levels, treatment can begin with diet and exercise, and medication can be added as needed. **Treat diabetes** and other concurrent metabolic syndrome risk factors if present.

KEY FACT

LDL control is the 1° cholesterol-related goal in patients with CAD or diabetes. Recommendations for LDL goals have recently changed from absolute target values to % reduction based on risk profile.

TABLE 3-10.   **Mechanisms and Features of Cholesterol-Lowering Medications**

MEDICATION	PRIMARY EFFECT	SIDE EFFECTS	COMMENTS
HMG-CoA reductase inhibitors ("statins")	↓ LDL	Hepatitis, myositis.	Potent LDL-lowering medication. The only medication to show a mortality benefit.
Cholesterol absorption inhibitors (ezetimibe)	↓ LDL	Generally well tolerated, but can cause diarrhea and arthralgias.	Introduced in 2003; no mortality benefit.
Fibrates (gemfibrozil)	↓ triglycerides, slightly ↑ HDL	Potentiates myositis with statins.	—
Bile acid–binding resins	↓ LDL	Bloating and cramping.	Many patients cannot tolerate GI side effects.
Nicotinic acid (niacin)	↓ LDL, ↑ HDL	Hepatitis, flushing.	Causes flushing, which can be ↓ by taking aspirin beforehand.

Q

A 73-year-old man with a history of diabetes mellitus, but with no history of clinical CAD, comes to your office for the results of his recent bloodwork. His fasting lipid panel is significant for an LDL of 130 mg/dL, and his 10-year risk of atherosclerotic cardiovascular disease is 7%. In addition to educating him on diet and lifestyle changes, what action should you take?

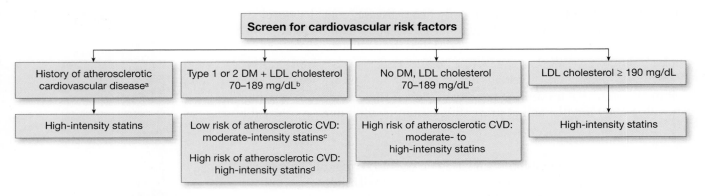

ᵃ Atherosclerotic cardiovascular disease = acute coronary syndrome, MI, stable/unstable angina, revascularization procedures, stroke/TIA, atherosclerotic peripheral arterial disease.
ᵇ In patients 40–75 years of age.
ᶜ Moderate-intensity statins = atorvastatin, 10–20 mg; rosuvastatin, 5–10 mg; simvastatin, 20–40 mg; pravastatin, 40–80 mg; lovastatin, 40 mg; extended-release fluvastatin, 80 mg; fluvastatin, 40 mg BID; pitavastatin, 2–4 mg (lower LDL cholesterol by 30–50%).
ᵈ High-intensity statins = atorvastatin, 40–80 mg; rosuvastatin, 20–40 mg (lower LDL cholesterol by ≥ 50%).

F I G U R E   3 - 7 .   Guidelines for the treatment of hyperlipidemia with statin therapy.

Endocarditis

Inflammation of the heart valves. Can be infective or noninfective. Infective endocarditis (IE) is commonly seen in IV drug abusers, hemodialysis patients, and those with valvular lesions or prosthetic heart valves. Valvular thrombi are composed of bacteria and platelets and are devoid of WBCs. IE is further distinguished as follows:

- **Acute IE (days):** Usually affects **normal heart valves** and is most often caused by *S aureus*, group A streptococci, or other β-hemolytic streptococci, such as *Streptococcus pneumoniae.* IV drug users typically have *S aureus* organisms and right heart involvement.
- **Subacute IE (weeks to months):** Usually colonizes a **previously damaged valve** in the setting of bacteremia from oral surgery or poor dentition. It is most often caused by the viridans group of streptococci. The aortic and mitral valves are most commonly affected.

SYMPTOMS

- **Acute IE:** Presents with fever, rigors, heart failure from valve destruction, and symptoms related to systemic emboli (neurologic impairment, back pain, pulmonary symptoms).
- **Subacute IE:** Characterized by weeks to months of fever, malaise, and weight loss. Also presents with symptoms of systemic emboli.
- **Noninfective endocarditis:** Generally asymptomatic. Can cause heart failure by destroying valves.

EXAM

- Listen for a new **murmur.**
- Multiple organs can be affected in IE (see Table 3-11).

DIFFERENTIAL

The differential diagnosis of endocarditis is outlined below and in Table 3-12.

- **Differential for a vegetation found on echocardiography:** IE, nonbacterial thrombotic endocarditis (NBTE, also known as marantic endocardi-

KEY FACT

Streptococcus bovis bacterial endocarditis should raise suspicion for occult GI malignancy. These patients need a colonoscopy.

A

Start moderate-intensity statin therapy with a goal LDL reduction of 30–50%.

TABLE 3-11.   Exam Findings and Organ Systems Affected in Infective Endocarditis

ORGAN SYSTEM/ POSITION	FINDINGS
Neurologic	Focal neurologic deficits; tenderness to percussion or palpation of the spine.
Ophthalmologic	Retinal exudates **(Roth's spots).**
Extremities	Deep-seated, painful hand/foot nodules **(Osler's nodes);** small skin infarctions **(Janeway lesions)** (see Figure 3-8).

tis), verrucous endocarditis (Libman-Sacks endocarditis), valve degeneration.
- **Differential for bacteremia:** IE, infected hardware (eg, from a central line), abscess, osteomyelitis.

DIAGNOSIS

- Noninfective endocarditis is usually an incidental finding on echocardiography. It may be found during the workup of systemic emboli.
- IE is diagnosed by a combination of lab and clinical data. If suspicious, obtain **at least 3 sets of blood cultures** and an echocardiogram. If TTE is ⊖, proceed to **TEE** (more sensitive). ⊕ blood cultures and echocardiogram findings together are strongly suggestive of IE. The modified Duke criteria are often used for diagnosis (see Table 3-13).

TREATMENT

- Treat with **prolonged antibiotic therapy,** generally for 4–6 weeks (can be as short as 2 weeks for small subgroups of patients; > 6 weeks for patients with highly virulent organisms). Begin empiric therapy with gentamicin and antistaphylococcal penicillin **(oxacillin or nafcillin).** If there is a risk of MRSA, treat empirically with vancomycin instead of oxacillin/nafcillin.
- **Valve replacement** is appropriate for fungal endocarditis, **heart failure** from valve destruction, valve ring abscess, cardiac conduction abnormalities, persistently ⊕ blood cultures despite antibiotic treatment, large or

KEY FACT

Any patient with *S aureus* bacteremia should be evaluated for endocarditis with echocardiography.

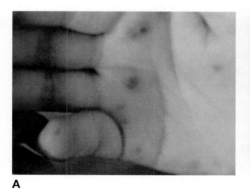
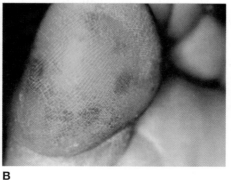

A   **B**

FIGURE 3-8.   Exam findings in infective endocarditis. (A) Osler's nodes. Randomly distributed, tender nodules are seen on the palm of the hand. **(B) Janeway lesions.** Note the nontender, purpuric macules with irregular borders scattered on the toes. (Reproduced with permission from Hall JB et al. *Principles of Critical Care,* 3rd ed. New York: McGraw-Hill, 2005, Figs. 49-1 and 49-2.)

Q

A 26-year-old IV drug user is admitted to the hospital with fevers and chills. Despite broad antibiotic therapy, blood cultures remain persistently ⊕, but transthoracic echocardiography (TTE) is normal. Given your suspicion of infective endocarditis, what is your next step?

TABLE 3-12.   Causes of Endocarditis

ACUTE	SUBACUTE	CULTURE NEGATIVE	NBTE (MARANTIC ENDOCARDITIS)	VERRUCOUS (LIBMAN-SACKS)
Most commonly *S aureus*	Viridans streptococci *Enterococcus* *Staphylococcus epidermidis* Gram-$\ominus$ rods *Candida*	HACEK organisms[a] *Coxiella burnetii* Noncandidal fungi	Thrombus formation on the valve is seen in many cancers	Seen in lupus; vegetation is composed of fibrin, platelets, immune complexes, and inflammatory cells

[a] **HACEK** organisms: **H**aemophilus aphrophilus and **H** parainfluenzae, **A**ctinobacillus actinomycetemcomitans, **C**ardiobacterium hominis, **E**ikenella corrodens, **K**ingella kingae.

KEY FACT

Surgery is indicated in the setting of hemodynamic instability, heart failure symptoms, valvular destruction, conduction abnormalities, perivalvular extension, fungal endocarditis, or persistently $\oplus$ blood cultures. Surgery should not be delayed while the acute infection is cleared with antibiotics.

Order a TEE, which is more sensitive than TTE for visualizing vegetations and diagnosing endocarditis. When endocarditis is suspected clinically but TTE is normal, a TEE is indicated to better confirm or rule out infection.

mobile vegetations, or systemic emboli despite adequate antibiotic therapy.
- Following treatment for IE, patients should receive endocarditis prophylaxis.
- For **NBTE**, treat the underlying disorder (often malignancy). Systemic anticoagulation (low-molecular-weight or unfractionated heparin) is useful for preventing recurrent emboli. Surgery is rarely indicated.
- For **verrucous endocarditis**, no treatment is required. Patients should receive endocarditis prophylaxis (see below).

PREVENTION

Endocarditis prophylaxis is indicated only in patients whose cardiac conditions are associated with the **highest risk of an adverse outcome from endocarditis**. These include:

- **Congenital cardiac disease:**
  - Unrepaired cyanotic disease, including those with palliative shunts and devices.
  - Congenital cardiac defects that have been completely repaired during the first 6 months after the repair (endothelialization occurs after 6 months).
  - Repaired congenital cardiac disease with residual defects that may inhibit endothelialization.
- **Other:**
  - Prosthetic heart valves (both homograft and bioprosthetic).
  - A patient history of prior IE.
  - Cardiac transplant patients with cardiac valvulopathy.
- **Guidelines for antibiotic prophylaxis:**
  - **Dental procedures:** All dental procedures that involve the manipulation of gingival tissue or the periapical region of teeth, as well as procedures involving perforation of the oral mucosa (**not** for routine anesthetic infections through noninfected tissue, dental radiographs, bleeding from trauma, adjustment of orthodontic devices, or shedding of deciduous teeth).
  - **Respiratory tract procedures:** Any of the above-mentioned cardiac patients who are undergoing an invasive procedure of the respiratory tract that involves incision (eg, tonsillectomy) or biopsy of the respiratory mucosa (includes bronchoscopy **with** biopsy).
  - **Skin procedures:** Any of the above-mentioned cardiac patients who are undergoing procedures involving infected skin or musculoskeletal tissue.
  - **GI and GU procedures:** Prophylaxis is not recommended even for

TABLE 3-13.   Modified Duke Criteria for the Diagnosis of Infective Endocarditis[a,b]

DUKE CRITERION	DEFINITION
MAJOR CRITERIA	
1. Microbiologic evidence of IE	■ Typical organisms isolated from 2 separate blood cultures: 　■ Viridans streptococci, *S aureus,* HACEK organisms, or *S bovis* OR 　■ Community-acquired enterococci in the absence of an alternative 1° site of infection ■ Persistently ⊕ blood cultures with other organisms: 　■ At least 2 ⊕ cultures drawn > 12 hours apart OR 　■ All of 3 or a majority of 4 ⊕ cultures, with the first and last drawn > 1 hour apart ■ One ⊕ culture (or phase I IgG > 1:800) for *Coxiella burnetii*
2. Evidence of endocardial involvement	Echocardiogram showing 1 of the following: ■ An oscillating intracardiac mass with no alternative explanation ■ An abscess ■ New partial dehiscence of a prosthetic valve ■ New valvular regurgitation
MINOR CRITERIA	
1. Predisposition to IE	Previous IE, IV drug use, a prosthetic heart valve, or a cardiac lesion causing turbulent blood flow.
2. Fever > 38°C	—
3. Vascular phenomena	Arterial emboli, pulmonary infarcts, mycotic aneurysms, intracranial or conjunctival hemorrhage, Janeway lesions.
4. Immunologic phenomena	Glomerulonephritis, Osler's nodes, Roth's spots, ⊕ RF.
5. Microbiologic findings not meeting major criteria	—

[a] The definitive diagnosis of IE requires 2 major criteria, 1 major and 3 minor criteria, or 5 minor criteria.

[b] The diagnosis of possible IE requires 1 major and 1 minor criterion or 3 minor criteria.

high-risk patients but may be considered in special scenarios involving the above-mentioned cardiac patients.

- **Prophylactic regimens:** Amoxicillin (or clindamycin, azithromycin, or cephalexin for those with penicillin allergy) 30–60 minutes before the procedure.

COMPLICATIONS

Spinal osteomyelitis, valve destruction and heart failure, stroke and renal damage (from septic emboli), metastatic abscesses, mycotic aneurysms.

KEY FACT

Don't forget—IE generally requires prolonged antibiotic therapy for 4–6 weeks.

NOTES

CHAPTER 4

EMERGENCY MEDICINE

Trauma

The acute management of trauma victims follows a linear algorithm that should be performed in the same order every time: **AcBCDE** (1° survey) followed by **FAST** (**F**ocused **A**ssessment with **S**onography in **T**rauma) and the 2° survey. An algorithm ensures that no important steps in the initial assessment and resuscitation will be skipped.

In actual practice, multiple steps occur simultaneously (eg, IV fluids are administered as an airway is being secured). However, the USMLE often asks about the "next step," thereby testing your understanding of the algorithm rather than your ability to manage multiple therapeutic approaches at the same time. It is the team leader's responsibility to ensure that the 1° survey is completed before the 2° survey is begun.

THE 1° SURVEY

Trauma treatment should proceed in accordance with the **AcBCDE** algorithm:

- **Ac**—Airway maintenance with cervical spine control. **Indications for a definitive airway (eg, intubation, cricothyroidotomy):**
  - The patient cannot protect his airway.
  - The patient cannot be ventilated by bag-valve mask.
  - Either condition is expected in the immediate future (eg, inhalational burn).
- **B**—Breathing with ventilation. Quickly evaluate for and treat **causes of impending cardiopulmonary death**—eg, tension pneumothorax, cardiac tamponade, open pneumothorax, massive hemothorax, or airway obstruction.
- **C**—Circulation with hemorrhage control.
  - **Resuscitation:** Think short and fat IV lines—eg, 2 large-bore (16- or 18-gauge) IVs. Triple-lumen central lines have high flow resistance and take too long to insert.
  - Crystalloids are the 1° resuscitation fluids. However, patients with significant blood loss will require a blood transfusion.
- **D**—Disability.
  - Determined by a brief neurologic exam; assess mental status and size of pupils.
  - **Glasgow Coma Scale (GCS):** Based on the **best** response of E + V + M (see Figure 4-1).
- **E**—Exposure/Environmental control: Completely undress the patient to assess for injury, but avoid hypothermia.

KEY FACT

Because hemodilution has not yet occurred, hematocrit will initially be normal in acute hemorrhage—so don't be falsely reassured. Patients don't bleed normal saline, so limit crystalloid resuscitation and administer blood products.

KEY FACT

When assessing disability in trauma, put your tuning fork away. Is the patient moving, and can he feel his arms and legs? Good!

Eye Opening (E)	Verbal Response (V)	Motor Response (M)
4 Spontaneous	**5** Oriented	**6** Obeys commands
3 Responds to voice	**4** Confused speech	**5** Localizes pain
2 Responds to pain	**3** Inappropriate speech	**4** Withdraws to pain
1 No response	**2** Incomprehensible	**3** Abnormal flexion
	1 No response	**2** Abnormal extension
		1 No response

FIGURE 4-1. **Scoring of the Glasgow Coma Scale.**

THE 2° SURVEY

The 2° survey consists of total patient evaluation as outlined below. This is also the time to order appropriate lab tests and radiographs based on the mechanism of injury, past medical history, and the like.

- **Obtain an AMPLE history:** Inquire about **A**llergies, **M**edications, **P**ast medical history, **L**ast oral intake, and **E**vents/Environmental factors related to the injury. If the patient can speak, ask about other symptoms that may not be obvious on exam. Obtain as much information as possible from EMTs/paramedics about the circumstances of the trauma.
- **Conduct a focused physical exam:**
  - **Head and skull:** Inspect for trauma, pupils, and loss of consciousness. Look for ecchymosis around the eyes (**"raccoon eyes"**) and hemotympanum, which point to a **basilar skull fracture.** Inspect the ears and nose for CSF leakage. If a septal hematoma is present, it will need to be drained once the patient is stabilized. Assess for midface instability, ocular/orbital trauma, or intraoral injuries. Ecchymosis of the mastoid process (**Battle's sign**) is a late sign of basilar skull fracture and is rarely found on initial presentation.
  - **Neck:** Look for trauma or a pulsatile/expanding hematoma; palpate for midline tenderness, crepitus, and tracheal deformity.
  - **Chest:** Inspect for irregular or paradoxical breathing patterns resulting from multiple rib fractures—ie, flail chest. Listen for equal and bilateral breath sounds. (If absent/asymmetric or if there is crepitus on palpation of the chest, suspect **pneumothorax;** however, be aware that absent breath sounds are only 80% sensitive.) Listen for clear heart sounds (if muffled and accompanied by JVD, suspect **cardiac tamponade**). A new diastolic murmur after trauma suggests **aortic dissection.**
  - **Abdomen:** Inspect the abdomen and flanks for signs of trauma. Palpate the pelvis for tenderness or instability. Do not compress the pelvis anteriorly/posteriorly; if the patient has an "open book" fracture, doing so will make it significantly worse.
  - **Perineum/rectum/vagina:** Assess for trauma, including urethral bleeding (suggests urethral tear). Check for prostate position, rectal tone, and rectal blood. Check women for vaginal trauma and blood in the vaginal vault.
  - **Musculoskeletal system:** Look for evidence of trauma, including contusions, lacerations, and deformities. Inspect the extremities for tenderness, crepitus, abnormal range of motion, and sensation. An externally rotated, shortened leg suggests **hip fracture.**
- **Imaging:**
  - **Head and skull:** Obtain a CT of the head and face if there is evidence of trauma. Maintain a low threshold for scanning intoxicated patients, elderly patients, and those on blood thinners.
  - **Neck:** Maintain in-line immobilization and protection with a hard cervical collar. Obtain radiographs if the cervical spine cannot be cleared clinically. If indeterminate, consider CT of the cervical spine (see Figure 4-2).
  - **Chest:** Rapidly assess for pneumothorax with ultrasound. Obtain a CXR in all patients with significant trauma. Penetrating thoracic wounds or clinical concern for major intrathoracic trauma often requires a chest CT.
  - **Abdomen:** Obtain a pelvic x-ray; arrange for a **FAST** scan and/or an abdominal CT if indicated. Diagnostic peritoneal lavage is rarely done anymore.
  - **Urinary system:** If there is blood at the urethral meatus or a "high-riding"

KEY FACT

Rules for clinical clearance of the cervical spine include the NEXUS criteria: the patient is alert and not intoxicated; no posterior midline C-spine tenderness; no neurologic deficit; and no painful distracting injuries.

KEY FACT

The spleen is the most commonly injured solid organ in blunt abdominal trauma.

KEY FACT

Cushing's triad (systolic hypertension, bradycardia, and irregular breathing) indicates ↑ ICP, as from a closed-head injury.

KEY FACT

Beck's triad (JVD, muffled heart tones, and hypotension) indicates cardiac tamponade. Pulsus paradoxus is rarely assessed in the trauma setting (low sensitivity, time consuming).

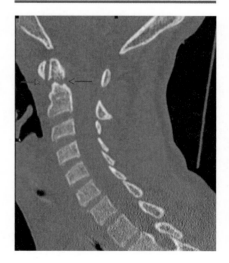

FIGURE 4-2. Cervical spine fracture. A sagittal reformation of a cervical spine CT shows a fracture through the base of the dens, a type 2 odontoid fracture (red arrows). (Reproduced with permission from USMLE-Rx.com.)

prostate, consult urology for a urethrogram. Do not insert a Foley. See Figure 4-3.

- **Musculoskeletal system:** Obtain an arteriogram if vascular injury is suspected (eg, pulsating or expanding hematoma, distal perfusion deficit). Obtain radiographs as needed for extremity injuries. Knee dislocations (**not** patellar dislocations) require a CT angiogram to rule out popliteal artery injury.

Management of Emergent Procedures

You should be familiar with the indications for a variety of emergent procedures.

- **Cricothyroidotomy:** Can't ventilate? Can't intubate? It's time to get out the scalpel.
- **Flail chest:** Serial rib fractures in at least 2 places create a paradoxically moving chest wall. The patient will likely require intubation to assist with breathing.
- **Needle thoracostomy:** Inserting a chest tube takes several minutes. A 14-gauge needle to the second intercostal space midclavicular line takes seconds.
- **Cardiac tamponade:** If seen on ultrasound with tamponade physiology, perform pericardiocentesis. If possible, insert a "pigtail" into the pericardium, as the bleeding will likely reaccumulate.
- **Tube thoracostomy** (aka "chest tube"): The treatment for pneumothorax and hemothorax.
- **Emergent thoracotomy:** For patients in extremis with suspected penetrating injury to the heart or disruption of major vessels (aorta, pulmonary artery).

Shock

Shock is a major complication of both medical and surgical emergencies. Rapid clinical assessment of circulatory status includes pulse, skin color, and level of consciousness. The evolution of the symptoms of shock is shown in Figure 4-4.

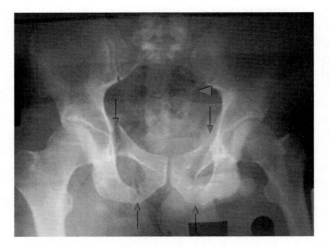

FIGURE 4-3. **Pelvic fractures.** Frontal pelvic radiograph in a trauma patient shows bilateral superior and inferior pubic ramus fractures (red arrows) and a left sacral fracture (red arrowhead). (Reproduced with permission from Brunicardi FC et al. *Schwartz's Principles of Surgery*, 9th ed. New York: McGraw-Hill, 2010, Fig. 7-30A.)

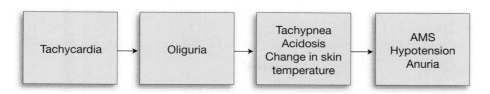

FIGURE 4-4.   Symptoms of shock over time.

- Low blood pressure does not in itself represent shock. Shock is a physiologic **O₂ supply/demand mismatch.** ↓ tissue perfusion leads to cell hypoxia with subsequent dysfunction and eventual tissue death. Consequently, LFTs, creatinine, and troponin may be ↑ in severe shock. Lactic acid is a useful marker for tissue hypoperfusion.
- Classically, shock has been divided into 4 types on the basis of physiologic response: **hypovolemic, cardiogenic, distributive,** and **obstructive.** Distributive shock is further subdivided into septic, anaphylactic, and neurogenic shock. These types are reviewed in Table 4-1.

KEY FACT

With increasing blood loss, a patient's mental status progresses from anxiety to agitation to confusion and then to lethargy/unconsciousness.

TREATMENT

- Treat shock by correcting the underlying cause. A good first step is to administer O₂ and IV fluids (use caution in cardiogenic shock). Urine

TABLE 4-1.   Hemodynamic Characteristics of Shock

TYPE	MAJOR CAUSES	CARDIAC OUTPUT	PCWP (≈ LEFT ATRIAL PRESSURE)	SVR (VASOCONSTRICTION)	SVO₂	TREATMENT
Hypovolemic	Trauma, blood loss, inadequate fluid repletion, third spacing, burns.	↓	↓ [a]	↑	↓	Crystalloid/blood.
Cardiogenic	MI, CHF, arrhythmia, structural heart disease (eg, severe mitral regurgitation, VSD).	↓ [a]	↑	↑	↓	Treat the cause and give pressors (dopamine; norepinephrine or dobutamine if necessary).
Distributive	**Septic:** Bacteremia (especially gram ⊖). **Anaphylactic:** Bee stings; food/medication allergies. **Neurogenic:** Trauma to the spinal cord (leading to loss of autonomic/motor reflexes).	↑	Normal	↓ [a]	↑	For **septic shock,** obtain cultures; then give antibiotics, fluid, and pressors (norepinephrine, dopamine). For **anaphylactic shock,** give diphenhydramine and steroids (and epinephrine if severe).
Obstructive	Cardiac tamponade, tension pneumothorax, pulmonary embolism (PE).	↓	↑/↓ [b]	↑	↓	For tamponade, needle pericardiocentesis. For PE, thrombolytics.

[a] Driving force.

[b] ↑ PCWP for tamponade; ↓ PCWP for PE.

output and lactate are surrogate markers to guide the clinician's treatment approach.

- Keep in mind that shock is a symptom of a disease process, not the disease itself.

Orthopedic Injuries

Patients present to the ED with a variety of orthopedic complaints, a detailed discussion of which is beyond the scope of this book. This section provides a high-yield summary of common and dangerous conditions, their diagnostic workup, and their initial management. In general, any compromise of blood flow or nerve function due to fracture/dislocation is an indication for an emergent reduction.

ANKLE INJURIES

- **Traumatic ankle injuries** are among the most common orthopedic complaints encountered in the ED. The spectrum of injury ranges from sprains (microscopic damage to a ligament) to significant fracture requiring operative intervention.
- In general, the **Ottawa ankle rules** (see Figure 4-5) guide the clinician in determining which patients need radiographic imaging. X-rays of the ankle and/or foot are indicated in the presence of:
  - Tenderness over the distal 6 cm of the posterior tibia or fibula
  - Tenderness over either malleolus
  - Inability to bear weight over 4 steps
  - Tenderness over the base of the fifth metatarsal
  - Tenderness over the navicular bone
- If there is concern for syndesmotic disruption between the tibia and fibula, rupture of the deltoid ligament, or ankle instability due to fractures, stress views of the ankle should also be added (x-ray in supination/external rotation).

KNEE INJURIES

- **Knee pain** is another common reason patients present to the ED. Several exam maneuvers should be performed to assess for certain injuries.

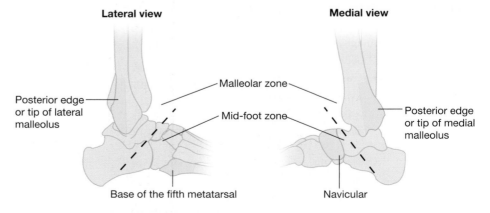

FIGURE 4-5. **Ottawa ankle rules.** If there is tenderness over these areas, x-rays are indicated. (Reproduced with permission from Tintinalli JE et al. *Tintinalli's Emergency Medicine: A Comprehensive Study Guide,* 7th ed. New York: McGraw-Hill, 2011, Fig. 273-4.)

- A locking sensation on **passive range of motion** may be a sign of meniscal injury.
- **Active range of motion** not resulting in full extension can indicate quadriceps tendon rupture.
- The **anterior/posterior drawer test** assesses ACL and PCL integrity.
- **Varus/valgus stress** assesses the integrity of the medial/lateral collateral ligaments.
- Knee dislocation in obese patients may occur after only minor trauma and may self-reduce before presentation to the ED.

HIP INJURIES

- The differential for **hip pain** is highly dependent on the age of the patient.
  - Children and adolescents (particularly if they are obese) are at risk for a **slipped capital femoral epiphysis** (see Figure 4-6) or **Legg-Calvé-Perthes disease** (avascular necrosis of the femoral head; typically affects children 4–8 years of age). If the hip pain was preceded by a recent URI, the patient may be suffering from **toxic synovitis.** Keep in mind that the presenting complaint for hip issues in children may be knee pain.
  - Older patients are at high risk for "hip fractures" (technically a proximal femur fracture) 2° to osteopenia. Classically, the affected limb is shortened and externally rotated.
- Other causes of hip pain include osteoarthritis and trochanteric bursitis. In addition, patients of all ages are at risk for hip dislocation.
  - A tremendous amount of force is required to dislocate the hip joint, and dislocation typically occurs only when the hip is flexed at the moment of impact (eg, knee vs dashboard in an MVA).
  - Typically the ligamentum teres artery is severed in the process, placing the patient at risk of developing avascular necrosis of the femoral head as a delayed complication.

KEY FACT

A fracture line will alter sound conduction (osteophony). Place a stethoscope on the pubic symphysis and tap each patella with a reflex hammer.

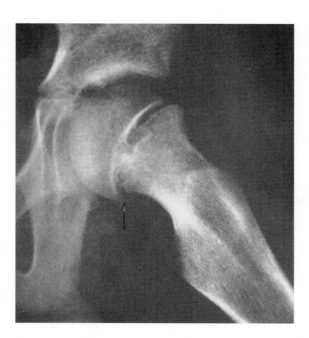

FIGURE 4-6. **Slipped capital femoral epiphysis.** Note the appearance of "ice cream about to fall off the cone" (arrow). (Reproduced with permission from Chen MY et al. *Basic Radiology*, 2nd ed. New York: McGraw-Hill, 2011, Fig. 6-1B.)

- All joints in the body are at risk for septic arthritis, which involves direct inoculation of the joint or hematogenous spread of pathogens.
  - Patients may be febrile with exquisite tenderness on ranging the joint.
  - Labs show an ↑ WBC count, CRP, and ESR.
  - Joint aspirate with a WBC count > 100,000/mm³ is compatible with septic arthritis.
  - Treatment consists of IV antibiotics and joint washout by an orthopedic surgeon.

ORTHOPEDIC PEARLS

- Tenderness over the scaphoid bone requires splinting even if initial x-rays are ⊖. A scaphoid fracture may take several days to become visible on x-rays.
- Compartment syndrome typically features good pulses and sensation until it reaches an advanced state. Excruciating pain with passive movement is the earliest clinical sign.
- An ankle injury may lead to a knee injury (Maisonneuve fracture).
- Shoulder dislocations may lead to axillary nerve injury.
- Supracondylar fractures in children may lead to radial nerve injury.
- Clavicle fractures are typically treated conservatively with a sling.
- The first rib, proximal clavicle, sternum, scapula, and femur require significant force to fracture. Look for other injuries.

Common Dysrhythmias

Tables 4-2 and 4-3 illustrate a variety of important dysrhythmias. In general, these can be subdivided into **narrow-complex arrhythmias** (eg, reentry supraventricular tachycardia [SVT], pulseless electrical activity [PEA]) and **wide-complex arrhythmias** (eg, ventricular tachycardia and ventricular fibrillation).

Advanced Cardiac Life Support (ACLS)

ACLS provides a framework for resuscitating a critically ill medical patient. There have recently been some changes to the protocol; most notably, circulation is now being addressed before airway and breathing. It was found that CPR was often significantly delayed as intubation was attempted. In addition, several drugs have been taken out of the algorithm. Even epinephrine barely made the cut, as it ↑ the rate of return of spontaneous circulation but has been found to have no effect on survival to discharge.

UNSTABLE BRADYCARDIA

Symptomatic bradycardia is usually due to 1 of the following:

- High vagal tone (cholinergic toxicity, inferior MI, digoxin toxicity).
- Conduction abnormalities (sick sinus syndrome, AV-nodal blocks, diseases such as Lyme carditis or multiple myeloma).
- Medication effects (β-blockers, calcium channel blockers [CCBs]).

The underlying cause influences the efficacy of the treatment approach:

- High vagal tone responds to atropine.
- Conduction abnormalities often require a manual override of the conduction system (eg, pacing).

MNEMONIC

ABC is now CAB—

Circulation
Airway
Breathing
Drugs
Electricity (shock)
Fluids

KEY FACT

After a premature ventricular contraction (PVC), the sinus rhythm resumes as if the PVC never occurred. After a premature atrial contraction (PAC), however, the sinus rhythm resets as if the PAC were a normal beat.

KEY FACT

"Geminy" refers to the sequence of normal beats with PVCs. Bigeminy is a pattern of 1 normal beat followed by a PVC; trigeminy is a pattern with 2 normal beats followed by a PVC.

TABLE 4-2.   **Common Bradyarrhythmias**

BRADYARRHYTHMIA	EXAMPLE
Sinus bradycardia	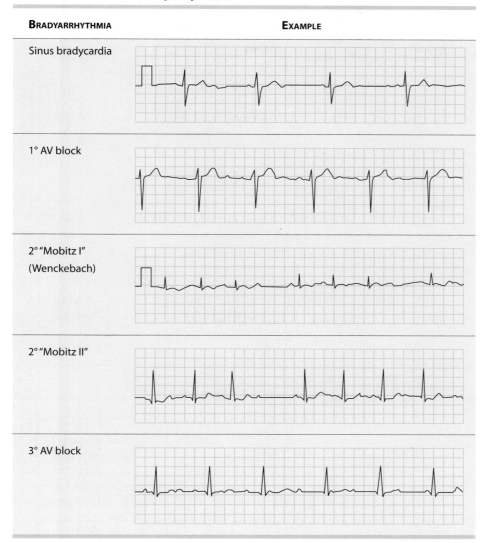
1° AV block	
2° "Mobitz I" (Wenckebach)	
2° "Mobitz II"	
3° AV block	

- Unfortunately, conditions such as β-blocker overdose lead to ⊖ chronotropy and ⊖ inotropy. In many cases, even pacing remains ineffective.

TREATMENT

- A patient found to be in unstable bradycardia (HR < 60) with symptomatic hypotension (eg, chest pain, changes in mental status, or other signs/symptoms of shock) requires treatment. While preparing for pacing, administer **atropine** 0.5 mg IV q 3–5 min × 3.
- There are 3 ways to pace a patient:
  - **Transcutaneously:** Place pads on the chest/back, set to the desired rate, and ↑ amperage until you have **mechanical** capture. If possible, sedate.
  - **Transvenously:** Place a cordis central line and float a pacing wire to the heart. This takes about 15 minutes but provides the most definitive management until a permanent pacemaker can be placed.
  - **Chemically:** Dopamine 2–10 µg/kg/min or epinephrine 2–10 µg/min.

 KEY FACT

Transcutaneous pacing will lead to contraction of the chest wall and sternocleidomastoid muscles. This pulsation is easily mistaken for a carotid pulse. Check femoral pulses instead.

TABLE 4-3. **Common Tachyarrhythmias**

TACHYARRHYTHMIA	EXAMPLE
SUPRAVENTRICULAR TACHYARRHYTHMIAS	
Sinus tachycardia	
Atrial fibrillation (AF)	
Atrial flutter	
Premature atrial contraction (PAC)	
Multifocal atrial tachycardia (MAT)	
Atrioventricular nodal reentrant tachycardia (AVNRT)	
Wolff-Parkinson-White syndrome (slurred upstroke; delta wave)	III aVF V₃

TABLE 4-3. **Common Tachyarrhythmias** *(continued)*

TACHYARRHYTHMIA	EXAMPLE
VENTRICULAR TACHYARRHYTHMIAS	
Premature ventricular contraction (PVC) (unifocal vs multifocal)	
Ventricular tachycardia (VT) (monomorphic vs polymorphic)	
Torsades de pointes (a type of VT that can lead to VF as well)	
Ventricular fibrillation (VF)	

CARDIAC ARREST

In the event of cardiac arrest, start CPR immediately using end-tidal CO_2 to monitor quality. As CPR is being performed, begin bag-valve-mask ventilation, rapidly obtain vascular access (or interosseous access), and attach defibrillator pads to the patient. At the first rhythm check, you will find 1 of 4 electrical patterns: VF, pulseless VT, asystole, or PEA.

- **Asystole or PEA:** CPR and epinephrine. No defibrillation, atropine, or pacing.
- **VF or pulseless VT:**
  - CPR with epinephrine q 3–5 minutes + **defibrillation** with 200 J (biphasic) or 360 J (monophasic) + an **antiarrhythmic agent (amiodarone** 300 mg IV once followed by a 150-mg dose in 3–5 minutes if still in a shockable rhythm).
  - If torsades de pointes develops, give magnesium 1–2 g IV.
- Identify and treat the **H's and T's:**
  - Hypothermia → warm them up.
  - H^+ (acidosis) → reverse acidosis.

Q **1**

A 73-year-old woman who has had palpitations for 4 days presents with AF with rapid ventricular response. Other than mild shortness of breath, she is hemodynamically stable. What is the best management approach?

Q **2**

An 80-year-old woman presents with dizziness. Her BP is 138/52 and her heart rate 28 bpm. She has a pacemaker, but no pacer spikes are visible on ECG. What is the first therapeutic intervention?

- Hypo-/**H**yperkalemia → either give or remove K^+.
- **H**ypoxia → 100% O_2; secure/establish airway.
- **H**ypovolemia → fluid replacement.
- **T**hrombosis (PE, MI) → thrombolytics.
- **T**amponade → pericardiocentesis.
- **T**ension pneumothorax → needle decompression.
- **T**oxins → antidote (eg, hydroxocobalamin in cyanide toxicity).

TACHYCARDIA

Tachycardia is defined as a heart rate > 100 bpm. Sinus tachycardia has an underlying cause that must be addressed (eg, dehydration, fever, pain) and will not be reviewed here in detail. The treatment of sinus tachycardia with rate-limiting agents is likely harmful, as the heart rate was compensatory to an underlying process and the compensatory mechanism is removed. Tachydysrhythmias can result from:

- Self-sustained conduction pathways (eg, SVT)
- Multiple foci of automaticity (atrial flutter, AF)
- Ventricular focus (VT)

TREATMENT

- A patient with unstable tachycardia (eg, shortness of breath, chest pain, hypotension, ischemic ECG changes) requires immediate synchronized cardioversion. Stable patients can be treated medically.
- In **stable** tachycardia, attempt vagal maneuvers first, and then escalate therapy as follows:
  - **Narrow, regular complex** (eg, SVT): Adenosine.
  - **Narrow, irregular complex** (eg, AF): Rate control (metoprolol, diltiazem).
  - **Wide complex** (eg, VT): Amiodarone.
  - All of the above rhythms can be electrically cardioverted if medical therapy fails.
- Special cases:
  - Do **not** cardiovert stable AF that has been present for > 48 hours. Get a transesophageal echocardiogram first to assess for an atrial thrombus.
  - In torsades de pointes, give magnesium 1–2 g IV and provide either chemical or electrical overdrive pacing (may resolve with ↑ heart rate).

Toxicology

In general, there are several things you need to inquire about or obtain when treating a poisoned patient:

- Time and type of ingestion
- Quantity and route of ingestion
- Comorbidities
- Vitals
- ECG
- Pupils, bowel sounds, skin exam, reflexes, and clonus
- Respiratory/heart rate, mental status

Also bear in mind that while patients on the USMLE are always truthful, "real" patients may intentionally provide you with false information out of concern for the legal implications of substance abuse.

1 **A**

Rate control. Paroxysmal AF may also lead to atrial clot formation. Cardioversion should be attempted only if a mural thrombus has been ruled out.

2 **A**

The pacemaker may be oversensing and may "think" that the patient has a higher heart rate than she actually does, thereby withholding pacing signals. Apply a magnet over the pacemaker to force it into asynchronous default pacing.

TOXIDROMES

Table 4-4 lists symptoms and signs associated with common toxin-induced syndromes ("toxidromes"). Table 4-5 outlines several hypothetical scenarios involving toxidromes. Some additional toxicology pearls are as follows:

- Do not intubate patients with aspirin toxicity unless you absolutely must. Because the mechanical ventilator will never match these patients' high minute volume, they will become more acidotic and die.
- In all overdoses, send an acetaminophen level.
- In smoke inhalation, consider carbon monoxide and cyanide toxicity.
- Serotonin syndrome kills (see Chapter 17).
- Neuroleptic malignant syndrome can look like serotonin syndrome but develops more slowly (> 24 hours) and features rigidity rather than clonus (see Chapter 17).
- If a patient appears altered or intoxicated, don't forget to check a blood sugar.
- Make sure you know how to treat different toxic alcohols (methanol, isopropanol, ethylene glycol).
- Lithium toxicity may require dialysis.
- Digoxin toxicity may require antibody fragment administration (Digibind).
- Charcoal is useful only in ingestions that occurred < 60 minutes ago. Mul-

KEY FACT

With a paucity of data to support their theoretical benefits, emesis and gastric lavage have fallen out of favor. Gastric lavage is rarely performed in practice today, and emesis not at all.

MNEMONIC

Indications for emergent hemodialysis—

AEIOU

Metabolic **A**cidosis that cannot be corrected with $NaHCO_3$
Severe **E**lectrolyte imbalances (eg, hyperkalemia)
Toxic **I**ngestions (eg, lithium or aspirin)
Fluid **O**verload that is resistant to treatment with diuretics
Uremia (eg, uremic encephalopathy, uremic serositis)

TABLE 4-4.   Classic Toxidromes

TOXIDROME	SYMPTOMS/SIGNS	EXAMPLES
Cholinergic	**SLUDGE: S**alivation, **L**acrimation, **U**rination, **D**iarrhea, **G**I distress, and **E**mesis.	Muscarine-containing mushrooms, organophosphates, pilocarpine, pyridostigmine.
Anticholinergic	"Hot as a hare, red as a beet, dry as a bone, mad as a hatter, blind as a bat": fever, skin flushing, dry mucous membranes, psychosis, mydriasis. Also tachycardia and urinary retention.	Antihistamines, antipsychotics, atropine, Jimson weed, scopolamine, TCAs.
Opioid	Triad of coma, respiratory depression, and miosis. Also bradycardia, hypothermia, and diminished bowel sounds.	Heroin, morphine, oxycodone.
Sedative-hypnotic	CNS depression, respiratory depression, and coma.	Alcohol, barbiturates, benzodiazepines.
Sympathomimetic	Disorientation, panic, seizures, hypertension, tachycardia, and tachypnea.	Amphetamines, cocaine, PCP.
Extrapyramidal	Parkinsonian symptoms: tremor, torticollis, trismus, rigidity, oculogyric crisis, opisthotonos, dysphonia, and dysphagia.	Haloperidol, metoclopramide, phenothiazines.

TABLE 4-5.   **Scenarios Involving Toxidromes**

VIGNETTE	TOXIDROME	TREATMENT
A 25-year-old man is pushed out of the back seat of a car in front of the ED before the car takes off speeding. The triage nurse finds the patient apneic and cyanotic with a thready pulse. He is tachycardic and hypoxic, and his pupils are constricted and minimally reactive. The patient has multiple scars on his arms and neck. Bag-valve-mask ventilations are provided.	This patient has likely overdosed on an opiate such as oxycodone or heroin and is suffering from **opioid toxidrome.** Given the scars on his arms (track marks) and neck (from "jugging"), he likely injected the opiate.	Administer naloxone. Long-acting opiates (eg, methadone) need repeat doses and hence will likely require admission. Pulmonary edema may occur in some cases.
A 17-year-old girl is brought to the ED by her parents for acting erratically. She is unable to give a history and is speaking nonsensically while picking at her clothing. Her pupils are 6 mm and reactive, and no nystagmus is present. She has no axillary moisture. Palpation of her abdomen reveals a suprapubic mass. Her reflexes are normal. She is tachycardic and has a temperature of 38.1°C (100.4°F).	This patient appears to have ingested an **anticholinergic,** as evidenced by her dry skin, mydriasis, ↑ temperature, mental status changes, and urinary retention (distended bladder). The repetitive picking behavior is typical. ECG shows a QRS of 108 msec with a sloped R′ in aVR.	Most patients require only observation and benzodiazepines for symptom control. Improvement with physostigmine confirms the diagnosis. Watch for QRS widening and subsequent seizures or arrhythmia. Antihistamines have sodium channel–blocking properties similar to TCAs. Administer sodium bicarbonate to narrow the QRS.
A 42-year-old man is brought in for erratic behavior after partying all night. He is diaphoretic and must be restrained by security. A limited physical exam reveals mydriasis but no other significant abnormalities. After administration of lorazepam 2 mg IM, the patient becomes more cooperative and states that he has chest pain. An ECG shows sinus tachycardia with concerning ST-segment changes in the lateral leads.	The **sympathomimetic** toxidrome can be triggered by drugs like PCP, methamphetamine, or, as in this case, cocaine. Chemical restraints are always preferred over physical ones, as physically restrained patients will remain agitated, fight the restraints, and develop hyperthermia and rhabdomyolysis.	Treat cocaine-associated chest pain as you would regular chest pain. Six percent of cocaine chest pain cases will result in MI. The use of β-blockers to treat cocaine overdose remains controversial. Benzodiazepines are the mainstay of treatment in light of concern over unopposed α-adrenergic stimulation.
A 40-year-old man finds his father pulseless in the garden shed with a letter by his side 2 days after his mother's death. The son's attempts at mouth-to-mouth resuscitation and chest compressions prove futile. Shortly thereafter, the son loses control of his bowel and bladder, develops rhinorrhea, and coughs up copious amounts of sputum. His heart rate is found to be 38 bpm.	Exposure to **cholinergic** toxins results in **SLUDGE** (**S**alivation, **L**acrimation, **U**rination, **D**iarrhea, **G**I distress, and **E**mesis). Exposure can be intentional but may also be accidental (as in carbamate [insecticide] exposure).	The antidote is atropine. In organophosphate poisoning, early administration of pralidoxime prevents maturation of the chemical bond that inhibits cholinesterase.
Three young men are stopped near the Canadian border for driving 63 mph in a 65-mph zone. Before a search of the car can be conducted, 1 of the occupants eats an entire bag of their contraband. Shortly thereafter, he tells his friends that he is "freaking out." While under arrest, the patient finds that parts of the police cruiser taste like his favorite fruit.	The patient is experiencing a **hallucinogenic toxidrome.** A variety of substances can induce this state, most commonly LSD and marijuana.	Although hemodynamic instability can occur with high drug doses, most patients just need control of agitation if present. Give benzodiazepines as needed.
A 5-year-old boy is brought to the ED obtunded and tachypneic. His younger brother reports that the boy had been drinking "candy juice" that he found in the garage. A blood glucose level is normal.	The **sedative-hypnotic** toxidrome is frequently seen in the ED, often in the form of benzodiazepine abuse or alcohol intoxication—or, in this case, ethylene glycol from antifreeze.	Patients with sedative-hypnotic toxidrome often require only supportive care. However, in the setting of ethylene glycol ingestion, the patient may need fomepizole or ethanol and potentially dialysis.

tidose activated charcoal can be given for "gut dialysis" (removal of toxins from the enterohepatic circulation).

- Whole bowel irrigation (similar to a colonoscopy prep) is indicated for "body packers" and for children with visible lead paint chips on x-ray, as well as for certain other ingestions.

Abdominal Pain

Pain is poorly localized by patients, and many conditions have symptoms that substantially overlap. Approximately 50% of patients presenting to the ED will not receive a diagnosis for their discomfort. Common abdominal conditions are discussed in Chapter 7 of this book. What follows is a discussion of conditions that require emergent treatment.

EPIGASTRIC PAIN

Discomfort in this region may be due to intraabdominal or intrathoracic processes (eg, lower lobe pneumonia or an inferior MI). Broaden the differential appropriately in the elderly, in women, and in patients with diabetes.

DIFFERENTIAL

Pneumonia, pancreatitis (alcohol, gallstones), MI, gastritis/PUD (heavy EtOH, NSAID use).

TREATMENT

- Withdrawal/removal of the offending agent (alcohol, NSAIDs, gallstones) is the first step in the management of both gastritis and pancreatitis.
- Both conditions are then treated conservatively with pain control and NPO/IV fluids (in the case of pancreatitis). The Ranson criteria allow the clinician to estimate the mortality of pancreatitis and help determine disposition.

RUQ PAIN

The source of discomfort in this area is often the gallbladder or the liver. Remember the **5 F's** that place a patient at ↑ risk for gallstones: Fat, Female, Forty, Fair (Caucasian), and Fertile.

SYMPTOMS/EXAM

Physical exam may show a ⊕ Murphy's sign. Referred pain in the ipsilateral shoulder may stem from diaphragmatic irritation.

DIAGNOSIS

- LFTs are ↑.
- Ultrasonography shows gallbladder wall thickening or, in the case of acute cholecystitis, pericholecystic fluid.
- The presence of gallstones is not sufficient for a diagnosis of cholecystitis, but the patient may be experiencing biliary colic (which, contrary to its name, typically features constant pain, especially after eating).

TREATMENT

- Most patients with cholecystitis require delayed operative management.
- Antibiotics are given to allow the gallbladder to "cool down" (ie, to allow

KEY FACT

Body packers are professional drug smugglers with drug packages prepared to withstand the GI tract.
Body stuffers swallow/stuff drug bags in a panic when they are confronted by police. The latter are at much greater risk of experiencing toxicity from bag rupture.

Q

A 24-year-old man is found to have overdosed on an unknown medication. He is comatose on arrival with a heart rate of 29 bpm, a BP of 80/42, and a blood glucose level of 458 mg/dL. What was the likely ingested medication?

the infection to subside). This can often be done on an outpatient basis followed by elective surgery.

RLQ PAIN

RLQ pain can indicate a variety of conditions, especially in young women. The history often does not suffice to establish a diagnosis. The differential includes:

- Appendicitis
- Ovarian torsion (requires emergent pelvic ultrasound)
- Ruptured ovarian cyst
- Ectopic pregnancy
- Tubo-ovarian abscess (PID)
- Renal calculus at the ureterovesical junction

Appendicitis

Has a bimodal distribution, affecting teenagers/young adults and those ~ 60 years of age. Caused by a fecalith or occlusion of the appendix by swollen lymphoid tissue, leading to bacterial overgrowth. Left untreated, the infection may lead to rupture of the appendix.

SYMPTOMS/EXAM

- Classic signs and symptoms include pain in the periumbilical area that migrates to the RLQ; anorexia; and pain with jumping.
- Physical exam maneuvers such as Rovsing's sign or the obturator sign are not sensitive or specific enough to confirm or rule out the diagnosis.

DIAGNOSIS/TREATMENT

- CT of the abdomen with IV contrast may quickly rule the diagnosis in or out.
- In children, ultrasound is preferred. MRI is a reasonable diagnostic modality in pregnancy.
- Antibiotics for GI flora and immediate surgical consultation.

Abdominal Aortic Aneurysm (AAA)

Risk factors include age > 60, atherosclerosis, and smoking. Underlying mechanisms are as follows:

- Weakness in the connective tissue of the tunica muscularis leads to bulging out of the vessel, typically inferior to the origin for the renal arteries.
- Wall stress is directly correlated to diameter (Laplace's law); once a critical threshold is passed, the aneurysm will rupture. Rupture occurs into the retroperitoneal space, which can hold enough blood volume to cause the patient to exsanguinate within minutes.

SYMPTOMS/EXAM

- Presents with back pain/abdominal pain and syncope.
- Leg pain/paresthesias 2° to occlusion of the artery of Adamkiewicz leads to spinal cord infarcts.

CCBs. You can distinguish CCB from β-blocker overdose by assessing blood glucose. Because insulin release is Ca^{++} mediated, CCB overdose leads to hyperglycemia.

DIAGNOSIS

- Physical exam may show an abdominal bruit or a palpable pulsatile abdominal mass.
- Ultrasound can assess for the presence of AAA but not rupture.
- CT angiography of the abdomen/pelvis can detect rupture.

TREATMENT

- A ruptured AAA requires immediate resuscitation and emergent operative repair.
- Several large-bore (14- to 16-gauge) IVs should be inserted with type O blood running via a level-1 transfuser (can administer 1 unit of blood over 30 seconds).
- Reverse coagulopathy.
- Do not manipulate BP with pressors (more pressure = more bleeding).

Sexual Assault

Begin by diagnosing and treating the victim's **physical and emotional injuries.** Then collect legal evidence and document that evidence carefully. Your main concern should always be the well-being of the patient. Information should include the following:

- Ascertain any injuries sustained during the assault.
- Determine the **risk of pregnancy.** When was the last menstrual period? Any birth control?
- Find out **where, when, and how** the assault occurred. What happened during the assault? Determine the **number** of assailants; the use of force, weapons, objects, or restraints; which **orifices** were penetrated; and whether alcohol and/or drugs were involved.
- Determine what happened **after the assault.** Are there any specific symptoms or pains? Did the patient bathe, defecate, urinate, brush teeth, or change clothes? Has the patient had **sexual intercourse in the last 72 hours?**

DIAGNOSIS

- Assess for pelvic trauma that may require immediate intervention.
- The collection of **physical evidence** (eg, debris, fingernail scrapings, dried secretions from the skin, pubic hairs) is often restricted to certified personnel.
- Medically indicated tests include a pregnancy test; nucleic acid amplification testing for gonorrhea and chlamydia; a wet mount and culture for trichomoniasis, bacterial vaginosis, and candidiasis; serology for syphilis; and HBV/HIV testing. These tests will be ⊖ in patients who present early after the assault and may need to be repeated later.

TREATMENT

- Treat traumatic injuries.
- **Infection prevention:**
  - Gonorrhea and chlamydia prophylaxis.
  - HIV prophylaxis in high-risk populations.
- **Pregnancy prevention:**
  - Administer 2 ethinyl estradiol/norgestrel (Ovral) tablets PO immediately and again 12 hours later.
  - Offer counseling.

KEY FACT

Tearing dog bites cause considerably more physical trauma, but puncture-like cat bites are more likely to become infected.

KEY FACT

Scorpion stings are treated with antivenom and benzodiazepines to control agitation and involuntary muscle movements. Monitor for hypertension, arrhythmias, and pancreatitis.

KEY FACT

For monkey bites, add postexposure prophylactic valacyclovir or acyclovir × 14 days. Herpes B virus from monkeys has an 80% fatality rate.

KEY FACT

Although "rusty nails" are associated with tetanus, any anaerobic wound with soil contamination can lead to the disease.

Animal and Insect Bites

Animal bites are a common reason patients present to the ED. The management of bite wounds requires a fine balance between reducing the risk of infection and achieving cosmesis. Patients are often surprised when they do not receive sutures for wounds that they feel should be closed.

- Animal bites result in tissue destruction and inoculation of the wound with oral flora. Depending on the animal, the patient may be at risk for a variety of complications.
- Dog bites produce large, torn wounds (bite and then shake/pull).
- Dogs have relatively clean mouths, so wounds may be sutured unless they are on the hand.
- Cat bites cause deep penetrative wounds (high anaerobic infection risk).
- The kicking action of a cat's hind legs may lead to inoculation with *Bartonella henselae*.

TREATMENT

- Antibiotic prophylaxis should be provided even if the wound is not repaired. Amoxicillin/clavulanate or a similar agent that covers oral flora is preferred.
- Wounds should be irrigated at high pressure with copious amounts of fluid. A wound may be loosely approximated rather than sutured tightly to prevent further wound contamination without creating an anaerobic environment.
- New CDC recommendations on the treatment of rabies are as follows:
  - If the animal can be observed and does not display symptoms of rabies after 10 days, no vaccine is necessary.
  - If the patient slept in the same room as a bat, vaccinate.
  - There have been no documented cases of rabies transmitted by a rodent (including squirrels).
  - Don't forget to address wound care and tetanus status.
  - Give immunoglobulin (HRIG) to all patients who were not previously immunized. If possible, inject half around the bite and half IM elsewhere.
  - Vaccine should be administered in 4 doses on days 0, 3, 7, and 14.
  - Those previously vaccinated need only 2 vaccine doses.
  - Immunocompromised patients still get 5 doses of the vaccine (as in the previous recommendations).
- Table 4-6 summarizes bite types (including human), associated infecting organisms, and appropriate treatment.

Tetanus

Trismus (ie, lockjaw), glottic spasm, and convulsive spasms caused by *Clostridium tetani*. High-risk patients include the elderly (due to inadequate immunization), IV drug users, and skin ulcer patients.

- The tetanus toxin affects modulatory motor neurons that normally secrete GABA to suppress motor impulses. As GABA levels in the synaptic cleft decline, even small, accidental impulses will produce muscle contractions. This results in a generalized tonic state in which all striated muscles begin to contract (see Figure 4-7).
- Because the posterior muscle groups of the torso are stronger than the anterior groups, patients in the most advanced disease states are often

TABLE 4-6.   Bite Types, Infecting Organisms, and Treatment

BITE TYPE	LIKELY ORGANISMS/TOXINS	TREATMENT
Dog	α-hemolytic streptococci, *S aureus*, *Pasteurella multocida*, and anaerobes.	**Amoxicillin/clavulanate** or a first-generation cephalosporin +/– tetanus and rabies prophylaxis.
Cat	*P multocida* (high rate of infection), anaerobes.	**Amoxicillin/clavulanate** +/– tetanus prophylaxis.
Human	Polymicrobial. Viridans streptococci are most frequently implicated.	Second- or third-generation cephalosporins, dicloxacillin + penicillin, **amoxicillin/clavulanate** or clarithromycin +/– tetanus prophylaxis, HBV vaccine, HBIG, and postexposure HIV prophylaxis.
Rodent	*Streptobacillus moniliformis*, *P multocida*, *Leptospira* spp.	**Penicillin VK** or doxycycline.
Bat	Rabies and other viruses.	Vaccination against rabies.
Snake	*Pseudomonas aeruginosa*, *Proteus* spp., *Bacteroides fragilis*, *Clostridium* spp., venom.	Antivenom as appropriate. Venomous snakes (eg, coral snake, pit viper, rattlesnake) may not require antibiotics; ampicillin/sulbactam (or, alternatively, a fluoroquinolone or clindamycin + TMP-SMX) is given to combat the snake's oral flora. Monitor for rhabdomyolysis, neurologic impairment, coagulopathy, and serum sickness.
Spider	Venom (can cause tissue necrosis and/or rigid paralysis, depending on species).	Antivenom as appropriate; otherwise supportive care (analgesics, antihistamines, wound irrigation/debridement). Tetanus prophylaxis.

arched with contracted arms (the biceps is stronger than the triceps). This is called opisthotonos.

■ Although the heart muscle is not affected, tetanus may lead to respiratory arrest, hyperthermia and rhabdomyolysis, and subsequent death.

TREATMENT

■ Benzodiazepines to control muscle spasms; neuromuscular blockade if needed to control the airway.
■ **Metronidazole** is the antibiotic of choice.
■ Administer tetanus immune globulin (TIG) and/or adsorbed tetanus and diphtheria toxoid (Td) vaccine as indicated in Table 4-7.

Anaphylaxis

Patients who are presensitized to certain antigens may develop a significant type I hypersensitivity (allergic) reaction on exposure. True anaphylaxis is associated with significant mortality, usually from airway occlusion rather than from anaphylactic shock (which is easily treated with IV fluids and pressors).

■ IgE-mediated cytokine release in response to an antigen triggers a variety of reactions. The predominant cytokine is histamine. Histamine can also be released independent of IgE by direct mast cell stimulation (eg, morphine, IV contrast dye).

Q 1

A 25-year-old man becomes involved in a bar fight and sustains a "fight bite" (closed-fist injury) to his hand. The wound culture grows gram-⊝ rods. What is the most likely pathogen, and how should it be treated?

Q 2

A 37-year-old known IV drug user is brought to the ED with trismus and facial grimacing 30 minutes after using heroin. What is the most likely diagnosis?

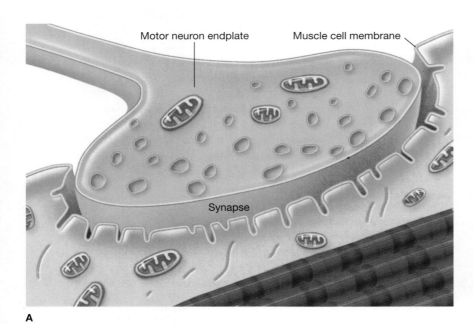
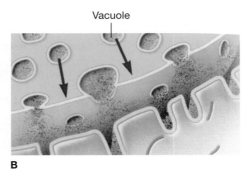
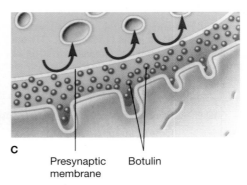

FIGURE 4-7. **Tetanus and botulinum neurotoxins.** (A) The motor neuron endplate, synapse, and neuromuscular junction. For tetanus toxin, the neurons have an inhibitory function. (B) Vesicles release neurotransmitters across the synapse to the muscle cell membrane. (C) For tetanus toxin, the release of neurotransmitters that activate inhibitory neurons is blocked, resulting in spasmodic contractions. (Reproduced with permission from Ryan KJ, Ray CG. *Sherris Medical Microbiology,* 6th ed. New York: McGraw-Hill, 2014, Fig. 29-3.)

- In addition to vasodilation, the capillary bed becomes leaky and significant edema ensues. Edema may occur superficially (facial swelling), in the gut (leading to nausea/vomiting/abdominal pain), and in the airway (placing the patient at risk for airway occlusion). The latter is exacerbated by induced bronchospasm as well as bronchorrhea.
- Anaphylaxis also leads to systemic vasodilation, resulting in hypotension despite high cardiac output (distributive shock).

DIAGNOSIS

- A clinical diagnosis. Patients often present with significant hives and obvious swelling along with a history of allergic reactions.

TABLE 4-7. **Tetanus Prophylaxis Schedule**

HISTORY OF ADSORBED TETANUS TOXOID (DOSES)	NON-TETANUS-PRONE WOUNDS	TETANUS-PRONE WOUNDS[a]	
	Td	Td	TIG
Unknown or < 3 doses	√	√	√
Three doses:			
Last dose ≥ 5 years		√	
Last dose ≥ 10 years	√	√	

[a] Tetanus-prone wounds are those that are present for > 6 hours; are nonlinear; are > 1 cm deep; and show signs of infection, devitalized tissue, and contamination.

---

1 **A**

Eikenella corrodens, the most likely pathogen, is common in human bite infections that are sustained in closed-fist injuries. Treat with amoxicillin/clavulanate.

2 **A**

Strychnine poisoning, which can look just like tetanus. When heroin is "cut," drug dealers often use white, bitter chemicals so that the drug still tastes pure. Strychnine antagonizes glycine (an inhibitory neurotransmitter) in the spinal cord. Give benzodiazepines.

- To meet the diagnostic criteria for anaphylaxis, 2 organ system must be involved (eg, hives and abdominal pain or vomiting). No lab tests or imaging studies aid in diagnosis.

TREATMENT

Several treatment modalities are available for patients with an allergic reaction or anaphylaxis:

- IM epinephrine.
- Histamine blockade (diphenhydramine for H_1 blockade; famotidine for H_2 blockade).
- Steroids.
- Nebulized albuterol (for wheezing).
- Early intubation if necessary.

KEY FACT

Type I: Anaphylactic/immediate (IgE).
Type II: Cytotoxic (antibody mediated).
Type III: Immune complex.
Type IV: Delayed (CD4 mediated).

Angioedema

There are 2 types of angioedema: hereditary and acquired (eg, related to ACEIs). The condition becomes an emergency if it involves the tongue or upper airway. Underlying mechanisms include the following:

- The complement system is a cascade that ends in the formation of the "membrane attack complex" (MAC), which disrupts the cell walls of pathogens. C1 is the first step in this cascade. In hereditary angioedema, C1 is not inhibited, so it may inappropriately trigger the cascade.
- An autosomal dominant mutation leads to a deficiency of C1 esterase (aka C1 inhibitor). C1 then becomes overactive, leading to the production of kallikrein. Subsequently, kininogen and therefore bradykinin levels can be ↑.
- Bradykinin enhances vascular permeability, which in turn produces significant tissue edema. ACEIs also ↑ bradykinin.

DIAGNOSIS

- Diagnosis is clinical.
- C1 esterase inhibitor levels confirm the diagnosis but are not available for immediate decision making in the ED.

TREATMENT

- Most treatment modalities available for anaphylaxis have no effect on the course of angioedema.
- Provide airway protection.
- Fresh frozen plasma (FFP) contains C1 esterase inhibitor and may ↓ the severity of hereditary angioedema.
- Concentrated C1 esterase inhibitor (Cinryze) is available but is costly.

Environmental Emergencies

COLD EMERGENCIES

Frostbite

- Cold injury with pallor and loss of cold sensation resulting from exposure to cold air or direct contact with cold materials. Nonviable structures demarcate and slough off. May be superficial or deep.

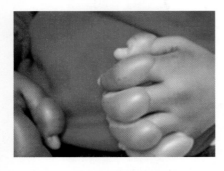

FIGURE 4-8. Frostbite injury in a child. (Used with permission of Mark Sochor, MD.)

KEY FACT

Do not rewarm frostbite until refreezing can be prevented.

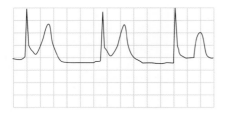

FIGURE 4-9. Sinus bradycardia, Osborn wave. J-point elevation with ST-segment elevation and a prolonged QT interval (0.56 sec) is seen in a patient with hypothermia.

KEY FACT

The "J" in J waves refers not only to the approximate shape of these waves but also to the initials of the man who first described them: John J. Osborn.

KEY FACT

"No one is dead until they're warm and dead."

KEY FACT

Heat stroke presents with altered mental status and ↑ temperature, often with no sweating.

- **Superficial:** Injury to cutaneous and subcutaneous tissue. Skin is soft under a frozen surface. Large, clear, fluid-filled vesicles develop within 2 days (indicating a good prognosis); sloughing leaves new skin that is pink and hypersensitive (see Figure 4-8).
  - **Deep:** Injury to the above tissues plus deep structures (muscle, bone). Skin is hard under a frozen surface.
- **Tx:** Rapidly rewarm once refreezing can be prevented. Circulating water at 40°C (104°F); wound care; tetanus prophylaxis.

Hypothermia

- Defined as a core body temperature of < 35°C (< 95°F).
- Caused by environmental exposure, **alcohol ingestion,** drugs (barbiturates, benzodiazepines, narcotics), hypoglycemia, CNS or hypothalamic dysfunction (via loss of stimulus of shivering response and adrenal activity), hypothyroidism, skin disorders, and sepsis.
- **Dx:** Look for arrhythmias and/or **Osborn/J waves** (positive deflection in the QRS complex) on ECG (see Figure 4-9).
- **Tx:**
  - ABCs, CPR (in the event of cardiac arrest), and stabilization.
  - **Rewarming:**
    - **Passive external:** Blankets should be used only in patients who shiver. Once shivering stops, the patient no longer generates heat, and additional methods of rewarming must be used.
    - **Active external:** Warmed blankets, warm-air circulatory blankets, hot-water bottles.
    - **Active internal:** Warm humidified O_2; heated IV fluids; gastric, colonic, bladder, or peritoneal lavage; thoracic lavage; extracorporeal rewarming.
  - Do not pronounce patients dead until they have been rewarmed to 35°C (95°F); full recovery is not uncommon.
  - Associated with a risk of dysrhythmias, especially VF at core temperatures of < 30°C (86°F).

HEAT EMERGENCIES

Heat Exhaustion

- Extreme fatigue with **profuse sweating.** Also presents with nausea/vomiting and a dull headache.
- **Sx/Exam:** Body temperature is **normal** or slightly ↑. Patients are tachypneic, tachycardic, and hypotensive.
- **Tx:** Treat with IV normal saline and a cool environment.

Heat Stroke

- Elevation of body temperature above normal as a result of temperature dysregulation (> 40°C [104°F]). **A true emergency.** Monitor for convulsions and cardiovascular collapse.
- **Sx/Exam:** Presents with ↑ **body temperature,** altered mental status, and possibly paradoxical shivering. Patients have hot, dry skin, often with no sweating. Ataxia may be seen.
- **Tx:**
  - Treat with **aggressive cooling.** Remove from the heat source and undress. Use an atomized tepid water spray in combination with fans (can cool as fast as 0.5°C/min), and apply ice packs to the groin/axillae (some facilities use cooled IV fluids run through a central line).
  - Treat neuroleptic malignant syndrome and drug fever with **dantrolene.** Treat seizures with **diazepam.**

Burns

Burn victims pose highly complex challenges. Not only are they prone to dehydration, hypothermia, and infection from their compromised skin barrier, but they are also at risk for airway compromise (inhalational burn), trauma (when attempting to escape fire), and toxicity from inhaled gases (primarily carbon monoxide and cyanide).

EXAM

- **Airway, airway, airway.** Whether the patient has perioral or intraoral burns, carbonaceous sputum, or a hoarse voice, intubate early. Intubation is a reversible procedure; death from airway edema is not.
- Gauge the body surface area (BSA) involved. Observe the **rule of 9's: 9% BSA** for the head and each arm; **18% BSA** for the back torso, the front torso, and each leg.
- In **children,** the rule is 9% BSA for each arm; 18% BSA for the head, back torso, and front torso; and 14% BSA for each leg.
- Determine the **depth of the burn** (see Table 4-8 and Figure 4-10).

TREATMENT

- **Prehospital treatment:**
  - Administer IV fluids and high-flow O_2.
  - Remove the patient's clothes and cover with clean sheets or dressings.
  - Give pain medications.
- **In-hospital treatment:**
  - **Early airway control** is critical.
  - **Fluid resuscitation:** Appropriate for patients with > 20% BSA second-degree burns.
    - Give 4 cc/kg per % total BSA (**Parkland formula**) over 24 hours—the first half over the first 8 hours and the second half over the next 16 hours. Keep in mind that the clock starts at the time of the burn. Don't fall behind with fluid resuscitation; you will never catch up in these patients.
    - Maintain a urine output of 1 cc/kg/hr.
  - Tetanus prophylaxis; pain control. Prophylactic antibiotics are of no benefit.

TABLE 4-8.   Burn Classification

SEVERITY OF BURN	TISSUE INVOLVEMENT	FINDINGS
First degree	Epidermis only.	Red and painful.
Second degree (superficial)	Epidermis and superficial dermis.	Red, wet, and painful with **blisters.**
Second degree (deep)	Epidermis and deep dermis.	White, dry, and painful.
Third degree	Epidermis and **entire dermis.**	Charred/leathery, pearly white, and **nontender.**
Fourth degree	Below the dermis to bone, muscle, and fascia.	—

Q 1

A 20-year-old woman is pulled unconscious from a cold lake 5 minutes after her sailboat capsized. Despite the problems associated with hypothermia, her near-drowning is likely to have a better outcome than other causes of hypoxia. Why is this the case?

Q 2

A 35-year-old migrant worker with no past medical history has a syncopal episode while harvesting tobacco. Exam reveals diminished mentation, tachypnea, and rales. His bloodwork reveals hypovolemic hyponatremia, hypoglycemia, leukocytosis, and ↑ LFTs. What diagnosis can account for all these abnormalities?

Q 3

A 20-year-old, 154-lb (70-kg) college student was attempting to light a campfire when his shirt caught on fire. Because of the remote location, it took EMS 2 hours to bring the patient to the ED. On exam, you estimate a 30% body surface full-thickness burn. What is the initial fluid administration rate?

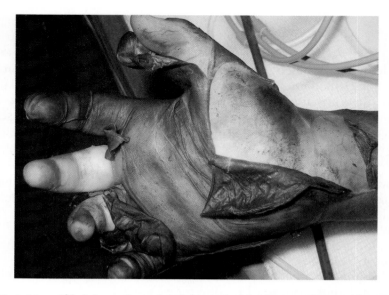

FIGURE 4-10. **Third-degree burns involving underlying bone and/or muscle.** (Reproduced with permission from Goldsmith LA et al. *Fitzpatrick's Dermatology in General Medicine*, 8th ed. New York: McGraw-Hill, 2012, Fig. 95-1D.)

- **Disposition:**
  - **Minor burns:** Discharge with pain medications.
  - **Moderate burns** (partial-thickness 15–25% BSA or full-thickness < 10% BSA): Admit to the hospital.
  - **Major burns** (partial-thickness > 25% BSA or full-thickness > 10% BSA; burns to the face, hands, joints, feet, or perineum; electrical or circumferential burns): Refer to a burn center.

Electrical Injuries

Electrical current flows most easily through tissues of low resistance, such as nerves, blood vessels, mucous membranes, and muscles. The current pathway determines which organs are affected. External injuries **do not** predict internal injuries.

Symptoms/Exam

Symptoms vary with the nature of the current.

- **Alternating current (household and commercial):**
  - Associated with explosive exit wounds (see Figure 4-11).
  - Effects are worse with AC than with DC current at the same voltage.
  - VF is common.
- **Direct current (industrial, batteries, lightning):**
  - Causes discrete exit wounds.
  - Asystole is common.

Treatment

- CABs as above; IV fluids for severe burns.
- Administer pain medications and treat burns.
- In mass casualty events (eg, a lightning strike into a crowd), perform **reverse** triage and prioritize pulseless patients, as return of spontaneous circulation (ROSC) is very likely.

---

1 **A**

Activation of the diving reflex (reflex bradycardia and breath holding), which reduces metabolic demands and the effects of hypoxemia, shunts blood to the vital organs and limits aspiration of water.

2 **A**

Exertional heat stroke.

3 **A**

The rate should be 0.5 × 70 kg × 4 cc/kg × 30% ÷ 6 hours = 700 cc/hr. The Parkland formula requires that half the volume be given in the first 8 hours (0.5), is weight based (70 kg × 4 cc/kg), and depends on the surface area burned (30%). Why divide by 6 hours and not 8? Because we're already 2 hours in from the initial burn.

- Treat **myoglobinuria** with IV fluids to maintain a urine output of 1.5–2.0 cc/kg/hr.
- Tetanus prophylaxis.
- Asymptomatic patients with low-voltage (< 1000-V) burns can be discharged.

Ophthalmology

OCULAR TRAUMA

Corneal Abrasion

- **Sx/Exam:** Presents with pain out of proportion to the exam as well as with a foreign-body sensation and photophobia.
- **Dx: Fluorescein staining** (cobalt-blue light source via slit-lamp or Wood's lamp examination) reveals an abraded area.
- **Tx:** Treat with topical broad-spectrum antibiotics (eg, gentamicin, sulfacetamide, bacitracin), tetanus prophylaxis, and oral analgesics.

Ruptured Globe

- **Sx/Exam:** Presents with trauma and loss of vision. Exam may reveal a vitreous humor leak leading to a **teardrop-shaped pupil** and a marked ↓ in visual acuity.
- **Dx:** Diagnosis can often be made only by clinical means. Ocular ultrasound or tonometry will worsen the injury.
- **Tx:** Manage with a rigid eye shield to prevent pressure on the globe. An immediate ophthalmologic consultation is necessary.

Ocular Foreign Body

- **Sx/Exam:** Presents with a foreign-body sensation.
- **Dx:**
  - Superficial foreign bodies can often be seen on slit-lamp exam; deep foreign bodies may be seen on ultrasound.
  - **Seidel's test:** Apply fluorescein to the cornea; if the anterior chamber begins to glow with a Wood's lamp, globe perforation has occurred.
- **Tx:** Remove superficial foreign bodies with a wet cotton tip or needle (embedded). Call ophthalmology for deep foreign bodies or perforated globes.

Retinal Detachment

- **Sx/Exam:** Patients present with "flashing lights" in vision. Painless, and may occur spontaneously or after trauma.
- **Dx:** Ocular ultrasound shows a detached retina.
- **Tx:** Urgent ophthalmology consult.

CONJUNCTIVITIS

Allergic Conjunctivitis

- Intensely **pruritic, watery eyes.** Most commonly affects males with a family history of atopy.
- **Sx/Exam/Dx:** Look for diffuse conjunctival injection with normal visual acuity. Lid edema and cobblestone papillae may be seen under the upper lid.
- **Tx:** Treat with topical antihistamine/vasoconstrictor preparations such as naphazoline/pheniramine. Cool compresses are also of benefit.

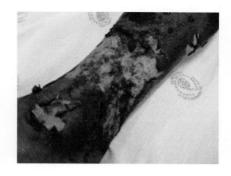

FIGURE 4-11. **Circumferential electrical burn of the right lower extremity.** (Used with permission of Benjamin Silverberg, MD.)

KEY FACT

A CT scan of the orbit, though sometimes helpful, usually reveals more about damage to the temporal bone than about injury to the eyeball itself.

Bacterial Conjunctivitis

- Painful, red eye that is usually unilateral. Causative organisms include *Staphylococcus, Streptococcus, Neisseria gonorrhoeae,* and *Chlamydia trachomatis* (in newborns and sexually active adults).
- **Sx/Exam:** Presents with photophobia, a gritty foreign-body sensation, and a **purulent exudate.**
- **Dx:** Diffuse conjunctival injection with normal visual acuity. Bacteria can be seen on Gram stain.
- **Tx:**
  - Treat staphylococcal and streptococcal infection with topical 10% sulfacetamide or aminoglycoside.
  - Treat suspected *N gonorrhoeae* with IV ceftriaxone and topical erythromycin or tetracycline (if left untreated, can lead to blindness and sepsis).
  - PO doxycycline or PO/topical erythromycin is appropriate for chlamydial infection (if left untreated, can lead to corneal scarring and/or *C trachomatis* pneumonia).
  - Warm compresses and frequent flushes are also of benefit.

Viral Conjunctivitis ("Pink Eye")

- **Sx/Exam:** Presents as an irritated, red eye with **watery discharge** and crusting. Frequently bilateral, and often occurs in conjunction with cold symptoms (eg, rhinorrhea, sore throat, cough).
- **Dx:** Diffuse conjunctival injection with normal vision and **preauricular lymphadenopathy.** Multiple superficial punctate corneal lesions are seen on fluorescein staining.
- **Tx:** Generally no treatment is necessary.

Chemical Conjunctivitis

- Caused by acid or alkali exposure.
- **Dx:** Determine pH from litmus paper. Coagulation necrosis is associated with acid burns, liquefaction necrosis with alkali burns.
- **Tx:** Treat with copious irrigation with a Morgan lens until pH approaches neutral (keep in mind that the pH of normal saline is about 5.5, so you will never get the pH to be 7 no matter how much you irrigate).

OTHER CONDITIONS OF THE EYE

- **Dacryostenosis:** Congenital nasolacrimal duct obstruction (can lead to conjunctivitis).
- **Hordeolum:** Infection of the meibomian glands; most frequently caused by *S aureus.*
- **Periorbital/preseptal cellulitis:** Infection of the tissue around the eye/eyelid, usually caused by *S aureus.* If there is pain on eye movement or proptosis, treat as orbital cellulitis, a vision-threatening emergency. IV antibiotics (vancomycin, piperacillin/tazobactam) and **an emergent ophthalmology consult** are needed.
- **Blepharoconjunctivitis:** Concurrent inflammation of the conjunctiva and eyelid.
- **Keratitis:** Inflammation of the cornea; may be caused by syphilis, HSV, or UV light exposure.
- **Uveitis:** Inflammation of the inner eye (iris or retina); usually 2° to inflammatory diseases (eg, SLE).
- **Hyphema:** Blood in the anterior chamber of the eye; usually 2° to trauma.
- **Xerophthalmia:** Dry eyes.
- **Strabismus ("lazy eye"):** Can lead to blindness (amblyopia) if not treated during childhood.

KEY FACT

Timeline of neonatal conjunctivitis (ophthalmia neonatorum):
- Within 24 hours = chemical.
- 2–5 days = gonorrheal.
- 5–14 days = chlamydial.

KEY FACT

Alkali burns do far more damage than acid burns.

- **Presbyopia:** Normal age-related reduction in accommodation.
- **Cataracts:** Painless, progressive loss of vision; absent red reflex.
- **Glaucoma:** Refer to Chapter 2 for a detailed discussion of open- and closed-angle glaucoma.

Dental Emergencies

The numbering system for 1° and permanent teeth is shown in Figure 4-12.

DENTAL AVULSION

Fractures of the teeth are classified by the deepest layer violated (enamel, dentin, or pulp). They should be evaluated by a dentist within 24 hours. Complete removal of the tooth from its socket, or an avulsion, represents a **dental emergency,** and reimplantation should occur within 2–3 hours of injury.

TREATMENT

- Wash the tooth in clean water to remove debris. **Do not scrub;** doing so will also remove the periodontal ligaments. Then attempt to reimplant the tooth in its socket.
- If this is not possible (eg, if the tooth doesn't fit or the patient is unconscious and likely to swallow it), place the tooth in an isotonic solution such as sterile saline or milk. There are also commercially available solutions for this purpose.
- Further treatment depends on the amount of time the tooth has been "dry." The patient should be referred to a dentist or an oral surgeon.

MANDIBULAR FRACTURE

Consider fracture of the mandible in any patient with blunt-force trauma to the face with subsequent jaw pain, asymmetry, and/or difficulty speaking/eating. Because of the semiannular shape of the mandible, **contrecoup fractures** (fractures at a site other than the point of impact) are likely (see Figure 4-13). Be sure to stabilize the patient's airway before focusing on his facial injuries.

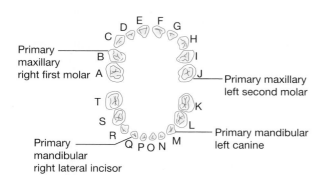

A

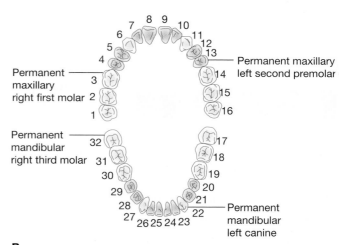

B

FIGURE 4-12. **Numbering system and types of teeth in children and adults.** (Adapted with permission from Tintinalli JE et al. *Tintinalli's Emergency Medicine: A Comprehensive Study Guide,* 7th ed. New York: McGraw-Hill, 2011, Fig. 240-2.)

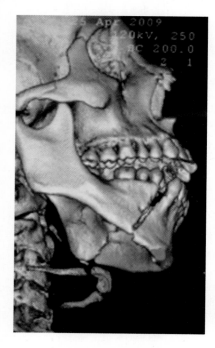

FIGURE 4-13. **CT reconstruction of a double fracture through the right body and left mandibular angle.** (Used with permission of Benjamin Silverberg, MD.)

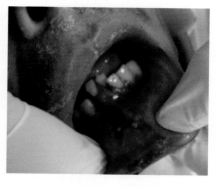

FIGURE 4-14. **Likely mandibular fracture.** Note the dislocation of teeth 25 and 26 while still tethered in the gum line. (Used with permission of Benjamin Silverberg, MD.)

 KEY FACT

Water-soluble contrast (Gastrografin) leads to chemical pneumonitis if aspirated. Barium contrast leads to peritonitis if a perforation is present. Choose your contrast agent carefully!

SYMPTOMS/EXAM

Malalignment of the teeth (malocclusion), **ecchymosis of the floor of the mouth,** intraoral lacerations (including open fractures into the mouth), dental fractures, inferior alveolar or mental nerve paresthesia, trismus. See Figure 4-14.

DIAGNOSIS

Diagnosis is confirmed with a panoramic dental x-ray, AP/oblique plain films, or a CT of the face.

TREATMENT

- Clindamycin or amoxicillin/clavulanate against anaerobic oral flora. Tetanus prophylaxis if needed.
- Analgesia; immobilization of the jaw.
- Refer to an oral surgeon.

Radiology

Appropriate radiology screening modalities and confirmation for various diagnoses are listed by test below:

- **CT with contrast:** Abdominal abscess, abdominal trauma, aortic aneurysm/dissection, appendicitis, bowel perforation, chest mass/trauma, colitis, diverticulitis, hemoptysis, hydronephrosis, intestinal obstruction, persistent hematuria, PE, tumor diagnosis/staging.
- **CT without contrast:** Head trauma (including skull fracture), intracranial bleed, nephrolithiasis, suspected spinal trauma/fracture.
- **MRI with contrast:** Brain/spinal tumor/infection, joint imaging, MS, osteomyelitis, vascular imaging, spinal cord compression.
- **Plain film:** Chest mass/trauma, hemoptysis, intestinal obstruction/perforation, most orthopedic problems, pneumonia.
- **Duplex ultrasound:** Carotid stenosis, DVT.
- **Ultrasound:** AAA screening, appendicitis (in pediatric/pregnant patients), gallstones/cholecystitis, hydronephrosis, intussusception, liver screening, pregnancy/most gynecologic pathology, pyloric stenosis, scrotal pathology (torsion, hydrocele, epididymitis/orchitis, scrotal mass).
- **Barium swallow:** Esophageal obstruction.
- **Barium enema:** Colonic masses (single contrast), IBD/diverticulosis (double contrast).
- **Upper (or lower) endoscopy:** Esophageal obstruction, hematemesis, PUD, upper (or lower) GI bleeding.
- **Cystoscopy:** Persistent hematuria.
- **HIDA scan:** Cholecystitis.
- **V/Q scan:** PE.

ENDOCRINOLOGY

Diabetes Mellitus (DM)

DM results from ↓ insulin secretion (type 1) or from tissue resistance to insulin (type 2), leading to hyperglycemia. Complications include microvascular disease (retinopathy, nephropathy, neuropathy) and macrovascular disease (atherosclerosis).

TYPE 1 DIABETES MELLITUS

In type 1 DM, destruction of insulin-producing pancreatic β cells leads to insulin deficiency (see Table 5-1). Type 1 DM is generally immune mediated and may be triggered by environmental agents. It accounts for < 10% of all cases of DM. Diabetic ketoacidosis (DKA) is often the initial presentation.

SYMPTOMS/EXAM

- Presents with the classic symptoms of **P**olyuria (including nocturia), **P**olydipsia, and **P**olyphagia (the **3 P's**).
- Patients may also have rapid or unexplained weight loss, blurry vision, or recurrent infections (eg, candidiasis).

DIFFERENTIAL

Pancreatic disease (eg, chronic pancreatitis), glucagonoma, Cushing's disease, iatrogenic factors (eg, high-dose glucocorticoids), gestational diabetes, diabetes insipidus.

MNEMONIC

The 3 P's of type 1 DM:

Polyuria
Polydipsia
Polyphagia

TABLE 5-1. **Type 1 vs Type 2 DM**

	TYPE 1 (INSULIN-DEPENDENT DM)	TYPE 2 (NON-INSULIN-DEPENDENT DM)
Pathophysiology	Failure of the pancreas to secrete insulin as a result of autoimmune destruction of β cells.	Insulin resistance and inadequate insulin secretion by the pancreas to compensate.
Incidence	15%.	85%.
Age (exceptions are common)	< 30 years.	> 40 years.
Association with obesity	No.	Yes.
"Classic symptoms"	Common.	Sometimes.
DKA	Common.	Rare.
Genetic predisposition	Weak, polygenic.	Strong, polygenic.
Association with HLA system	Yes (HLA-DR3 and -DR4).	No.
Serum C-peptide	↓; can be normal during the "honeymoon period."	↓ late in the disease.

DIAGNOSIS

At least 1 of the following is required to make the diagnosis:

- A random plasma glucose concentration of ≥ 200 mg/dL with classic symptoms of diabetes.
- A fasting plasma glucose level of ≥ 126 mg/dL on > 1 occasion.
- A 2-hour postprandial glucose level of ≥ 200 mg/dL after a 75-g oral glucose tolerance test on 2 separate occasions.
- A **hemoglobin A$_{1c}$ (HbA$_{1c}$) > 6.5%.**

TREATMENT

- Start insulin (see Table 5-2). Both basal and bolus insulin is required. Oral hypoglycemic agents are ineffective.
- Most patients with type 1 DM are on a multiple-daily-injection (MDI) regimen consisting of a premeal short-acting insulin (eg, lispro or aspart) and a bedtime long-acting insulin (glargine) or twice-daily NPH or detemir.
- Insulin pumps use only short- or rapid-acting insulins, which provide improved glycemic control.
- Long-term management should include the following:
  - Check an **HbA$_{1c}$ level** every 3 months.
  - Maintain a low-fat, reduced-carbohydrate diet, and refer to a dietitian.
  - Manage **CAD risk factors** (hypertension, smoking, obesity, hyperlipidemia).
  - Check the eyes annually for retinopathy or cataracts. An ophthalmologic exam is also indicated if the patient is planning a pregnancy.
  - Consider screening newly diagnosed type 1 diabetics for **thyroid disease,** particularly autoimmune hypothyroidism, and for celiac disease.
  - Order an annual BUN/creatinine and a spot urine sample for measurement of the urine microalbumin/creatinine ratio to screen for diabetic nephropathy.
  - Check the **feet** annually for neuropathy, ulcers, and peripheral vascular disease. Patients should inspect their feet daily and wear comfortable shoes.
  - Administer an annual flu shot and keep pneumococcal vaccinations up to date.

KEY FACT

The rate of destruction is slow in some patients (primarily adults) who are afflicted with late-onset autoimmune diabetes.

TABLE 5-2. **Types of Insulin[a]**

INSULIN	ONSET	PEAK EFFECT	DURATION
Regular	30–60 minutes	2–4 hours	5–8 hours
Humalog (lispro)	5–10 minutes	0.5–1.5 hours	6–8 hours
NovoLog (aspart)	10–20 minutes	1–3 hours	3–5 hours
NPH	2–4 hours	6–10 hours	18–28 hours
Levemir (detemir)	2 hours	No discernible peak	20 hours
Lantus (glargine)	1–4 hours	No discernible peak	20–24 hours

[a] Combination preparations mix longer- and shorter-acting types of insulin together to provide immediate and extended coverage in the same injection, eg, 70 NPH/30 regular = 70% NPH + 30% regular.

Reproduced with permission from Le T et al. *First Aid for the USMLE Step 2 CK,* 7th ed. New York: McGraw-Hill, 2007: 114.

TYPE 2 DIABETES MELLITUS

Type 2 DM is a common disorder with 2 etiologies: insufficient insulin secretion and ↑ insulin resistance (see Table 5-1). Prevalence rises with increasing degrees of obesity.

- Characterized by impaired insulin secretion, insulin resistance, and excessive hepatic glucose production.
- In its early stages, glucose tolerance remains near normal despite insulin resistance. After an initial period of insulin resistance and ↑ insulin secretion, pancreatic β-cell function falters and fails to meet peripheral demand.

SYMPTOMS/EXAM

- The 3 P's (**P**olyuria, **P**olydipsia, **P**olyphagia), recurrent blurred vision, paresthesias, and fatigue are found in both type 1 and type 2 DM.
- Because of the insidious onset of hyperglycemia, patients may be asymptomatic at the time of diagnosis and may present with both macrovascular and microvascular complications.
- **Macrovascular complications:**
    - **Atherosclerosis:** Advanced glycosylation end products produce changes in collagen composition in arterial walls, trapping LDL and resulting in ↑ lipid deposition.
    - **CAD;** peripheral vascular disease.
    - **Stroke:** Commonly due to carotid artery stenosis or arteriolosclerosis of the lenticulostriate arteries.
- **Microvascular complications** (see also Table 5-3):
    - **Diabetic nephropathy:** Hyalinization of glomerular arterioles (Kimmelstiel-Wilson nodules); proteinuria/microalbuminuria.
    - **Diabetic retinopathy.**
    - **Diabetic neuropathy:** Peripheral neuropathy (loss of pain and vibratory sensation in the legs in the characteristic "stocking" distribution); autonomic neuropathy (sexual impotence, delayed gastric emptying).

DIFFERENTIAL

- **Pancreatic insufficiency:** Chronic pancreatitis, hemosiderosis, subtotal pancreatectomy, hemochromatosis.
- **Endocrinopathies:** Cushing's syndrome, acromegaly, glucagonoma, gestational diabetes, diabetes insipidus.
- **Drugs:** Glucocorticoids, thiazides, niacin.

DIAGNOSIS

Similar to that of type 1 DM.

TREATMENT

- Diet, weight loss, and exercise are critical in that they ↓ insulin resistance and blood glucose levels.
- Start oral therapy in patients whose diabetes is not controlled by weight loss, diet, or exercise (see Table 5-4).
- Typical stepwise pharmacologic management includes metformin (the best initial medical therapy). If diabetes is not controlled, add a second medication (usually a sulfonylurea such as glyburide).
- If the patient continues to have inadequate control on oral antidiabetic drugs, insulin is either added to the oral regimen or used to replace it.
    - Insulin is administered subcutaneously, typically in the abdomen, arms, or legs. It can be given intravenously in emergencies (eg, DKA).

KEY FACT

Metabolic syndrome refers to clinical combinations of hypertension, ↑ LDL, ↓ HDL, and type 2 diabetes.

KEY FACT

The risk of microvascular complications in DM is ↓ by tight glycemic control.

KEY FACT

Step 3 loves to ask about lifestyle changes in diseases like diabetes!

KEY FACT

Metformin should not be administered with renal failure, conditions predisposing to lactic acidosis, or concurrent use of a contrast agent.

TABLE 5-3.   Common Microvascular Complications of Type 2 Diabetes Mellitus

	NEPHROPATHY	RETINOPATHY	NEUROPATHY
Symptoms/ exam	Usually asymptomatic, but may present with bilateral lower extremity edema (from nephrotic syndrome).	Correlates with the duration of DM and glycemic control. Patients may have retinopathy at the time of diagnosis. **Nonproliferative:** Characterized by retinal vascular microaneurysms, blot hemorrhages, and cotton-wool spots. Macular edema may be seen. **Proliferative:** Neovascularization in response to retinal hypoxia is the hallmark.	Primarily a symmetrical sensory polyneuropathy affecting the distal lower extremities. May also present as a mononeuropathy and/or autonomic neuropathy. Patients are at ↑ risk for the development of diabetic foot ulcers (see Figure 5-1).
Diagnosis	Kimmelstiel-Wilson lesions (nodular glomerulosclerosis) may be seen on kidney biopsy. Look for **coexisting retinopathy.**	Diagnosed through a comprehensive eye exam, supplemented by retinal tomography and fluorescein angiography.	Diagnosed clinically.
Treatment	Start patients with microalbuminuria or proteinuria on an ACEI to keep BP < 140/90. End-stage nephropathy requires chronic hemodialysis or transplantation.	Prevention, regular eye exams, and laser therapy are the mainstays.	Strict glycemic control improves nerve conduction. TCAs, carbamazepine, and gabapentin to treat sensory dysfunction.

- Dosing depends on the type of insulin (eg, short- vs long-acting). New inhaled forms are also available. Consider long-acting insulin (NPH, detemir, or glargine) if insulin is added to oral hypoglycemic therapy (given in the morning or at bedtime).
- For those who require more intense therapy, a split/mixed regimen of regular or short-acting and NPH or glargine insulin may be used (usually a basal-bolus regimen of glargine with premeal aspart or lispro).
  - **Pre-breakfast glucose level:** Reflects pre-dinner NPH dose.
  - **Pre-lunch glucose level:** Reflects pre-breakfast regular insulin dose.
  - **Pre-dinner glucose level:** Reflects pre-breakfast NPH dose.
  - **Bedtime glucose level:** Reflects pre-dinner regular insulin dose.
- Long-term management includes **monitoring blood glucose** (see Table 5-5) and checking a fasting glucose level once a day. Otherwise, management is similar to that of type 1.

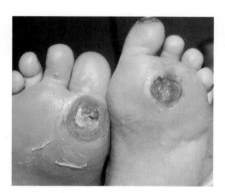

FIGURE 5-1.   Neuropathic ulcers in a diabetic. (Reproduced with permission from Tintinalli JE et al. *Tintinalli's Emergency Medicine,* 7th ed. New York: McGraw-Hill, 2011, Fig. 247-3.)

COMPLICATIONS OF DIABETES MELLITUS

Diabetic Ketoacidosis (DKA)

DKA may be the initial manifestation of **type 1 DM** and is usually precipitated by a stressor (eg, infection, surgery, MI). ↑ catabolism due to lack of insulin action combined with ↑ counterregulatory hormones results in life-threatening metabolic acidosis. Hyperkalemia is due to ↓ insulin and hyperosmolality, **not** to H^+-K^+ shifts.

Q

A 45-year-old obese man presents with polyuria and weight loss. What level of serum glucose is diagnostic of diabetes mellitus?

TABLE 5-4.   Oral Diabetes Medications

MEDICATION	EXAMPLES	MECHANISM OF ACTION	SIDE EFFECTS	CONTRAINDICATIONS
Biguanides	Metformin	Inhibit hepatic gluconeogenesis, ↑ glucose utilization, ↓ insulin resistance, ↓ postprandial glucose levels.	Lactic acidosis, diarrhea, GI discomfort, metallic taste, weight loss. Does not cause hypoglycemia.	Renal insufficiency, any form of acidosis, liver disease, severe hypoxia.
Sulfonylureas	**First generation:** Chlorpropamide **Second generation:** Glipizide, glyburide	Inhibit K⁺ channels that prevent hyperpolarization, leading to an influx of Ca^{2+}, insulin secretion, and glucagon release; ↑ insulin sensitivity.	Hypoglycemia, weight gain, type IV hypersensitivity reactions.	Renal/liver disease.
Meglitinides	Repaglinide	↑ insulin secretion. (Work like sulfonylureas by stimulating the release of insulin from the pancreas.)	Hypoglycemia.	Renal/liver disease.
α-glucosidase inhibitors	Acarbose	↓ glucose absorption. (↓ carbohydrate absorption from the GI tract; ↓ insulin demand.)	↑ flatulence, GI discomfort, ↑ LFTs.	Renal/liver disease.
Thiazolidinediones ("glitazones")	Rosiglitazone, pioglitazone	↓ insulin resistance; ↑ glucose utilization. (↑ insulin sensitization; ↓ hepatic gluconeogenesis and insulin receptor upregulation.)	Hepatocellular injury, anemia, pedal edema, CHF.	Liver disease, CHF (class III/IV), LFTs > 2 times normal.
Glucagon-like peptide-1 (GLP-1) agonists	Exenatide	↑ postprandial glucose utilization.	Nausea, vomiting, weight loss, hypoglycemia.	Renal disease.
Dipeptidyl peptidase (DPP-4) inhibitors	Sitagliptin, vildagliptin	Same as that of GLP-1 agonists.	Same as those of GLP-1 agonists.	Same as that of GLP-1 agonists.

TABLE 5-5.   Target Glucose Levels in Diabetics

	NORMAL GLUCOSE LEVEL (mg/dL)	TARGET LEVEL WITH DRUG TREATMENT (mg/dL)	ADJUST DOSAGE OF DRUG WHEN LEVEL IS:
Preprandial glucose	< 110	80–120	< 80 or > 140
Bedtime glucose	< 120	100–140	< 100 or > 160

A serum glucose level of ≥ 200 mg/dL is diagnostic of DM in a symptomatic patient.

SYMPTOMS/EXAM

"Fruity" breath odor, Kussmaul hyperpnea (an abnormal ↑ in the depth and rate of breathing), dehydration, abdominal pain, an ↑ anion gap, hyperkalemia, hyperglycemia, and ketones in the blood and urine.

DIAGNOSIS

- Order a CBC, electrolytes, BUN/creatinine, glucose, ABGs, serum ketones, a CXR, a blood culture, a UA and urine culture, and an ECG.
- Labs reveal hyperglycemia (blood glucose > 250 mg/dL), acidosis with a blood pH < 7.3, serum bicarbonate < 15 mEq/L, and ↑ serum/urine ketones.

TREATMENT

- Inpatient admission is usually necessary (depends on the patient's clinical status).
- Fluid resuscitate (3–4 L in 8 hours) with NS and IV insulin.
- Sodium, potassium, phosphate, and glucose must be monitored and replaced every 2 hours (change NS fluids to D_5NS when glucose levels are < 250 mg/L).
- Change IV insulin to SQ insulin by combining a basal-bolus regimen with a sliding scale once the anion gap normalizes.
- Continue IV insulin for at least 30 minutes following the administration of the first dose of SQ insulin.
- Consider administering bicarbonate if the arterial pH is < 6.90.

Hyperglycemic Hyperosmolar State (HHS)

Typically occurs in **type 2 DM.** Can be precipitated by dehydration, infection, or medications (eg, β-blockers, steroids, thiazides); marked by elevated serum osmolality. In the absence of ketosis, the presence of small amounts of insulin inhibits lipolysis, ketosis, and acidosis. Patients often have ↑ serum glucose levels and ↑ serum volume depletion.

SYMPTOMS/EXAM

Patients are acutely ill and dehydrated with altered mental status.

DIAGNOSIS

Diagnostic criteria are as follows:

- Serum glucose > 600 mg/dL (hyperglycemia)
- Serum pH > 7.3
- Serum bicarbonate > 15 mEq/L
- Anion gap < 14 mEq/L (normal)
- Serum osmolality > 310 mOsm/kg

TREATMENT

- Fluid resuscitate with 4–6 L NS within the first 8 hours.
- Identify the precipitating cause and treat.
- Monitor and replete sodium, potassium, phosphate, and glucose every 2 hours. Give IV insulin only if glucose levels remain elevated after sufficient fluid resuscitation.

KEY FACT

Symptoms and signs of DKA:
- "Fruity" breath
- Kussmaul hyperpnea
- Dehydration
- Abdominal pain
- ↑ anion gap
- Hyperkalemia
- Hyperglycemia
- Ketones in blood/urine

KEY FACT

Despite the total body potassium deficit in DKA, serum potassium concentration is usually normal or ↑ at presentation because of insulin deficiency and potassium shift out of the cells due to acidemia.

KEY FACT

In DKA, improvement is monitored via anion gap, not blood glucose levels.

KEY FACT

In patients with HHS, neurologic symptoms such as lethargy, focal signs, and obtundation are common. In patients with DKA, hyperventilation and abdominal pain are most frequently seen.

Q

An 8-year-old boy presents with a 2-day history of a productive cough and a fever of 38.4°C (101.1°F). Labs reveal leukocytosis, a blood glucose level of 341 mg/dL, a serum bicarbonate level of 13 mEq/L, and a UA positive for 2+ ketones. CXR reveals lobar pneumonia. Which serum ketone is likely elevated?

Thyroid Disorders

FUNCTIONAL THYROID DISORDERS

Classified as hyperthyroidism or hypothyroidism.

SYMPTOMS/EXAM

Table 5-6 lists distinguishing features of hypo- and hyperthyroidism.

DIAGNOSIS

- Order a TSH and a free T_4 to distinguish hyperthyroidism from hypothyroidism.
    - **Hyperthyroid patients ($\downarrow$ TSH and $\uparrow$ T_4):** Order a radioactive iodine (RAI) uptake and scan. If the patient has contraindications or is pregnant, measure thyroid-stimulating immunoglobulin.
    - **Hypothyroid patients ($\uparrow$ TSH and $\downarrow$ T_4):** Order an anti–thyroid peroxidase (anti-TPO) antibody assay.
- Figure 5-2 and Table 5-7 outline the workup, differential, and treatment of functional thyroid disease.

TREATMENT

- **Symptomatic hyperthyroidism:**
    - Treat with **propranolol** (to address symptoms such as tremors and palpitations), hydration, rest, and adequate nutrition.
    - Mild cases of hyperthyroidism can be treated with **propylthiouracil** or **methimazole,** which **block thyroid hormone synthesis.** Then use radioactive ^{131}I thyroid ablation.

KEY FACT

Methimazole should **not** be given during pregnancy because it can cause congenital anomalies.

A

β-hydroxybutyrate.

TABLE 5-6. **Clinical Presentation of Functional Thyroid Disease**

	HYPOTHYROIDISM	**HYPERTHYROIDISM**
General	Fatigue, lethargy.	Hyperactivity, nervousness, fatigue.
Temperature	Cold intolerance.	Heat intolerance.
GI	Constipation leading to ileus; weight gain despite a poor appetite.	Diarrhea; weight loss despite a good appetite.
Cardiac	Bradycardia, pericardial effusion, hyperlipidemia.	Tachycardia, atrial fibrillation, CHF; systolic hypertension, $\uparrow$ pulse pressure.
Neurologic	Delayed DTRs.	Fine resting tremor; apathetic hyperthyroidism (elderly).
Menstruation	Heavy.	Irregular.
Dermatologic	Dry, coarse skin; thinning hair; thin, brittle nails; myxedema.	Warm, sweaty skin; fine, oily hair; nail separation from matrix.
Other	Arthralgias/myalgias.	**Osteoporosis.**

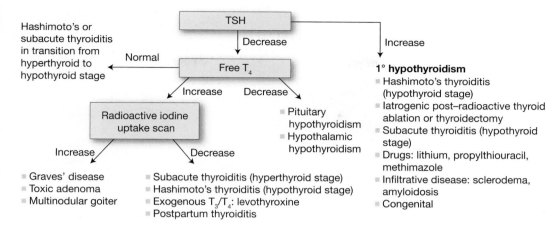

FIGURE 5-2. **Workup of functional thyroid disease.**

TABLE 5-7. **Differential and Treatment of Functional Thyroid Disease**

	GRAVES' DISEASE	SUBACUTE THYROIDITIS	HASHIMOTO'S THYROIDITIS
Etiology/ pathophysiology	Antibody directed at TSH receptor. More prevalent in females.	Viral (possibly mumps or coxsackievirus).	Autoimmune disorder.
Symptoms/exam	Hyperthyroidism; diffuse, painless goiter. Proptosis (also called exophthalmos; see Figure 5-3A), lid lag, diplopia, conjunctival injection. Pretibial myxedema (see Figure 5-3B).	Hyperthyroidism followed by hypothyroidism. Tender thyroid. Malaise, upper respiratory tract symptoms, fever early on.	Occasionally presents with hyperthyroidism (hashitoxicosis) followed by hypothyroidism; painless thyroid enlargement.
Diagnosis	↑ radioactive uptake scan, ⊕ thyroid-stimulating immunoglobulin.	↓ radioactive uptake scan, ↑ ESR.	⊕ anti-TPO antibody.
Disease-specific treatment	Propylthiouracil, methimazole, thyroid ablation with ^{131}I, thyroidectomy. Ophthalmopathy may require surgical decompression, steroids, or orbital radiation.	NSAIDs for pain control; steroids for severe pain. Self-limited.	Levothyroxine.

Q

A 30-year-old woman presenting with weight loss and heat intolerance is found to be tachycardic. Labs reveal a suppressed TSH and an ↑ T_4 level. What is the most common cause of these findings?

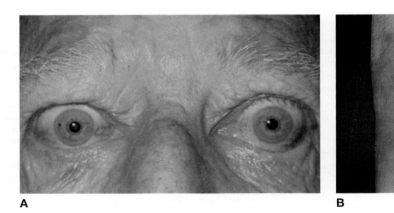

FIGURE 5-3. **Physical signs of Graves' disease.** (A) Grave's ophthalmopathy. (B) Pretibial myxedema. (Reproduced with permission from USMLE-Rx.com.)

- **Thyroidectomy** is indicated for large goiters, pregnant patients, or obstruction of the trachea. Patients who have undergone radioactive ablation or thyroidectomy become hypothyroid and are treated with levothyroxine.
- **Thyroid storm** is a form of severe hyperthyroidism that is characterized by high fever, dehydration, tachycardia, coma, and high-output cardiac failure.
- **Subacute thyroiditis** presents with tender diffuse goiter. Hyperthyroidism is followed by euthyroidism and hypothyroidism.
- **Hypothyroidism:**
  - Treat with **levothyroxine.** Patients with myxedema coma require IV levothyroxine and IV hydrocortisone to preemptively treat for possible coexisting adrenal insufficiency.
  - Mechanical ventilation and warming blankets are required for hypoventilation and hypothermia, respectively.
  - **Myxedema coma** is a form of severe hypothyroidism characterized by altered mental status and hypothermia.

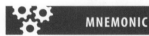

MNEMONIC

Characteristics of thyroid nodules—

90% of nodules are benign.
90% of nodules are cold (nonfunctioning) on RAI uptake scan; 15–20% of these are malignant (vs 1% of hot, or functioning, nodules).
90% of thyroid malignancies present as a thyroid nodule.
> **90%** of thyroid cancers are either papillary or follicular.

Graves' disease.

THYROID NODULES

More common in older women; can be benign or malignant. Hyperfunctioning ("hot") nodules are rarely malignant; therefore, checking TSH levels is the first step in evaluation. Risk factors for malignancy include male gender, a history of head and neck irradiation, a ⊕ family history of thyroid disease or multiple endocrine neoplasia (MEN), and a rapidly growing nodule.

- Head and neck irradiation predisposes patients to chromosomal breaks and thus to genetic rearrangements and loss of tumor suppressor gene, increasing the risk of malignancy.
- Thyroglobulin is a good marker for the presence of thyroid tissue and can be used to determine if malignancy has recurred or if residual cancer remains after treatment.

SYMPTOMS/EXAM

- May be asymptomatic or present as a single firm, palpable nodule.
- Often found incidentally on radiologic studies that are ordered for other purposes.
- Cervical lymphadenopathy, dysphagia, and hoarseness should raise concern.

DIFFERENTIAL

- The differential for thyroid nodules includes:
    - **Benign:** Adenomatous thyroid nodule; thyroglossal duct cyst.
    - **Malignant:** 1° thyroid cancer, thyroid lymphoma, metastatic cancer.
- Subtypes of **malignant lesions** include:
    - **Papillary: Most common;** spreads lymphatically. Has an **excellent prognosis,** with a 10-year survival rate of > 95%.
    - **Follicular:** The second most common subtype; spreads locally and hematogenously. Can metastasize to the bone, lungs, and brain. Has a 10-year survival rate of ~ 90%.
    - **Medullary:** A tumor of parafollicular C cells. May secrete calcitonin. Fifteen percent are familial or associated with MEN 2A or 2B.
    - **Anaplastic:** Undifferentiated. Has a **poor prognosis;** usually occurs in older patients.

DIAGNOSIS

- **Check TSH.**
    - **Normal or high:** Obtain an **ultrasound** to select a nodule for **biopsy with FNA**—the **most accurate** method for evaluating thyroid nodules.
    - **Low:** Conduct an RAI uptake and scan to identify whether the nodule is functioning ("hot") or nonfunctioning ("cold"). Functioning nodules are almost always benign, whereas those that are nonfunctioning are associated with a 5% chance of malignancy and may require biopsy.
- Figure 5-4 outlines subsequent steps in the evaluation and treatment of thyroid nodules.

TREATMENT

Treatment is contingent on FNA or RAI uptake results (see Figure 5-4):

- **Follicular cells or malignancy:** Surgery.
- **Benign:** Serial follow-up.
- **Indeterminate:** Repeat FNA under ultrasound guidance.
- **Hot nodules:** Ablation/resection or medical management.

KEY FACT

Papillary and follicular thyroid cancer are the most common 1° thyroid cancers and carry the best prognosis.

KEY FACT

Medullary thyroid cancer can produce ↑ levels of calcitonin and is often associated with MEN 2A or 2B.

KEY FACT

Ultrasound features suggestive of malignancy include hypoechogenicity, microcalcification, irregular margins, ↑ vascular flow, and size > 3 cm.

KEY FACT

If a thyroid nodule is associated with low TSH, the next best diagnostic exam is an RAI uptake and scan to determine if the nodule is functioning (hot) or nonfunctioning (cold). Functioning nodules are almost always benign.

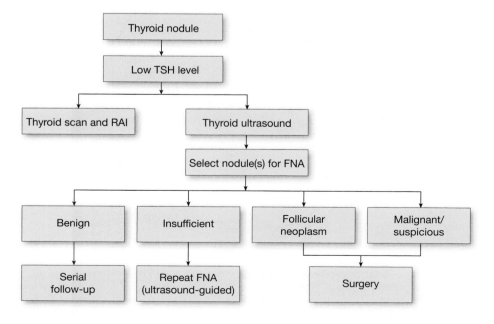

FIGURE 5-4. Workup and treatment of a thyroid nodule.

Q

A 55-year-old man complains of hoarseness and difficulty swallowing. As a teenager, he received external radiation to treat his severe acne. Exam reveals a palpable thyroid nodule. His TSH level is 1.5 mIU/L. What is the next step in diagnosis?

KEY FACT

Hypercalcemic crisis (Ca²⁺ > 13) presents with altered mental status, polyuria, short QT syndrome, and severe dehydration.

Hypercalcemia

Most cases of 1° hyperparathyroidism are caused by a parathyroid adenoma. Initial treatment is focused on correcting the underlying hypercalcemia (see Figure 5-5). Table 5-8 lists the clinical characteristics of 1° hyperparathyroidism and other causes of hypercalcemia.

Osteoporosis

A common metabolic bone disease characterized by ↓ bone strength, low bone mass, and skeletal fragility, resulting in an ↑ risk of fracture. More com-

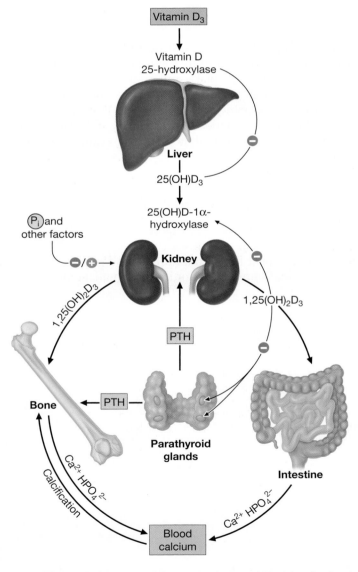

FIGURE 5-5. **Relationship between calcium, vitamin D, and PTH.** A reduction in serum calcium prompts a proportional increase in the secretion of PTH and mobilizes additional calcium from the bone. PTH promotes the synthesis of 1,25(OH)$_2$D in the kidney, which stimulates the mobilization of calcium from bone and intestine and regulates the synthesis of PTH by negative feedback. (Reproduced with permission from Longo DL et al. *Harrison's Principles of Internal Medicine,* 18th ed. New York: McGraw-Hill, 2012, Fig. 352-5.)

The patient's clinical presentation, history of irradiation, and normal TSH level raise suspicion for malignancy. Order an ultrasound of the thyroid to isolate the nodule or nodules to be screened for thyroid cancer by FNA.

TABLE 5-8.   Clinical Characteristics of Hypercalcemia

	1° HYPERPARATHYROIDISM	OTHER CAUSES
Etiology	Adenoma, multiglandular disease.	Malignancy that produces PTH-related peptide, multiple myeloma, granulomatous disease (sarcoidosis 2° to ↑ vitamin D), vitamin D excess, vitamin A excess, thiazide diuretics, bone metastasis.
Symptoms/exam	Fatigue, constipation, polyuria, polydipsia, bone pain, nausea.	Presentation is the same as that of 1° disease.
Diagnosis	↑ calcium and PTH; ↓ PO_4.	↑ calcium; ↓ PTH; sometimes ↑ PO_4.
Treatment	Parathyroidectomy. Hydrate with IV fluids; give furosemide after volume deficit is corrected; bisphosphonates for severe hypercalcemia.	Management of the underlying disorder (eg, chemotherapy for cancer). Low-calcium diet. Hydrate with IV fluids; give furosemide after volume deficit is corrected; bisphosphonates for severe hypercalcemia.
Complications	Nephrolithiasis, nephrocalcinosis, osteopenia, osteoporosis, pancreatitis, cardiac valve calcifications.	Same as those for 1° disease.

mon among inactive, **postmenopausal Caucasian women;** other risk factors include a ⊕ family history, steroid use, smoking, and alcohol.

SYMPTOMS/EXAM

Commonly asymptomatic. Patients may present with **hip fractures, vertebral compression fractures** (resulting in loss of height and progressive thoracic kyphosis), and/or distal radius fractures following minimal trauma.

DIFFERENTIAL

Osteomalacia (inadequate bone mineralization), hyperparathyroidism, multiple myeloma, metastatic carcinoma (pathologic fracture).

DIAGNOSIS

- All patients > 65 years of age, as well as those 40–60 years of age with at least 1 risk factor for osteoporotic fractures after menopause, should be screened with a DEXA scan of the spine and hip. DEXA results are categorized as follows:
    - **T-score ≥ –1.0:** Normal.
    - **T-score –1.0 to –2.5:** Osteopenia ("low bone density").
    - **T-score < –2.5:** Osteoporosis.
    - **T-score < –2.5 with a fracture:** Severe osteoporosis.
- Rule out 2° causes, including smoking, alcoholism, renal failure, hyperthyroidism, multiple myeloma, 1° hyperparathyroidism, vitamin D deficiency, hypercortisolism, heparin use, and chronic steroid use.

TREATMENT

- Treat when the T-score is < –2.5 or when the T-score is < –1.0 in a patient with high risk factors for osteoporotic fractures.
- Drugs of choice include **bisphosphonates,** which inhibit osteoclastic

Q

A 68-year-old woman presents to her primary care physician for a routine checkup. The physician orders a DEXA scan of the spine and hip. What T-score value denotes osteoporosis?

activity (alendronate, risedronate, etidronate, ibandronate); selective estrogen receptor modulators (SERMs) such as tamoxifen and raloxifene; and denosumab (Prolia), a RANK ligand inhibitor.

■ Eliminate or treat 2° causes, and add weight-bearing exercises and calcium/vitamin D supplementation.

■ A DEXA scan should be repeated 1–2 years after the initiation of drug therapy. If the T-score is found to have worsened, combination therapy (eg, a SERM and a bisphosphonate) or a change in therapy should be initiated, with consideration given to ruling out 2° causes.

Cushing's Syndrome (Hypercortisolism)

Results from excess levels of exogenously administered glucocorticoids or endogenous overproduction of cortisol. The most common cause is iatrogenic Cushing's due to exogenous glucocorticoids. The second most common form is Cushing's disease, which results from pituitary hypersecretion of ACTH.

SYMPTOMS/EXAM

■ Presents with skin atrophy and proximal muscle weakness.
■ Also look for psychiatric disturbances, hypertension, hyperglycemia, oligomenorrhea, growth retardation, and hirsutism.
■ Muscle wasting, easy bruising, and striae are characteristic.

DIFFERENTIAL

DM, chronic alcoholism, depression, obesity due to other causes, chronic steroid use, adrenogenital syndrome, acute stress.

DIAGNOSIS

■ When Cushing's is suspected, establish whether the hypercortisolism is ACTH dependent (ie, due to a pituitary or nonpituitary ACTH-secreting tumor) or ACTH independent (ie, due to an adrenal source). See Figure 5-6.
■ The overnight test consists of administration of 1 mg of dexamethasone at 11 PM and measurement of serum cortisol at 8 AM the next morning. Most normal individuals have an 8 AM serum cortisol value of < 2 µg/dL.
■ To diagnose the location of Cushing's syndrome, measure the ACTH level:
  ■ **AM serum ACTH < 5 pg/mL:** Obtain an adrenal CT scan or an MRI to look for an adrenal adenoma or carcinoma (unilateral) or adrenal hyperplasia (bilateral).
  ■ **AM serum ACTH > 5 pg/mL:** Administer a high-dose dexamethasone suppression test. If the high-dose dexamethasone suppresses ACTH, the origin is pituitary; if ACTH is not suppressed, the origin is ectopic production of ACTH.

TREATMENT

■ The most favorable treatment involves localization and total removal of an ACTH-secreting or cortisol-secreting adrenal tumor.
■ Patients with Cushing's disease are usually treated by transsphenoidal microsurgical excision of the pituitary adenomas.
■ Adenomas are always cured with unilateral adrenalectomy.
■ Bilateral total adrenalectomy with lifelong daily glucocorticoid and mineralocorticoid replacement therapy is the definitive cure.
■ **Ectopic ACTH-secreting tumor:** Surgical resection of the tumor.

KEY FACT

Excess ACTH may be produced by pituitary adenomas (Cushing's disease) or by extrapituitary ACTH-producing tumors (ectopic ACTH syndrome, eg, small-cell lung cancer).

KEY FACT

The first step in the diagnosis of Cushing's syndrome is an overnight dexamethasone suppression test or measurement of 24-hour urinary free cortisol. Both tests are highly sensitive, and a normal value excludes the diagnosis.

T-score < -2.5.

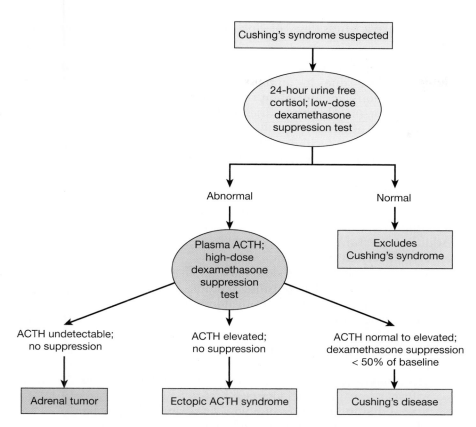

FIGURE 5-6. **Diagnostic evaluation of Cushing's syndrome.** (Reproduced with permission from McPhee SJ, Hammer GD. *Pathophysiology of Disease: An Introduction to Clinical Medicine,* 6th ed. New York: McGraw-Hill, 2010, Fig. 21-4.)

▪ **Exogenous steroids:** Minimize use.
▪ Table 5-9 lists the laboratory characteristics of Cushing's syndrome according to etiology.

Adrenal Insufficiency

1° adrenal insufficiency, or Addison's disease, is most commonly caused by autoimmune adrenalitis. Acute adrenal insufficiency may occur in previously undiagnosed patients with 1° adrenal insufficiency in the setting of serious infection or other acute stressors and in patients with 1° adrenal insufficiency

TABLE 5-9. **Laboratory Characteristics of Endogenous Cushing's Syndrome**

	ACTH DEPENDENT	**ACTH INDEPENDENT**
Plasma cortisol	↑	↑
Urinary cortisol	↑	↑
ACTH	↑	↓
Source	Pituitary (suppressible) Ectopic (nonsuppressible)	Adenoma (↓ DHEA) Carcinoma (↑ DHEA)

Q 1

A 30-year-old woman with a history of SLE presents with ↑ truncal obesity, a fatty hump between her shoulders, and a round face. She is on chronic steroids. What is the first step in diagnosis?

Q 2

A 65-year-old man with a known recent diagnosis of melanoma presents with vague complaints of dizziness, weakness, fatigue, and weight loss. Basic lab testing reveals hyponatremia. What testing will help determine the diagnosis?

who do not take a "stress dose" of glucocorticoid during an infection or other major illness.

- **1° adrenal insufficiency:** Adrenocortical hypofunction resulting from adrenal failure due to autoimmune disease (idiopathic), metastatic tumors, hemorrhagic infarction (from coagulopathy or septicemia), adrenalectomy, or granulomatous disease (TB, sarcoid).
- **2° adrenal insufficiency:** Results from ↓ ACTH production from the pituitary resulting from withdrawal of exogenous steroids or hypothalamic/pituitary pathology (tumor, infarct, trauma, infection, iatrogenic).

SYMPTOMS/EXAM

- **Common features:** Chronic malaise; fatigue that is worsened by exertion and improved with bed rest; generalized weakness.
- **Additional features:**
    - **Hypoglycemia** and weight loss.
    - **GI:** Nausea, vomiting, abdominal pain, diarrhea.
    - **Cardiovascular: Hypotension;** postural dizziness or syncope due to volume depletion resulting from aldosterone deficiency.
    - **Electrolyte abnormalities:** Hyponatremia and hyperkalemia (mild hyperchloremic acidosis) due to mineralocorticoid deficiency (affect 60–65% of patients, primarily those with 1° adrenal insufficiency).
    - **Hyperpigmentation** due to cortisol deficiency and ↑ production of proopiomelanocortin (brown hyperpigmentation); occurs primarily with 1° adrenal insufficiency (see Figure 5-7).
    - **Sexual dysfunction:** Loss of libido, ↓ axillary and pubic hair.
    - **Musculoskeletal symptoms:** Diffuse myalgias and arthralgias.

DIAGNOSIS

- Measure 8 AM serum cortisol and plasma ACTH as well as a cosyntropin stimulation test (synthetic ACTH). An AM serum cortisol < 5 μg/dL or a serum cortisol < 20 μg/dL after an ACTH stimulation test makes the diagnosis more likely.

KEY FACT

Infection, surgery, or other stressors can trigger an addisonian crisis with symptomatic adrenal insufficiency, confusion, and vasodilatory shock.

---

1   **A**

A 24-hour urine collection should reveal an ↑ cortisol level, which is diagnostic for Cushing's syndrome.

2   **A**

AM serum cortisol and AM serum ACTH.

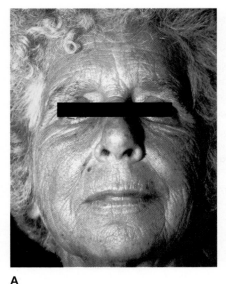
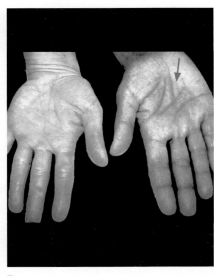

A   **B**

FIGURE 5-7.   Addison's disease. (**A**) Note the characteristic hyperpigmentation in sun-exposed areas. (**B**) Contrast the hyperpigmented palmar creases (arrow) with the normal hand of a different patient. (Reproduced with permission from Goldsmith LA et al. *Fitzpatrick's Dermatology in General Medicine*, 8th ed. New York: McGraw-Hill, 2012, Fig. 151-12.)

- If the cause is unclear, the plasma ACTH level distinguishes 1° from 2° adrenal failure (see Table 5-10).

TREATMENT

- Adrenal crisis is a life-threatening emergency that requires immediate treatment. Check serum electrolytes and glucose, plasma cortisol, and ACTH.
- Start immediate fluid resuscitation. If the diagnosis of adrenal failure has not been established, start with dexamethasone (does not interfere with the measurement of plasma cortisol). If the diagnosis of adrenal failure is known, treat with hydrocortisone.
- Add **fludrocortisone** for persistent orthostatic hypotension, hyponatremia, or hyperkalemia.
- Glucocorticoid doses should be ↑ in times of illness, trauma, or surgery.
- Patients in **adrenal crisis** need immediate fluid resuscitation and IV hydrocortisone.

> **KEY FACT**
>
> Mineralocorticoid administration is not necessary in an acute setting.

Hyperaldosteronism

May be 1° or 2°:

- **1° hyperaldosteronism:** Due to excess secretion of aldosterone, resulting in ↑ sodium reabsorption and potassium secretion. Most commonly caused by an aldosterone-producing adenoma.
- **2° hyperaldosteronism:** Caused by renin-secreting tumors, renovascular disease such as renal artery stenosis and malignant hypertension, and edematous states with ↓ arterial volume (CHF, cirrhosis, nephrotic syndrome).

SYMPTOMS/EXAM

Presents with hypertension, hypokalemia (causes symptoms of muscle weakness and can cause arrhythmia), metabolic alkalosis, and mild hypernatremia.

DIAGNOSIS

- Look for low plasma renin activity (PRA), resistant hypertension, and a plasma aldosterone concentration (PAC) that is inappropriately high for the plasma renin activity (PAC/PRA ratio > 20).
- The diagnosis is confirmed by a saline infusion test and is localized with a CT scan or an MRI of the adrenal gland. Abnormality in both glands suggests adrenal hyperplasia.

TREATMENT

Surgery to remove the adenoma for unilateral adrenal aldosterone hypersecretion; medical therapy for bilateral adrenal hyperplasia; spironolactone.

TABLE 5-10. 1° vs 2° Adrenal Insufficiency

	ADDISON'S DISEASE	2° ADRENAL INSUFFICIENCY
ACTH	↑	↓
Cortisol after ACTH challenge	↓	↑

Reproduced with permission from Le T et al. *First Aid for the USMLE Step 2 CK,* 4th ed. New York: McGraw-Hill, 2004: 121.

Q 1

A 60-year-old man with a history of erectile dysfunction presents with headaches and associated temporal field visual loss. Lab testing reveals ↑ prolactin levels. What is the imaging test of choice?

Q 2

A 40-year-old woman with a history of difficult-to-control hypertension presents with a headache. A review of systems reveals associated palpitations and diaphoresis. On exam, she is found to have a BP of 200/100. What lab test will yield the suspected diagnosis?

Prolactinoma

The most common functioning pituitary tumor; characterized by hypersecretion of prolactin.

SYMPTOMS/EXAM

- ↓ GnRH leads to ↓ FSH and LH, which ↓ progesterone and estrogen levels (testosterone in males).
- Presents differently in men and women; usually appears later in men.
    - Women typically present with galactorrhea and amenorrhea in the absence of pregnancy and with osteopenia due to ↓ estrogen.
    - Men develop impotence, ↓ libido, and often, with larger adenomas, symptoms related to mass effect (eg, CN III palsy, diplopia, temporal field visual loss, headache).

DIAGNOSIS

- Rule out 2° causes by screening for hypothyroidism, pregnancy, confounding antiemetic/antipsychotic medications, renal failure, and cirrhosis. Marked psychological stress can also ↑ prolactin levels.
- MRI to identify mass lesions (see Figure 5-8).

TREATMENT

- **Dopamine agonists (bromocriptine, cabergoline)** are first-line treatment for hyperprolactinemia and ↓ the size and secretion of > 90% of lactotroph adenomas.
- If medical therapy is not tolerated or if the tumor is large, transsphenoidal surgery followed by irradiation is indicated.
- Asymptomatic patients without hypogonadism can be followed with **serial prolactin levels.**

Multiple Endocrine Neoplasia (MEN)

A group of familial, autosomal dominant syndromes (see Table 5-11).

KEY FACT

MRI is the best imaging method with which to identify mass lesions.

1 ➤ **A**

MRI to assess the pituitary for possible prolactinoma.

2 ➤ **A**

Urine or plasma free metanephrines and normetanephrines.

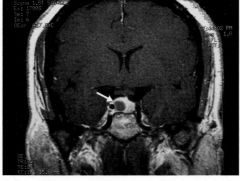

A

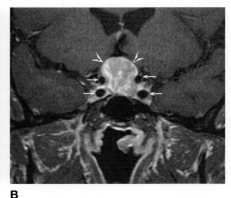

B

FIGURE 5-8. **Pituitary adenomas.** Coronal gadolinium-enhanced MR images demonstrating **(A)** a microadenoma (arrow), which enhances less than the adjacent pituitary tissue, and **(B)** a pituitary macroadenoma (arrowheads) extending superiorly from the sella turcica to the suprasellar region. Arrows denote the internal carotid arteries. (Image A reproduced with permission from Hoffman BL et al. *Williams Gynecology,* 2nd ed. New York: McGraw-Hill, 2012, Fig. 15-14A. Image B reproduced with permission from Longo DL et al. *Harrison's Principles of Internal Medicine,* 18th ed. New York: McGraw-Hill, 2012, Fig. 339-4.)

TABLE 5-11. **Characteristics of MEN Syndromes**

Syndrome	Type	Characteristics
Wermer's syndrome	MEN 1	**P**arathyroid hyperplasia
		Pancreatic islet cell tumor
		Pituitary adenoma
Sipple's syndrome	MEN 2A	Parathyroid hyperplasia
		Thyroid medullary cancer
		Pheochromocytoma
	MEN 2B	**T**hyroid medullary cancer
		Pheochromocytoma
		Mucocutaneous neuromas
		Ganglioneuromatosis of the colon
		Marfan-like habitus

PHEOCHROMOCYTOMA

- Pheochromocytoma (adrenal medullary tumor) is a catecholamine-secreting tumor that secretes epinephrine, norepinephrine, and dopamine. It is a clinical syndrome that typically presents with hypertension, headaches, palpitations, and sweating.
- **Dx:** The diagnosis is confirmed with lab testing for urine or plasma free metanephrines and normetanephrines along with a CT/MRI.
- **Tx:** Treat preoperatively with irreversible α-blockade (phenoxybenzamine) to ↓ intraoperative hypertensive crisis followed by surgical resection.

KEY FACT

Screen for pheochromocytoma with 24-hour urinary fractionated metanephrines.

MNEMONIC

The 3 P's of primary MEN:

Parathyroid hyperplasia
Pancreatic islet cell tumor
Pituitary adenoma

MNEMONIC

MEN 2A and 2B—2 common characteristics:

Thyroid medullary cancer
Pheochromocytoma

NOTES

ETHICS AND STATISTICS

Basic Principles

Be familiar with the following principles:

- **Autonomy:** The right to make decisions for oneself in accordance with one's own system of morals and beliefs.
- **Paternalism:** Providing for your perception of patients' needs without their input.
- **Beneficence:** Action intended to bring about a good outcome.
- **Nonmaleficence:** Action not intended to bring about harm.
- **Truth telling:** Revealing all pertinent information to patients.
- **Proportionality:** Ensuring that a medical treatment or plan is commensurate with the illness and with the goals of treatment.
- **Distributive justice:** Allocation of resources in a manner that is fair and just, though not necessarily equal.

Autonomy

INFORMED CONSENT

Involves discussing diagnoses and prognoses with patients as well as any proposed treatment, its risks and benefits, and its alternatives. Only with such information can a patient reach an informed decision. **Do not conceal a diagnosis from a patient,** as doing so would violate the principle of truth telling. However, respect your patients' wishes if they ask you to share only certain things with them.

RIGHTS OF MINORS

The treatment of patients < 18 years of age requires parental consent unless:

- They are emancipated (ie, financially independent, married, pregnant, raising children, living on their own, or serving in the armed forces).
- They are requesting contraception or treatment of pregnancy, STDs, or psychiatric illness. Note that many states require parental consent or notice for termination of pregnancy in a minor.

Most Step 3 exam questions on parental consent will deal with situations such as those cited above. In general, this means that for the Step 3 exam, the governing principle should be to let minors make their own decisions.

Competency

COMPETENCY vs CAPACITY

The terms **competency** and **capacity** should not be used interchangeably. Competency is a **legal** determination made only by a court, whereas capacity is a **clinical** assessment. Each involves the assessment of a patient's ability to think and act rationally (though not necessarily wisely). Incompetence is permanent (eg, severe dementia), and incompetent patients are generally assigned a surrogate by the court. Incapacity may be temporary (eg, delirium), and careful decision making is important when considering therapeutic interventions for patients with questionable capacity.

DETENTION AND USE OF RESTRAINTS

Psychiatric patients may be held against their will only if they are a danger to themselves or to others (in accordance with the principle of beneficence). The use of restraints can be considered if a patient is at risk of doing harm to self or others, but such use must be evaluated on at least a daily basis.

DURABLE POWER OF ATTORNEY (DPOA) FOR HEALTH CARE

DPoA has 2 related meanings. First, it can refer to a document signed by the patient assigning a surrogate decision maker in the event that he or she becomes incapacitated. Second, it can refer to the person to whom that authority has been granted.

SURROGATE/PROXY

Defined as an alternate decision maker, designated by the patient (DPoA), by law, or by convention. If no person has been formally designated to represent the patient, surrogacy falls to relatives in accordance with a hierarchy that may vary from state to state (typically, a spouse is at the top of this hierarchy).

Confidentiality

IMPORTANCE OF CONFIDENTIALITY (AND HIPAA)

Maintaining the confidentiality of patient information is critical. Violations are unethical, may have legal implications, and may irreparably harm the patient-physician relationship. HIPAA outlines rules and guidelines for preserving patient privacy.

WHEN TO VIOLATE CONFIDENTIALITY

If a physician learns about a threat to an individual's life or well-being (ie, a danger to self or to others), violating confidentiality is mandatory. In a similar manner, information about child abuse or elder abuse must be reported.

REPORTABLE CONDITIONS

Most contagious, rare, and incurable infections, as well as other threats to public health, are reportable. The list of reportable conditions varies by state but often includes HIV/AIDS, syphilis, gonorrhea, chlamydia, TB, mumps, measles, rubella, smallpox, and suspected bioterrorist events. Such reporting is mandatory, is anonymous, and does not constitute a violation of patient confidentiality.

ASKING FOLLOW-UP QUESTIONS

Follow-up questions should be used to clarify unclear issues such as which family members can be included in discussions of care, who is the primary surrogate, and what patients want to know about their own conditions.

Q

A 22-year-old Jehovah's Witness presents with GI bleeding but states that he does not want a blood transfusion. His hematocrit falls from 40 to 22, and his BP falls as well. The patient is urged to accept lifesaving treatments but refuses. When his BP reaches a critical level, one of his physicians initiates plans to transfuse. The rest of the team vetoes the plan. What ethical principles are involved, and which principle trumps the other?

End-of-Life Care

Patients in the end stages of a terminal illness have the right to obtain medical treatment that is intended to preserve human dignity in dying. The best means of reaching an agreement with the patient and family regarding end-of-life care is to continue to talk about the patient's condition and to resolve decision-making conflicts. Ultimately, this is the same task that an ethics consultant would attempt to perform for the physician and the patient.

There is a growing body of literature addressing the importance of cultural issues in end-of-life care. In the United States, emphasis is placed on patient autonomy, full disclosure of medical information, and the primacy of objective over subjective medical findings. However, members of other cultures may lend more credibility to family-based decisions, particular methods of diagnosis communication, and the importance of subjective aspects of illness. It is important to elicit and respect these cultural frameworks and interactional dynamics in end-of-life care.

ADVANCE DIRECTIVES

Defined as oral or written instructions regarding what a patient would want in the event that intensive resuscitative intervention became necessary to sustain life. These instructions can be detailed—which is obviously preferable—or broad. Oral statements are ethically binding but are not legally binding in all states. Remember that an informed, competent adult can refuse treatment even if it means that doing so would lead to death. Such instructions must be honored.

DO NOT RESUSCITATE (DNR) ORDERS/CODE STATUS

The express wishes of a patient (eg, "I do not want to be intubated") supersede the wishes of family members or surrogates. Physicians should inquire about and follow DNR orders during each hospitalization. If code status has not been addressed and the matter becomes relevant, defer to the surrogate.

PAIN IN TERMINALLY ILL PATIENTS

Terminally ill patients are often inadequately treated for pain. Prescribe as much narcotic and non-narcotic medication as needed to relieve patients' pain and suffering. Do not worry about addiction in this setting. Two-thirds of terminally ill patients reported moderate to severe pain in the last 3 days of life.

This is a conflict between beneficence and autonomy. The physician aims to bring a good outcome for the patient, but the patient is making a decision in accordance with his belief system. The principle of autonomy trumps beneficence in this situation.

THE PRINCIPLE OF "DOUBLE EFFECT"

Actions can have more than one consequence, some intended, others not. Unintended medical consequences are acceptable if the intended consequences are legitimate and the harm proportionately smaller than the benefit. For example, a dying patient can be given high doses of analgesics even if it may unintentionally shorten life.

PERSISTENT VEGETATIVE STATE (PVS)

Defined as a state in which the brainstem is intact and the patient has sleep-wake cycles, but there is no awareness, voluntary activity, or ability to interact with the environment. Reflexes may be normal or abnormal. Some patients survive this way for 5 years or more, with the aggregate annual cost reaching into the billions of dollars.

QUALITY OF LIFE

A subjective evaluation of a patient's current physical, emotional, and social well-being. This must be evaluated from the perspective of the patient.

EUTHANASIA

Euthanasia involves helping an informed, competent, terminally ill patient end life, usually through the administration of a lethal dose of medication. Euthanasia differs from physician-assisted suicide, in which the physician prescribes a medication that the patient administers to himself to end life. Neither is the same as withdrawal of care. Currently, euthanasia is illegal in all states, and physician-assisted suicide is legal only in Washington, Oregon, Montana, and Vermont.

PALLIATION AND HOSPICE

These related concepts involve the provision of end-of-life care within (palliation) or outside (hospice) a traditional medical system. Each is an attempt to manage the patient's psychosocial and physical well-being in a manner that preserves dignity and maximizes comfort. Both involve interdisciplinary collaboration (MD, RN, chaplain, social worker, nurses' aides), focusing on patient-defined goals of care.

WITHDRAWAL OF TREATMENT

Withdrawal of treatment is the removal of life-sustaining treatment and is legally and ethically no different from never starting treatment. The decision to withdraw treatment may come from the patient, an advance directive, a DPoA, or, absent any of these, the patient's closest relative and/or a physician. It is easiest when all parties are in agreement, although this is not required. When there is conflict, the patient's wishes take precedence. In futile cases or those involving extreme suffering, a physician may withdraw or withhold treatment; if the family disagrees, the physician should seek input from an ethics committee or a court's approval.

Biostatistics

Not everyone with a given disease will test positive for that disease, and not everyone with a positive test result has the disease.

SENSITIVITY AND SPECIFICITY

Sensitivity is the probability that a person with a disease will have a positive result on a given test. High sensitivity is useful in a screening test, as the goal is to identify everyone with a given disease. **Specificity** is the probability that a person without a disease will have a negative result on a test. High specificity is desirable for a confirmatory test.

Ideally, a test will be highly sensitive and specific, but this is rare. A test

KEY FACT

The Elisabeth Kübler-Ross psychological stages at the end of life are denial, anger, bargaining, depression, and acceptance.

Q

You have a test that has a sensitivity of 0.95 and a specificity of 0.95. How helpful is this test in your diagnostic reasoning for the following scenarios?

1. Disease prevalence of 1%
2. Disease prevalence of 10%
3. Disease prevalence of 50%
4. Disease prevalence of 90%

KEY FACT

Sense (sensitivity) who does have a disease. **Specify (specificity)** who does not.

that is highly sensitive but not specific will yield many false positives, whereas one that is highly specific but not sensitive will yield many false negatives.

PREDICTIVE VALUES

Positive predictive value (PPV) is the probability that a person with a positive test result has the disease (true positives/all positives; see Table 6-1). If a disease has a greater prevalence, then the PPV is higher. **Negative predictive value (NPV)** is the probability that a person with a negative test result is disease free (see Table 6-1). A test has a higher NPV value when a disease has a lower prevalence. It is important to note that PPV and NPV can be determined only if the incidence in the sample is representative of the population. For example, if the data for Table 6-1 are derived from a case-control study, then the PPV and NPV cannot be calculated. Generally, one needs a cohort study design to get PPV or NPV.

INCIDENCE

Defined as the number of **new** cases of a given disease per year—for example, 4 cases of X per year.

PREVALENCE

Defined as the total number of **existing** cases of a given disease in the entire population; for example, 20 people have X (right now).

ABSOLUTE RISK

The **probability** of an event in a given time period; for example, 0.1% chance of developing X in 10 years.

RELATIVE RISK (RR)

Used to evaluate the results of cohort (prospective) studies. The RR compares the incidence of a disease in a group exposed to a particular risk factor with the incidence in those not exposed to the risk factor (see Table 6-2). An RR < 1 means that the event is less likely in the exposed group; conversely, an RR > 1 signifies that the event is more likely in that group.

ODDS RATIO (OR)

Used in case-control (retrospective) studies. The OR compares the rate of exposure among those with and without a disease (see Table 6-2). It is considered less accurate than RR, but in rare diseases the OR approximates the RR.

1. Not helpful. Most of the positives will be false positives, so further evaluation will be necessary.
2. Somewhat helpful. A negative test reduces the probability of disease below a threshold for further testing, while a positive test helps stratify a high-risk population that requires further testing.
3. Very helpful. Both positive and negative results make significant changes in disease probability and can confirm or disprove a diagnosis. This is the situation in which a laboratory test is most helpful.
4. Not helpful. The positive result adds nothing to your clinical suspicion, and a negative test is likely to be a false negative.

TABLE 6-1.   **Determination of PPV and NPV**

	DISEASE PRESENT	**NO DISEASE**	
Positive test	a	b	PPV = a/(a + b)
Negative test	c	d	NPV = d/(c + d)
	Sensitivity = a/(a + c)	Specificity = d/(b + d)	

TABLE 6-2.   Determination of RR and OR

	DISEASE DEVELOPS	NO DISEASE	
Exposure	a	b	RR = [a/(a + b)]/[c/(c + d)]
No exposure	c	d	OR = ad/bc

ABSOLUTE RISK REDUCTION (ARR) OR ATTRIBUTABLE RISK

Measures the risk accounted for by exposure to a given factor, taking into account the background of the disease. Useful in randomized controlled trials. Numerically, ARR = the absolute risk (rate of adverse events) in the placebo group minus the absolute risk in treated patients.

RELATIVE RISK REDUCTION (RRR)

Also used in randomized controlled trials, this is the ratio between 2 risks. Numerically, RRR = [the event rate in control patients minus the event rate in experimental patients] ÷ the event rate in control patients.

RRR can be deceptive and is clinically far less important than ARR. Consider a costly intervention that reduces the risk of an adverse event from 0.01% to 0.004%. ARR is 0.01 − 0.004 = 0.006%, but RRR is (0.01 − 0.004)/0.01 = 0.6, or 60%! Would you order this intervention?

NUMBER NEEDED TO TREAT (NNT)

The number of patients who would need to be treated to prevent 1 event. NNT = 1/ARR. In the example above, the NNT is 167.

STATISTICAL SIGNIFICANCE/p-VALUE

The p-value expresses the likelihood that an observed outcome was due to random chance. A p-value < 0.05 is generally accepted as indicating that an outcome is statistically significant.

CONFIDENCE INTERVAL (CI)

Like the p-value, the CI expresses the certainty that the observation is real or is a product of random chance. Used with ORs and RR, the 95% CI says that the observed risk or odds have a 95% chance of being within the interval. Thus, in Figure 6-1, the relative risk of cancer with smoking is 2.0 with a 95% CI of 1.3–3.5—meaning that the **observed** RR of cancer was 2.0, and that there is a 95% certainty that the **actual** RR of cancer from smoking falls somewhere between 1.3 and 3.5.

Study Design

Statistical analyses are used as a means of assessing relationships between events and outcomes. They do not prove irrefutably that a relationship exists but point to the likelihood of this being the case. The validity of the results depends on the strength of the design.

KEY FACT

ARR and RRR give different values and should not be confused. ARR is a much better measure of benefit; because it is a ratio, RRR can look deceptively large. Watch out for drug advertising that touts RRR.

KEY FACT

If a 95% CI includes 1.0, the results are not significant. So if an RR is 1.9 but the 95% CI is 0.8–3.0, the RR is not significant.

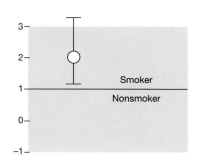

FIGURE 6-1.   Relative risk of cancer.

SURVEYS

These are self-reporting of symptoms, exposures, feelings, and other subjective data. Such data may be analyzed with descriptive statistics or qualitative methodologies.

PROSPECTIVE AND RETROSPECTIVE STUDIES

Prospective studies assess future outcomes relating to present or future events; this enables the study designer to control for biases and to modify inputs/exposures. **Retrospective studies** relate to outcomes from past events. They may be less reliable than prospective studies.

COHORT STUDIES

In a **cohort study** (see Figure 6-2), a population is observed over time, grouped on the basis of exposure to a particular factor, and watched for a specific outcome. Such studies are not good for rare conditions. Studies can be prospective or retrospective. Use RR to interpret results. Examples include the Nurses' Health Study and the Framingham Heart Study.

CASE-CONTROL STUDIES

A **case-control study** (see Figure 6-3) is a retrospective study involving a group of people with a given disease and an otherwise similar group of people without the disease who are compared for exposure to risk factors. Good for rare diseases. Use OR to interpret results.

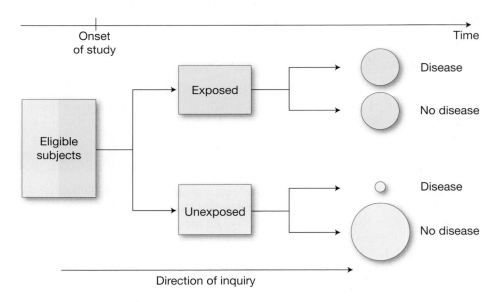

FIGURE 6-2. Schematic diagram of a cohort study. Shaded areas in the diagram represent exposed persons; unshaded areas represent unexposed persons. (Reproduced with permission from Greenberg RS et al. *Medical Epidemiology*, 4th ed. New York: McGraw-Hill, 2005, Fig. 8-2.)

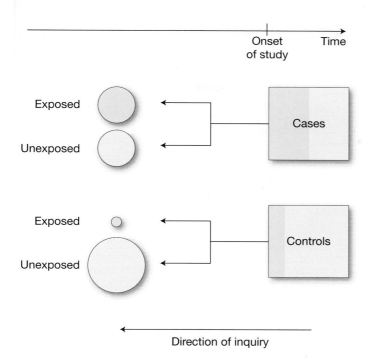

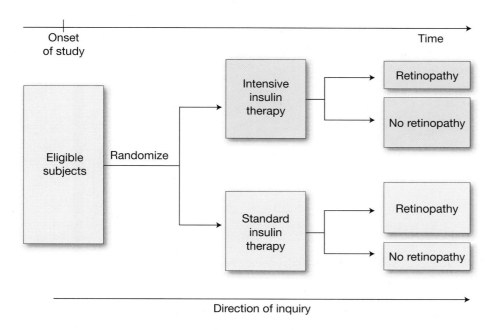

FIGURE 6-3. Schematic diagram of a case-control study. Shaded areas represent subjects who were exposed to the risk factor of interest. (Reproduced with permission from Greenberg RS et al. *Medical Epidemiology*, 4th ed. New York: McGraw-Hill, 2005, Fig. 9-1.)

RANDOMIZED CONTROLLED TRIALS (RCTs)

A prospective study that randomly assigns participants to a treatment group or to a placebo group (see Figure 6-4). The placebo group and the treatment group are then compared to determine if the treatment made a difference. The double-blind RCT is the gold standard of experimental design.

FIGURE 6-4. Schematic diagram of a randomized controlled clinical trial. The study above compares standard therapy with intensive insulin therapy for the treatment of diabetes mellitus. Shaded areas correspond to patients randomized to intensive insulin therapy. (Reproduced with permission from Greenberg RS et al. *Medical Epidemiology*, 4th ed. New York: McGraw-Hill, 2005, Fig. 7-2.)

NOTES

GASTROENTEROLOGY

Esophageal Pathology

Broadly defined as **dysphagia,** or difficulty swallowing food.

SYMPTOMS/EXAM

- Patients may complain of food that "sticks" or "hangs up."
- Dysphagia may be accompanied by **odynophagia,** or pain with swallowing.

DIFFERENTIAL

- If difficulty is with **solids alone,** consider the following:
  - **Lower esophageal ring (Schatzki's ring):** Characterized by intermittent symptoms or sudden obstruction with a food bolus ("**steakhouse syndrome**") due to a ring located at the gastroesophageal junction.
  - **Zenker's diverticulum:** Outpouching of the upper esophagus. Presents with foul-smelling breath and food regurgitation as well as with difficulty initiating swallowing.
  - **Plummer-Vinson syndrome:** Cervical esophageal web and iron-deficiency anemia. Associated with esophageal cancer.
  - **Peptic stricture:** Progressive symptoms with long-standing heartburn (see Figure 7-1A).
  - **Carcinoma:** Progressive symptoms in an older patient, often with weight loss.
  - **Esophagitis:** Inflammation can be 2° to a number of causes:
    - **Gastroesophageal reflux:** Reflux of acid and stomach contents through the lower esophageal sphincter (LES).
    - **Pill esophagitis:** Usually caused by taking a pill with little or no fluid before lying down. Common medications that are known to cause esophageal damage are doxycycline, NSAIDs, and bisphosphonates.
    - **Opportunistic infections:** Include *Candida*, HSV, and CMV. Usually occur in immunocompromised patients (eg, HIV, chemotherapy).
    - **Eosinophilic esophagitis:** Chronic inflammatory disease mediated by IL-5. Usually found in young men with a history of respiratory allergies. Thirty percent of cases have peripheral eosinophilia.
- If difficulty is with **both solids and liquids,** consider:
  - **Achalasia:** Progressive symptoms that worsen at night with no heartburn. Presents with a **"bird's beak"** on barium swallow (see Figure 7-1B).
  - **Esophageal spasm:** Intermittent symptoms with chest pain. Triggered by acid, stress, and hot and cold liquids. Diagnosed by esophageal manometry; presents with **"corkscrew esophagus"** on barium swallow (see Figure 7-1C).
  - **Scleroderma:** Progressive symptoms with heartburn and Raynaud's phenomenon. Patients have lower esophageal pressure and aperistalsis of the distal esophagus leading to reflux (**CREST** syndrome: **C**alcinosis cutis, **R**aynaud's phenomenon, **E**sophageal dysmotility, **S**clerodactyly, and **T**elangiectasia).

DIAGNOSIS

Workup includes barium swallow and/or EGD.

KEY FACT

Think cancer in older patients with worsening dysphagia, weight loss, and heme-⊕ stools.

KEY FACT

Think food impaction when a patient has sudden difficulty swallowing—even swallowing saliva.

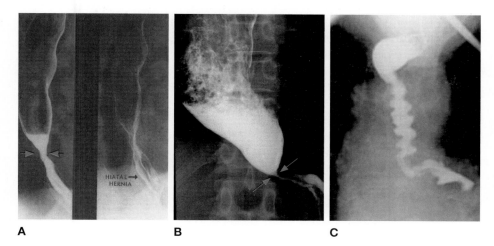

A   **B**   **C**

FIGURE 7-1. **Esophageal disease on barium esophagram.** **(A)** Peptic stricture (arrow) secondary to GERD above a hiatal hernia (right). **(B)** Achalasia. Note the dilated esophagus tapering to a "bird's-beak" narrowing at the LES. **(C)** Esophageal spasm. (Image A reproduced with permission from Chen MY et al. *Basic Radiology,* 2nd ed. New York: McGraw-Hill, 2011, Fig. 10-14. Image B reproduced with permission from Doherty GM. *Current Diagnosis & Treatment: Surgery,* 13th ed. New York: McGraw-Hill, 2010, Fig. 20-5. Image C reproduced with permission from USMLE-Rx.com.)

Gastroesophageal Reflux Disease (GERD)

Results when the LES is weakened by ↑ pressure or ↓ tone. Risk factors include:

- ↑ **pressure:** Hiatal hernia, obesity, collagen vascular disease, pregnancy.
- ↓ **tone:** Alcohol, caffeine, nicotine, chocolate, fatty foods.

SYMPTOMS/EXAM

- Presents with an uncomfortable hot and burning sensation beneath the sternum.
- Symptoms usually worsen after meals, on reclining, and with tight clothes.

DIFFERENTIAL

Cardiovascular causes of chest pain, esophageal motility disorders, peptic ulcer.

DIAGNOSIS

For classic symptoms, diagnosis is usually based on response to treatment. EGD and ambulatory pH monitoring are warranted only if therapy fails.

TREATMENT

- **Lifestyle modification:** Elevate the head of the bed; avoid bedtime snacks, trigger foods (fatty foods, chocolate, mint, alcohol), cigarettes, and NSAIDs; promote weight loss.
- **Drugs:** Antacids, H$_2$ blockers, or PPIs. If symptomatic relief is achieved with an H$_2$ blocker or a PPI, discontinuation of treatment after 8–12 weeks may be successful.
- **Other:**
  - If refractory to medical therapy, consider evaluation for Nissen fundoplication or hiatal hernia repair.

KEY FACT

GERD is a common cause of hoarseness and chronic cough and can exacerbate or mimic asthma.

Q

A 56-year-old man presenting for a routine physical mentions that he has had increasing difficulty swallowing over the past 6 months, more with solids than with liquids. He adds that he has never smoked or consumed alcohol. What is the likely diagnosis?

KEY FACT

H_2 blockers act as competitive antagonists of histamine on the H_2 receptor of parietal cells, thereby preventing parietal cells from secreting acid.

KEY FACT

PPIs irreversibly block proton pumps of gastric parietal cells, which form the last stage of gastric acid secretion.

- Further workup (usually with endoscopy) is warranted for signs or symptoms of more serious disease—eg, weight loss, anemia, heme-⊕ stools, or signs of anatomic obstruction.

Peptic Ulcer Disease (PUD)

The most common sites of PUD are the **stomach** and **duodenum**. *H pylori* infection and **NSAID/aspirin use** are the principal causes; Zollinger-Ellison syndrome, HSV infection, CMV, and cocaine use are less common etiologies.

SYMPTOMS/EXAM

- Presents with **epigastric** pain that patients describe as a **"gnawing"** or **"aching"** sensation that comes in waves.
- Advanced disease may present as upper GI bleeding or perforation and/or penetration into adjacent structures (eg, the pancreas, vascular structures such as the SMA, and the bile ducts), leading to hemodynamic instability and associated symptoms such as pancreatitis.
- Symptoms are often distinguished by disease site:
    - **Duodenal ulcers:** Pain is relieved by food and comes on **postprandially.**
    - **Gastric ulcers:** Pain worsens with food (**pain with eating**).
- **Red flags:** With diarrhea, weight loss, and excessive gastric acid (↑ basal acid output), think of more uncommon causes (eg, Zollinger-Ellison syndrome, systemic mastocytosis, hyperparathyroidism, extensive small bowel resection, gastric cancer).

DIAGNOSIS

- For young, healthy patients, assess response to treatment.
- **Measure gastrin levels.** If gastrin levels are inconclusive, perform a secretin stimulation test to rule out Zollinger-Ellison syndrome.
- **Look for *H pylori* infection** in patients < 55 years of age with a history of peptic ulcers or MALT lymphoma or a family history of gastric cancer.
    - **Urea breath test:** Good for detecting active infection or resolution after treatment, but patients must be off PPIs for 2 weeks and off antibiotics and bismuth for 4 weeks.
    - **Fecal antigen test:** Useful in the 1° diagnosis of *H pylori*, but as above, patients must be off antibiotics, PPIs, and bismuth. False positives and false negatives can occur after treatment.
    - **Serum antibody:** Easy to obtain, but has relatively poor accuracy in relation to other available tests. Antibody can remain ⊕ even after treatment.
- In high-risk patients—ie, older patients, those unresponsive to treatment, and those with melena or heme-⊕ stools—perform **endoscopy** with rapid urease testing for *H pylori*, and biopsy any gastric ulcers to rule out malignancy (see Figure 7-2).

TREATMENT

- **Discontinue aspirin and NSAIDs;** promote smoking cessation and encourage weight loss.
- Give PPIs to control symptoms, ↓ acid secretion, and heal the ulcer (4 weeks for duodenal ulcers; 8–12 weeks for gastric ulcers).
- For *H pylori* infection, initiate multidrug therapy. Two of the following

A

Esophageal adenocarcinoma. Unlike squamous cell carcinoma of the esophagus, esophageal adenocarcinoma is not associated with alcohol or tobacco use. It usually presents as an obstructive lesion that causes progressive difficulty swallowing solid foods and then liquids.

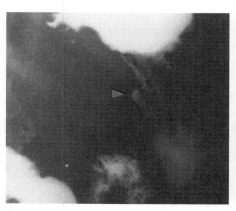
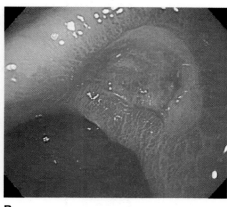

A   **B**

FIGURE 7-2. Gastric ulcer. (A) Gastric ulcer on barium upper GI. A benign gastric ulcer can be seen as pooling of contrast (arrowhead) extending beyond the adjacent gastric wall. **(B)** Benign gastric ulcer on endoscopy. (Image A reproduced with permission from Longo DL et al. *Harrison's Principles of Internal Medicine,* 18th ed. New York: McGraw-Hill, 2012, Fig. 291-2A. Image B reproduced with permission from Chen MY et al. *Basic Radiology.* New York: McGraw-Hill, 2004, Fig. 10-21.)

drugs may be used—amoxicillin, clarithromycin, or metronidazole—along with a PPI (omeprazole, lansoprazole) for 10–14 days.
- Indications for surgery include recurrent/refractory upper GI bleed, gastric outlet obstruction, recurrent/refractory ulcers, perforation, and Zollinger-Ellison syndrome.

Inflammatory Bowel Disease (IBD)

Describes 2 distinct chronic idiopathic inflammatory diseases: **Crohn's disease** and **ulcerative colitis** (see Table 7-1 and Figures 7-3 through 7-5).

Irritable Bowel Syndrome (IBS)

A GI disorder characterized by abdominal pain and altered bowel function (diarrhea or constipation) with or without bloating. Possible etiologies include altered gut motor function, **autonomic nervous system abnormalities,** and **psychological factors.**

SYMPTOMS/EXAM

- Presents with **abdominal pain** with complete or incomplete relief with defecation. Pain is poorly localized, migratory, and variable in nature.
- **Intermittent diarrhea or constipation.**
- May also present with a feeling of incomplete rectal evacuation, urgency, passage of mucus, and bloating.

DIAGNOSIS

- A **diagnosis of exclusion** based primarily on the history and physical exam. Basic labs to exclude other causes should include CBC, BMP, calcium, TSH, and stool O&P.
- The **Rome III criteria** can aid in diagnosis. Look for recurrent abdominal pain or discomfort for at least 3 days a month for the last 3 months plus 2 or more of the following symptoms:
  - Improvement of pain with bowel movements.

KEY FACT

Pain that is unrelated to defecation or is induced with activity, menstruation, or urination is unlikely to be IBS.

A 56-year-old woman was recently diagnosed with osteoarthritis. Two months later she started having abdominal pain that worsens with the consumption of food. What is the likely diagnosis?

TABLE 7-1.   Crohn's Disease vs Ulcerative Colitis

	CROHN'S DISEASE	ULCERATIVE COLITIS
Pathology	**Transmural** inflammation. **Skip** lesions. Noncaseating **granulomas** are found in 30% of cases and are diagnostic if infectious causes are excluded.	Limited to mucosal involvement. Continuous, uniform involvement with a **"lead pipe"** appearance. Crypt abscesses and microulcerations but no granulomas.
Anatomic location	Anywhere from the mouth to the anus. Most commonly affects the **terminal ileum,** small bowel (80%), and colon.	Usually involves the **rectum,** but can involve all or part of the colon. Does not involve the small bowel or above in the GI tract.
Epidemiology	Bimodal distribution (20s and 50–70). More common among those of Jewish ancestry.	Bimodal distribution (15–30 and 60–80). More common among those of Jewish ancestry.
Symptoms	**GI symptoms:** Colicky RLQ pain, diarrhea (often with mucus and usually nonbloody), **perirectal abscess/fistula, oral ulcers.** **Other symptoms:** Fever, weight loss, erythema nodosum, pyoderma gangrenosum (see Figure 7-6), iritis and episcleritis, arthritis, gallstones, kidney stones.	**GI symptoms:** Cramping abdominal pain, urgency, and **bloody diarrhea.** **Other symptoms:** Weight loss, fatigue, arthritis, uveitis and episcleritis, erythema nodosum, pyoderma gangrenosum.
Diagnosis	**Labs:** ▪ Anemia: Chronic disease or iron, vitamin B_{12}, or folate deficiency. ▪ ESR or CRP may be ↑. ▪ **ASCA** ⊕. **Imaging:** ▪ Cobblestoning and fistulas on barium enema. ▪ CT may show abscesses, fistulas, and strictures. ▪ Confirmed with pathologic diagnosis via colonoscopy.	**Labs:** ▪ Anemia: Normocytic or iron deficiency. ▪ ESR or CRP may be ↑. ▪ **p-ANCA** ⊕. **Imaging:** ▪ Lead-pipe colon and loss of haustra on barium enema. ▪ Confirmed with pathologic diagnosis via colonoscopy.
Treatment	**Mild:** 5-ASA compounds. **Moderate:** Oral corticosteroids +/− azathioprine, 6-mercaptopurine, or methotrexate. **Refractory disease:** IV steroids +/− **anti-TNF** therapy. Rule out perforations, **fistulas,** megacolon, or **abscesses.** Resection may be needed.	**Mild:** 5-ASA compounds. **Moderate:** Oral corticosteroids +/− azathioprine, 6-mercaptopurine, or methotrexate. **Refractory disease:** IV steroids +/− cyclosporine +/− anti-TNF therapy. Rule out **toxic megacolon.** Resection may be needed.
Other	Surveillance colonoscopy 8 years after diagnosis and then at least annually thereafter.	Associated with **1° sclerosing cholangitis** and autoimmune liver disease. Surveillance colonoscopy 8–12 years after diagnosis (unless limited to the rectum) and then at least annually thereafter.

A

Gastric ulcer 2° to the use of NSAIDs for joint pain.

▪ Often associated with a change in frequency of bowel movements.
▪ Onset associated with a change in the form/appearance of stool.

TREATMENT

▪ **High-fiber diet** (20–30 g/day), **exercise,** and adequate fluid intake.
▪ TCAs are often used even in the absence of depression, especially in the setting of chronic pain and diarrhea.

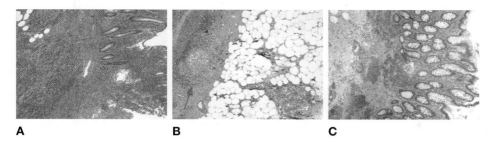

A   **B**   **C**

FIGURE 7-3. **Inflammatory bowel disease.** (A)–(B) Crohn's disease. Transmural inflammation with noncaseating granulomas (arrow) is seen deep in the serosal fat on pathology. (C) Ulcerative colitis. Inflammation is confined to the mucosa and submucosa, with a crypt abscess (arrow). (Reproduced with permission from USMLE-Rx.com.)

- Additional treatment options depend on symptom predominance.
  - **If constipation predominates:** Bulking agents (psyllium), lactulose, PEG, or enemas.
  - **If diarrhea predominates:** Loperamide, cholestyramine, or TCAs.
  - **If bloating predominates:** Simethicone or probiotics (eg, *Lactobacillus*).
  - **Postprandial symptoms:** Anticholinergic agents, dicyclomine, or hyoscyamine.

Diarrhea

Described as watery consistency and/or ↑ frequency of bowel movements. Typically characterized as acute or chronic.

- **Acute diarrhea:** Duration of < 2 weeks; usually infectious.
- **Chronic diarrhea:** Lasting > 4–6 weeks.

Tables 7-2 and 7-3 outline the etiology, presentation, and treatment of acute and chronic diarrhea.

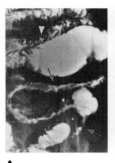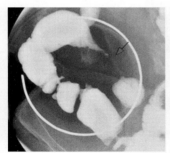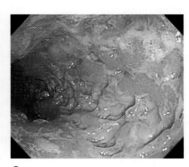

A   **B**   **C**

FIGURE 7-4. **Crohn's disease.** (A) Small bowel follow-through (SBFT) barium study shows skip areas of narrowed small bowel with nodular mucosa (arrows) and ulceration. Compare with normal bowel (arrowhead). (B) Spot compression image from SBFT shows "string sign" narrowing (arrow) due to stricture. (C) Deep ulcers in the colon of a patient with Crohn's disease, seen at colonoscopy. (Image A reproduced with permission from Chen MY et al. *Basic Radiology.* New York: McGraw-Hill, 2004, Fig. 10-30. Image B reproduced with permission from USMLE-Rx.com. Image C reproduced with permission from Longo DL et al. *Harrison's Principles of Internal Medicine,* 18th ed. New York: McGraw-Hill, 2012, Fig. 291-4B.)

KEY FACT

If a patient with diarrhea is on antibiotics, think *C difficile*.

Q **1**

A 27-year-old man comes to your office complaining of diarrhea and weight loss. He states that his diarrhea often contains mucus but denies any blood in his stool. He also describes having difficulty eating food because of ulcers in his mouth. What is the next step in management?

Q **2**

A 30-year-old woman complains of vague, crampy abdominal pain that is mitigated with defecation. The patient is concerned that her illness may be serious and is worried that her children may be taken away from her, as she recently divorced and is now a single mother. What is the likely diagnosis?

TABLE 7-2.   **Characteristics of Acute Diarrhea**

CAUSE	HISTORY	SYMPTOMS/SIGNS	LABS	TREATMENT
Bacterial	History may be unremarkable. Look for a history of foreign travel or consumption of raw, undercooked, or unpasteurized products. A history of recent antibiotic use suggests *C difficile*.	Symptoms are often severe. Bloody diarrhea suggests enterohemorrhagic *E coli* (EHEC). Patients may complain of fever.	↑ fecal WBCs. Guaiac-⊕ stool in the case of hemorrhagic disease. Culture and sensitivity may reveal the pathogen (be sure to ask specifically to test for EHEC when appropriate). Request a *C difficile* toxin assay when appropriate.	Most cases of bacterial diarrhea will resolve with symptomatic treatment (fluids, electrolytes). Avoid antibiotics if possible in light of potentially ↑ release of endotoxin. TMP-SMX or macrolides can be used to treat most cases of invasive diarrhea. Antibiotics are contraindicated in EHEC. Metronidazole or oral vancomycin is used to treat *C difficile*. Avoid loperamide.
Viral	Family or friends may have similar symptoms.	Symptoms are usually milder and of shorter duration than bacterial illness. Fever is unusual.	Labs are generally nonspecific.	Supportive care with loperamide, bismuth, and probiotics may be helpful.
Parasitic	*Giardia* is associated with day care outbreaks and foreign travel. *Entamoeba* is associated with foreign travel.	Can cause prolonged symptoms if left untreated.	↑ fecal WBCs. Check stool O&P smear. Consider checking HIV status.	Metronidazole is the treatment of choice for most parasitic illnesses.

1   **A**

In light of his age and presenting symptoms, this patient needs a colonoscopy and an evaluation for possible Crohn's disease.

2   **A**

Irritable bowel syndrome. The patient has pain associated with defecation, and her background points to recent stressors and a possible anxiety disorder.

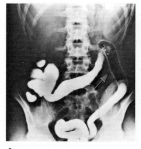
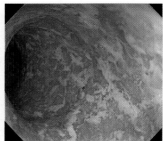
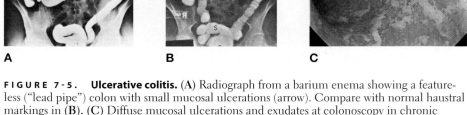

A   **B**   **C**

FIGURE 7-5. **Ulcerative colitis.** (**A**) Radiograph from a barium enema showing a featureless ("lead pipe") colon with small mucosal ulcerations (arrow). Compare with normal haustral markings in (**B**). (**C**) Diffuse mucosal ulcerations and exudates at colonoscopy in chronic ulcerative colitis. (Image A reproduced with permission from Doherty GM. *Current Diagnosis & Treatment: Surgery,* 13th ed. New York: McGraw-Hill, 2010, Fig. 30-17. Image B reproduced with permission from Chen MY et al. *Basic Radiology.* New York: McGraw-Hill, 2004, Fig. 10-10A. Image C reproduced with permission from Longo DL et al. *Harrison's Principles of Internal Medicine,* 18th ed. New York: McGraw-Hill, 2012, Fig. 291-4A.)

TABLE 7-3.   Characteristics of Chronic Diarrhea

Type	Characteristics	Causes	Diagnosis	Treatment
Osmotic	↑ stool osmotic gap. Malabsorption associated with bloating and gas.	Lactose intolerance Magnesium supplements Sorbitol, lactulose, or mannitol ingestion	Usually made by the history.	Stop the offending agent. Lactose enzyme tablets can be helpful in those with lactose intolerance.
Secretory	Caused by mucosal oversecretion. Normal stool osmotic gap.	Hormonal stimulation (gastrin, VIP) Viruses Bacterial toxins	Serum gastrin level and secretin stimulation test if a hormonal cause is suspected.	Varies with the cause.
Exudative	Associated with mucosal inflammation.	IBD or celiac disease TB Colon cancer	↑ ESR or CRP. Colonoscopy.	Treat the underlying cause.
Rapid transit	↑ gut motility.	Hyperthyroidism IBS Laxative abuse Carcinoid Antibiotics (erythromycin)	Check TSH. Take a thorough history.	Treat the underlying cause.
Slow transit	↓ gut motility.	Microscopic colitis Diabetes Radiation damage Scleroderma Small bowel bacterial overgrowth	Colonoscopy in addition to history.	Treat the underlying cause. A short course of antibiotics can be given to patients with bacterial overgrowth.

Celiac Sprue

An autoimmune malabsorptive disorder in which the body's reaction to dietary gluten causes small bowel villous atrophy and crypt hypertrophy. More common in those with **northern European** ancestry; affects approximately 1% of the population.

SYMPTOMS/EXAM

- Celiac sprue leads to **malabsorption** with **chronic diarrhea.** Patients complain of **steatorrhea** and **weight loss.**
- Can also present with nonspecific symptoms (nausea, abdominal pain, weight loss), iron-deficiency anemia, ↑ LFTs, muscle wasting, and osteoporosis.
- Associated with **dermatitis herpetiformis** and an ↑ risk of GI malignancies.

DIAGNOSIS

- Biopsy reveals **flattening or loss of villi** and inflammation.
- Antibody assays are ⊕ for **anti–tissue transglutaminase antibodies** and are falsely ⊖ only with IgA deficiency.
- A gluten-free diet improves symptoms and the histology of the small bowel.

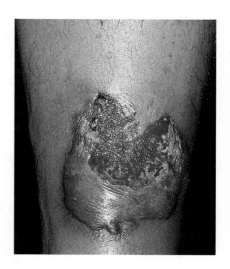

FIGURE 7-6.   Pyoderma gangrenosum. (Reproduced with permission from Wolff K et al. *Fitzpatrick's Color Atlas & Synopsis of Clinical Dermatology,* 5th ed. New York: McGraw-Hill, 2005: 153.)

TREATMENT

Institute a **gluten-free diet.** Gluten is found in most grains in the Western world (eg, wheat, barley, rye, some oats, additives, many prepared foods).

Upper GI Bleed

Bleeding in the section of the GI tract extending from the upper esophagus to the duodenum to the **ligament of Treitz.** The most common causes include **PUD, gastritis, varices** (caused by cirrhosis with portal hypertension), and **Mallory-Weiss syndrome** (caused by excessive vomiting) (see Figure 7-7).

SYMPTOMS

- May present with **dizziness,** lightheadedness, weakness, and nausea.
- Patients may also report vomiting of blood or dark brown contents (**hematemesis**—vomiting of fresh blood, clots, or coffee-ground-like material) or passing of black stool (**melena**—dark, tarry stools composed of degraded blood from the upper GI tract). Severe upper GI bleeds can present as bright red blood in stool (**hematochezia**).

EXAM

- Associated with pallor +/− abdominal pain, tachycardia, and hypotension; rectal exam reveals blood.
- If patients show signs of **cirrhosis** (telangiectasias, spider angiomata, gynecomastia, testicular atrophy, palmar erythema, caput medusae), think varices.
- **Vital signs** reveal **tachycardia** at 10% volume loss, orthostatic **hypotension** at 20% blood loss, and **shock** at 30% loss.

DIAGNOSIS

- Assess the severity of the bleed beginning with **patient stabilization.**
- Check **hematocrit** (may be normal in acute blood loss), **platelet count,** PT/PTT, and LFTs. ↑ BUN indicates digestion of blood.
- If perforation is suspected, obtain upright and abdominal x-rays or a CT scan.
- Endoscopy can be both diagnostic and therapeutic.

TREATMENT

- Start by **stabilizing the patient.** Use at least **2 large-bore** peripheral IV catheters. **Transfusion** and intravascular volume replacement can be initi-

KEY FACT

Melena by definition points to an upper GI bleed. There is no other location in the GI tract that is acidic enough to result in melena.

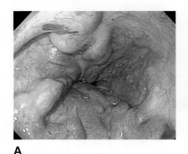
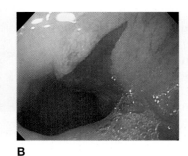
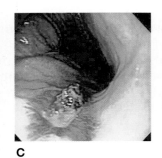
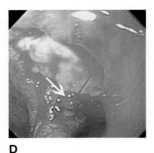

A   **B**   **C**   **D**

FIGURE 7-7. **Causes of upper GI bleed at endoscopy.** (**A**) Esophageal varices. (**B**) Mallory-Weiss tear. (**C**) Gastric ulcer with protuberant vessel. (**D**) Duodenal ulcer with active bleeding (arrow). (Reproduced with permission from Longo DL et al. *Harrison's Principles of Internal Medicine,* 18th ed. New York: McGraw-Hill, 2012, Figs. 291-17, 291-20, and 291-16D and E.)

ated if indicated. Treat empirically with a PPI (can be stopped later if not appropriate).

- Consult GI and surgery if bleeding does not stop or if difficulty is encountered with resuscitation 2° to a brisk bleed.
- Treat **variceal bleeds** with **octreotide**, PPIs, endoscopic **sclerotherapy, or band ligation.** If the bleed is severe, balloon tamponade is appropriate, followed by embolization, transjugular intrahepatic portosystemic shunt **(TIPS)**, or a surgical shunt if endoscopic therapy fails.
- To prevent variceal bleeds, treat with **nonselective** β-blockers (eg, propranolol), obliterative endoscopic therapy, **shunting,** and, if the patient is an appropriate candidate, liver transplantation.
- For **PUD,** use **PPIs, endoscopic** epinephrine injection, thermal contact, and ligation with clip placement. Begin *H pylori* eradication measures.
- **Mallory-Weiss tears** usually stop bleeding **spontaneously.**
- Treat **esophagitis/gastritis** with PPIs. Avoid aspirin and NSAIDs.

Lower GI Bleed

Bleeding that is distal to the ligament of Treitz. Causes include hemorrhoids, diverticulosis, angiodysplasia, carcinoma, enteritis, IBD, polyps, ischemic colitis, infectious colitis, postpolypectomy bleeding, and Meckel's diverticulum.

SYMPTOMS/EXAM

- Presents with **hematochezia.**
- Diarrhea, tenesmus, bright red blood per rectum, and maroon-colored stools are also seen.
- As with upper GI bleeds, check vital signs to assess the severity of the bleed. Obtain orthostatics; perform a rectal exam for hemorrhoids, fissures, or a mass.

DIAGNOSIS

- Bleeding usually **stops spontaneously.** However, colonoscopy should be performed; in the majority of cases, the diagnosis can be made at the time of visualization.
- If the bleed continues, a bleeding scan (⁹⁹Tc-tagged RBC scan) can be done to detect bleeding if it is > 1.0 mL/min.
- If the bleed is refractory, **arteriography** or **exploratory laparotomy** may be done.

TREATMENT

- Although bleeding generally ceases spontaneously, resuscitative efforts should be initiated, as with upper GI bleeds, until the source is found and the bleeding stops.
- With diverticular disease, bleeding usually stops spontaneously, but **epinephrine injection,** catheter-directed **vasopressin,** or **embolization** can be used. In some cases, surgery may be needed.

Pancreatitis

Inflammation of the pancreas that is thought to be caused by the release of excessive pancreatic enzymes. Can be acute or chronic. Chronic pancreatitis can result in diabetes and steatorrhea. Etiologies include:

KEY FACT

A small number of GI bleeds (3.5%) are called "obscure GI bleeds" because they are associated with a ⊖ EGD and colonoscopy followed by a ⊖ small bowel pill camera.

KEY FACT

Think diverticulosis with painless lower GI bleeding. Think diverticulitis in the presence of pain without bleeding.

Q **1**

A 74-year-old woman is transported from a rehabilitation facility where she was being treated for osteomyelitis. She was sent to the hospital after having many foul-smelling bowel movements over the past 2 days. What is the likely cause of her diarrhea, and what is the treatment of choice?

Q **2**

A 32-year-old man presents to the ED with sharp abdominal pain. He states that the pain radiates to his back and is constant in nature. He adds that the pain started after he attended a barbecue at which he drank 14 beers. What is your diagnosis, and how should the patient be managed?

MNEMONIC

Causes of acute pancreatitis—

GET SMASH'D

Gallstones
Ethanol, **E**RCP
Trauma
Steroids
Mumps
Autoimmune
Scorpion bites
Hyperlipidemia
Drugs

- **Acute disease:**
  - **Gallstones and alcohol:** Account for 70–80% of acute cases.
  - **Other causes: Obstruction** (pancreatic or ampullary tumors), **metabolic** factors (severe hypertriglyceridemia, hypercalcemia), abdominal **trauma,** endoscopic retrograde cholangiopancreatography (**ERCP**), **infection** (mumps, CMV, clonorchiasis, ascariasis), **drugs** (thiazides, azathioprine, pentamidine, sulfonamides).
- **Chronic disease:** Alcohol, cystic fibrosis, a history of severe pancreatitis, idiopathic causes (excluding gallstones).

SYMPTOMS

- Presents with abdominal pain—typically in the **midepigastric** region—that **radiates to the back,** may be relieved by sitting forward, and lasts hours to days.
- Nausea, vomiting, and fever are also common.

EXAM

- Exam reveals **midepigastric tenderness,** guarding, occasionally jaundice, and fever.
- **Cullen's sign** (periumbilical ecchymoses) and **Grey Turner's sign** (flank ecchymoses) reflect hemorrhage and severe pancreatitis, although they are often seen long after symptoms manifest and the diagnosis has been made.

DIAGNOSIS

- The hallmark of the disease is ↑ **lipase** (although lipase levels can be normal in chronic pancreatitis as a result of pancreatic burnout).
- **Abdominal CT** is especially useful in detecting complications of pancreatitis (eg, necrotic or hemorrhagic pancreatitis). In **chronic pancreatitis (especially alcohol induced), calcifications** may be seen (see Figure 7-8). However, CT scans are not required if the patient is improving.
- ↑ ALT, AST, or alkaline phosphatase levels suggest **gallstone pancreatitis.**
- Ultrasound may show gallstones, a dilated common bile duct, or sludge in the gallbladder.

TREATMENT

- **Acute:**
  - **Supportive:** NPO, IV fluids (patients may need large quantities), pain management.
  - In the setting of **gallstone pancreatitis,** ERCP with sphincterotomy

This patient was likely receiving long-term antibiotics for osteomyelitis, placing her at risk for *Clostridium difficile* infection. She needs to be treated with metronidazole.

The patient likely has alcoholic pancreatitis. Initial management should consist of bowel rest, IV hydration, and pain control.

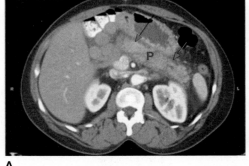 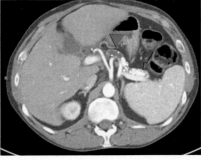

A   B

FIGURE 7-8. Pancreatitis. Transaxial contrast-enhanced CT images. **(A) Uncomplicated acute pancreatitis.** Peripancreatic fluid and fat stranding can be seen (arrows). P = pancreas. **(B) Chronic pancreatitis.** Note the dilated pancreatic duct (arrowhead) and pancreatic calcifications (arrow). (Reproduced with permission from USMLE-Rx.com.)

is appropriate with common bile duct obstruction or with evidence of cholangitis. If the gallstone has passed, perform a cholecystectomy once the patient is sufficiently stable for surgery.

- **Antibiotics** are useful only when there is suspicion for an infected necrotic pancreas (10% of cases; can be seen on CT). Treat with imipenem monotherapy or with a fluoroquinolone + metronidazole.
- Resume diet once pain and nausea have abated. Enteral feeding is preferable to TPN if nutritional support is needed in patients with protracted pancreatitis.

- **Chronic:**
  - Treat malabsorption with pancreatic enzyme and B_{12} replacement.
  - Treat glucose intolerance or diabetes; encourage alcohol abstinence.
  - Manage chronic pain.

COMPLICATIONS

- **Acute: Pseudocyst,** peripancreatic effusions, **necrosis,** abscess, ARDS, hypotension, splenic vein thrombosis.
- **Chronic: Malabsorption,** osteoporosis, diabetes mellitus (DM), **pancreatic cancer.**

Approach to Liver Function Tests

The algorithm in Figure 7-9 outlines a general approach toward the interpretation of LFTs.

Gallstone Disease

Gallstones can be symptomatic or asymptomatic; in the United States, they are usually due to cholesterol stones. They can also result in **cholecystitis** (inflammation of the gallbladder) or **cholangitis** (inflammation of the com-

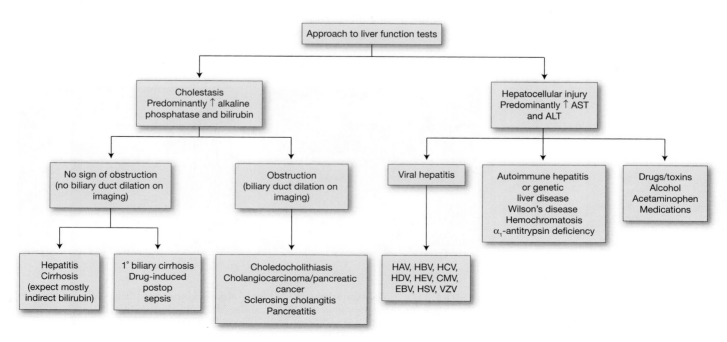

FIGURE 7-9. **Abnormal liver function tests.**

KEY FACT

Symptoms of cholangitis:
- RUQ pain
- Fever
- Jaundice

MNEMONIC

Risk factors for cholecystitis—

The 5 F's

Fat
Female
Forty
Fair
Fertile

mon bile duct). In trauma patients, burn patients, or those on TPN, acute cholecystitis may occur in the absence of stones (**acalculous cholecystitis**).

SYMPTOMS/EXAM

- Most patients with gallstones are **asymptomatic** (80%).
- May also present as follows:
  - **Biliary colic:** Characterized by episodes of **RUQ** or epigastric pain that may radiate to the right shoulder. Pain is usually **postprandial**, lasts about 30 minutes, and is occasionally accompanied by vomiting. **Nocturnal** pain that awakens the patient is common. Associated with **fatty food** intolerance and **Murphy's sign** (inspiratory arrest during deep palpation of the RUQ).
  - **Cholangitis:** Suggested by fever, jaundice (a sign of common bile duct obstruction), and persistent RUQ pain (**Charcot's triad**).
  - **Reynolds' pentad:** Charcot's triad plus shock and altered mental status may be seen in **suppurative cholangitis**.

DIAGNOSIS

- Labs reveal **leukocytosis** and ↑ LFTs.
- **Ultrasound** is 85–90% sensitive for gallbladder gallstones and cholecystitis (**echogenic focus that casts a shadow**; pericholecystic fluid = acute cholecystitis). A thickened gallbladder wall and biliary sludge are less specific findings (see Figure 7-10).
- If ultrasound is equivocal and suspicion for acute cholecystitis is high, proceed to a **HIDA** scan. A ⊖ HIDA indicates that there is no obstruction in the gallbladder. False positives are common.

TREATMENT

- **Acute cholecystitis:**
  - IV antibiotics (generally a third-generation cephalosporin plus metronidazole in severe cases); IV fluids, electrolyte repletion.
  - Early cholecystectomy within 72 hours with an intraoperative cholangiogram to look for common bile duct stones. For patients who are high-risk surgical candidates, elective surgery may be appropriate if the clinical condition allows.
  - For patients who are not candidates for surgery, consider a percutaneous biliary drain.

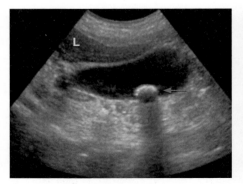
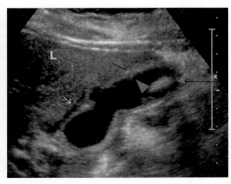

A **B**

FIGURE 7-10. **Gallstone disease.** (A) **Cholelithiasis.** Ultrasound image of the gallbladder shows a gallstone (arrow) with posterior shadowing. (B) **Acute cholecystitis.** Ultrasound image shows a gallstone (red arrow), a thickened gallbladder wall (arrowheads), and pericholecystic fluid (white arrow). L = liver. (Reproduced with permission from USMLE-Rx.com.)

- Cholangitis:
  - Admission, NPO, hydration, pressors if needed, **IV antibiotics** (ciprofloxacin is preferred).
  - **For very ill patients who are not responsive to medical treatment, urgent next-day ERCP with endoscopic sphincterotomy** may be needed. Other emergency options are ERCP with stent placement, percutaneous transhepatic drainage, and operative decompression.

Viral and Nonviral Hepatitis

May be acute and self-limited or chronic and symptomatic. May not be detected until years after the initial infection.

SYMPTOMS/EXAM

- In **acute** cases, patients may present with anorexia, **nausea,** vomiting, malaise, and fever but are frequently **asymptomatic.**
- Exam is often normal but may reveal an enlarged and tender liver, dark urine, and jaundice.

DIFFERENTIAL

- With a **high level of transaminase elevation (> 10–20 times the upper limit of normal),** consider acute viral infection as well as ischemia ("shock liver"), acute choledocholithiasis, autoimmune hepatitis, or toxins (acetaminophen).
- With **moderate transaminase elevation,** consider the most common cause, nonalcoholic fatty liver disease. Also consider chronic viral infection, mononucleosis, CMV, 2° syphilis, drug-induced illness, alcohol, Budd-Chiari syndrome, hemochromatosis, celiac disease, IBD, right-sided heart failure, and muscle damage (eg, rhabdomyolysis).

DIAGNOSIS

- Diagnose on the basis of:
  - The presence of hepatitis based on clinical presentation as well as ↑ transaminases.
  - Serology and/or PCR testing confirming a specific virus (see Tables 7-4 and 7-5 and Figure 7-11).
- If the cause cannot be determined, liver biopsy may be helpful.
- RUQ ultrasound may be performed to see if the liver is enlarged in acute hepatitis (vs cirrhotic nodular liver in the advanced disease state).

TREATMENT

- Treat according to subtype as outlined in Table 7-5. Additional guidelines are as follows:
  - Rest during the acute phase.
  - Avoid hepatotoxic agents and elective surgery. Use hepatically metabolized drugs with caution (eg, opiates).
- Although most symptoms resolve in 3–16 weeks, LFTs may remain ↑ for much longer.

KEY FACT

There is an ↑ (25–40%) risk of cirrhosis and hepatocellular carcinoma with chronic HBV.

Q **1**

A 48-year-old woman with a history of diabetes, obesity, and hyperlipidemia comes to your clinic for a routine physical and lab work. Labs show a normal bilirubin level with an AST and ALT of 58 and 72 U/L, respectively; alkaline phosphatase is within normal limits. What is the likely cause of her transaminitis?

Q **2**

A 59-year-old man comes to your clinic for a checkup. He lived in Vietnam until age 32 and has not seen a primary care physician since that time. He is concerned that many of the people in his community have had hepatitis B. Which labs should be ⊕ if this patient has chronic hepatitis B?

TABLE 7-4. Viral Hepatitis and Serologic Tests

Type of Viral Hepatitis	⊕ Serology [a]
Acute HAV	Anti-HAV IgM.
Previous HAV	Anti-HAV IgG.
Acute HBV	HBsAg; HBeAg; HBcAb IgM.
Acute HBV, window period	HBcAb IgM only.
Chronic active HBV	HBsAg, HBeAg, HBcAb IgG.
Recovery HBV	HBsAb IgG, HBcAb IgG, normal ALT.
Immunized HBV	HBsAb IgG.
Chronic HCV infection	HCV RNA, anti-HCV Ab, elevated/normal ALT.
Recovery HCV	Anti-HCV Ab and ⊖ HCV RNA.

[a] Anti-HAV IgM = anti–hepatitis A IgM antibody; anti-HAV IgG = anti–hepatitis A IgG antibody; HBsAg = hepatitis B surface antigen; HBeAg = hepatitis B core antigen; HBcAb IgM = hepatitis B core IgM antibody; HBcAb IgG = hepatitis B core IgG antibody; HBsAb IgG = hepatitis B surface IgG antibody; HCV RNA = hepatitis C RNA (can be quantitative to determine disease severity); anti-HCV Ab = hepatitis C antibody.

Cirrhosis and Ascites

Chronic irreversible changes of the hepatic parenchyma, including fibrosis and regenerative nodules. The most common cause in the United States is alcohol abuse, followed by chronic viral hepatitis.

SYMPTOMS/EXAM

- Cirrhosis can be asymptomatic for long periods. Symptoms reflect the **severity** of hepatic damage, not the underlying etiology of the liver disease (see Figure 7-12).
- ↓ hepatic function leads to jaundice, edema, coagulopathy, and metabolic abnormalities.
- Fibrosis and distorted vasculature results in portal hypertension, which leads to gastroesophageal varices and splenomegaly.
- ↓ hepatic function and portal hypertension result in ascites and hepatic encephalopathy.

DIAGNOSIS

Cirrhosis is diagnosed as follows:

- **Labs:**
  - Laboratory abnormalities may be absent in quiescent cirrhosis.
  - ALT/AST levels are ↑ during active hepatocellular injury. However, levels may not be ↑ in cirrhosis because a large portion of the liver is replaced by fibrous tissue, and little new cell injury may be occurring.
  - Additional lab findings include anemia from suppressed erythropoiesis; leukopenia from hypersplenism or leukocytosis from infection; throm-

---

1 Ⓐ

Nonalcoholic fatty liver disease, a common cause of liver disease in patients with obesity and diabetes. Other causes of liver disease, such as hepatitis and alcoholism, should be excluded.

2 Ⓐ

HBsAg, HBeAg, and HBcAb IgG.

TABLE 7-5. Etiologies, Diagnosis, and Treatment of Viral Hepatitis

Subtype	Transmission	Clinical/Lab Findings	Treatment	Other Key Facts
HAV	Transmitted via contaminated food, water, milk, and shellfish. Known day-care-center outbreaks have been identified. **Fecal-oral transmission;** has a 6-day to 6-week incubation period. Virus is shed in stool up to 2 weeks before symptom onset.	No chronic infection.	Supportive; generally no sequelae.	Give **immunoglobulin** to close contacts without HAV infection or vaccination.
HBV	Transmitted by **infected blood,** through **sexual contact,** or **perinatally.** Incubation is 6 weeks to 6 months. HDV can coinfect those with HBV.	High prevalence in men who have sex with men, prostitutes, and IV drug users. Fewer than 1% of cases are fulminant. Adult acquired infection usually does not become chronic. Much more common in Asian countries and among immigrants from that region.	Interferon and other nucleotide/nucleoside analogs. (The goal is to ↓ viral load and improve liver histology; cure is uncommon.)	Vaccinate against HAV. Associated with arthritis, glomerulonephritis, and **polyarteritis nodosa.** Chronic infection can result in hepatocellular carcinoma (even without cirrhosis).
HCV	Transmitted through **blood transfusion or IV drug use,** tattoos, or body piercing. Incubation is 6–7 weeks.	Acute illness is often mild or asymptomatic. Characterized by **waxing and waning aminotransferases.** HCV antibody is not protective. Antibody appears 6 weeks to 9 months after infection. More than 70% of infections become chronic.	Interferon + **ribavirin** + sofosbuvir +/– simeprevir (only for genotype 1).	Vaccinate against HAV and HBV. Complications include **cryoglobulinemia,** membranoproliferative glomerulonephritis, and hepatocellular carcinoma in patients with cirrhosis. Check for HIV. Screen all people born in the United States between 1945 and 1965 for HCV.
HDV	Requires a coexistent **HBV** infection. Percutaneous exposure. Usually found in **IV drug users** and high-risk **HBsAg carriers.**	Anti-HDV IgM is present in acute cases. Immunity to HBV implies immunity to HDV.	Similar to HBV infection.	If acquired as a superinfection in chronic HBV, there is ↑ severity of infection. Fulminant hepatitis or severe chronic hepatitis with rapid progression to cirrhosis can occur. Associated with an ↑ risk of **hepatocellular carcinoma.**
HEV	Fecal-oral transmission.	Will test ⊕ on serology for HEV.	Supportive.	Self-limited; endemic to India, Afghanistan, Mexico, and Algeria. Carries a 10–20% mortality rate in **pregnant** women.

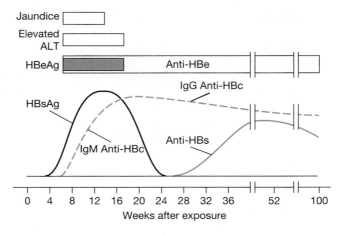

FIGURE 7-11. **Natural history of HBV infection.** (Reproduced with permission from Stern SD et al. *Symptom to Diagnosis: An Evidence-Based Guide,* 2nd ed. New York: McGraw-Hill, 2010, Fig. 22-2.)

bocytopenia from alcoholic marrow suppression; ↓ hepatic thrombopoietin production and splenic sequestration; and a prolonged PT from failure of hepatic synthesis of clotting factors.

■ **Imaging:**
  ■ **Ultrasound:** Used to assess liver size and surface contour and to **detect ascites or hepatic nodules.** Doppler ultrasound can establish the patency of the splenic, portal, and hepatic veins. Commonly used in

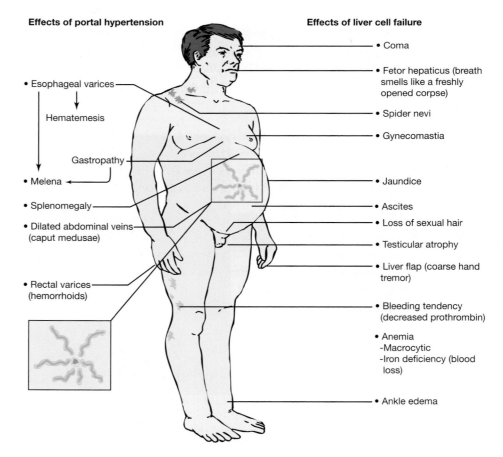

FIGURE 7-12. **Clinical effects of cirrhosis.** (Modified with permission from Chandrasoma P, Taylor CE. *Concise Pathology,* 3rd ed. Originally published by Appleton & Lange. Copyright © 1998 by The McGraw-Hill Companies, Inc.)

the setting of chronic liver disease without known cirrhosis (see Figure 7-13).

- **CT or MRI with contrast:** Used to characterize hepatic nodules. A biopsy may be needed to rule out malignancy.
- Liver biopsy is the most accurate means of assessing disease severity.

Ascites is diagnosed as follows:

- **Paracentesis:** Check cell count, differential, albumin, and bacterial cultures +/− acid-fast stain and +/− cytology. The etiology of the ascites can be further characterized as follows:
  - **Related to portal hypertension (serum-ascites albumin gradient [SAAG] ≥ 1.1):** Cirrhosis, heart failure, Budd-Chiari syndrome (hepatic vein thrombosis).
  - **Unrelated to portal hypertension (SAAG < 1.1):** Peritonitis (eg, TB), cancer, pancreatitis, trauma, nephrotic syndrome.
- If a patient with cirrhosis and established ascites presents with worsening ascites, fever, altered mental status, renal dysfunction, or abdominal pain, think of **spontaneous bacterial peritonitis (SBP).**

TREATMENT

- Treatment for **cirrhosis** is as follows:
  - Abstinence from alcohol.
  - Restrict fluid intake to 800–1000 mL/day if the patient is hyponatremic.
  - Treat anemia with iron (in iron-deficiency anemia) or folic acid (in alcoholics).
  - Liver transplantation is required in the setting of progressive liver disease.
- Treatment for **ascites** includes the following:
  - **Sodium restriction** to < 2 g/day.
  - **Diuretics:** Furosemide and spironolactone in combination.
  - Large-volume paracentesis for ascites that is refractory to diuretics.

KEY FACT

Diagnose spontaneous bacterial peritonitis with ⊕ cultures or a peritoneal fluid neutrophil count > 250 cells/mm³.

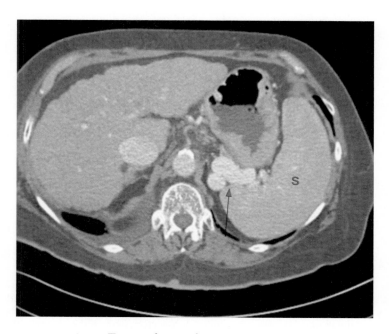

FIGURE 7-13.   Cirrhosis. Transaxial image from contrast-enhanced CT shows a nodular liver contour (arrowheads) and the stigmata of portal hypertension, including splenomegaly (S) and perisplenic varices (arrow). (Reproduced with permission from USMLE-Rx.com.)

- TIPS can be used in refractory cases caused by portal hypertension, but this will ↑ the rate of encephalopathy.
- Ultimately, liver transplantation will be needed if the patient is a candidate.
- Treat SBP with a **third-generation cephalosporin** (first-line therapy) or a fluoroquinolone. Often recurs.

Acetaminophen Toxicity

Within 2–4 hours of an acute acetaminophen overdose, patients present with nausea, vomiting, diaphoresis, and pallor. Within 24–48 hours, hepatotoxicity is manifested by RUQ tenderness, hepatomegaly, and ↑ transaminases. Figure 7-14 describes the underlying pathophysiologic mechanisms.

TREATMENT

- Supportive measures; oral administration of activated charcoal or cholestyramine within 30 minutes of ingestion to prevent absorption of residual drug.
- Begin **N-acetylcysteine** administration up to 36 hours after ingestion if the acetaminophen level is > 150 μg/mL measured at 4 hours or > 18.8 μg/mL at 16 hours after ingestion, or if the time of ingestion is unknown and ↑ levels are seen. Even late treatment can be helpful.

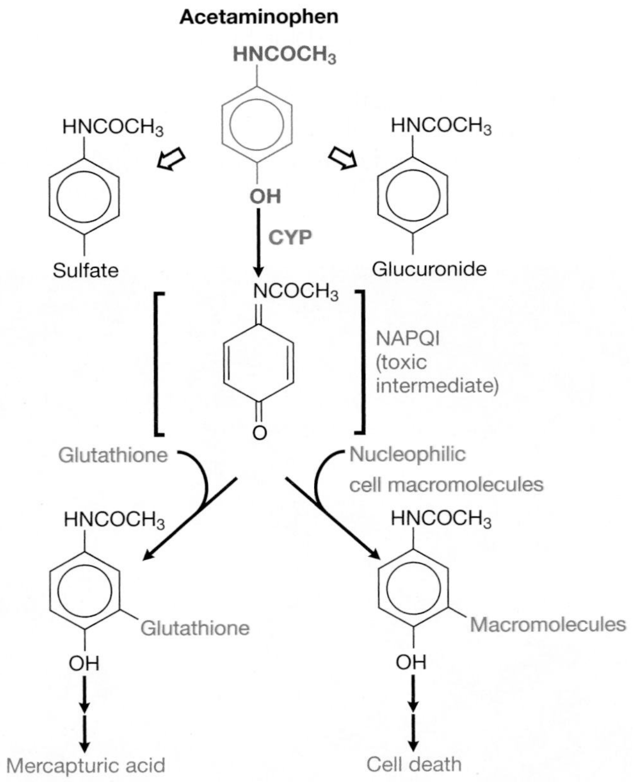

FIGURE 7-14. **Mechanism of acetaminophen toxicity.** Acetaminophen is converted to NAPQI, which is toxic. Glutathione converts NAPQI to a nontoxic substance. In acetaminophen toxicity, glutathione becomes overwhelmed. N-acetylcysteine is the precursor to glutathione and can replete the body so that it can continue to detoxify NAPQI. (Reproduced with permission from Brunton LL et al. *Goodman & Gilman's The Pharmacological Basis of Therapeutics,* 12th ed. New York: McGraw-Hill, 2011, Fig. 4-5).

Hereditary Hemochromatosis

- An **autosomal recessive** disorder of **iron overload.** Usually affects **middle-aged Caucasian men** at a rate of 1 in 300. (Women carry the disorder in equal number but are generally unaffected owing to iron loss from menstrual bleeding.)
- **Sx/Exam:** Presents with **mild transaminitis, DM, arthritis, infertility,** and heart failure. Patients can develop cirrhosis.
- **Dx:** Diagnosis is made with ↑ iron saturation (> 60% in men and > 50% in women), ↑ ferritin, ↑ transferrin saturation, and the presence of the **HFE gene mutation.**
- **Tx:** Treat with **phlebotomy** to ↓ the iron burden. Genetic counseling is useful to assess the likelihood of transmission.

Wilson's Disease

- An **autosomal recessive** disorder of **copper overload.**
- **Sx/Exam:** Exam may reveal **Kayser-Fleischer rings** and **neuropsychiatric disorders.**
- **Dx:** Labs reveal ↑ urinary copper, ↓ serum **ceruloplasmin,** and ↑ hepatic copper content on liver biopsy.
- **Tx:** Treatment consists of **chelation** with penicillamine and trientine or liver transplantation.

α_1-Antitrypsin Disorder

- Usually affects the **liver** (cirrhosis) and the **lung** (emphysema). In the liver, intrahepatic accumulation of variant α_1-antitrypsin molecules accumulate, causing hepatocyte injury. In the lung, excessive protease causes destruction of elastase.
- **Dx:** Diagnosed by the quantitative absence of α_1-antitrypsin on serum protein electrophoresis (SPEP) as well as by genotype analysis (autosomal recessive).
- **Tx:**
  - **Liver transplantation** is curative for both liver and lung disease.
  - α_1-antitrypsin replacement for the lung while awaiting transplant.

Autoimmune Hepatitis

- Primarily affects **young women;** usually suspected when transaminases are elevated.
- **Dx:** Hypergammaglobulinemia is seen on SPEP; autoantibodies are sometimes seen (**ANA,** anti–smooth muscle antibody [**ASMA**], liver/kidney microsomal antibody [**LKMA**]). Ultimately a **liver biopsy** is needed to confirm the diagnosis.
- **Tx:** Treat with **corticosteroids and azathioprine.** A significant number of patients relapse when off therapy and thus require long-term treatment.

Q

A 46-year-old woman presents to your clinic with scleral icterus, pruritus, and abnormal LFTs. Her AST, ALT, and alkaline phosphatase levels are 48, 56, and 603 U/L, respectively. What lab test will reveal the likely diagnosis?

1° Biliary Cirrhosis

- **Autoimmune** destruction of microscopic **intrahepatic** bile ducts. Usually associated with other autoimmune diseases. More common in **women.**
- **Sx/Exam:** Presents with fatigue, **pruritus, jaundice,** fat **malabsorption,** and **osteoporosis.**
- **Dx:** Suggested by markedly ↑ alkaline phosphatase, ↑ bilirubin (late), and **antimitochondrial antibody (AMA).** Confirmed by biopsy.
- **Tx:** Ursodeoxycholic acid, fat-soluble vitamins, cholestyramine for pruritus, and transplantation.

1° Sclerosing Cholangitis

- **Idiopathic intra-** and **extrahepatic** fibrosis of the bile ducts. Affects **men** 20–50 years of age; associated with **IBD (usually ulcerative colitis).**
- **Sx/Exam:** Can present with **RUQ pain** and pruritus but is often **asymptomatic.**
- **Dx:** Look for ↑ bilirubin and alkaline phosphatase; ⊕ **ASMA;** ⊕ **p-ANCA;** and multiple areas of beaded bile duct strictures on ERCP (see Figure 7-15).
- **Tx:** Treat with ursodeoxycholic acid, cholestyramine, fat-soluble vitamins, balloon dilation and, less commonly, stenting of the strictures, and ultimately liver transplantation.

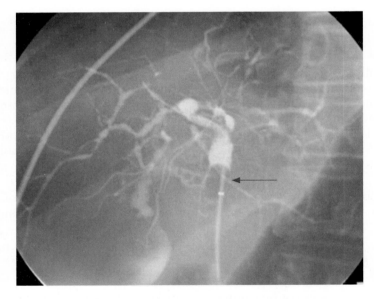

FIGURE 7-15. **Primary sclerosing cholangitis.** ERCP image following contrast injection through a catheter in the common bile duct with the balloon (blue arrow) inflated. Multifocal structuring and dilation of the intrahepatic bile ducts can be seen. (Reproduced with permission from USMLE-Rx.com.)

A ⊕ antimitochondrial antibody will reveal the likely diagnosis of 1° biliary cirrhosis.

CHAPTER 8

HEMATOLOGY

Hematology Definitions

- **Ferritin:** A measure of iron stores ($\downarrow$ in iron-deficiency anemia but $\uparrow$ in infection and inflammation).
- **Haptoglobin:** A protein that binds free hemoglobin (in intravascular hemolysis, free hemoglobin is released, haptoglobin binds to the hemoglobin, and levels of haptoglobin $\downarrow$).
- **Mean corpuscular volume (MCV):** Also known as mean cell volume; a measure of the *average volume* of the RBCs.
- **Mean corpuscular hemoglobin concentration (MCHC):** Measure of hemoglobin in a given volume of RBCs.
- **Red blood cell distribution width (RDW):** Measure of the *variation in volume* of the RBCs ("width" refers to the volume curve or distribution width, not the actual width of the individual cells).
- **Reticulocyte count (RC):** Percentage (not technically a count) of reticulocytes (or immature blood cells) in the blood.
- **Reticulocyte index (RI):** Reticulocyte count multiplied by the patient's hematocrit/normal hematocrit; also known as corrected reticulocyte count.
- **Total iron-binding capacity (TIBC):** Measures the capacity of transferrin to bind with iron (or how much iron is carried throughout the body).
- **Transferrin:** Protein that reversibly binds and carries iron.
- **Direct Coombs' test:** An antiglobulin test to determine if antibodies are bound to the RBC membrane; indicative of hemolytic anemia.

Anemia

Anemia can be caused by (1) blood loss, (2) underproduction, or (3) $\uparrow$ destruction (hemolysis). It can be categorized by the volume of the RBC (see Figure 8-1) or by MCV as microcytic, normocytic, or macrocytic:

- **Microcytic:** MCV < 80 fL.
- **Normocytic:** MCV 80–100 fL.
- **Macrocytic:** MCV > 100 fL.

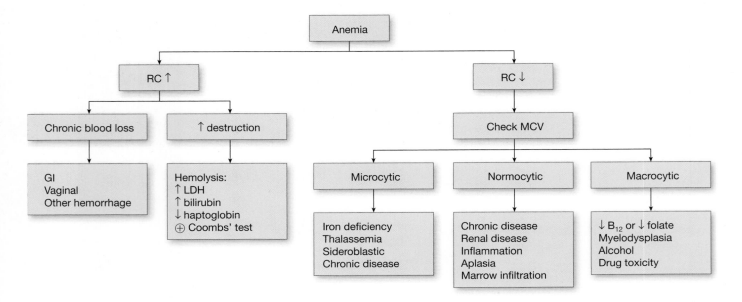

FIGURE 8-1.   Classification of anemia.

DIAGNOSIS

- Initially, look for a bleeding source. Order a CBC, an MCV, an RC, and a peripheral blood smear (see Table 8-1).
- Determine if other cell lines are down (eg, WBCs and platelets).
- If there is **pancytopenia,** think drugs, infection, myelodysplasia, malignancy, radiation, vitamin B_{12}/folate deficiency, SLE, or congenital causes.

TREATMENT

Patients who are symptomatic require fluid resuscitation and RBC transfusion. Transfuse to keep serum hemoglobin > 7 **g/dL.** Identify the cause of the anemia and treat the underlying disorder.

MICROCYTIC ANEMIA

Anemia with an **MCV of < 80 fL** is due to either iron deficiency or thalassemia. Other causes of microcytic anemia include anemia of chronic disease and sideroblastic anemia (see the mnemonic **TICS**).

SYMPTOMS/EXAM

- Patients may report fatigue or dyspnea on exertion. Iron-deficient patients may have **pica.**
- Ask about melena and blood in the stool, and check for fecal occult blood. Ask female patients about heavy menstrual periods. A ⊕ family history of anemia should raise suspicion for thalassemia.
- Possible exam findings include pallor, **fatigue,** jaundice, postural hypotension, and tachycardia.

DIAGNOSIS

- Examine iron studies and a blood smear to identify the cause of the microcytic anemia (see Table 8-2 and Figure 8-2).
- Suspect **colorectal cancer** in elderly patients with microcytic anemia, and refer these patients for a colonoscopy.
- The Mentzer index can help distinguish iron-deficiency anemia from thalassemia.

KEY FACT

If possible, check all necessary lab studies pertaining to anemia (eg, iron, ferritin, RC) **before** transfusion.

MNEMONIC

Causes of microcytic anemia—

TICS

Thalassemia
Iron deficiency
Chronic disease
Sideroblastic anemia

KEY FACT

In iron-deficiency anemia, first RDW widens and then MCV ↓.

Q 1

A 70-year-old woman presents with fatigue, dyspnea on exertion, and dizziness. She has a hemoglobin level of 9 g/dL (from a baseline of 12 g/dL); ↑ indirect bilirubin, RC, and LDH; and a ↓ haptoglobin level. What type of anemia do you suspect, and which test do you order next?

Q 2

A 75-year-old man presents with fatigue, new constipation, weight loss, and an anemia with an MCV of < 80 fL. Which type of anemia does this suggest, and what should you include in your diagnostic tests?

TABLE 8-1. Common Peripheral Blood Smear Findings

FINDING	DIAGNOSIS
Microcytosis	Iron deficiency.
Target cells	Hemoglobinopathy, liver disease, splenectomy.
Schistocytes	TTP, HUS, DIC.
Spherocytes	Hereditary spherocytosis, warm autoimmune hemolytic anemia.
Bite cells	G6PD deficiency.
Sickle cells	Sickle cell anemia.
Macrocytes	B_{12} or folate deficiency.
Teardrop cells	Fibrosis, marrow infiltration.

TABLE 8-2. **Causes of Microcytic Anemia**

	IRON-DEFICIENCY ANEMIA	THALASSEMIA	ANEMIA OF CHRONIC DISEASE (LATE)	SIDEROBLASTIC ANEMIA
Pathology	↓ iron in marrow, ↓ heme synthesis.	↓ synthesis of α- or β-globin subunits.	↓ ability to use iron and response to erythropoietin from ↑ inflammatory markers.	RBC precursors have defective heme synthesis.
Serum ferritin	↓[a]	Normal to ↑	↑↑	↑
Serum iron	↓	Normal to ↑	Slightly ↓	↑
TIBC	↑	Normal to ↑	Normal to ↓	Normal or ↓
Other tests	**Wide RDW.** Thrombocytosis is common. Mentzer index > 13.	**Normal RDW.** Confirm the diagnosis with hemoglobin electrophoresis. Presence of basophilic stippling; typically MCV < 70. ↑ MCHC and a Mentzer index of < 13.		Smear shows normal and dimorphic RBCs with basophilic stippling (see Figure 8-3). Confirm the diagnosis with bone marrow biopsy (shows erythroid hyperplasia and ringed sideroblasts). Check lead levels if suspected.

[a] May be normal in inflammatory states and cancer.

- Mentzer index = MCV/RBC count.
- If the Mentzer index is > 13, the condition is more likely to be iron-deficiency anemia.

TREATMENT

- If iron-deficiency anemia is the cause, initiate oral iron (patients intolerant of oral therapy and those with GI disease may need parenteral therapy).

1 **A**

Hemolytic anemia; check a blood smear and a direct Coombs' test. The patient's indirect bilirubin level and LDH are elevated as a result of ↑ RBC destruction. A blood smear and a ⊕ direct Coombs' test can give you a clue as to the etiology—eg, spherocytes in congenital or autoimmune hemolytic anemia.

2 **A**

Microcytic anemia from iron deficiency. Check a colonoscopy to rule out colon cancer given the patient's age and history of weight loss.

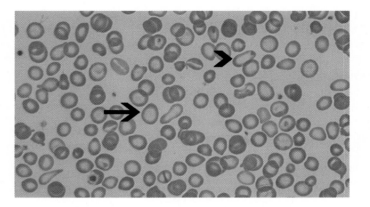

FIGURE 8-2. **Microscopic smear showing iron-deficiency anemia.** Most of the RBCs exhibit central pallor (arrow). Also seen is a characteristic "pencil cell" (arrowhead). (Reproduced with permission from Kemp WL et al. *Pathology: The Big Picture.* New York: McGraw-Hill, 2008, Fig. 12-1.)

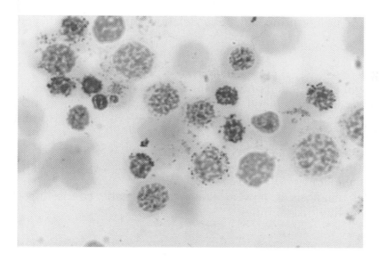

FIGURE 8-3. **Basophilic stippling characteristic of sideroblastic anemia.** (Reproduced with permission from Lichtman MA et al. *Williams Hematology*, 8th ed. New York: McGraw-Hill, 2010, Fig. 58-1B.)

To help replenish stores, treatment should be continued 3–6 months after lab values have normalized.
- Erythropoietin (**Epogen**) should be considered in patients with anemia of chronic disease, particularly those with chronic kidney disease when the hemoglobin level is < 10 g/dL.

Thalassemia

A group of disorders resulting from ↓ synthesis of α- or β-globin protein subunits. α-thalassemia is most common among **Asians** and African Americans; β-thalassemia is most frequently found in people of **Mediterranean** origin, Asians, and African Americans.

SYMPTOMS/EXAM

Clinical presentation varies according to subtype:

- α-thalassemia:
    - **All 4 α-alleles** are affected; babies are stillborn with **hydrops fetalis** or die shortly after birth.
    - **HbH** (α-thalassemia intermedia): **Three** alleles are affected; leads to **chronic hemolytic microcytic anemia** and **splenomegaly.**
    - **Carriers:** One or two alleles are affected; usually asymptomatic.
- β-thalassemia:
    - **β-thalassemia major** (homozygous; no β-globin production and hence no HbA): Presents in the **first year of life** as fetal hemoglobin declines. Manifestations include growth retardation, **bony deformities**, hepatosplenomegaly, and jaundice.
    - **β-thalassemia intermedia:** A ↓ in (but not absence of) both β-globins. The phenotype is in between β-major and β-minor.
    - **β-thalassemia minor/trait** (heterozygous): Usually less severe because the patient has ↓ expression of a single β gene. Usually diagnosed by an ↑ HbA_2 on electrophoresis.

DIAGNOSIS

- Severe microcytic anemia presents with a **normal RDW** (vs iron deficiency, in which RDW is ↑).
- Hemoglobin electrophoresis is the definitive diagnostic test (except in α-thalassemia trait, which has normal hemoglobin electrophoresis results;

KEY FACT

The RDW is a measure of the variation in RBC volume, which changes as microcytic RBCs mix with normocytic RBCs. Over time, the MCV ↓ as more of the RBCs are microcytic.

KEY FACT

Clinically significant α-thalassemia can present at birth because the α chain is made in fetal/neonatal hematopoiesis, but β-thalassemia won't present until the α-chain predominance (present in fetal hemoglobin) changes to the β chain.

MNEMONIC

Features of β-thalassemia major—

BETA THAL D

Basophilic stippling
Excess iron from transfusions
Transplant, bone marrow
Hb**A** decreased
Tower skull and bony abnormalities
Heart failure
Anisocytosis
Liver and spleen enlargement
Deferoxamine

KEY FACT

With a severely low MCV, a Mentzer index of < 13, microcytic anemia that is unresponsive to iron supplementation, or familial anemia, suspect thalassemia and order a hemoglobin electrophoresis.

this must be confirmed by gene deletion studies if the diagnosis is suspected).

TREATMENT

- Although allogeneic bone marrow transplantation may be curative in severe thalassemia, blood transfusions should be given as necessary for symptomatic control, and patients must receive folate. Monitor for iron overload.
- Treatment measures vary by subtype (see Table 8-3).
- To prevent 2° hemosiderosis due to iron overload, consider deferoxamine, an iron chelator.
- Prenatal diagnosis is now available, and genetic counseling should be offered to high-risk families.

KEY FACT

An MCV of > 110 fL is usually due to vitamin B_{12} or folate deficiency.

MACROCYTIC ANEMIA

Anemia with an MCV of > 100 fL. Characterized by impaired DNA synthesis with normal cytoplasm maturation and delayed nucleus development that results in macrocytosis. The most common etiologies include:

- **Folate deficiency:** Poor dietary intake (including **alcoholism**) and **drugs** (eg, phenytoin, zidovudine, TMP-SMX, methotrexate and other chemotherapeutic agents).
- **B_{12} deficiency:** Commonly caused by a strict vegan diet, **pernicious anemia** (a ↓ in intrinsic factor by gastric parietal cells and therefore ↓ absorption), gastrectomy, PPIs (which inhibit B_{12} absorption), and ileal dysfunction (IBD, surgical resection). B_{12} deficiency can cause **neurologic deficits** (paresthesias, gait disturbance, and mental status changes).
- **Other:** Liver disease, hypothyroidism, alcohol abuse, myelodysplasia, fish tapeworm.

DIAGNOSIS

- Check serum B_{12}, folate, and a **blood smear** to look for megaloblastic anemia, which shows **oval macrocytes** and hypersegmented neutrophils (see Figure 8-4).
- If B_{12} deficiency is suspected, check **intrinsic factor antibody** and **anti–parietal cell antibody** for pernicious anemia.
- Homocysteine and methylmalonic acid (MMA) levels can distinguish folate from B_{12} deficiency:
  - **Folate deficient:** ↑ homocysteine but normal MMA.
  - **B_{12} deficient:** ↑ homocysteine and ↑ MMA.

KEY FACT

- F**O**late deficiency: ↑ in h**O**mocysteine; normal MMA.
- B_{12} deficiency: ↑ in **B**oth.

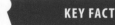

TABLE 8-3.   **Treatment of Thalassemia**

SUBTYPE	TREATMENT
β-thalassemia minor	Observe.
β-thalassemia intermedia	Transfusion, chelation therapy, close observation.
β-thalassemia major	Transfusion, chelation, consider stem cell transplant.
HbH (α-thalassemia intermedia)	Treatment is similar to that of β-thalassemia intermedia.
α-thalassemia	No specific treatment.

TREATMENT

- Treat B$_{12}$ deficiency with monthly B$_{12}$ shots or oral replacement (in a normal GI tract, oral replacement has been shown to be as effective as IV); treat folate deficiency with oral replacement.
- Discontinue any medications that could be contributing to megaloblastic anemia; minimize alcohol use.

NORMOCYTIC NORMOCHROMIC ANEMIA

Anemia with an MCV of 80–100 fL. Can be due to **blood loss (hemorrhage)**, **hemolysis**, or ↓ **production**.

SYMPTOMS/EXAM

Look for evidence of acute bleeding. Patients with **hemolytic anemia** may present with jaundice and dark urine from unconjugated hyperbilirubinemia as well as with pigment gallstones and splenomegaly.

DIAGNOSIS

The initial workup includes RC, creatinine, hemolysis labs, and blood smear.

- **Normal RC:** Anemia of chronic disease or chronic kidney disease.
- **↑ RC with normal hemolysis labs:** Hemorrhage.
- **↑ RC, ↑ LDH, ↑ unconjugated bilirubin, and ↓ haptoglobin:** Hemolysis.

Hemolytic Anemia

The causes of hemolytic anemia are outlined in Table 8-4.

TREATMENT

- Patients who are hemorrhaging must be resuscitated with fluids and RBC transfusions. Identify and treat the cause.
- **Hereditary spherocytosis** usually responds to **splenectomy.** Remember to vaccinate against encapsulated organisms (*Neisseria meningitidis, Streptococcus pneumoniae, Haemophilus influenzae* type b).
- Treatment for **autoimmune hemolytic anemia** include **steroids,** immunosuppressive agents, IVIG, and, if necessary, splenectomy.

Microangiopathic Hemolytic Anemia

Presence of **intravascular hemolysis with fragmented RBCs (schistocytes and helmet cells** on blood smear). This is a **medical emergency.** See also Table 8-5.

- **Disseminated intravascular coagulation (DIC):** Overwhelming systemic activation of the coagulation system stimulated by serious illness. Causes include sepsis, shock, malignancy, obstetric complications, and trauma. This results in thrombosis in the microvasculature and consumption of platelets and coagulation factors, leading to bleeding. There is an ↑ in D-dimer (due to ↑ fibrin split products).
- **Hemolytic-uremic syndrome (HUS):** The triad of hemolytic anemia, thrombocytopenia, and acute kidney injury (AKI). Causes include viral illness and *E coli* O157:H7. **Most common in children.**
- **Thrombotic thrombocytopenic purpura (TTP):** Presents as a **pentad** of the HUS triad plus **fever** and fluctuating **neurologic** signs, although patients may not have all 5 signs. Causes include HIV, pregnancy, and OCP use. There is ↓ ADAMTS13 activity (a protease that cleaves vWF; high levels of vWF multimers accumulate, leading to abnormal platelets).

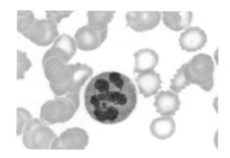

FIGURE 8-4. Hypersegmented neutrophil seen in megaloblastic anemia.
(Reproduced with permission from USMLE-Rx.com.)

MNEMONIC

The pentad of TTP, a medical emergency—

Run FAST!

Renal failure
Fever
Anemia (microangiopathic hemolytic anemia)
Seizure (CNS dysfunction)
Thrombocytopenia

TABLE 8-4.   Types and Characteristics of Hemolytic Anemia

SUBTYPE	PATHOLOGY	SPECIAL FEATURES
HEREDITARY SPHEROCYTOSIS		
	Mutations in RBC anchoring proteins lead to destabilization in the membrane.	**Smear:** Spherocytes. ⊕ family history, ⊖ Coombs' test.
AUTOIMMUNE HEMOLYTIC ANEMIA		
Cold agglutinin disease	Ig**M** binds to RBC antigens, causing intravascular lysis.	**Smear:** Spherocytes, ⊕ Coombs' test. Acrocyanosis in cold. Cold agglutinin test is ⊕. Seen with *Mycoplasma* infection and **M**ononucleosis.
Warm autoimmune hemolytic anemia	Ig**G** binds to RBC antigens and is cleared by the spleen.	**Smear:** Spherocytes, ⊕ Coombs' test. Can present with jaundice/splenomegaly.
G6PD DEFICIENCY		
	Deficiency in metabolic enzyme. Hemolysis in the presence of infection or drugs (eg, sulfa).	**Smear:** Bite cells (see Figure 8-5). G6PD may be normal during hemolytic episodes but ↓ after.
SICKLE CELL ANEMIA		
	Point mutation leading to sickling of RBCs and subsequent hemolysis and vaso-occlusive crisis.	**Smear:** Sickled cells (see Figure 8-6).
MICROANGIOPATHIC HEMOLYTIC ANEMIA		
	RBC fragments due to shearing through partially coagulated capillaries.	**Smear:** Schistocytes and helmet cells (see Figure 8-7).
OTHER NORMOCYTIC ANEMIA		
Myelofibrosis	Myeloproliferative disorder with abnormally activated fibroblasts. Leads to medullary fibrosis and anemia.	Idiopathic or 2° to polycythemia vera. Can have splenomegaly. Labs: Reticulocytes, teardrop RBCs, ↑ LDH. Dx: Bone marrow; see the discussion of myeloproliferative disorders below.
Paroxysmal nocturnal hemoglobinuria (PNH)	Acquired disorder with intravascular hemolysis and hemoglobinuria.	Recurrent thrombosis and pancytopenia. Dx: Flow cytometry.

KEY FACT

Distinguish HUS from TTP by the presence of neurologic signs in TTP. The treatment of choice for TTP is plasma exchange; for HUS it is dialysis.

TREATMENT

- **DIC:** Treat the underlying condition; transfuse platelets; give protein C concentrate or cryoprecipitate (to replace fibrinogen) and FFP (to replace coagulation factors).
- **TTP:** It is sometimes difficult to distinguish **TTP** from **HUS**. HUS generally has less thrombocytopenia (rarely < 30,000/μL). **Plasma exchange** is given emergently for TTP, and even with treatment, patients can die within the first 24 hours. If clinical decline or neurologic symptoms occur

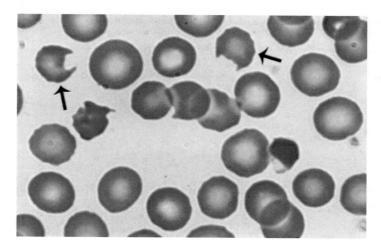

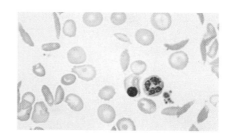

FIGURE 8-6. **Sickled red blood cells.** The elongated and crescent-shaped RBCs seen on this smear represent circulating irreversibly sickled cells. Target cells and a nucleated RBC are also seen. (Reproduced with permission from Fauci AS et al. *Harrison's Principles of Internal Medicine,* 17th ed. New York: McGraw-Hill, 2008, Fig. 99-4.)

FIGURE 8-5. **Bite cells associated with G6PD deficiency.** Bite cells can be distinguished from schizocytes by their normal volume and by the retention of their biconcave shape. (Reproduced with permission from Lichtman MA et al. *Lichtman's Atlas of Hematology.* New York: McGraw-Hill, 2007, Plate I.A.6.)

before plasma exchange, **FFP** should be given. **Do not give platelets,** as this may exacerbate the TTP.

- **HUS:** Treat with dialysis for AKI.

Sickle Cell Anemia

An autosomal recessive disease resulting from the substitution of valine for glutamic acid at the sixth position in the globin chain.

SYMPTOMS/EXAM

Seen predominantly among African Americans, who often have a family history. Clinical features include:

- Chronic hemolysis resulting in gallstones, poorly healing ulcers, jaundice, splenomegaly (usually during childhood), and CHF.
- **Pain** due to vaso-occlusion (most commonly musculoskeletal).

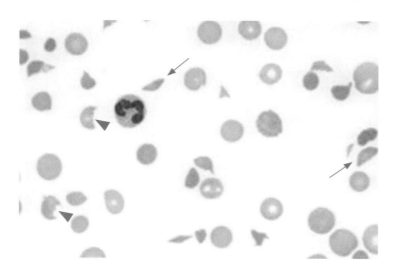

FIGURE 8-7. **Schistocytes (arrows) and helmet cells (arrowheads) in a patient with DIC.** (Reproduced with permission from USMLERx.com.)

KEY FACT

Hydroxyurea is a chemotherapeutic agent that ↓ HbS and ↑ fetal hemoglobin (HbF). It should be considered in sickle cell patients with frequent pain crises and a history of strokes or other serious complications.

Q 1

A 32-year-old woman with Crohn's disease and a history of partial bowel resection, including resection of the terminal ileum, presents with fatigue and is found to have a hematocrit of 29% and an MCV of 104 fL. Why is she at risk for vitamin B_{12} deficiency?

Q 2

A 59-year-old woman presents for dyspnea on exertion. You find that she has a hematocrit of 31% with an MCV of 89 fL. What are your next steps?

TABLE 8-5. Differential of Microangiopathic Hemolytic Anemia

	PLATELETS	PT/PTT	D-DIMER	OTHER FINDINGS
TTP or HUS	↓↓↓	Normal	Normal	AKI, CNS dysfunction.
DIC	↓↓	↑	↑↑	↑ fibrin split products, ↓ fibrinogen.
Mechanical valve	Normal	Normal	Normal	Heart murmur.
Severe vasculitis, severe hypertension, HELLP	↓	Normal	Normal	Elevated liver enzymes in HELLP.

KEY FACT

As in thalassemia, sickle cell patients who receive frequent transfusions need prophylactic treatment of hemosiderosis with iron chelators such as deferoxamine.

MNEMONIC

Treatment of acute chest syndrome—

TO AID

Transfusion
Oxygen
Antibiotics
Incentive spirometry
Dilators (bronchodilators)

1 · **A**

Intrinsic factor receptors are located in the terminal ileum. Patients with B_{12} absorption deficiencies, such as those with intestinal disease, partial bowel resection, or pernicious anemia, should be treated with injected vitamin B_{12}.

2 · **A**

Check a blood smear, an RC, creatinine, LDH, haptoglobin, and indirect bilirubin, and look for possible bleeding sites. The most common cause of normocytic anemia is anemia of chronic disease. Also consider hemolytic anemia.

DIAGNOSIS

Blood smear shows sickled cells (see Figure 8-6), Howell-Jolly bodies, and evidence of hemolysis. **Hemoglobin electrophoresis** is the definitive diagnostic test.

TREATMENT

- Vaccinate all patients for *S pneumoniae, H influenzae, N meningitidis*, HBV, and the influenza virus.
- Give folic acid.
- Consider transfusions for severe anemia, sickle cell crisis, and priapism.
- Instruct patients to avoid dehydration, hypoxia, intense exercise, and high altitudes.
- In patients with frequent pain crises, hydroxyurea or bone marrow transplantation should be considered.

COMPLICATIONS

The complications of sickle cell disease (see also Figure 8-8) include:

- **Pain (vaso-occlusive) crisis:**
  - Sickled cells cause occlusion of arterioles, leading to tissue ischemia and/or infarction.
  - Characterized by pain in the back, limbs, abdomen, and ribs; precipitated by dehydration, acidosis, infection, fever, or hypoxia.
  - Treat with hydration, analgesia, and supplemental O_2.
- **Aplastic crisis:** A sudden ↓ in hemoglobin and RC caused by parvovirus B19. Support with transfusions.
- **Acute chest syndrome:**
  - A combination of factors, including infection, infarction, and pulmonary fat embolism.
  - Clinical findings include fever, chest pain, cough, wheezing, tachypnea, and new pulmonary infiltrate on CXR.
  - Treat with O_2, analgesia, transfusions, and antibiotics (a second- or third-generation cephalosporin with a macrolide such as erythromycin).
- **Lungs:** Pulmonary infarcts can lead to pulmonary hypertension. This is caused by chronic intravascular hemolysis, which ↓ nitric oxide and leads to pulmonary artery vasoconstriction.
- **Heart:** Sickle cell cardiomyopathy may lead to heart failure.
- **GI tract:** Cholecystitis, which may lead to cholecystectomy; splenic infarcts.

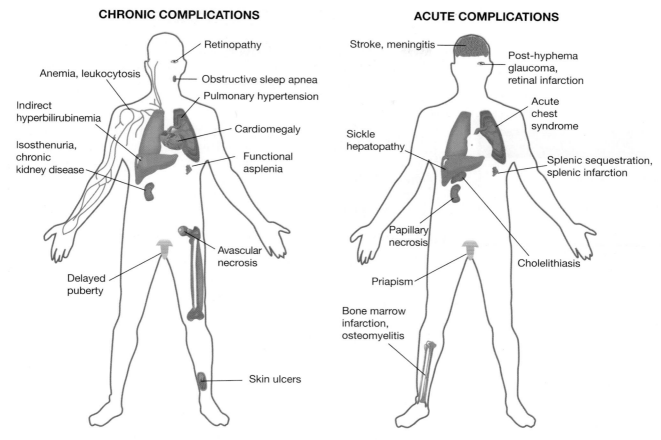

FIGURE 8-8. **Complications of sickle cell disease.** (Adapted with permission from Hall JB et al. *Principles of Critical Care,* 3rd ed. New York: McGraw-Hill, 2005, Fig. 108-1.)

- **Kidneys:** Sickling of cells can cause infarcts, leading to papillary necrosis and AKI (particularly in sickle cell trait).
- **Genital:** Priapism, impotence in males.
- **Infections:** The absence of a functional spleen predisposes patients to encapsulated organisms, including S *pneumoniae,* H *influenzae,* N *meningitidis,* and gram-⊖ bacterial infections.
- **Bones:** Avascular necrosis, *Salmonella* osteomyelitis.
- **CNS:** Stroke is one of the most devastating complications.
- **Pregnancy:** Patients are at ↑ risk of spontaneous abortions.

Myeloproliferative Disorders

A group of conditions—including polycythemia vera (PCV), essential thrombocytosis, 1° myelofibrosis, and chronic myelogenous leukemia (CML)—characterized by abnormal cell growth in the bone marrow. Figure 8-9 shows the relationship of each condition to another.

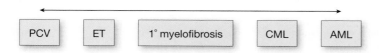

FIGURE 8-9. **Spectrum of myeloproliferative disorders and risk of progression to AML.**

Q **1**

An 8-year-old boy eats at a fast-food restaurant. Two days later he develops bloody diarrhea and is hospitalized. On day 4 he is noted to have dark urine. Labs reveal a hemoglobin level of 8.5 g/dL, a platelet count of 41,000/µL, a creatinine level of 5.6 mg/dL, and schistocytes on blood smear. You diagnose HUS. What is the treatment for his renal failure?

Q **2**

A 5-year-old girl with sickle cell disease is in a kindergarten class with a child who recently developed a facial rash and was diagnosed with fifth disease. The girl's mother calls you for advice. What complication is a concern?

POLYCYTHEMIA VERA (PCV)

A myeloproliferative syndrome in which the predominant abnormality is ↑ RBCs. Classically affects males > 60 years of age. The most common cause of erythrocytosis is **chronic hypoxia** 2° to lung disease rather than 1° PCV.

KEY FACT

Distinguish PCV from other causes of 2° polycythemia through an erythropoietin level. An ↑ erythropoietin level excludes the diagnosis of PCV.

Symptoms/Exam

- Presents with malaise, fever, pruritus (especially after a warm shower involving ↑ histamine release from basophils), and signs of vascular sludging (eg, **stroke**, angina, MI, claudication, hepatic vein thrombosis, **headache**, and **blurred vision**).
- Exam may reveal hypertension, **plethora**, large retinal veins on funduscopy, and **splenomegaly.**

Diagnosis

- Labs show ↑ **hematocrit** (≥ 50%), ↑ RBC mass, and a normal **erythropoietin** level (↑ in chronic hypoxia-induced polycythemia). Basophilia suggests myeloproliferative disorder. JAK-2 ⊕.
- Establish the diagnosis by bone marrow biopsy, which shows a hypercellular marrow.
- Table 8-6 outlines the laboratory features of PCV in contrast to those of other myeloproliferative disorders.

Treatment

- Treatment includes **serial phlebotomy** until hematocrit is < 45% (men) and < 42% (women) along with **daily aspirin.**
- Hydroxyurea is appropriate for those at high risk of thrombosis (age > 60, prior thrombosis, platelet count > 1,500,000/μL, presence of cardiovascular risk factors).

Complications

Like other myeloproliferative syndromes, PCV is associated with an ↑ **risk of conversion** to other myeloproliferative syndromes or AML.

ESSENTIAL THROMBOCYTOSIS

An ↑ platelet count with no Philadelphia chromosome to suggest CML.

1 **A**

Hemodialysis. HUS was likely caused by *E coli* O157:H7 beef contamination.

2 **A**

Aplastic crisis (a sudden ↓ in hemoglobin and RC) due to parvovirus B19, which causes fifth disease. The girl can have a serious aplastic crisis from parvovirus infection because she already has a reduced lifespan of RBCs.

TABLE 8-6. Laboratory Features of Myeloproliferative Disorders

	WBC Count	Hematocrit	Platelet Count	RBC Morphology
CML	↑↑	Normal	Normal or ↑	Normal
Myelofibrosis	Normal or ↓/↑	Normal or ↓	Normal or ↓/↑	**Abnormal**
PCV	Normal or ↑	↑	Normal or ↑	Normal
Essential thrombocytosis	Normal or ↑	Normal	↑	Normal

Reproduced with permission from Tierney LM et al (eds). *Current Medical Diagnosis & Treatment: 2004.* New York: McGraw-Hill, 2004: 481.

SYMPTOMS/EXAM

Many patients are asymptomatic, but symptoms can include digital ischemia (from microvascular thrombi) and erythromelalgia.

DIAGNOSIS

Labs show a platelet count of > 600,000/μL on 2 separate occasions at least 1 month apart. JAK-2 is ⊕ in 50% of patients.

TREATMENT

Thrombosis and bleeding are the principal complications. Therefore, consider platelet-lowering agents in those who are high risk (eg, on hydroxyurea or low-dose aspirin).

1° MYELOFIBROSIS

An abnormal myeloid proliferation with impaired marrow function and extramedullary hematopoiesis.

SYMPTOMS/EXAM

Presents with fever, sweats, weight loss, and hepatosplenomegaly.

DIAGNOSIS

Bone marrow is difficult to aspirate ("dry tap"). Labs show ↑ LDH, alkaline phosphatase, and uric acid.

TREATMENT

- Asymptomatic patients should be followed.
- If symptomatic, treat supportively with transfusions, hydroxyurea, and occasionally splenectomy or radiation. Allogeneic stem cell transplantation may be considered in younger patients.

Bleeding Disorders

Disorders in **coagulation or platelets** that predispose patients to bleed (see Table 8-7 and Figure 8-10).

TABLE 8-7.   **Clinical Features of Coagulopathies and Platelet Disorders**

CLINICAL FEATURE	PLATELET DISORDERS	COAGULOPATHIES
Amount of bleeding after surface cuts	Excessive, prolonged ↑↑↑.	Normal to slightly ↑.
Onset of bleeding after injury	Immediate.	Delayed after surgery or trauma. Spontaneous bleeding into joints or hematoma.
Clinical presentation	Superficial and mucosal bleeding (GI tract, gingival, nasal). Petechiae, ecchymosis.	Deep and excessive bleeding into joints, muscles, GI tract, and GU tract.

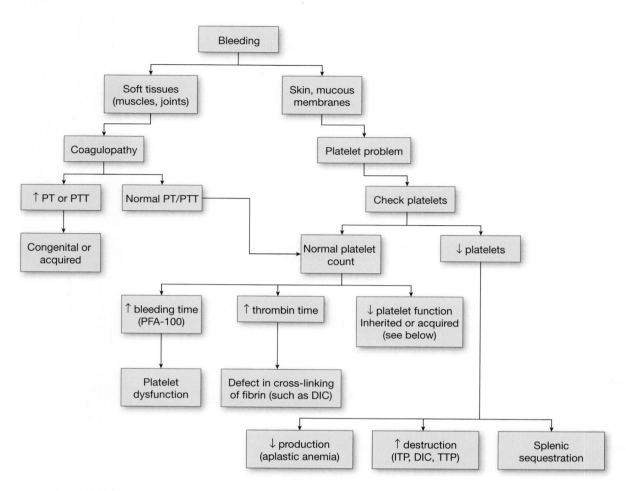

FIGURE 8-10.   **Diagnosis of coagulopathies and platelet disorders.**

KEY FACT

Petechiae = **P**latelet deficiency.
Cavity/joint bleeding = **C**lotting factor
  deficiency.

KEY FACT

Idiopathic **T**hrombocytopenic **P**urpura:
Treat with **P**rednisone.

DIAGNOSIS

- Think **thrombocytopenia** when the platelet count is < 90,000/μL.
- Think **coagulopathy** if the PT or PTT is ↑ (see the discussion of coagulopathies). See Figure 8-10.

TREATMENT

- Patients who are hemodynamically unstable need immediate resuscitation with IV fluids. The source of hemorrhage should be treated.
- Blood transfusions should be given to maintain a hemoglobin level of > 7 g/dL. FFP should be given to normalize PTT and PT. Platelets should be given as needed.

PLATELET DISORDERS

A ↓ in the *number* of platelets (**thrombocytopenia**) or a ↓ in the *functioning* of platelets predisposes patients to bleed (**platelet dysfunction**). Look for petechiae and easy bruising. In addition to TTP and HUS, common platelet disorders include:

- ↑ **platelet destruction:**
  - **ITP/autoimmune thrombocytopenia:** Severe thrombocytopenia due to **platelet-associated IgG** antibodies. A diagnosis of exclusion. DIC panel is ⊖ (see Table 8-5). Treatment involves **prednisone** and, if the patient is unresponsive to steroids, splenectomy.

- **HIT: Immune-mediated thrombocytopenia** occurring 5–14 days after the initiation of heparin (or < 24 hours if previously exposed). Platelet factor-4 (PF-4) antibodies and the serotonin release assay are used for diagnosis. Stop heparin immediately and start an alternative anticoagulant such as fondaparinux, lepirudin, argatroban, or danaparoid sodium (**not** warfarin).
- **Platelet dysfunction—acquired:**
  - **Acquired disease:** Platelet function can be impaired as a result of severe liver disease (from splenic sequestration), severe renal disease, or multiple myeloma. Treat with desmopressin, OCPs (if the patient has resulting menorrhagia), and FFP or cryoprecipitate for major bleeding. Do not use aspirin (inhibits platelet function).
  - **Drug-induced thrombocytopenia:** One of the most common causes of mild asymptomatic thrombocytopenia. Common medications include quinine, antibiotics, sulfa drugs, and glycoprotein IIb/IIIa inhibitors. Usually resolves within 1 week of stopping the implicated drug.
- **Platelet dysfunction—inherited:** Include **Bernard-Soulier syndrome** (a problem with adhesion), **Glanzmann's thrombasthenia** (a problem with aggregation), and **storage pool disease** (problems with platelet granule release). Treatment is the same as that for acquired disease.

DIAGNOSIS

- Confirm the presence of thrombocytopenia (ie, recheck platelets in citrated blood).
- Check a peripheral blood smear and a 1-hour posttransfusion platelet count to distinguish ↓ **platelet production** (pancytopenia; small platelets; ↑ platelet count following platelet transfusion) from ↑ **platelet destruction** (large platelets; no significant ↑ in platelet count after platelet transfusion).
- Obtain a bone marrow biopsy in cases of severe thrombocytopenia.

TREATMENT

See above.

COAGULOPATHIES

A defective clotting cascade predisposes patients to bleeding. Ask about medications that predispose to bleeding (eg, warfarin, enoxaparin, heparin); note factors that predispose to **vitamin K** deficiency (eg, liver disease, malnutrition, antibiotic use, alcoholism).

- Recurrent **spontaneous** bleeding suggests a **factor deficiency** (eg, factor VIII [hemophilia A] or factor IX [hemophilia B]).
- **Delayed** bleeding after trauma or surgery (classically after the umbilical cord falls off) suggests factor **XIII** deficiency.

DIAGNOSIS

- Look for evidence of liver disease on exam and order LFTs and PT/PTT.
- Defects in the clotting cascade can be due to defects in the intrinsic pathway, the extrinsic pathway, or the common pathway.
  - **Intrinsic pathway:** Involves **factors VIII, IX, XI, and XII.** Abnormality results in an ↑ in aPTT. Impaired in patients with **hemophilia A (factor VIII)** or **B (factor IX).**
  - **Extrinsic pathway:** Involves **factor VII.** Abnormality leads to an ↑ in **PT (INR). Prolonged by warfarin.**
  - **Common pathway:** Involves **factors V, X, and II (prothrombin).** An ↑ is seen in **both aPTT and PT (INR).**
- A diagnostic approach toward patients with coagulation disorders is summarized in Figure 8-11.

KEY FACT

Generally, treat with platelet transfusion if platelet count is:

- < 100,000 before neurosurgery
- < 50,000 before a general procedure or symptomatic
- < 20,000 in an asymptomatic patient who has fever/sepsis, is receiving heparin, or will be outpatient soon
- < 10,000 in an asymptomatic patient

Q **1**

You are called to the ICU to evaluate a 64-year-old woman who was admitted 6 days ago, following cardiac surgery, for a "black" rash. Exam reveals necrotic patches of skin on the distal extremities. Her medications include furosemide, enoxaparin, enalapril, amlodipine, insulin, and aspirin. Her platelet count is 36,000/μL with ⊕ PF-4 antibodies. What condition accounts for her skin necrosis?

Q **2**

A 19-year-old man with hemophilia A comes to the ED after having fallen on his knee 2 hours ago. His knee is now red, warm, and held in partial flexion as a result of an effusion. What medication should be used to reverse his coagulopathy?

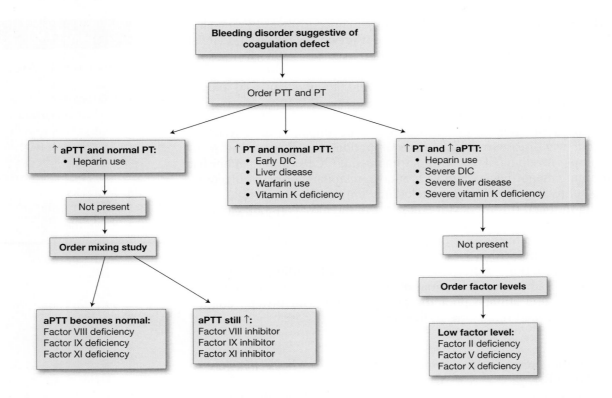

FIGURE 8-11. **Approach to patients with bleeding disorders suggestive of a coagulation defect.**

TREATMENT

- Coagulopathic patients who are actively bleeding need **FFP** to normalize their PT and PTT levels. Heparin and warfarin must be stopped.
- If vitamin K deficiency is suspected, it is reasonable to empirically give 10 mg of oral vitamin K for 3 days to see if PT normalizes.
- Patients with hemophilia A or B require **factor VIII** (either recombinant factor VIII or as cryoprecipitate) or **factor IX** replacement, respectively.

von Willebrand's Disease (vWD)

An autosomal dominant condition that is the most common bleeding disorder. It is characterized by low levels of von Willebrand's factor (vWF), which is involved in the transport of **factor VIII** and also helps platelets form a hemostatic plug.

SYMPTOMS/EXAM

Clinical features can mimic platelet dysfunction (causing mucocutaneous bleeds and ↑ bleeding time) as well as hemophilia (joint bleeds, ↑ aPTT) depending on the subtype.

DIAGNOSIS

Diagnosed by ↓ levels of vWF antigen and/or by abnormal vWF activity (ristocetin cofactor activity).

TREATMENT

- Generally, **no treatment is routinely required except before surgical procedures or in the setting of bleeding.**

---

1 **A**

Heparin-induced thrombocytopenia (HIT) platelet activation and thrombosis causing heparin-induced skin necrosis. The immune system forms antibodies to heparin when it is bound to platelet factor 4.

2 **A**

Recombinant factor VIII. Adjunctive treatments include joint rest, ice, analgesia (but avoid salicylates and NSAIDs), and sometimes joint aspiration.

- **Desmopressin** (increases endothelial release of vWF) is first-line therapy in symptomatic cases.

Hypercoagulable State (Thrombophilia)

Thrombophilias are a group of conditions that predispose patients to blood clotting. May be inherited or acquired (see Table 8-8).

Symptoms/Exam

Look for possible 1° **causes of hypercoagulability** in the following patients:

- Those with a history of a first venous thrombotic event before age 50.
- Those with recurrent thrombotic episodes.
- Those who have had a thrombotic event as well as a first-degree relative who experienced a thromboembolic event before age 50.

TABLE 8-8. Inherited vs Acquired Thrombophilias

CONDITION	PATHOLOGY	DIAGNOSIS/COMMENTS
INHERITED		
Factor V Leiden	Mutation disrupts activated protein C (APC), which slows the breakdown of Va and ultimately VIIIa.	Most common.
Prothrombin G20210A mutation	Mutation stabilizes and thus ↑ prothrombin.	Confirm with DNA testing. Second most common.
Protein C or S deficiency	Protein C normally inactivates Va and VIIIa. Mutation affects protein C synthesis. Protein S is a cofactor for protein C.	Warfarin carries a risk of skin necrosis.
Anti–thrombin III deficiency	Antithrombin typically inhibits thrombin and factor Xa.	Can result in heparin resistance.
Hyperhomocysteinemia	Inherited or acquired.	
ACQUIRED[a]		
Antiphospholipid syndrome	Any thrombosis and > 3 miscarriages before 10 weeks or 1 after 10 weeks.	⊕ anticardiolipin or lupus anticoagulant antibodies.
Cancer	Expresses tissue factor on surfaces and leads to a prothrombotic state.	Cancer screening.

[a] Acquired thrombophilia is associated with prolonged rest, immobilization, smoking, OCP use, pregnancy, nephrotic syndrome, cancer, DIC, and lupus anticoagulant (antiphospholipid syndrome).

 KEY FACT

Desmopressin, also known as ADH, ↑ circulating concentrations of factor VIII and vWF while also improving platelet adhesion. Classic uses are to reverse coagulopathic hemorrhage in vWD and hemophilia.

 KEY FACT

von **W**illebrand's **D**isease: Treat **W**ith **D**esmopressin.

 KEY FACT

Factor V Leiden deficiency, the most common inherited hypercoagulable disorder, is screened with an APC resistance assay and is confirmed with DNA testing. Factor V Leiden mutation disrupts the activated protein C cleavage sites.

 KEY FACT

Remember: Factor **Vee**—check AP**C.**

 Q

A 28-year-old G2P1 at 28 weeks' gestation comes to a routine pregnancy check complaining of unilateral ankle swelling. Her left leg is > 2 cm larger than her right, and ultrasound shows a noncompressible left popliteal vein. Which anticoagulant will you start, and for what duration?

DIAGNOSIS

- Screening should include APC resistance, prothrombin gene mutation, antiphospholipid antibody, plasma homocysteine, antithrombin deficiency, protein C deficiency, and protein S deficiency.
- Protein C, protein S, and antithrombin III are affected by acute thrombosis or anticoagulation. Check levels for at least 2–4 weeks after completing anticoagulation.

TREATMENT

- Acute thrombosis must be treated with at least 6 months of anticoagulation with warfarin.
- Indications for **lifelong anticoagulation** include > 2 spontaneous thromboses, antithrombin deficiency, antiphospholipid syndrome, spontaneous life-threatening thrombosis, and thrombosis in an unusual site (eg, the mesenteric or cerebral vein).
- Warfarin takes 3–5 days to reach its therapeutic effect, can lead to serious skin necrosis in those with protein C deficiency, and can initially be thrombotic. Thus, **bridge with heparin.**
- Pregnant women with a history of hypercoagulable state need to be treated with LMWH.
- Hyperhomocysteinemia can be treated with vitamin B_{12} and folate.

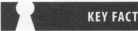

Transfusion Reactions

The complications of transfusion-related reactions are listed in Table 8-9.

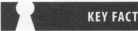
KEY FACT

Virchow's triad: vessel wall trauma, venous stasis, and alterations in coagulation.

KEY FACT

Bridge the initiation of warfarin therapy with IV heparin for at least 5 days until INR rises to the therapeutic goal. (Factor II and X levels require at least 5 days to decline.)

A

Start LMWH, and continue until 24 hours before delivery (more easily done if you are inducing). Restart after delivery, and continue anticoagulation for 6 weeks. Although a known teratogen, warfarin is considered safe for nursing mothers and remains an option postpartum.

TABLE 8-9.   Transfusion Complications

	CLINICAL	PATHOLOGY	TESTS	MANAGEMENT
Acute hemolytic reaction (< 24 hours)	Chills, fever, shortness of breath, nausea, chest/flank pain, hypotension, flushing. Complications: AKI (from hemoglobinuria), DIC.	Caused by ABO incompatibility between donor and recipient.	⊕ Coombs' test, agglutination of RBC on smear, low haptoglobin (best test). UA for hemoglobinuria (⊕ urine dip for hematuria in the setting of few RBCs on microscopy).	Stop transfusion. Maintain BP and urine output with IV fluids; give furosemide if urine output is < 100 mL/hr. Type and cross RBCs just transfused.
Delayed hemolysis	Onset 4–14 days posttransfusion. Jaundice, anemia, hemoglobinuria, fever.	Previous exposure to erythrocyte antigen outside the ABO system; can develop alloantibodies after transfusion.	↑ LDH, unconjugated hyperbilirubinemia, ↓ haptoglobin.	Type and screen blood before future transfusions. Acetaminophen for fever. Patients with sickle cell disease may have a worsening pain crisis.
Febrile, nonhemolytic reaction	Onset within 2 hours posttransfusion. Fever, rigors, nausea, vomiting, chills.	Interaction between recipient leukoreactive antibodies and donor cytokines.	Rule out acute hemolytic reaction or infectious cause of hemolysis.	For future transfusions, use **leukocyte-reduced** RBCs. Avoid transfusion when febrile.
Allergic: urticaria	Rash, pruritus.			Stop transfusion; monitor for anaphylaxis. Give diphenhydramine or other antihistamines. Resume transfusion at a slower rate when symptoms resolve.
Transfusion-related acute lung injury (TRALI)	Occurs 1–6 hours posttransfusion. Like ARDS of the lung. Acute respiratory distress, cyanosis, fever; gone in 24 hours. DDx: Fluid overload.	Reaction between donor antibodies against recipient neutrophil antigens.	CXR shows bilateral pulmonary infiltrates without CHF.	Ventilation (O_2, intubation), diuretics, steroids.
Bacterial infection	More likely with platelets (because they are stored at room temperature). Fever, hypotension; onset within 4 hours.		Culture remaining blood product.	Antibiotics.

Reproduced with permission from Le T et al. *First Aid for the USMLE Step 2,* 4th ed. New York: McGraw-Hill, 2003: 202.

NOTES

CHAPTER 9

ONCOLOGY

Hematologic Malignancies

LEUKEMIA

Defined as malignant proliferations of hematopoietic cells. Leukemias may be myelogenous or lymphocytic and may have an acute or chronic course, but all are typically characterized by marrow failure that produces anemia, infections, and bleeding by reducing RBCs, WBCs, and platelets, respectively (see Table 9-1). Characterized as follows:

- **Acute leukemia:**
    - **Immature** cells (myeloblasts, lymphoblasts).
    - At least 20% blasts in bone marrow (cases with < 20% blasts are defined as *myelodysplastic syndrome*).
    - Typically affects the very young or the elderly with a short and potentially life-threatening course.
- **Chronic leukemia:**
    - More **mature** differentiated cells (metamyelocytes/myelocytes and lymphocytes).
    - Affects the middle-aged and has a longer and less destructive course.

LYMPHOMA

Lymphomas result from monoclonal proliferation of cells of lymphocyte lineage. Approximately 90% are derived from B cells, 9% from T cells, and 1% from monocytes or natural killer (NK) cells. There are 2 main types: Hodgkin's and non-Hodgkin's lymphoma (see Table 9-2).

Hodgkin's Lymphoma

A malignancy that is thought to arise from B cells and is associated with neoplastic Reed-Sternberg cells (see Figure 9-1). EBV infection may play a role in its pathogenesis. Usually affects young adults, but has a bimodal distribution.

SYMPTOMS/EXAM

- Usually presents with **cervical or mediastinal lymphadenopathy** and spreads in a contiguous manner along the lymph nodes. The **spleen** is the most commonly involved intra-abdominal site.
- **B symptoms** are defined as **10% weight loss in 6 months, night sweats requiring a change of clothes/sheets, and fever > 38.5°C (101.3°F).** These symptoms indicate bulky disease and a worse prognosis.

DIAGNOSIS

- Excisional lymph node biopsy shows Reed-Sternberg cells.
- Staging is based on anatomic lymph node involvement; prognosis depends on stage and other risk factors. PET/CT of the chest, abdomen, and pelvis are routinely done; bone marrow biopsies may also be considered.

TREATMENT

Chemotherapy with doxorubicin (Adriamycin), bleomycin, vinblastine, and dacarbazine (**ABVD cocktail**) +/− radiation of the involved field.

Non-Hodgkin's Lymphoma

A proliferation of B and occasionally T cells; classified as indolent or aggressive on the basis of histologic type (see Table 9-3). Extranodal involvement

KEY FACT

- T and B lymphocytes and natural killer cells are derived from a common **lymphoid** progenitor.
- Megakaryocytes, neutrophils, eosinophils, basophils, monocytes, erythrocytes, and mast cells are derived from a common **myeloid** progenitor.

KEY FACT

Lymphadenopathy, splenomegaly, and CNS involvement are common in ALL but rare in AML.

KEY FACT

Cytoplasmic Auer rods are diagnostic for AML.

KEY FACT

Stem cell transplantation is used for a variety of hematologic malignancies and has 2 types:

- **Autologous:** The patient serves as the source of stem cells.
- **Allogeneic:** Stem cells are acquired from a matched donor.

KEY FACT

Stem cell transplantation has many treatment-related toxicities, including **graft-versus-host disease,** in which lymphocytes from the donor mount an immune response to the patient's organs, potentially affecting the skin, GI tract, liver, lungs, bone marrow, and soft tissues. Immunosuppressive agents mitigate the risk.

is common. Associated with infections—EBV with Burkitt's lymphoma; HIV with CNS lymphoma; HTLV with T-cell lymphoma; and *H pylori* with gastric MALToma. **Diffuse large B-cell lymphoma** is the most common type.

SYMPTOMS

Similar to other lymphomas. Lymphadenopathy typically occurs in groups of peripheral nodes, and patients may have **fewer B symptoms.**

DIAGNOSIS

Similar to that of Hodgkin's lymphoma (see above). LDH is a prognostic marker. Excisional biopsy is preferred to FNA for the evaluation of lymph node architecture.

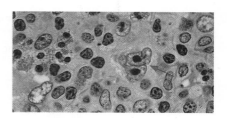

FIGURE 9-1. Hodgkin's lymphoma. A Reed-Sternberg cell shows a characteristic "owl's eye" appearance (arrow). (Reproduced with permission from Longo DL et al. *Harrison's Principles of Internal Medicine*, 18th ed. New York: McGraw-Hill, 2012, Fig. 110-11.)

TABLE 9-1. Characteristics of Acute and Chronic Leukemias

	ACUTE LYMPHOCYTIC LEUKEMIA (ALL)	ACUTE MYELOGENOUS LEUKEMIA (AML)	CHRONIC LYMPHOCYTIC LEUKEMIA (CLL)	CHRONIC MYELOGENOUS LEUKEMIA (CML)
Epidemiology	Most common in **children;** ↑ risk in Down syndrome.	Median age 65. Risk ↑ with **age** and with **previous chemotherapy** or radiation.	The **most common** adult leukemia; affects those > 65 years of age.	Affects the **middle-aged.** Risk ↑ with previous radiation.
Symptoms	**Viral-like syndrome; bone pain** and bruising.	**Fever,** bruising, fatigue, **anemia,** or frequent **infections.**	Often asymptomatic; may be an incidental finding on CBC. Can present with fatigue and B symptoms.	**Chronic phase:** Asymptomatic or presents with fatigue, weight loss, night sweats (B symptoms), and **splenomegaly. Accelerated or blastic phase:** Worsening symptoms; **bone pain, bleeding** (platelet dysfunction), infections.
Exam	Pallor, petechiae/purpura (see Figure 9-2), bleeding. Adenopathy, hepatomegaly, splenomegaly, testicular and CNS involvement. T-cell ALL often presents with an **anterior mediastinal mass.**	Petechiae/purpura (see Figure 9-2), lethargy, **leukemia cutis** (small, raised, painless skin lesions). Gingival hyperplasia, CNS involvement, **DIC,** or **tumor lysis syndrome.**	**Lymphadenopathy** and hepatosplenomegaly in addition to leukemic cells.	**Splenomegaly,** early satiety, purpura.
Differential	**AML.**	**ALL. Acute promyelocytic leukemia** (APL/AML M3): A different variant of AML; ⊕ (15;17) gene translocation.	**Mantle cell lymphoma:** Typically more aggressive, with extranodal involvement in the small intestine, colon, and bone marrow. ⊕ cyclin D1 and t(11;14) translocation.	**Hairy cell leukemia:** B lymphocytes with hairy cytoplasmic projections (see Figure 9-3); **CD11c, TRAP** ⊕, CD103 ⊕. In addition to aplastic anemia and myelofibrosis, it is a common cause of a "dry" bone marrow aspiration or tap.

TABLE 9-1. **Characteristics of Acute and Chronic Leukemias** *(continued)*

	ACUTE LYMPHOCYTIC LEUKEMIA (ALL)	ACUTE MYELOGENOUS LEUKEMIA (AML)	CHRONIC LYMPHOCYTIC LEUKEMIA (CLL)	CHRONIC MYELOGENOUS LEUKEMIA (CML)

Diagnosis	• ↑ or ↓ leukocytes; ↓↓ platelets.
	• ↑ **LDH**, ↑ **uric acid** (from tumor lysis).
	• **Smear:** Lymphoblasts.
	• **Bone marrow:** More than 20% lymphoblasts.
	• Order CXR, LP, and CT for mediastinal or brain involvement.
		• ↑ **uric acid** from ↑ cell turnover.
		• **Smear:** Predominance of myeloblasts with Auer rods (see Figure 9-4).
		• **Bone marrow:** More than 20% blasts, hypercellular (⊕ **myelo-peroxidase staining**) and cytogenetics.
			• **Lymphocytosis.**
			• **Smear:** Predominance of small lymphocytes.
			• **Smudge cells** may be present (see Figure 9-5).
			• **Bone marrow:** Lymphocytes, **CD5** (T-cell marker) and CD23 ⊕.
				• ↑↑ WBC count (median 150,000 cells/μL).
				• **Smear:** ↑ WBCs (mature and immature, primarily neutrophils or granulocytes) and basophilia.
				• **Bone marrow:**
				  • **Chronic:** Fewer than 10% blasts.
				  • **Accelerated:** 10–19% blasts.
				  • **Blastic:** More than 20% blasts.
				• Confirm t(9;22) Philadelphia chromosome bcr-abl gene.

Treatment	**Chemotherapy induction:** To **induce remission** (destroy all blasts). Usually **cyclophosphamide +** vincristine + prednisone + daunorubicin. Use prophylactic CNS therapy (intrathecal chemotherapy). **Consolidation:** To **kill any residual leukemia.** **Maintenance: Maintain remission.** Daily methotrexate, 6-mercaptopurine, or both.	**Chemotherapy induction:** Cytosine arabinoside (Ara-C) + anthracycline and consolidation chemotherapy. **APL treatment:** Add *all*-trans-retinoic acid (ATRA). **Allogeneic bone marrow transplantation (BMT):** If poor prognostic factors. **Tumor lysis prevention/ treatment:** IV fluid; allopurinol +/– rasburicase.	**No treatment is indicated for asymptomatic patients; often indolent disease.** Anemia and thrombocytopenia have ↓ survival. Symptomatic patients are treated with a fludarabine-based regimen. May be associated with **autoimmune hemolytic anemia** and **ITP,** which can be treated with splenectomy and/or steroids.	**Treat even if asymptomatic.** **Imatinib (Gleevec)** specifically targets and inhibits **bcr-abl** tyrosine kinase and eliminates the CML clone. **Allogeneic BMT** can be curative in select patients and should be more strongly considered for patients in the accelerated or blast phase.
Prognosis/ complications	**Children:** Nearly all achieve complete remission; 80% achieve long-term leukemia-free survival. **Adults:** 25–40% cure rate.	Depending on risk factor profile, 5-year survival rates range from 15% to 60%. Treatment of transplant patients can be complicated by graft-versus-host disease.	Stage dependent; prognosis can range from 18 months to > 10 years. ↑ risk of 2° malignancies and transformation to more aggressive disease, including large cell lymphoma (Richter transformation).	Stage dependent. Since the introduction of tyrosine kinase inhibitors (eg, imatinib), 5-year survival rates have ↑ to 70–80% (lower in the elderly). Many patients eventually progress to blast crisis/acute leukemia.

TREATMENT

- Chemotherapy with rituximab (monoclonal anti-CD20) plus cyclophosphamide, hydroxydoxorubicin, vincristine (Oncovin), and prednisone (**R-CHOP**).
- Treatment of **high-grade** non-Hodgkin's lymphoma may be complicated by **tumor lysis syndrome** (see below). Treat with **aggressive hydration** and **allopurinol.**
- Gastric MALTomas can be treated with antibiotics for *H pylori* as initial therapy.
- All HIV-related non-Hodgkin's lymphoma requires initiation of antiretroviral therapy.

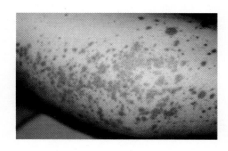

FIGURE 9-2.   Scattered nonblanchable petechiae coalescing into purpura on the lower limb. (Reproduced with permission from Lichtman MA et al. *Williams Hematology,* 8th ed. New York: McGraw-Hill, 2010, Fig. 123-5.)

TUMOR LYSIS SYNDROME

A metabolic disturbance that may follow the initiation of cancer therapy. Most often associated with high-grade lymphomas or ALL. An **oncologic emergency!**

SYMPTOMS/EXAM

- Tumor cell lysis results in severe **hyperkalemia, hyperphosphatemia, hyperuricemia, and hypocalcemia. Hyperuricemia** results from the release of large amounts of serum nucleic acids, and hypocalcemia is 2° to calcium phosphate deposition. Can quickly lead to renal failure from uric acid crystal and calcium phosphate deposition.
- Clinical manifestations may also include **seizure, cardiac arrhythmia, or sudden death.**

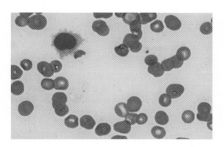

FIGURE 9-3.   Hairy cell in peripheral blood with cytoplasmic projections. Note the single neoplastic cell with fine, hairlike projections extending from its surface. (Reproduced with permission from Kemp WL et al. *Pathology: The Big Picture.* New York: McGraw-Hill, 2008, Figure 12-22.)

TREATMENT

- **Prevent** with adequate IV hydration and the reduction of uric acid with allopurinol or rasburicase (the drug of choice if uric acid levels are high before the initiation of chemotherapy).
- Correct electrolyte abnormalities using phosphate binders, calcium gluconate, sodium polystyrene sulfonate, insulin, and sodium bicarbonate.
- Consider dialysis if abnormalities are severe or do not respond to therapies.

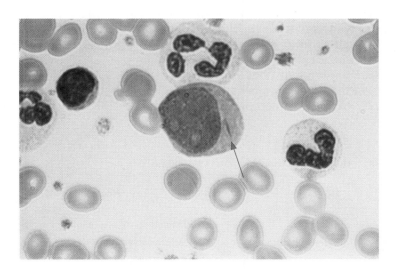

FIGURE 9-4.   Leukemic myeloblast with an Auer rod. Note the large, prominent nucleoli. (Reproduced with permission from Longo DL et al. *Harrison's Principles of Internal Medicine,* 18th ed. New York: McGraw-Hill, 2012, Fig. 109-1B.)

Q   1

A 70-year-old man presents with fatigue. His physical exam is unrevealing, but a routine CBC shows lymphocytosis with a normal hematocrit and platelet count. What is the next step in diagnosis?

Q   2

A 30-year-old man presents with a temperature of 38.7°C (101.7°F), drenching night sweats, and weight loss of 6 months' duration. Exam reveals cervical lymphadenopathy. He is not incarcerated and has no travel history or exposure to sick contacts. What diagnosis do you consider, and what is the next step in diagnosis?

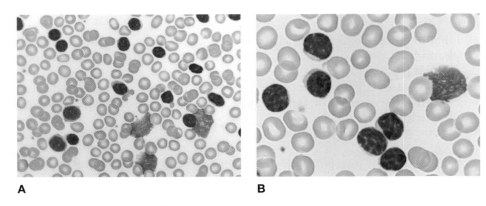

A   **B**

FIGURE 9-5.   Smudge cells in CLL. (A) Classic presentation composed predominantly of small lymphocytes with scant cytoplasm along with three smudge cells. (B) Small lymphocytes with a thin rim of cytoplasm, dense chromatin, and generally unapparent nucleoli are seen along with a smudge cell. (Reproduced with permission from Lichtman MA et al. *Williams Hematology,* 8th ed. New York: McGraw-Hill, 2010, Fig. 94-1A and B.)

KEY FACT

- **Hodgkin's lymphoma:** Cervical/mediastinal lymphadenopathy; centrifugal spread.
- **Non-Hodgkin's lymphoma:** Noncontiguous spread; can present with diffuse lymphadenopathy.

KEY FACT

EBV is associated with aggressive lymphomas (eg, Burkitt's) in patients with immune deficiencies such as HIV.

1   A

Obtain a peripheral smear to check for smudge cells. Chronic lymphocytic leukemia is the most common type of leukemia encountered in adults.

2   A

Given the patient's history, an infectious etiology such as TB or HIV is unlikely. An excisional lymph node biopsy should be done to rule out lymphoma in a young patient with B symptoms (weight loss, night sweats, fever).

MULTIPLE MYELOMA

A malignancy of monoclonal **plasma cells** within bone marrow, often with unbalanced, excessive production of immunoglobulin protein. Typically seen in **older adults.**

SYMPTOMS/EXAM

- **Bone pain, hypercalcemic symptoms** ("stones, bones, abdominal groans, and psychiatric overtones"), **pathologic fractures,** fatigue, and frequent infections (2° to dysregulation of antibody production).
- Pallor, fever, bone tenderness (see Table 9-4), and lethargy.

DIFFERENTIAL

The differential includes the following (see also Table 9-5):

- **Waldenström's macroglobulinemia:** Similar to multiple myeloma, but with ↑ **IgM.**
  - ↑ cold agglutinins (can cause autoimmune hemolysis, lymphadenopathy, and hepatosplenomegaly).
  - Hyperviscosity syndrome (visual disturbance, dizziness, headache). Treat with urgent plasmapheresis.
- **Monoclonal gammopathy of undetermined significance (MGUS):**
  - Found incidentally on protein electrophoresis.
  - M protein < 3 g/dL.
  - Fewer than 10% plasma cells on bone marrow.
  - No **CRAB**s (see mnemonic).

TABLE 9-2.   Hodgkin's vs Non-Hodgkin's Lymphoma

HODGKIN'S	NON-HODGKIN'S
Reed-Sternberg cells	No Reed-Sternberg cells
Mediastinal mass/lymph nodes	**Peripheral lymph nodes**
B symptoms	Fewer B symptoms
Contiguous spread	Typically noncontiguous
Young (but bimodal)	Old/middle-age

TABLE 9-3. Indolent vs Aggressive Non-Hodgkin's Lymphoma

INDOLENT	AGGRESSIVE
Follicular	Diffuse large B-cell lymphoma
MALT	Mantle cell
Marginal zone	Peripheral T cell
Small lymphocytic lymphoma	Anaplastic
	Burkitt's lymphoma

DIAGNOSIS

- Critical tests to evaluate for the presence of multiple myeloma (and to distinguish it from Waldenström's) include UPEP/UIFE and SPEP/SIFE.
- Bone marrow shows **clonal plasma cells** (> 10%), and a **full-body skeletal survey** may demonstrate **"punched-out" osteolytic lesions** of the skull and long bones (see Figure 9-6A and B).

TREATMENT

- Determine if the patient is a candidate for high-dose chemotherapy and stem cell transplantation. β-microglobulin and albumin are prognostic markers.
    - **Transplant candidates:** Bortezomib- or lenalidomide-based regimens. Autologous stem cell transplantation improves disease-free and overall survival.
    - **Non–transplant candidates:** Melphalan-based therapy +/– lenalidomide or bortezomib.
- Symptom relief and prevention:
    - **Hypercalcemia:** Hydration, bisphosphonates, and diuresis.
    - **Bone pain/destruction/fractures:** Bisphosphonates, radiation, and kyphoplasty.
    - **Renal failure:** Hydration to help prevent myeloma cast nephropathy due to high concentration/precipitation in the renal tubules.
    - **Infections:** Vaccinate, diagnose early, and treat appropriately.
    - **Anemia:** Erythropoietin, transfusions.
    - **Thrombosis:** Monitor closely.

AMYLOIDOSIS

There are many types of amyloidosis, but all are characterized by tissue deposition of abnormal protein fibrils. AL amyloidosis, one of the most common types, is a disorder of plasma cells that leads to deposition of monoclonal light

TABLE 9-4. Bone Lesions and Associated Malignancies

BONE LESIONS	ASSOCIATED CANCER
OsteoLytic	Myeloma, kidney, lung, breast, GI (can see on plain films).
OsteoBlastic	Prostate, breast (may be mixed), germ cell, ovary, uterus (less likely to be seen on plain films).

KEY FACT

- **Leukemia:** Can be detected in circulating cells.
- **Lymphoma:** Produces tumor masses.
- **Lymphoma/leukemia:** Can be detected in circulating cells; produce tumor masses (eg, CLL).

MNEMONIC

Myeloma symptoms—

CRAB

hyper**C**alcemia
Renal failure
Anemia
Bone lesions (lytic)

Q **1**

A 65-year-old woman presents with back pain and fatigue. Routine lab testing reveals anemia, hypercalcemia, and renal failure. A bone scan shows multiple lytic lesions. What is your diagnosis, and which other tests should you order?

Q **2**

A 68-year-old man presents with lower extremity edema, dyspnea on exertion, periorbital bruising, and ↑ tongue size. He is found to have nephrotic-range proteinuria and a low-voltage ECG. What is a possible diagnosis, and which other minimally invasive test can help confirm the diagnosis?

TABLE 9-5.   Differential Diagnosis of Multiple Myeloma

	Multiple Myeloma	Waldenstrom's Macroglobulinemia	MGUS
Plasma cells	> 10%	> 10%	< 10%
M protein	> 3 g/dL	> 3 g/dL, IgM	< 3 g/dL
Other	**CRAB** symptoms (see mnemonic)	Lymphadenopathy, hepatosplenomegaly, hyperviscosity	Incidental finding, asymptomatic

chains in organs such as the kidney and heart, resulting in proteinuria and restrictive cardiomyopathy (see Table 9-6).

DIAGNOSIS

- **Fat aspirate:** When amyloid proteins are stained with Congo red, they demonstrate an **apple-green** birefringence under polarized light (see Figure 9-7).
- Without treatment, the prognosis for AL amyloidosis is poor. The key is to think about the diagnosis earlier in the differential to prevent further organ dysfunction from delayed treatment.

Breast Cancer

The most commonly diagnosed cancer and the second most common cause of cancer death in women in the United States (after lung cancer). Annual or biennial screening mammography is recommended after age 50 (or earlier for high-risk cases and patients with a ⊕ family history). Screening mammography for those who are 40–50 years of age and not at high risk is controversial.

---

1   **A**

With renal failure, anemia, hypercalcemia, and lytic bone lesions, think **multiple myeloma** and order:
- **SPEP:** To quantify M protein (most commonly **IgG, > 3 g/dL**).
- **SIFE:** To determine immunoglobulin type and monoclonality.
- **UPEP:** To determine the presence of Bence Jones protein in the urine.
- **UIFE:** To identify the types of light chains in the urine.

2   **A**

AL amyloidosis and fat pad aspirate. A fat pad aspirate is highly sensitive and specific for amyloidosis.

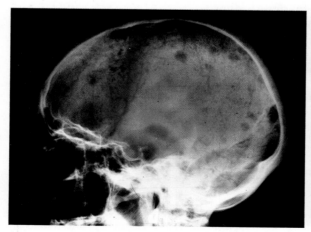
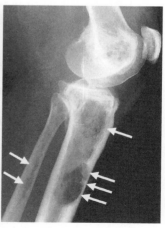

A   B

FIGURE 9-6.   **Multiple myeloma.** (**A**) Radiograph of the skull showing "punched out" osteolytic lesions characteristic of multiple myeloma. (**B**) Lateral view of the tibia and fibula showing focal lytic lesions (arrows). (Image A reproduced with permission from Kantarjian HM et al. *The MD Anderson Manual of Medical Oncology*, 2nd ed. New York: McGraw-Hill, 2011, Fig. 11-2. Image B reproduced with permission from Lichtman MA et al. *Williams Hematology*, 8th ed. New York: McGraw-Hill, 2010, Fig. 109-13A.)

TABLE 9-6.   **Types of Amyloidosis**

	AL	AA	ATTR (TRANSTHYRETIN)
Protein source	Bone marrow, clonal plasma cells.	2° inflammatory reaction to an infection or a rheumatologic disorder, creating an abundance of amyloid A (AA) protein.	Liver.
Most common organ involvement	Heart and kidneys.	Kidneys.	Heart, nerves.
Treatment	Chemotherapy, autologous stem cell transplant.	Treat the underlying infection or inflammation.	Determine if wild type or hereditary type. New drug stabilizing agents. Liver transplant for familial ATTR.

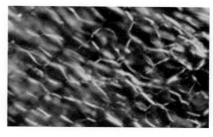

FIGURE 9-7.   **Subcutaneous fat aspirate in amyloidosis.** Note the apple-green birefringence when viewed under polarized light. (Reproduced with permission from Lichtman MA et al. *Williams Hematology*, 8th ed. New York: McGraw-Hill, 2010, Fig. 110-1C.)

Currently there is insufficient evidence to recommend screening in women > 75 years of age. Risk factors include:

- Female gender
- Older age
- Breast cancer in first-degree relatives
- BRCA1/2 mutation
- A history of atypical hyperplasia or carcinoma in situ
- Early menarche, late menopause, or first childbirth after 30 years
- HRT use for > 5 years
- Obesity
- ↑ alcohol intake (2–5 drinks per day)
- Prior radiation (eg, for treatment of Hodgkin's lymphoma)

Symptoms/Exam

- Most masses are discovered by the patient and present as a **hard, irregular, immobile, painless breast lump,** possibly with nipple discharge.
- **Skin changes** (dimpling, erythema, ulceration) and **axillary adenopathy** indicate more advanced disease.

Diagnosis

- Look for a palpable mass or check a mammogram for microcalcifications, hyperdense regions, and irregular borders. Confirm with biopsy.
- **Ultrasound** is appropriate in younger women with dense breasts or in those > 35 years of age with any breast lump, especially after a ⊖ mammogram (to check for cystic vs solid lesions).
- Consider **breast MRI,** FNA, or stereotactic core **biopsy** until the absence of cancer has been confirmed.

KEY FACT

The sensitivity of mammography for breast cancer is only 75–80%, so do not stop workup following a ⊖ mammogram in clinically suspicious cases.

KEY FACT

Women should be tested for BRCA1/2 mutations if they have a "genetic" risk—ie, a strong family history of breast or ovarian cancer and/or other cancers associated with the gene.

Q

A 62-year-old woman presents with a suspicious breast mass. Mammography reveals clusters of microcalcifications and stellate lesions. A biopsy confirms invasive cancer. What is the next step in management?

KEY FACT

Sentinel lymph node biopsy, not axillary lymph node dissection, is the current standard of care.

KEY FACT

Breast-conserving surgery is generally as effective as radical mastectomy in patients with a unifocal tumor size of < 5 cm.

KEY FACT

ER/PR-⊕ status is a good prognostic indicator; patients should be treated with hormonal therapy.

- Determine estrogen/progesterone receptor (**ER/PR**) and **HER2/neu** status to help guide treatment strategy.
- Special forms of breast cancer include:
    - **Inflammatory breast cancer:** Highly aggressive and rapidly growing; invades the lymphatics and causes skin inflammation (peau d'orange). Has a poor prognosis.
    - **Paget's disease:** Ductal carcinoma in situ or invasive cancer of the nipple with unilateral itching, burning, and nipple erosion. May be mistaken for infection or eczema; associated with another focus of invasive cancer elsewhere in the breast.

TREATMENT

- **Ductal carcinoma in situ (DCIS): Local therapy** (lumpectomy or wide excision plus radiation). If ER/PR ⊕, consider **tamoxifen** for 5 years to ↓ the risk of recurrence.
- **Lobular carcinoma in situ (LCIS):** Carries a high risk (up to 20%) of developing a subsequent infiltrating breast cancer, including cancer in the contralateral breast. Consider close monitoring, mastectomy, or tamoxifen for prophylaxis.
- **Invasive cancer:** The choice of treatment is based on **lymph node status, tumor size,** and **hormone receptor status** (see Table 9-7).
- **Adjuvant chemotherapy:** Indicated for larger tumors, those associated with a high risk of recurrence (based on genomic assay), hormone-⊖ tumors, and lymph node involvement. Several regimens are now used (eg, cyclophosphamide or doxorubicin followed by paclitaxel for 4–6 months).
- **Endocrine therapy:** Some types of breast cancer are dependent on estrogen for growth. Endocrine therapy is indicated for all patients with ER/PR-⊕ tumors (see Table 9-8).
    - In **premenopausal** women, estrogen is produced by the ovaries. **Tamoxifen** and **raloxifene** block estrogen effects on receptors.
    - In **postmenopausal** women, estrogen is produced by fat and muscles. Aromatase peripherally converts androgens to estrogen. Aromatase inhibitors such as anastrozole do not inhibit ovarian production of estrogen and are thus ineffective in premenopausal women.
- **Trastuzumab** (Herceptin) is beneficial for those with **HER2-neu-⊕** tumors.
- In BRCA-⊕ patients, prophylactic bilateral mastectomy and/or salpingo-oophorectomy significantly ↓ the risk of breast or ovarian cancer.

TABLE 9-7.   Treatment of Breast Cancer by Type

TYPE	TREATMENT
DCIS	Lumpectomy, mastectomy and radiation, endocrine therapy if ER/PR ⊕.
Infiltrating ductal carcinoma with ⊖ lymph nodes	Lumpectomy, breast-conserving surgery, and radiation may be considered depending on tumor size. Chemotherapy to shrink large tumors preoperatively; adjuvant chemotherapy if ↑ risk of recurrence; endocrine therapy if ER/PR ⊕.
Infiltrating ductal carcinoma with ⊕ lymph nodes	Breast-conserving surgery or modified radical mastectomy, axillary dissection, radiation, adjuvant chemotherapy, and endocrine therapy if ER/PR ⊕.

A

Testing for estrogen and progesterone receptor status and HER2/neu status.

TABLE 9-8. **Treatment of Breast Cancer Based on Hormone Receptor Status**

	SOURCE OF ESTROGEN	TREATMENT	ACTION
Premenopausal ER/PR ⊕	Ovaries	Tamoxifen	Blocks estrogen effects on receptors
Postmenopausal ER/PR ⊕	Fat and muscle	Aromatase inhibitors, sometimes preceded by tamoxifen therapy	Inhibits peripheral conversion

Lung Cancer

The **leading cause of cancer death.** The major risk factor is **tobacco** use. Other risk factors include radon and asbestos exposure. Subtypes are described in Table 9-9.

SYMPTOMS/EXAM

- Asymptomatic lesions are discovered incidentally on either CXR or chest CT (see Figure 9-8).
- Most patients develop signs that herald a problem—eg, **chronic cough, hemoptysis, weight loss,** or **postobstructive pneumonia.**
- Less frequently, patients may present late with **complications of a large tumor burden:**
  - **Pancoast's syndrome:** Presents with shoulder pain, Horner's syndrome (miosis, ptosis, anhidrosis), and lower brachial plexopathy.
  - **Superior vena cava syndrome:** Characterized by swelling of the face and arm, most often on the right side, and ↑ JVP. Treat urgently with radiation.
  - **Hoarseness:** Vocal cord paralysis from entrapment of the recurrent laryngeal nerve, most often on the left.

MNEMONIC

The 3 C's of squamous cell carcinoma of the lung:

Central
Cavitary
Hyper**C**alcemia

KEY FACT

Adenocarcinoma presents **A**way (peripheral).
Squamous cell presents **C**entrally with **C**avities and can have hyper**C**alcemia.

TABLE 9-9. **Classification of Lung Cancers**

SUBTYPE	CHARACTERISTICS	TREATMENT
Small cell lung cancer (SCLC)	Highly related to **cigarette exposure.** Usually **centrally** located; often presents as **disseminated disease.**	**Chemotherapy;** chemoradiation for limited-stage disease.
Non–small cell lung cancer (NSCLC)	**Adenocarcinoma:** The most common lung cancer; has a **peripheral** location. More common in women than in men. **Adenocarcinoma, bronchoalveolar subtype:** Multiple nodules, bilateral lung infiltrates, and metastases late in the disease course. **Squamous cell carcinoma:** Presents **centrally** and is often **cavitary. Large cell carcinoma:** Least common.	**Potentially curable with resection of localized disease, but only modestly responsive to chemotherapy.** Patients are classified into 1 of 3 clinical groups at the time of diagnosis: ■ **Stages I and II:** Early-stage disease. Candidacy for surgical resection. ■ **Locally or regionally advanced disease** (supraclavicular or mediastinal lymphadenopathy or chest wall/pleural/pericardial invasion): Combination chemotherapy and radiation; surgery is not indicated. ■ **Distant metastases:** The goal of chemotherapy or radiation is **palliation.**

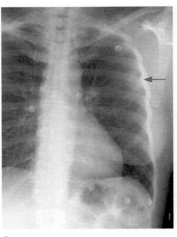
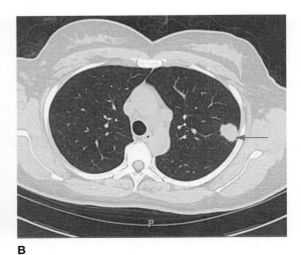

A   **B**

FIGURE 9-8.   **Lung cancer.** Lung cancer (arrows) on **(A)** frontal CXR and **(B)** transaxial CT. (Reproduced with permission from USMLE-Rx.com.)

KEY FACT

If a patient has recurrent pneumonia in the same spot with no improvement on appropriate antibiotics, look for cancer.

DIFFERENTIAL

- Patients with a history of exposure to asbestos are at ↑ risk of bronchogenic carcinoma and malignant mesothelioma.
- Serial CXRs are useful for distinguishing benign from malignant lesions. Lesions that remain stable over > 2 years are generally not cancerous.
- Other features suggestive of benign lesions include young age, smooth margins, and small size (< 2 cm). However, any lung nodule in a smoker or an ex-smoker should be evaluated for cancer.

DIAGNOSIS

- Biopsy of the lung mass is critical. If there is a palpable lymph node, consider biopsy of the node first. Order a CXR, and in doubtful or suspicious cases, obtain a **chest CT and, if necessary, bronchoscopy.**
- If mediastinal lymph nodes are enlarged, consider a PET scan and mediastinoscopy for proper staging.
- **Centrally** located cancers can be diagnosed by **bronchoscopy** or **sputum cytology.**
- Staging includes chest and abdominal CT with contrast, PET scan, bone scan, and CT or MRI of the brain.

TREATMENT

See Table 9-9.

Paraneoplastic Syndromes

Disorders or symptoms that result from an immune, hormonal, or cytokine response to a neoplasm. Often present before the diagnosis of cancer.

- **Hypercalcemia:** Most often seen with squamous cell carcinoma (NSCLC) from ↑ PTHrP production or bone metastases. Treat with bisphosphonates.
- **SIADH/hyponatremia:** Occurs more frequently with small cell carcinoma (cells make more ADH).
- **Cushing's disease:** Results from overproduction of ACTH secreted by small cell carcinoma. ACTH ↑ cortisol levels. Cushing's syndrome can also cause high blood pressure or new-onset diabetes.

MNEMONIC

Paraneoplastic syndromes—

CLASH

Carcinoid
Lambert-Eaton syndrome
ACTH
SIADH
Hypercalcemia

- **Lambert-Eaton syndrome:** Similar to myasthenia gravis except that **muscle fatigue improves with repeated stimulation** (vs myasthenia gravis, in which repeated stimulation yields no improvement). Found more often in small cell carcinoma.
- **Erythrocytosis:** Seen in renal cell carcinoma and hepatocellular carcinoma 2° to ectopic erythropoietin production.

GI Tumors

PANCREATIC CANCER

Seen in patients > 50 years of age. **Ductal adenocarcinoma** accounts for 85% of 1° tumors; > 60–70% arise in the head of the pancreas. Risk factors include smoking, chronic pancreatitis, and diabetes mellitus (DM). **Trousseau's syndrome** (migratory thrombophlebitis; hypercoagulable state with venous thrombosis associated with pancreatic adenocarcinoma) can occur.

SYMPTOMS/EXAM

Nausea, anorexia, weight loss, abdominal and lumbar back pain, new-onset DM, venous thromboembolism, and **painless obstructive jaundice** (cancer in the head of the pancreas).

DIAGNOSIS

- ↑ bilirubin, ↑ aminotransferases, and normocytic normochromic anemia.
- **Ultrasound** is useful as an initial diagnostic test. Abdominal/pelvic CT can evaluate the extent of disease; **CT** (see Figure 9-9) can determine if the mass is resectable.
- **Endoscopic ultrasonography** yields excellent anatomic detail and can help determine if the tumor is resectable.

TREATMENT

- **Pancreaticoduodenectomy** (Whipple procedure) is appropriate for patients with resectable tumors.

KEY FACT

Painless jaundice and/or a palpable gallbladder—think pancreatic cancer.

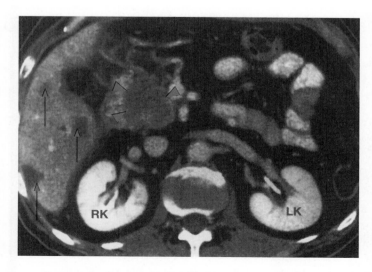

FIGURE 9-9. **Pancreatic adenocarcinoma.** Transaxial contrast-enhanced CT shows a mass in the head of the pancreas (arrowheads) and multiple liver metastases (arrows). RK = right kidney; LK = left kidney. (Reproduced with permission from Chen MY et al. *Basic Radiology*, 2nd ed. New York: McGraw-Hill, 2011, Fig. 11-71.)

Q

A 60-year-old woman presents with painless jaundice and weight loss. What is the most likely location of the obstructing mass?

- **Chemotherapy** or **radiation** is used for **palliative care** in patients with advanced or unresectable disease.

HEPATOCELLULAR CANCER (HEPATOMA)

Risk factors for hepatocellular cancer (HCC) include viral hepatitis (HBV, HCV), alcoholic cirrhosis, hemochromatosis, and α_1-antitrypsin deficiency. OCPs are associated with benign hepatic adenoma (vs HCC).

SYMPTOMS/EXAM/DIAGNOSIS

Abdominal discomfort with ↑ aminotransferases, ↑ bilirubin, and coagulopathy. Diagnosed on abdominal imaging (see Figure 9-10).

TREATMENT

- Surgical resection and liver transplantation can yield long-term survival.
- Alternatives for unresectable tumors include percutaneous alcohol injections, transarterial chemoembolization, radiofrequency ablation, and systemic therapy (eg, molecularly targeted agents such as sorafenib, chemotherapy).

COLORECTAL CANCER

Most cases occur after age 50. Suspect **hereditary nonpolyposis colorectal cancer** (HNPCC) in a younger person with colon cancer and a family history of colon, ovarian, and endometrial cancer. Table 9-10 outlines risk factors. Screen all average-risk patients > 50 years of age with annual fecal occult blood testing (FOBT) and flexible sigmoidoscopy every 5 years or colonoscopy every 10 years.

KEY FACT

2° liver tumors (metastases) are more common than 1° liver tumors.

KEY FACT

If there is a family history of polyps or colorectal cancer, start screening when the patient is 10 years younger than the age at which the affected relative was diagnosed or at age 50, whichever comes first.

A

The pancreatic head. A mass at the head of the pancreas obstructs the common bile duct as it runs through the pancreas, causing painless jaundice.

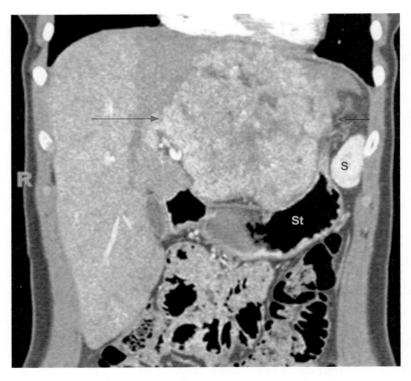

FIGURE 9-10.   Hepatocellular carcinoma. Coronal reformation from a contrast-enhanced CT shows a large HCC in the left hepatic lobe (arrows). St = stomach; S = spleen. (Reproduced with permission from USMLE-Rx.com.)

TABLE 9-10. Risk Factors for Colorectal Cancer

PATIENT AGE	PERSONAL HISTORY	COLORECTAL CANCER OR ADENOMATOUS POLYPS	HEREDITARY COLORECTAL CANCER SYNDROMES
> 50 years	Previous colorectal cancer Adenomatous polyp IBD, particularly ulcerative colitis	One first-degree relative < 60 years of age or 2 first-degree relatives of any age	HNPCC (Lynch syndrome) Familial adenomatous polyposis (FAP) Hamartomatous polyposis syndromes

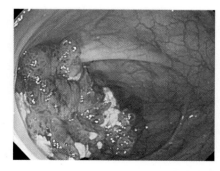

FIGURE 9-11. Colon cancer. Colonoscopy reveals an adenocarcinoma growing into the lumen of the colon. (Reproduced with permission from Fauci AS et al. *Harrison's Principles of Internal Medicine,* 17th ed. New York: McGraw-Hill, 2008, Fig. 285-6.)

SYMPTOMS/EXAM

Symptoms depend on the site of the 1° tumor and may include a change in bowel habits, melena, bright red blood per rectum, weight loss, fatigue, vomiting, and abdominal discomfort.

DIAGNOSIS

- Diagnosed by a mass palpated by DRE or detected by FOBT.
- Iron-deficiency anemia or ↑ transaminases may be seen.
- Often metastasizes to the **liver.**
- Confirm the diagnosis via colonoscopy and biopsy (see Figure 9-11).

TREATMENT

- Treatment decisions are influenced by tumor stage at diagnosis. 1° surgical resection involves resection of the bowel segment with adjacent mesentery and regional lymph nodes. Solitary liver/lung metastases can be resected.
- Stage I patients have an excellent prognosis with surgery alone (90% survival at 5 years).
- **Adjuvant chemotherapy (5-FU based)** is warranted for patients at stage III and above.

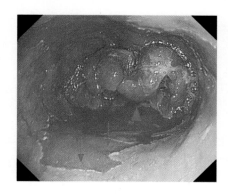

FIGURE 9-12. Esophageal cancer. An esophageal adenocarcinoma (arrowhead) is seen on endoscopy against a background of the pink tongues of Barrett's esophagus (arrows). (Reproduced with permission from Fauci AS et al. *Harrison's Principles of Internal Medicine,* 17th ed. New York: McGraw-Hill, 2008, Fig. 285-3D.)

MISCELLANEOUS GI TUMORS

Esophageal Tumors

- Risk factors include:
  - **Lower esophagus:** Obesity, GERD, and Barrett's esophagus (associated with adenocarcinoma).
  - **Upper esophagus:** Tobacco and alcohol use (associated with squamous cell carcinoma).
- **Sx/Exam: Dysphagia in the elderly.** Esophageal adenocarcinoma can arise from long-standing esophageal reflux with Barrett's esophagus.
- **Dx:** EGD with biopsy (see Figure 9-12).
- **Tx:** Resection for localized disease; radiation with chemotherapy for advanced disease.

Gastric Tumors

- Risk factors include *H pylori*, smoking, and a ⊕ family history. More common in Asia and South America.
- **Sx/Exam:** Classically presents as **iron-deficiency anemia with vague abdominal pain in the elderly.**

Q **1**

A 60-year-old man with a known diagnosis of colon cancer in remission is found to have a carcinoembryonic antigen (CEA) level that is ↑ from baseline. What does this indicate?

Q **2**

A 65-year-old man with a history of GERD presents with a 10-lb weight loss, dysphagia, and epigastric pain. What will biopsy results from EGD most likely reveal?

MNEMONIC

Esophageal cancer risk factors—

ABCDEF

Achalasia
Barrett's esophagus
Corrosive esophagitis
Diverticulitis
Esophageal web
Familial

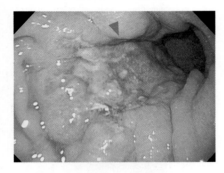

FIGURE 9-13. Gastric cancer.
A malignant gastric ulcer (arrow) involving the greater curvature of the stomach is seen on endoscopy. (Reproduced with permission from Fauci AS et al. *Harrison's Principles of Internal Medicine,* 17th ed. New York: McGraw-Hill, 2008, Fig. 285-2B.)

1 **A**

Cancer recurrence. CEA is normally produced in GI tissue during fetal development. An ↑ in CEA suggests colorectal cancer recurrence.

2 **A**

Esophageal adenocarcinoma. In the 1960s, most esophageal cancers were squamous cell and were associated with tobacco and alcohol use. Adenocarcinoma is now the main type in the United States and is thought to be associated with acid reflux (this patient has a history of GERD).

- **Dx:** EGD with biopsy (see Figure 9-13).
- **Tx:** Resection for localized disease and radiation therapy with chemotherapy for advanced disease.

Carcinoid Tumors (Neuroendocrine Tumors)

- Usually occur in the **appendix** or small bowel.
- **Sx/Exam:** Clinical features include flushing, abdominal pain, diarrhea, and tricuspid regurgitation (carcinoid syndrome; symptoms result from ↑ serotonin). Tumors may also be asymptomatic and may be discovered incidentally.
- **Dx:** Diagnosed by elevated levels of **5-HIAA** (the breakdown product of serotonin) or chromogranin A.
- **Tx:**
  - Surgical resection is curative in localized disease.
  - For symptomatic control, consider **octreotide,** a synthetic somatostatin analog that ↓ the secretion of serotonin.
  - Patients with well-differentiated tumors can be managed with close observation and serial imaging.

Islet Cell Tumors

- **Sx/Exam:** Presentation depends on type.
  - **Insulinoma (↑ proinsulin, C-peptide, and insulin levels):** Presents with the triad of hypoglycemic symptoms, a fasting blood glucose < 40 mg/dL, and immediate relief with glucose.
  - **VIPoma (↑ VIP levels):** Suspect in profuse, watery diarrhea that causes hypokalemia.
  - **Glucagonoma (↑ glucagon levels):** Persistent hyperglycemia with necrolytic erythema (intertriginous and perioral rash).
- **Dx:** Islet cell tumors and their metastases (liver is most common) can be localized by somatostatin receptor scintigraphy.
- **Tx:** Options vary according to type. Treatment includes surgical resection, debulking, chemotherapy, and somatostatin analogs with glucagonomas and VIPomas.

Genitourinary Tumors

BLADDER CANCER

The **most common** malignant tumor of the urinary tract; usually **transitional cell carcinoma.** Risk factors include **smoking,** exposure to aniline (rubber) dyes, and chronic bladder infections (eg, **schistosomiasis**).

SYMPTOMS/EXAM

Gross painless hematuria is the most common symptom. Other symptoms, such as frequency, urgency, and dysuria, may also be seen.

DIAGNOSIS

- UA often shows hematuria (macro- or microscopic). Lack of dysmorphic RBCs helps distinguish this from glomerular bleeding. Cytology may show dysplastic cells.
- **CT urography** or **IVP** can examine the upper urinary tract as well as defects in bladder filling.
- **Cystoscopy with biopsy is diagnostic.**

TREATMENT

Treatment depends on the extent of spread beyond the bladder mucosa.

- **Noninvasive stage I:** Transurethral resection of the bladder tumor **(TURBT).** If high risk (histologic grade or invasion), treat with intravesicular chemotherapy (eg, bacillus Calmette-Guérin). If very low risk, observe or give a single dose of intravesicular chemotherapy.
- **Invasive cancers without metastases:** Aggressive surgery, radiation therapy, or both.
- **Distant metastases:** Chemotherapy alone.

PROSTATE CANCER

The most common cancer in men. Ninety-five percent are adenocarcinomas. Risk ↑ linearly with age.

SYMPTOMS/EXAM

- Many patients are asymptomatic and are incidentally diagnosed either by **DRE** or by a **PSA** level that is obtained for screening purposes.
- If symptomatic, patients may present with **urinary urgency/frequency/ hesitancy** and, in late or aggressive disease, with anemia, hematuria, or low back pain.
- Routine screening in asymptomatic patients with **DRE** or **PSA is controversial.**
  - Some groups advocate that the side effects of aggressive treatment outweigh the benefits of detection; others recommend annual screening with both PSA and DRE in patients > 50 years of age.
  - It is often recommended that individualized discussions be held with men > 50 years of age whose life expectancy exceeds 10 years.
  - Screening is not routinely recommended in patients > 75 years of age.
  - However, if the patient is **symptomatic, test,** as you are no longer "screening."

DIAGNOSIS

- Ultrasound-guided needle biopsy of the prostate allows for both diagnosis and staging.
- The **Gleason score (2–10)** remains the best predictor of clinical behavior. It sums the scores of the 2 most prevalent differentiation patterns seen on biopsy on a scale of 1–5: well differentiated (low) to poorly differentiated (high).

TREATMENT

- Treatment choice is based on the aggressiveness of the tumor and on the patient's risk of dying from the disease.
- **Watchful waiting** may be the best approach for elderly patients with low Gleason scores.
- Consider **radical prostatectomy** or **radiation therapy** (eg, brachytherapy or external beam) for node-⊖ disease. Treatment is associated with an ↑ risk of incontinence and/or impotence.
- Treat node-⊕ and metastatic disease with **androgen deprivation therapy** (eg, GnRH agonists, orchiectomy, bicalutamide) +/– chemotherapy.

KEY FACT

- **Low risk:** Confined to the bladder mucosa or submucosa.
- **High risk:** Multifocal or recurrent lesions, carcinoma in situ, or invasion of the connective tissue, especially the muscularis mucosa.

KEY FACT

Incidental asymptomatic prostate cancer is especially common among men > 80 years of age and does not always need treatment.

Q

A 60-year-old man with a 35-pack-year smoking history presents with pink urine. UA shows macrohematuria; CT urography reveals no abnormalities of the kidneys or ureters. What is the diagnostic test of choice?

KEY FACT

- **Nonseminoma:** ↑ α-fetoprotein, ↑ β-hCG.
- **Seminoma:** Normal α-fetoprotein, ↑ β-hCG.

TESTICULAR CANCER

The most common solid malignant tumor in men 20–35 years of age. It is highly treatable and often curable. Risk factors include family history, **cryptorchid testis,** and Klinefelter's syndrome. Ninety-five percent are germ cell tumors (seminomas or nonseminomas). Pure seminomas have a better prognosis.

SYMPTOMS/EXAM

- **A unilateral scrotal mass is testicular cancer until proven otherwise.**
- Other symptoms include testicular discomfort or swelling suggestive of orchitis or epididymitis.

DIAGNOSIS

- Serum levels of **α-fetoprotein (AFP), LDH,** and **β-hCG** should be measured.
- Scrotal ultrasound is useful to differentiate nonneoplastic lesions (eg, hydrocele, spermatocele, infection) (see Figure 9-14).
- Definitive diagnosis is made by radical inguinal orchiectomy.
- Staging evaluation (TNM is widely used) should include serum LDH, AFP, β-hCG, and CT of the chest/abdomen and pelvis (the retroperitoneal lymph nodes and thorax are usually the first sites of metastasis).

TREATMENT

Radical inguinal orchiectomy +/− chemotherapy/radiation therapy.

KEY FACT

Do not do a scrotal biopsy to diagnose testicular cancer, as this may result in seeding of the biopsy tract.

RENAL CELL CARCINOMA

The cause is unknown, but risk factors include **cigarette smoking,** von Hippel–Lindau disease, tuberous sclerosis, and cystic kidney disease. **Clear cell** is the most common type.

Cystoscopy with possible biopsy.

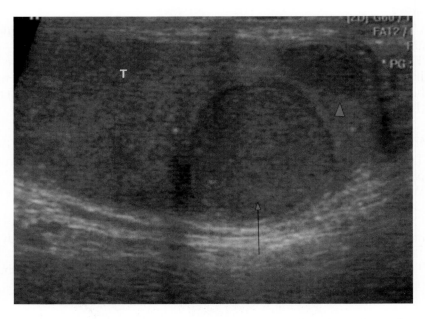

FIGURE 9-14.   Seminoma. Longitudinal ultrasound image of testicle (**T**) shows a homogeneous intratesticular mass (arrow) and an additional smaller focus of tumor (arrowhead). (Reproduced with permission from USMLE-Rx.com.)

SYMPTOMS/EXAM

- Generally asymptomatic in the early stages, but symptoms can include hematuria, flank pain, a palpable mass, fevers, night sweats, anemia, or symptoms of disseminated disease such as dyspnea and bone pain.
- Paraneoplastic effects such as erythrocytosis, hypercalcemia, and hypertension may be seen.

DIAGNOSIS

- Most are found incidentally (see Figure 9-15).
- Renal ultrasound can determine whether the mass is cystic or solid. CT-guided biopsies are usually not performed for masses > 3–4 cm because of the high likelihood of malignancy.

TREATMENT

- **Local disease: Partial vs radical nephrectomy** vs cryoablation/radiofrequency ablation.
- **Disseminated disease:** Nephrectomy may be recommended before chemotherapy even for patients with metastatic disease despite the goal of palliation. Treat with molecularly targeted agents (eg, sorafenib, sunitinib), mTOR inhibitors (eg, everolimus), immunotherapy, or chemotherapy.

KEY FACT

Biopsy should not be used to diagnose renal cell carcinoma unless disseminated disease or another 1° tumor is suspected. Risks include false negatives, bleeding, and tumor seeding.

OVARIAN CANCER

More than 90% are **adenocarcinomas.** Risk factors include age, infertility drugs, HNPCC, delayed menopause, and familial cancer syndromes (eg, BRCA1/2). Risk is ↓ with sustained use of OCPs, childbirth, breast-feeding, bilateral tubal ligation, and TAH-BSO.

SYMPTOMS/EXAM

- Usually **asymptomatic** until the disease has reached an advanced stage.
- Symptoms include abdominal pain, bloating, pelvic pressure, urinary frequency, early satiety, constipation, vaginal bleeding, and systemic symptoms (fatigue, malaise, weight loss).
- Exam reveals a palpable solid, fixed, nodular pelvic mass; ascites; and pleural effusion (Meigs' syndrome). **An ovarian mass in postmenopausal women is ovarian cancer until proven otherwise.**

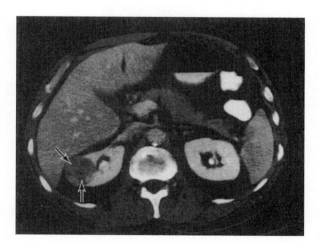

FIGURE 9-15.   CT with contrast of a renal cell carcinoma (arrows). (Reproduced with permission from McAninch JW, Lue TF. *Smith & Tanagho's General Urology,* 18th ed. New York: McGraw-Hill, 2013, Fig. 22-5.)

DIAGNOSIS/TREATMENT

- Evaluate adnexal masses with **pelvic ultrasound** and possibly CT; obtain serum **CA-125** and a **CXR**.
- Staging is surgical and includes **TAH-BSO, omentectomy**, and **tumor debulking**.

CERVICAL CANCER

The mean age at diagnosis is the mid-40s. Risk factors include **HPV infection** (see Figure 9-16), **tobacco use**, early onset of sexual activity, multiple sexual partners, immune compromise (eg, HIV), and STDs.

- **HPV vaccine** is recommended for cervical cancer prevention. It targets HPV 6, 11, 16, and 18.
- HPV **16** and **18** account for the majority of cervical cancers. HPV 6 and 11 cause most genital warts.

SYMPTOMS/EXAM

- Usually asymptomatic and diagnosed on routine **Pap smear**.
- If symptomatic, patients may present with menorrhagia and/or metrorrhagia, **postcoital bleeding**, pelvic pain, and vaginal discharge.

DIAGNOSIS

- **Colposcopy** and biopsy in patients with an abnormal Pap smear or visible cervical lesions.
- Cervical lesions are categorized as **cervical carcinoma** (depth > 3 mm, width > 7 mm) or **cervical intraepithelial neoplasia (CIN)**.

TREATMENT

- **CIN I (mild dysplasia or low-grade squamous intraepithelial lesion [LGSIL])**: Most regress spontaneously. Reliable patients can be observed with yearly Pap smears and colposcopy.
- **CIN II/III**: Treat with conization or the loop electrosurgical excision procedure (**LEEP**).

KEY FACT

The HPV vaccine targets HPV 6, 11, 16, and 18. HPV 16 and 18 account for most cervical cancers.

KEY FACT

In suspicious cases, the Pap smear should be followed by colposcopy and biopsy.

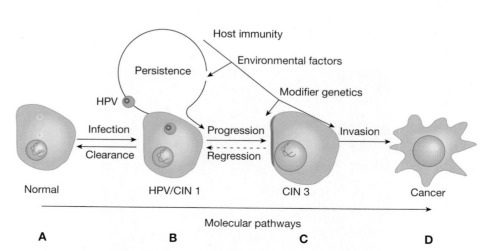

FIGURE 9-16. **Genesis of cervical cancer.** (A) Normal cell. (B) Cell at risk from active HPV infection. The HPV genome is a plasmid separate from the host DNA. (C) Cervical intraepithelial neoplasia 3 (CIN 3) or carcinoma in situ (CIS). The HPV genome has become integrated into the host DNA. (D) Interactive effects between environmental insults, host immunity, and somatic cell genomic variations lead to invasive cervical cancer. (Reproduced with permission from Hoffman BL et al. *Williams Gynecology*, 2nd ed. New York: McGraw-Hill, 2012, Fig. 30-1.)

- **Invasive cancer:** Early-stage disease can be treated with **radical hysterectomy and lymph node dissection.** Advanced disease can be treated with **radiation and chemotherapy.**

CNS Tumors

1° brain tumors make up < 2% of all tumors diagnosed. Meningioma, glioma, vestibular schwannoma, pituitary adenoma, and 1° CNS lymphoma are the most common CNS tumors in adults. There is an ↑ risk in immunocompromised states such as AIDS. Imaging findings can help distinguish the tumor from other intracranial lesions (see Table 9-11).

MENINGIOMA

- Accounts for one-third of all 1° brain tumors; usually benign.
- **Sx/Exam:** Most tumors are small, asymptomatic, and discovered incidentally. When symptoms are present, they usually consist of **progressive headache** or a **focal neurologic deficit** reflecting the location of the tumor. Symptoms can also include spastic paresis, urinary incontinence, or new-onset seizures.
- **Dx:** CT or MRI of the head typically demonstrates a partially **calcified, homogeneously enhancing extra-axial mass adherent to the dura** (see Figure 9-17 and Table 9-11). **Craniopharyngioma** is another highly calcified tumor in children but is present **around the pituitary gland** and can cause bitemporal hemianopia.
- **Tx:** Surgical resection is appropriate for large or symptomatic tumors; **observation with serial scans** is the preferred approach for **small or asymptomatic lesions.**

KEY FACT

MRI is superior to CT for viewing skull-base/cerebellar lesions but is less reliable for detecting calcifications.

GLIAL TUMORS

- Include astrocytomas, oligodendrogliomas, mixed gliomas, and ependymomas.
- **Sx/Exam:**
  - Headache is the most common symptom. It may be generalized or unilateral; often **awakens** the patient from sleep and induces **vomiting;** and worsens with the Valsalva maneuver.

TABLE 9-11. Imaging Findings Associated with Brain Tumors

TUMOR	IMAGING FINDING
Meningioma	Extradural, calcified.
Glioma—glioblastoma multiforme	Multifocal or "butterfly lesions"; possible hemorrhage; centrally necrotic lesion.
1° CNS lymphoma	Typically multifocal, diffusely enhancing, periventricular.
Metastatic tumor	Multifocal; ring enhancement with contrast; located at the gray/white matter junction. (The most common tumors that metastasize to the brain are lung, breast, and melanoma.)

Q **1**

A 25-year-old woman is noted to have dysplastic cells on a routine screening Pap smear. What test is required to confirm a diagnosis of cervical cancer?

Q **2**

A 60-year-old woman is involved in a motor vehicle accident in which she sustains head trauma. Aside from some minor bruising of the forehead, her exam, which includes a nonfocal neurologic exam, is unrevealing. Imaging shows an extradural 9-mm calcified lesion. What is the most likely diagnosis?

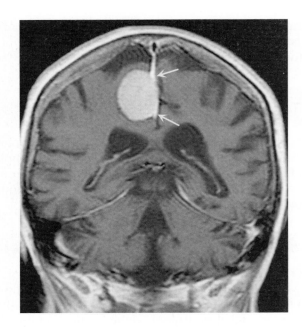

FIGURE 9-17. **Meningioma.** Coronal postcontrast T1-weighted MRI demonstrates an enhancing extra-axial mass arising from the falx cerebri (arrows). (Reproduced with permission from Fauci AS et al. *Harrison's Principles of Internal Medicine*, 17th ed. New York: McGraw-Hill, 2008, Fig. 374-5.)

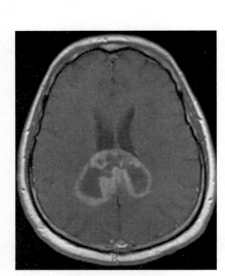

FIGURE 9-18. **Glioblastoma multiforme.** Transaxial contrast-enhanced image shows an enhancing intra-axial mass with central necrosis crossing the corpus callosum ("butterfly glioma"). (Reproduced with permission from USMLE-Rx.com.)

- Tumors are **diffusely infiltrating,** creating areas of low attenuation on CT or an ↑ T2 signal on MRI.
- **Astrocytomas** (specifically glioblastoma multiforme) are the most common 1° brain tumor. **Glioblastoma multiforme** is usually a **unifocal and centrally necrotic** enhancing lesion with surrounding edema and mass effect (see Figure 9-18).
- **Dx: Biopsy** is required for definitive diagnosis.
- **Tx: Surgical resection** followed by **external beam radiation** is used for high-grade tumors. Chemotherapy can be of benefit for some 1° CNS tumors.

Tumor Markers

Usually sensitive but not specific. Thus, they are most useful for monitoring recurrence and disease activity following resection. Tumor markers can also be useful in diagnosis if they are supported by clinical evidence. Common tumor markers and associated malignancies include the following:

- **CA-125:** Ovarian cancer.
- **CA 15-3:** Breast cancer.
- **CA 19-9:** Pancreatic cancer.
- **CEA:** GI cancer, particularly of the colon.
- **AFP:** Liver, yolk sac (testicular) cancer.
- **hCG:** Choriocarcinoma (testicular/ovarian).
- **PSA:** Prostate cancer.
- **LDH:** Lymphoma.
- **Calcitonin:** Medullary thyroid carcinoma.
- **Chromogranin A:** Carcinoid tumor.

1 **A**

Colposcopy and biopsy.

2 **A**

Benign meningioma. Calcified lesions that are extradural, or outside the brain, are typically benign and rarely limit life expectancy.

INFECTIOUS DISEASE

KEY FACT

- **Impetigo:** Infection of the epidermis.
- **Erysipelas:** Infection of the upper dermis.
- **Cellulitis:** Infection of the entire dermis and the subcutaneous fat.
- **Necrotizing fasciitis:** Infection of the subcutaneous fat and fascia.

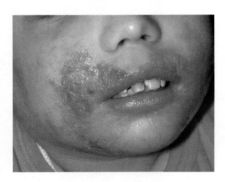

FIGURE 10-1. Impetigo. Classic honey-colored, crusted lesions are shown. (Reproduced with permission from Stern SD et al. *Symptom to Diagnosis: An Evidence-Based Guide,* 3rd ed. New York: McGraw-Hill, 2015, Fig. 29-6.)

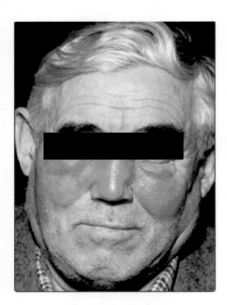

FIGURE 10-2. Erysipelas. Painful, edematous erythema with sharp margination is seen on both cheeks and on the nose. (Reproduced with permission from Goldsmith LA et al. *Fitzpatrick's Dermatology in General Medicine,* 8th ed. New York: McGraw-Hill, 2012, Fig. 178-4.)

Soft Tissue Infections

Infections of the epidermis, dermis, subcutaneous fat, and/or fascia. Patients with diabetes, HIV or other immunosuppressed states, peripheral vascular disease, and edema are at ↑ risk.

IMPETIGO

Infection of the epidermis, usually caused by β-hemolytic streptococci or by *S aureus.*

SYMPTOMS/EXAM

Presents with well-localized vesicles filled with serous fluid, usually in exposed areas of the skin. The vesicles rupture, leaving a thin yellow crust (see Figure 10-1).

TREATMENT

- Limited infections can be treated with topical mupirocin.
- More extensive infections should be treated with a penicillinase-resistant penicillin or a first-generation cephalosporin. Use TMP-SMX or doxycycline if there is concern for MRSA.

ERYSIPELAS

Infection of the upper dermis, usually caused by β-hemolytic streptococci or, rarely, by *S aureus.*

SYMPTOMS/EXAM

Presents with a well-demarcated, raised area of erythema, often on the face (see Figure 10-2).

TREATMENT

- Select the antimicrobial on the basis of patient risk factors and clinical severity.
- First-line treatment is penicillin; if *S aureus* is suspected, use a first-generation cephalosporin. For MRSA coverage, use TMP-SMX or doxycycline.

CELLULITIS

Infection of the dermis and subcutaneous fat that may be associated with an identifiable portal of entry—eg, cuts, tinea pedis, animal/insect bites, ulcers, or injection sites.

- Most commonly due to *S aureus* or *Streptococcus pyogenes.*
- In diabetics, consider *Pseudomonas aeruginosa* and other gram-⊖ rods (GNRs).
- In human bite infections, consider anaerobes such as *Eikenella* as well. In animal bites, consider anaerobes, *Pasteurella* (cats), and *Capnocytophaga* (dogs).

SYMPTOMS/EXAM

- Presents with **warm, erythematous, and tender skin** (see Figure 10-3).
- Patients may also have fever, chills, regional lymphadenopathy, lymphangitis (seen as red streaks), or associated abscess.

DIFFERENTIAL

- Cellulitis in the lower extremities may be difficult to distinguish from stasis dermatitis. Look for clues suggesting cellulitis, including new-onset erythema, unilateral findings, and systemic symptoms.
- Consider necrotizing fasciitis if the patient presents with pain out of proportion to the physical exam with or without evidence of systemic inflammatory response syndrome (SIRS).
- May be differentiated from hypersensitivity reactions, which usually present with discrete urticarial lesions (hives) that are itchy and in the distribution of the suspected allergen (eg, belt buckle).

DIAGNOSIS

- Primarily a clinical diagnosis.
- Consider obtaining blood cultures, CBC, ESR, and radiographs if there is a possibility of deeper infection such as necrotizing fasciitis or osteomyelitis.
- Lower extremity cellulitis can be associated with DVT. If clinically indicated, ultrasound may be useful for evaluation.

TREATMENT

- For most patients, a first-generation cephalosporin or an antistaphylococcal penicillin is appropriate.
- If there is concern for MRSA, clindamycin, doxycycline, or TMP-SMX may be given; for inpatients, vancomycin may be used.
- Choose an antibiotic with GNR coverage for diabetics.
- For human or animal bites, choose a penicillin/penicillinase combination (eg, amoxicillin/clavulanate) for coverage of anaerobes, *Pasteurella*, and *Capnocytophaga*. Consider tetanus vaccination.
- If associated with abscess, perform incision and drainage.

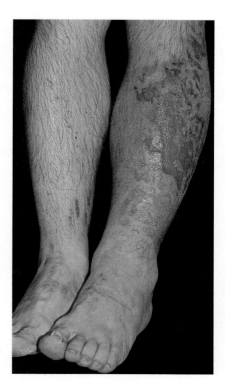

FIGURE 10-3. Cellulitis. Repeated excoriation of extremities led to MRSA cellulitis. Note the unilateral distribution. (Reproduced with permission from Wolff K et al. *Fitzpatrick's Color Atlas and Synopsis of Clinical Dermatology*, 7th ed. New York: McGraw-Hill, 2013, Fig. 25-38.)

NECROTIZING FASCIITIS

Rapidly spreading infection of the subcutaneous fat and fascia.

- **Type I necrotizing fasciitis:** Due to a polymicrobial infection with anaerobes and aerobes, including GNRs. Commonly seen in patients with risk factors such as diabetes and other immunosuppressed states, IV drug use, and peripheral vascular disease.
- **Type II necrotizing fasciitis:** Typically due to β-hemolytic streptococcus or S *aureus*.

SYMPTOMS/EXAM

- Presents with erythematous, warm, tender, and edematous skin that may rapidly progress to dark, indurated skin with bullae. Patients typically appear more toxic than those with simple cellulitis and may have significant pain in the involved area.
- A complication of necrotizing fasciitis is compartment syndrome due to edema, which causes elevated intracompartmental pressure that ultimately leads to hypoperfusion of the muscle. Symptoms of compartment syndrome include pain seemingly out of proportion to the infection, muscle weakness, and paresthesias/numbness.

DIFFERENTIAL

May be difficult to distinguish from cellulitis and requires a high degree of suspicion. Pain out of proportion to the physical exam distinguishes necrotiz-

KEY FACT

Compartment syndrome can present with a normal or unchanged arterial pulse.

Q

A 43-year-old diabetic man presents with 1 week of edema, erythema, and warmth of his anterior left lower leg. You start him on IV antibiotics for cellulitis. A few hours later he complains of 10/10 pain in his left leg. His leg is extremely painful to manipulation, and left foot dorsiflexion is 3/5. His left dorsalis pedis and posterior tibial pulses are 1+, unchanged from baseline. What is the next step?

ing fasciitis from cellulitis. An ↑ CK level can suggest the presence of myonecrosis or myositis in addition to necrotizing fasciitis.

DIAGNOSIS

Clinical diagnosis can be difficult. Obtain radiographs and a CT or an MRI to look for gas and soft tissue involvement.

TREATMENT

- A penicillin is best for coverage of group A streptococcus; clindamycin may be used to shut down toxin production. Vancomycin can be added for MRSA coverage.
- If mixed infection is possible, a broad-spectrum penicillin with anaerobic coverage (piperacillin/tazobactam) should be used.
- Obtain a surgery consult for debridement. Fasciotomy may be needed if compartment syndrome develops.

COMPLICATIONS

If it is not treated early, the condition may rapidly progress to compartment syndrome, shock, multiorgan failure, and death.

Periorbital/Orbital Infections

- Differentiating between periorbital (preseptal) and orbital infection is critical, as management differs significantly.
  - Although both present with erythema and ocular pain, orbital infections may also present with oculomotor dysfunction, proptosis, chemosis, worsening pain on eye movement, and ↓ visual acuity.
  - Because orbital infections involve postseptal structures, they can lead to **blindness, meningitis,** and **cavernous sinus thrombosis.**
- **Dx:** The diagnosis of preseptal cellulitis is typically clinical. If there is concern or suspicion for orbital infection, obtain a CT of the orbit (see Figure 10-4), blood cultures, and a CBC with differential.

KEY FACT

If necrotizing fasciitis is suspected, prompt medical **and** surgical management is imperative.

The patient's presentation raises concern for acute compartment syndrome, which suggests that his soft tissue infection has extended to the muscle fascia (ie, necrotizing fasciitis). Acute compartment syndrome requires immediate surgical consultation for possible fasciotomy.

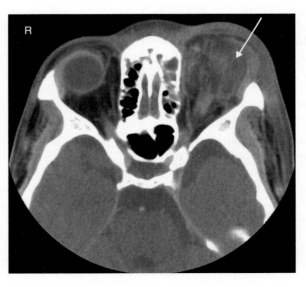

FIGURE 10-4. Left orbital abscess. (Reproduced with permission from Riordan-Eva P, Cunningham E. *Vaughan & Asbury's General Ophthalmology,* 18th ed. New York: McGraw-Hill, 2011, Fig. 13-6.)

Tx:
  - Preseptal cellulitis can be managed on an outpatient basis with antibiotics that cover skin flora (*S aureus*, *Streptococcus* spp.).
  - Orbital cellulitis requires broad-spectrum IV antimicrobials to cover GNRs (eg, ceftriaxone, ampicillin/sulbactam) and skin flora, including MRSA (vancomycin). Surgical consultation is an important part of management.

Acute Osteomyelitis

Infection of the bone that is spread hematogenously or, more commonly, by direct inoculation. Those with peripheral vascular disease, diabetes, and recent orthopedic surgery are at ↑ risk.

SYMPTOMS/EXAM

- Presents with pain with overlying erythema, edema, and tenderness. Patients may have an overlying ulcer or skin interruption.
- Systemic symptoms include fevers, chills, and fatigue.

DIFFERENTIAL

Cellulitis, necrotizing fasciitis.

DIAGNOSIS

- Obtain blood cultures, CBC, and ESR/CRP. ESR and CRP are usually ↑, but blood cultures may remain ⊖.
- Obtain plain films of the suspected area of infection. These may be normal, as infection must have been present for 10–14 days before changes are seen on x-ray.
  - If normal, proceed to MRI, a more sensitive modality for the detection of osteomyelitis.
  - In patients with a contraindication to MRI, a bone scan may be obtained (see Figure 10-5).
  - If plain films or MRI/bone scan are abnormal, obtain a bone biopsy with culture for definitive diagnosis.

TREATMENT

- Unless the patient is septic, delay antimicrobial therapy until a microbiologic specimen has been obtained through surgical debridement.
- Then start with broad coverage of the likely organisms, and narrow coverage once the organism has been identified. Treatment duration is 4–6 weeks of directed antimicrobial therapy.
- The most common organism is *S aureus*. Consider *Salmonella* if the patient has sickle cell anemia, and consider *Pseudomonas* in the setting of IV drug use, diabetes, and lower extremity ulcers.
- Axial skeleton osteomyelitis can resolve with antimicrobials alone, but all other cases require surgical debridement for cure.

Septic Arthritis

Infection of a joint. Risk factors include recent instrumentation of a joint (injection, arthroscopy, arthroplasty), joint damage (osteoarthritis, trauma, RA), a prosthetic joint, gonococcal infection, and bacteremia. Commonly caused by skin flora.

A 23-year-old female heroin user is diagnosed with osteomyelitis. Her history is significant for sickle cell anemia. While you are awaiting culture results, she needs to begin empiric antibiotic treatment. In addition to *S aureus*, for which additional organisms is this patient at risk?

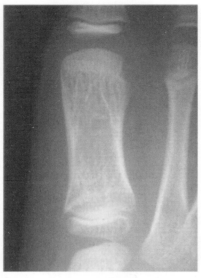

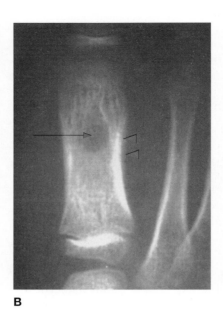

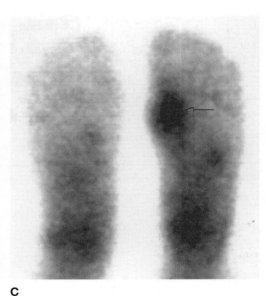

A   B   C

FIGURE 10-5. **Acute osteomyelitis. (A)** Radiograph of the right foot first metatarsal following puncture injury, with no foreign body and no evidence of osteomyelitis. **(B)** Follow-up radiograph reveals interval development of focal lucency (red arrow) and periosteal reaction (red arrowheads) consistent with acute osteomyelitis. **(C)** Planar image from a bone scan obtained at the same time as Image B shows increased radiotracer uptake in the region of the first metatarsal of the right foot (red arrow), confirming osteomyelitis. (Reproduced with permission from Skinner HB. *Current Diagnosis & Treatment in Orthopedics,* 4th ed. New York: McGraw-Hill, 2006, Fig. 8-8A, C, and D.)

- Think of disseminated gonococcal infections in sexually active young adults.
- *Staphylococcus epidermidis* is common in prosthetic joints.

SYMPTOMS/EXAM

Presents as an erythematous, warm, swollen, and painful joint with ↓ range of motion. **Gonococcal septic arthritis may present with multiple infected joints.** Systemic symptoms include fever and chills.

DIFFERENTIAL

- Trauma, hemarthrosis (spontaneous or traumatic), crystalline arthropathy, and autoimmune disease may all present with a similar joint exam.
- Autoimmune disease may present with systemic symptoms similar to those of septic arthritis.
- Septic arthritis may be concurrent with any of these processes; therefore, diagnosis relies on arthrocentesis.

DIAGNOSIS

- Arthrocentesis is required for definitive diagnosis. Send fluid for Gram stain, culture, cell count/differential, and crystal analysis. Synovial fluid in septic arthritis will typically have > 50,000 WBCs with > 90% neutrophilic predominance.
- Blood cultures.

TREATMENT

- Initiate empiric antibiotics promptly after joint aspiration based on Gram stain. Narrow coverage once the organism has been identified.
- **Surgical management with washout and 4–6 weeks of directed antimicrobials are necessary for appropriate management.**

COMPLICATIONS

Joint destruction, sepsis, and death.

Her IV drug use puts her at risk for *Pseudomonas* infection, and her sickle cell anemia puts her at risk for *Salmonella.*

Diverticulitis

Inflammation and microperforation of the diverticula.

SYMPTOMS/EXAM

Presents with fever, chills, nausea, vomiting, and abdominal pain, classically in the LLQ. Occasionally there may be a palpable mass in the LLQ.

DIFFERENTIAL

Ulcerative colitis, Crohn's disease, perforating colon cancer, ectopic pregnancy, PID, ovarian torsion, ovarian cyst rupture.

DIAGNOSIS

A clinical diagnosis that is nonetheless often made with CT (see Figure 10-6). Do not scope patients, as they are at high risk for perforation. Obtain a CBC and blood cultures.

TREATMENT

Bowel rest and antimicrobial coverage of gram-⊖ and anaerobic organisms (eg, ciprofloxacin and metronidazole). If a diverticular abscess is present, manage surgically with a drain or resection.

COMPLICATIONS

Abscess, obstruction, sepsis, death.

Encephalitis

Usually involves the brain parenchyma; HSV is the leading cause. Patients may have nonspecific complaints that are initially consistent with a viral prodrome (eg, fever, malaise, body aches) and may subsequently develop confusion, seizures, and focal neurologic deficits (eg, weakness, cranial nerve/sensory deficits). Headaches, photophobia, and meningeal signs may be seen in meningoencephalitis.

HERPES SIMPLEX VIRUS (HSV) ENCEPHALITIS

- Most cases are due to HSV-1 reactivation.
- **Sx/Exam:** Think of HSV encephalitis when patients present with bizarre behavior, speech disorders, gustatory or olfactory hallucinations, or acute hearing impairment.
- **Dx:** Key CSF studies include **HSV PCR tests and HSV culture.** MRI (see Figure 10-7) will show a characteristic pattern in the temporal lobes, usually bilaterally.
- **Tx:** Treat empirically with IV acyclovir.

WEST NILE ENCEPHALITIS

- Suspect in anyone presenting with fever and altered mental status in late spring, summer, or early autumn.
- **Sx/Exam:** In addition to fever and altered mental status, patients may have extrapyramidal symptoms or flaccid paralysis suggestive of transverse myelitis.

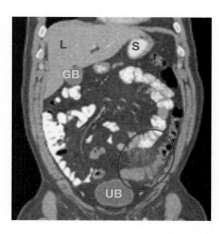

FIGURE 10-6. Acute diverticulitis. Coronal reconstruction from a contrast-enhanced CT demonstrates sigmoid diverticula with perisigmoid inflammatory "fat stranding." The area of abnormality is circled in red. (L = liver; S = stomach; GB = gallbladder; UB = urinary bladder.) (Reproduced with permission from USMLE-Rx.com.)

KEY FACT

If diverticulitis is suspected, do **not** perform lower endoscopy until the acute process resolves, as patients are at high risk for perforation.

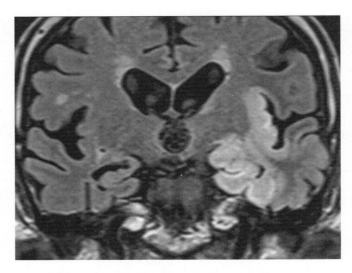

FIGURE 10-7. Herpes encephalitis. Coronal FLAIR MRI in a patient with acute herpes encephalitis shows increased T2 signal within the inferior and medial left temporal lobe. (Reproduced with permission from Ropper AH et al. *Adams & Victor's Principles of Neurology*, 10th ed. New York: McGraw-Hill, 2014, Fig. 33-1A.)

- **Dx:** CSF findings resemble those of **viral meningitis.** Test serum or CSF by ELISA for IgM antibody to West Nile virus. Viral PCR can be used in immunocompromised patients who may not be able to mount an antibody response.
- **Tx:** Treatment is supportive (eg, fluids).

Bacterial Meningitis

Common causative organisms vary with age (see Table 10-1).

SYMPTOMS/EXAM

- Typical symptoms include fever, malaise, headaches, photophobia, and neck stiffness. Patients may also complain of nausea and vomiting.
- Be sure to look for fever, nuchal rigidity, Kernig's sign, Brudzinski's sign, or "jolt sign."
- Funduscopic exam may reveal papilledema, indicating ↑ ICP.

DIAGNOSIS

- **Obtain an LP in any patient suspected of having meningitis.**
- When clinical features suggest a possible intracranial mass or ↑ ICP or if

TABLE 10-1. Common Causes of Bacterial Meningitis by Age

AGE GROUP	TYPICAL BACTERIAL PATHOGEN
Neonates (0–4 weeks)	**Group B streptococcus, *E coli*, *Listeria*.**
Infants (1–23 months)	***Streptococcus pneumoniae*,** *Neisseria meningitidis*, *H influenzae*.
Age 2–50 years	***S pneumoniae*, *N meningitidis*.**
Elderly (> 50 years)	*S pneumoniae*, *N meningitidis*, **Listeria monocytogenes.**

the patient has altered mental status or focal neurologic defects, obtain a head CT before LP.

- Obtain blood cultures before administering antibiotics. See Table 10-2 for CSF findings in meningitis.

TREATMENT

- **Begin empiric therapy immediately after obtaining blood cultures** in anyone suspected of having bacterial meningitis, as even a short delay will ↑ mortality. Antimicrobial therapy should not be delayed if LP cannot be performed immediately.
- Consider the patient's **risk factors** and then choose an antimicrobial regimen that will cover the most likely organisms (see Table 10-3).
- Administer dexamethasone before administering antibiotics if *S pneumoniae* is suspected, as this ↓ mortality.

KEY FACT

Treat suspected meningitis immediately; don't wait for CT or LP results! Therapy can always be tailored later.

Upper Respiratory Tract Infections

ACUTE SINUSITIS

- Inflammation of the mucosal lining of the paranasal sinuses. Viruses are the most common cause. The most common bacterial causes are *S pneumoniae*, *H influenzae*, and *Moraxella catarrhalis*. Anaerobes and rhinoviruses may also be implicated. Think of *Mucor* in diabetics with persistent/recurrent infections despite antibiotics.
- **Sx/Exam:** Look for acute onset of **fever, headache, facial pain,** or **swelling.** Most cases involve cough and purulent postnasal discharge. Patients with bacterial sinusitis are typically febrile and have unilateral tenderness over the affected sinus.
- **Dx:** Based on clinical findings. Radiographic imaging or CT may help (air-fluid level, inflammation of tissues).
- **Tx:** If symptoms persist after 10 days, are severe, or initially improve and then worsen, treat with a 7- to 10-day course of amoxicillin/clavulanate or doxycycline.

OTITIS MEDIA

- Causative agents are similar to those of acute sinusitis.
- **Sx/Exam:**
  - Typical features include **fever** and unilateral **ear pain.**
  - There may also be hearing loss, and children may be irritable or may tug at their ears.

TABLE 10-2.   Common CSF Findings in Meningitis

CSF PARAMETER	BACTERIAL	VIRAL	TB
Opening pressure (mmH₂O)	200–500	< 250	180–300
Cell type	PMNs	Lymphocytes	Lymphocytes
Glucose (mg/dL)	Low	Normal	Low to normal
Protein (mg/dL)	High	Normal	Normal to high

Q

A 55-year-old man with COPD and hypertension is admitted to the ED with a 12-hour history of fever, photophobia, and headache. LP cannot be performed immediately. Which antibiotics should be started empirically?

TABLE 10-3.   **Antibiotic Regimens for Bacterial Meningitis**

PATHOGEN	GRAM STAIN	RISK FACTORS	TREATMENT OF CHOICE
S pneumoniae	Gram-⊕ cocci in pairs and short chains	All patients.	Vancomycin + third-generation cephalosporin + dexamethasone.
N meningitidis	Gram-⊖ diplococci	Age < 50 years.	Ampicillin or third-generation cephalosporin.
L monocytogenes	Gram-⊕ rods	Age > 50 years.	Ampicillin (**not cephalosporins).**
Streptococcus agalactiae (group B strep)	Gram-⊕ cocci in pairs and short chains	Age > 50 years.	Ampicillin.
H influenzae type b	Gram-⊖ coccobacilli	Unvaccinated patients.	Third-generation cephalosporin.

- The tympanic membrane is typically erythematous, lacks a normal light reflex, and is bulging (see Figure 10-8). Look for perforation of the tympanic membrane along with pus in the ear canal.
- Tx:
  - First-line treatment is with amoxicillin/clavulanate × 10 days for children < 2 years of age, × 7 days for children 2–5 years of age, and × 7–10 days for children > 6 years of age. However, many recent studies suggest that a 5- to 7-day course may be adequate in children > 2 years of age with no history of recurrent otitis media.
  - Patients who do not respond to antimicrobial therapy and develop hearing loss should have tympanostomy tubes placed.

OTITIS EXTERNA

- Predisposing factors include **swimming**, eczema, hearing aid use, and mechanical trauma (eg, cotton swab insertion). In most patients, the

A

After blood cultures are obtained, vancomycin and ceftriaxone should be initiated to cover for *S pneumoniae, N meningitidis,* and *H influenzae.* In patients > 50 years of age, ampicillin should be started to cover for *L monocytogenes.*

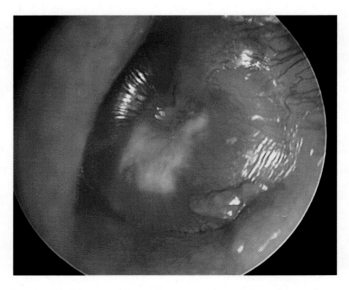

FIGURE 10-8.   Acute otitis media. Tympanic membrane of a patient with acute otitis media. (Reproduced with permission from Brunicardi FC et al. *Schwartz's Principles of Surgery,* 9th ed. New York: McGraw-Hill, 2010, Fig. 18-1.)

causative organism is *Pseudomonas. S aureus* is implicated in acute otitis externa.

- **Sx/Exam:**
  - Patients have a painful ear along with foul-smelling drainage. The **external ear canal** is typically swollen and erythematous. There may also be pus.
  - Patients have tenderness upon **movement of the pinna** or tragus.
- **Tx:** Remove any foreign material from the ear canal and start a topical antimicrobial (typically **ofloxacin**) with **steroids.**

PHARYNGITIS

Typically due to **viral causes** such as rhinovirus, adenovirus, or EBV. **Group A streptococcus** is implicated in up to 25% of cases. Untreated group A streptococcal infection can result in acute pyogenic complications and **rheumatic fever** (fever, arthritis, carditis, chorea, rash).

SYMPTOMS/EXAM

Symptoms include sore throat and fever +/– cough. Look for tonsillar exudates and tender anterior cervical adenopathy.

DIAGNOSIS

- Calculate the Centor score to determine the likelihood of streptococcal infection and the need for rapid streptococcal antigen testing (see Table 10-4).
- Think about infectious mononucleosis in patients with cervical lymphadenopathy, malaise, and/or splenomegaly.
- In adults with pharyngitis, always consider HIV infection and acute retroviral syndrome.
- In children, think about epiglottitis (febrile patients with complaints of severe sore throat and dysphagia with minimal findings on exam).

TREATMENT

- Treat group A streptococcal infections with penicillin. Use a macrolide for patients with penicillin allergy.
- Chronic carriers (ie, those who have a ⊕ throat culture or are asymptomatic) should be treated with clindamycin for eradication.

Pneumonia

Pneumonia still ranks as the sixth leading cause of death overall and is the leading cause of death from infection. Etiologies include:

- **Typical pathogens:** *S pneumoniae, H influenzae, S aureus* (in the setting of influenza virus).
- **Atypical pathogens:** *Mycoplasma, Chlamydia, Moraxella, Legionella.*

SYMPTOMS/EXAM

- Think of pneumonia in any patient with acute onset of **fever, productive cough, dyspnea,** and/or **pleuritic chest pain.**
- **Atypical organisms** may present with low-grade fever, nonproductive cough, and myalgias ("walking pneumonia").
- Look for evidence of consolidation (dullness to percussion, crackles, egophony) on lung exam.

TABLE 10-4. Centor Scoring for Streptococcal Infection[a]

FINDING	POINTS
Anterior cervical lymphadenopathy	1
Tonsillar exudate	1
History of fever	1
Absence of cough	1

[a] **0–1 point:** Low risk; no testing or antibiotics are required.

2–3 points: Intermediate risk; test and treat if ⊕.

4 points: High risk; treat empirically with antibiotics; no testing required.

Q 1

A 28-year-old man with a history of IV drug use presents with sore throat, myalgia, fever, and night sweats of 10 days' duration. He has cervical lymphadenopathy. In addition to being screened for group A streptococcal infection, for which condition should this patient be evaluated?

Q 2

A 75-year-old woman with a history of diabetes comes to the ED with shortness of breath and cough. She is breathing at a rate of 35 breaths per minute and has an O_2 saturation of 94% on room air. She has crackles in her right lower base. Should she be admitted to the hospital?

KEY FACT

Think of *Legionella* infection in a smoker with pneumonia, diarrhea, and elevated LDH.

KEY FACT

Use the CURB-65 score to determine the need for hospitalization in patients with pneumonia.

 A

Acute HIV infection. The symptoms of acute HIV are nonspecific but usually arise 2–4 weeks postexposure.

 A

Yes. Her clinical presentation is consistent with pneumonia. Her CURB-65 score is 2, indicating that she should be admitted to the hospital and started on a respiratory fluoroquinolone or ceftriaxone and azithromycin.

DIAGNOSIS

- There should be radiographic evidence of an infiltrate in all immunocompetent patients (see Figure 10-9) as well as recovery of a pathogenic organism from blood, sputum, or pleural fluid.
- **Urine *Legionella* antigen and urine *S pneumoniae* antigen** should be sent in patients who require ICU admission, fail outpatient antibiotic therapy, have alcohol use disorder, or have a pleural effusion. Asplenic patients and those with chronic liver disease should also be screened for *S pneumoniae*.
- Remember to check an ABG to determine the acid-base status of patients who appear to be in distress.
- If the patient is hospitalized, check blood cultures.

TREATMENT

- Use the CURB-65 score to determine the need for hospital admission. Patients get 1 point for each of the following: **C**onfusion, **U**rea > 19 mg/dL, **R**espiratory rate ≥ 30/min, **B**lood pressure (systolic < 90, diastolic ≤ 60), and age ≥ **65**. Patients with a score of 2 or more should be hospitalized.
- Initiate empiric antimicrobial therapy based on the patient's risk factors (eg, community-dwelling, healthy vs diabetic). **Think about MRSA** in patients with a history of colonization or in those who have been hospitalized (see Table 10-5).
- Treat community-acquired pneumonia for a minimum of 5 days. Treat health care–associated pneumonia for 7–8 days; if caused by MRSA or *Pseudomonas*, treat for 14 days.

PNEUMOCYSTIS JIROVECI PNEUMONIA

Formerly known as *Pneumocystis carinii* pneumonia (PCP). Can occur as an opportunistic infection in HIV-⊕ patients (usually when the CD4 count is < 200) as well as in anyone on immunosuppressive therapies such as high-dose steroids.

SYMPTOMS/EXAM

- Presents with fever, nonproductive cough, and dyspnea on minimal exertion that resolves quickly at rest.

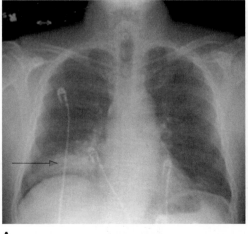 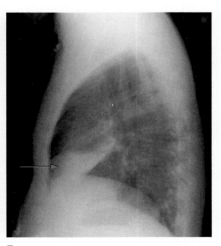

A **B**

FIGURE 10-9. Community-acquired pneumonia. Frontal (**A**) and lateral (**B**) radiographs show airspace consolidation in the right middle lobe (red arrows) in a patient with community-acquired pneumonia. (Reproduced with permission from USMLE-Rx.com.)

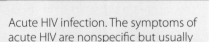

TABLE 10-5. **Empiric Antibiotic Treatment Strategies for Pneumonia**

PATIENT PROFILE	INCLUDE COVERAGE FOR	EMPIRIC ANTIBIOTIC CHOICE
Healthy community members	S pneumoniae, H influenzae, atypicals	Macrolide (azithromycin).
Community members with comorbidities (DM, alcoholism, asplenia, malignancies, chronic heart, lung, liver, or renal disease)	S pneumoniae, Klebsiella, Legionella	Respiratory fluoroquinolone (levofloxacin or moxifloxacin) OR Third-generation cephalosporin (ceftriaxone) + macrolide (azithromycin).
Community members requiring hospitalization	As above	β-lactam (ampicillin, ceftriaxone, cefotaxime) + macrolide (azithromycin) OR Respiratory fluoroquinolone.
Patients at ↑ risk for multi-drug-resistant organisms (MDROs)[a]	Gram-⊖ rods, Pseudomonas, MRSA	Vancomycin or linezolid + cefepime, imipenem, or piperacillin/tazobactam + respiratory fluoroquinolone or gentamicin.
Patients with cystic fibrosis	Pseudomonas	Ceftazidime + respiratory fluoroquinolone + aminoglycoside.
Community members with suspected aspiration	Anaerobes in addition to other organisms found in community members	Add clindamycin or metronidazole to the above regimen.
Suspicion for influenza		Oseltamivir if within 48 hours of symptom onset or in those who require hospitalization.
Ventilated patients	Pseudomonas, Klebsiella, Legionella, Acinetobacter, MRSA, other GNRs	Vancomycin or linezolid + cefepime, imipenem, or piperacillin/tazobactam + respiratory fluoroquinolone or gentamicin.

[a] Defined as patients who have been exposed to antimicrobials within the past 90 days, have been hospitalized for ≥ 5 days, are immunosuppressed, or have health care–associated exposure (hospitalization for ≥ 2 days within the past 90 days, residency in a long-term care facility, hemodialysis, home wound care, or a family member with a known MDR infection).

- Patients may have tachypnea or tachycardia with exertion, fever, or diffuse rales on exam, or there may be few physical exam findings.

DIAGNOSIS

- CXR ranges from normal to bilateral interstitial or alveolar infiltrates. The classic appearance is that of "ground-glass" infiltrates (see Figure 10-10). Look for pneumothorax.
- Other findings include ↑ LDH, often > 500 U/L.
- Obtain a fluorescence stain of sputum or bronchoalveolar lavage to look for Pneumocystis organisms.

TREATMENT

- First-line therapy is with IV TMP-SMX × 21 days. Alternatives include IV pentamidine.

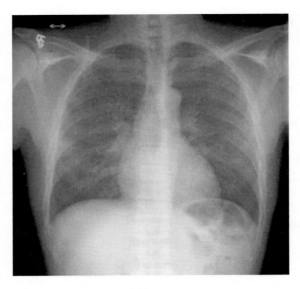

FIGURE 10-10. ***Pneumocystis jiroveci* pneumonia.** Frontal CXR shows diffuse "ground-glass" lung opacities characteristic of PCP in this patient with AIDS and a CD4 count of 26. (Reproduced with permission from USMLE-Rx.com.)

- Use **concomitant prednisone if Pao_2 is < 70 mm Hg** or if the patient has an alveolar-arterial oxygen gradient of > 35 mm Hg on room air.

Bronchitis

Infection of the upper airways (bronchi). Risk factors include cigarette smoking and COPD.

SYMPTOMS/EXAM

Presents with cough +/− sputum production, dyspnea, fever, and chills. The lungs are clear with possible upper airway noise.

DIFFERENTIAL

URI, pneumonia, allergic rhinitis.

DIAGNOSIS

CBC, CXR, sputum Gram stain and culture.

TREATMENT

- Depending on comorbidities and severity, patients may need hospitalization.
- If a bacterial etiology is suspected, give antimicrobials to cover *S pneumoniae* and atypicals.

Tuberculosis (TB)

Caused by *Mycobacterium tuberculosis*. May be 1°, latent, extrapulmonary, or reactivation (see Figure 10-11). Only about 10% of those infected with the bacterium develop active disease.

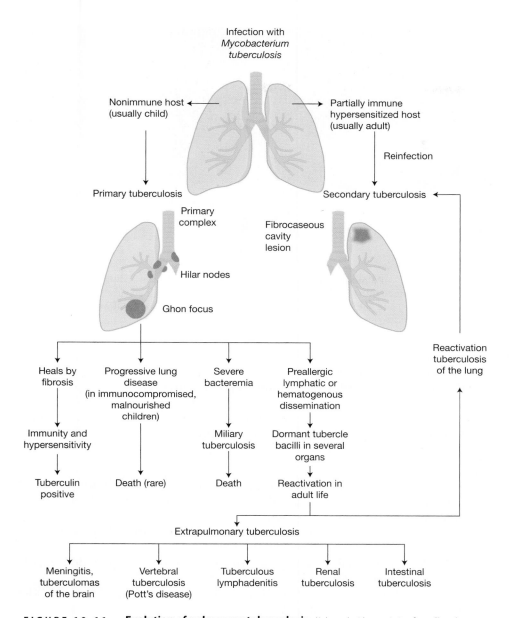

Infection with
Mycobacterium tuberculosis

Nonimmune host
(usually child)

Partially immune
hypersensitized host
(usually adult)

Reinfection

Primary tuberculosis

Secondary tuberculosis

Primary
complex

Fibrocaseous
cavity
lesion

Hilar nodes

Ghon focus

Reactivation
tuberculosis
of the lung

Heals by
fibrosis

Progressive lung
disease
(in immunocompromised,
malnourished
children)

Severe
bacteremia

Preallergic
lymphatic or
hematogenous
dissemination

Immunity and
hypersensitivity

Miliary
tuberculosis

Dormant tubercle
bacilli in several
organs

Tuberculin
positive

Death (rare)

Death

Reactivation in
adult life

Extrapulmonary tuberculosis

Meningitis,
tuberculomas
of the brain

Vertebral
tuberculosis
(Pott's disease)

Tuberculous
lymphadenitis

Renal
tuberculosis

Intestinal
tuberculosis

FIGURE 10-11. **Evolution of pulmonary tuberculosis.** (Adapted with permission from Chandrasoma P, Taylor CR. *Concise Pathology,* 2nd ed. Originally published by Appleton & Lange. Copyright © 1995 by The McGraw-Hill Companies, Inc.)

SYMPTOMS/EXAM

- **1° TB:** Symptoms include fevers and a dry cough. 1° TB usually involves the middle or lower lung zones and is associated with hilar adenopathy (Ghon complex) and radiographic abnormalities. The infection usually resolves, but reactivation occurs in 50–60% of patients.
- **Latent TB infection (LTBI):** Inactive and noninfectious, but reactivation occurs in about 10% of patients, typically involving the upper lungs and cavitation. Latent infection can be detected by a ⊕ PPD. If the PPD is ⊕, the next step is to evaluate for possible active disease with a CXR (see Figure 10-12).
- **Extrapulmonary TB:** Usually associated with HIV-⊕ patients. May involve any organ, but areas most commonly affected (in order of frequency) are the lymph nodes, pleura, GU tract, bones and joints, menin-

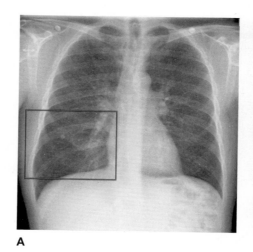
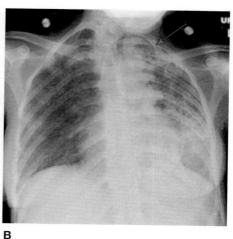

A   B

FIGURE 10-12. **Pulmonary tuberculosis.** **(A)** Frontal CXR demonstrating diffuse, 1- to 2-mm nodules due to miliary TB. **(B)** Frontal CXR demonstrating left apical cavitary consolidation (red arrow) and patchy infiltrates in the right and left lung in a patient with reactivation TB. (Reproduced with permission from USMLE-Rx.com.)

ges, peritoneum, and pericardium. Symptoms are related to the organ involved. Diagnosis is based on an AFB culture of affected tissue.

- **Reactivation TB:** After 1° infection, TB can cause reinfection. Symptoms include fevers, productive cough, hemoptysis, night sweats, and weight loss. Reactivation TB is characterized by fibrocaseous cavitary lesions. Diagnosis is based on an AFB sputum culture.

DIAGNOSIS

- Screening by PPD placement or QuantiFERON Gold should be conducted for LTBI in high-risk groups—eg, immigrants from endemic areas, HIV-⊕ patients, homeless persons, health care workers, IV drug users, and patients with chronic medical conditions (COPD, chronic kidney disease, DM, posttransplant, cancer).
- BCG vaccination status should be disregarded in the interpretation of test results (see Table 10-6).
- If initial testing is ⊕, obtain a CXR to evaluate for active infection. If CXR is ⊖, treat for LTBI as below.
- Active infection is diagnosed by AFB culture of sputum or tissue involved (see Figure 10-13).

TABLE 10-6. **PPD Interpretation**

POPULATION	⊕ TB SKIN TEST
Low risk of disease	≥ 15 mm
Patients with exposure risk (health care workers, immigrants, diabetics, homeless)	≥ 10 mm
HIV-⊕, immunocompromised, recent contact with TB, CXR consistent with previous TB infection	≥ 5 mm

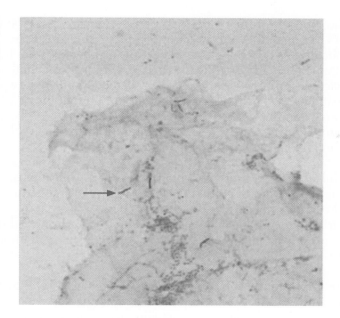

FIGURE 10-13. *Mycobacterium tuberculosis* **on AFB smear.** (Used with permission of the Centers for Disease Control and Prevention, Atlanta, GA, as published in Fauci AS et al. *Harrison's Principles of Internal Medicine,* 18th ed. New York: McGraw-Hill, 2012, Fig. 165-1.)

TREATMENT

- The most commonly used regimen consists of 4 drugs described by the mnemonic **RIPE**—**R**ifampin, **I**soniazid (INH), **P**yrazinamide, and **E**thambutol—given daily for 8 weeks, followed by INH and rifampin for an additional 16 weeks. Table 10-7 outlines the common side effects of these drugs.
- Treatment of LTBI requires 6–9 months of INH.

KEY FACT

Give vitamin B_6 to prevent INH-associated neuropathy.

Genitourinary Tract Infections

CYSTITIS

- **Uncomplicated infection of the lower urinary tract** (ie, cystitis): A symptomatic UTI in a patient with normal immunity and a normal GU tract

TABLE 10-7. **Common Side Effects of Tuberculosis Drugs**

DRUG	SIDE EFFECTS
Rifampin	Red-orange body fluids, hepatitis.
Isoniazid	Peripheral neuropathy (consider giving pyridoxine [vitamin B_6] with medication), hepatitis, lupus-like syndrome.
Pyrazinamide	Hyperuricemia, hepatitis.
Ethambutol	Optic neuritis.

with no prior instrumentation. Infections are common; approximately 10% of US women have at least 1 uncomplicated UTI each year.

- **Complicated UTIs:** Infections occurring in patients with functional or structural abnormalities of the GU tract, recent instrumentation of the urinary tract, or immune compromise (eg, diabetics, pregnant women, transplant patients). UTIs in which symptoms are present for > 7 days are also considered complicated.
- **Sx/Exam:** Dysuria, urgency, and frequency of urination are the most common complaints. Patients may or may not have a fever.
- **DDx:**
  - Think about urethritis/cervicitis in sexually active patients.
  - Renal stones may also present with colicky pain and dysuria.
- **Dx:** Check a UA for the presence of bacteria, WBCs, leukocyte esterase, and nitrites. Uncomplicated UTIs do not require a urine culture. A urine culture must be obtained in complicated UTIs because of the large variety and resistance patterns of organisms.
- **Tx:**
  - **Uncomplicated UTIs:** Give a 3-day course of TMP-SMX, a 5-day course of nitrofurantoin, or single-dose fosfomycin. Use fluoroquinolones or β-lactams only if the previous agents are contraindicated.
  - **Complicated UTIs:** May be treated with oral fluoroquinolones, but often require IV antibiotics for 5–14 days depending on the severity of the infection.

PYELONEPHRITIS

- Infection of the upper urinary tract/kidneys.
- **Sx/Exam:** Findings are similar to those of lower UTI, with systemic symptoms such as fever/chills, tachycardia/hypotension, back or flank pain, and CVA tenderness.
- **Dx:** Urine specimens usually demonstrate significant bacteriuria, pyuria, and occasional WBC casts. A urine culture should be sent on all patients. **Always obtain blood cultures on admission, as 15–20% of patients will be bacteremic.**
- **Tx:**
  - Mild infection may be treated on an outpatient basis with a fluoroquinolone. Otherwise, hospitalization for IV antibiotics is required. Treatment course is 7–14 days depending on the severity of the infection.
  - If there is no clinical response, order CT or ultrasound to look for an intrarenal or perinephric abscess or an obstruction such as a **renal calculus or stricture.**

PROSTATITIS

- **Sx/Exam:**
  - Presenting symptoms include spiking fevers, chills, dysuria, cloudy urine, and even obstructive symptoms if prostate swelling is significant.
  - In patients with chronic infection, low back pain or perineal/testicular discomfort may be present.
  - The gland is exquisitely tender on prostate DRE.
- **Dx:** Obtain urine cultures before and after a prostatic massage. In addition to typical organisms, think of atypical organisms such as *Chlamydia trachomatis* and *Neisseria gonorrhoeae.*
- **Tx:** Treat acute bacterial prostatitis with a fluoroquinolone or IV piperacillin/tazobactam or with a third-generation cephalosporin × 14 days. Treat

chronic bacterial prostatitis with a fluoroquinolone or TMP-SMX for 4–6 weeks.

Sexually Transmitted Diseases (STDs)

SYPHILIS

Caused by *Treponema pallidum*. Transmissible during early disease (1° and 2° syphilis) through exposure to open lesions (loaded with spirochetes!).

SYMPTOMS

- **1° syphilis:** Develops within several weeks of exposure; involves 1 or more painless, indurated, superficial ulcerations (chancre; see Figure 10-14).
- **2° syphilis:** After the chancre has resolved, patients may develop malaise, anorexia, headache, diffuse lymphadenopathy, or rash (involves the mucosal surfaces, palms, and soles).
- **3° syphilis:** Includes cardiovascular, neurologic, and gummatous disease (eg, general paresis, tabes dorsalis, aortitis, meningovascular syphilis).

EXAM

Findings depend on the stage of syphilis—a painless chancre for 1° disease; a maculopapular rash or diffuse lymphadenopathy for 2° disease; and multiple neurologic and/or cardiovascular signs for 3° disease.

DIAGNOSIS

- **1°:** Send a specific treponemal serologic test (FTA-ABS, MHA-TP, or syphilis enzyme immunoassay). Darkfield microscopy of the lesion's exudate will show the spirochetes. Nontreponemal tests (RPR or VDRL) are used for confirmation.
- **2°:** Diagnosed by the presence of clinical illness and ⊕ serologic tests.
- **3°:** Perform an LP in the presence of neurologic or ophthalmic signs and symptoms; in the setting of treatment failure; or with a VDRL of ≥ 1:32. Correlate with cardiovascular, neurologic, and systemic symptoms.

KEY FACT

Patients who have had HIV or syphilis for > 1 year should always undergo LP.

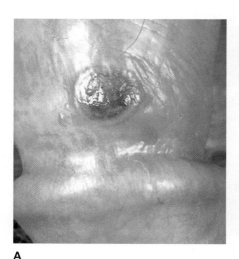
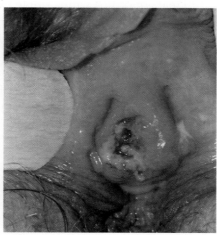
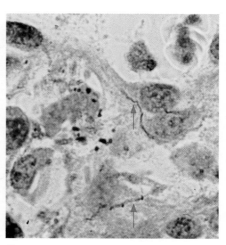

A   **B**   **C**

FIGURE 10-14. **Syphilis.** **(A)** Male and **(B)** female genital chancres, respectively, in primary syphilis infection. **(C)** Silver stain of sample from a chancre showing spiral-shaped spirochetes (arrows). (Reproduced with permission from Wolff K et al. *Fitzpatrick's Dermatology in General Medicine,* 7th ed. New York: McGraw-Hill, 2008, Figs. 200-2, 200-5, and 200-1.)

TREATMENT

- **1°/2°:** Penicillin G 2.4 MU in a single IM dose. Alternatives include doxycycline or erythromycin × 14 days. If the disease duration is > 1 year, give 3 doses of penicillin G IM 1 week apart.
- **Neurosyphilis:** Penicillin G IV × 14 days.

GENITAL HERPES

- Painful grouped vesicles in the anogenital region. Caused by the human herpes simplex virus, usually type 2.
- **Sx/Exam:** Frequently associated symptoms include tender inguinal lymphadenopathy, fever, myalgias, headaches, and aseptic meningitis. Symptoms are usually more pronounced during the initial episode and grow less frequent with recurrences.
- **Dx:** Diagnosis can be confirmed by viral PCR of the vesicle fluid or by direct fluorescent antibody stain.
- **Tx:**
  - Acyclovir × 7–10 days for 1° infections. Treatment should begin within 1 week of symptom onset.
  - Severe recurrences may necessitate repeat treatment with either acyclovir or valacyclovir × 5 days. Daily suppressive therapy can be used for frequent recurrences.

CERVICITIS/URETHRITIS

- Chlamydial and gonococcal infections often present as cervicitis or urethritis. *Mycoplasma genitalium* is an emerging pathogen in this syndrome.
- **Sx/Exam:** Dysuria, dyspareunia, and a mucopurulent vaginal discharge are frequent complaints in women. In men, dysuria and a purulent penile discharge predominate.
- **Dx:** A ⊕ endocervical or urethral culture or a ⊕ urine PCR for chlamydia/gonorrhea is diagnostic.
- **Tx:**
  - **Always treat for both infections simultaneously, and treat sexual partners.**
  - Treat chlamydia with a single PO dose of azithromycin.
  - Treat gonorrhea with a single IM dose of ceftriaxone.

HIV Infection

Acute retroviral syndrome occurs in 50–90% of cases. The incubation period is usually 2–6 weeks. Acute symptoms last 1–4 weeks, with an average of 2 weeks.

SYMPTOMS/EXAM

Patients have a typical viral prodrome (eg, malaise, low-grade fever) followed by the development of adenopathy. Unusual presentations include Bell's palsy, peripheral neuropathy, radiculopathy, cognitive impairment, and psychosis.

DIAGNOSIS

- The CDC recommends fourth-generation HIV serology (EIA) that detects both antibody to HIV and HIV antigen for HIV screening. Serology

KEY FACT

Counsel patients regarding safe-sex practices. HSV transmission can occur even in the absence of visible vesicles.

becomes ⊕ 2–3 weeks after exposure. A confirmatory Western blot is no longer used.

- For patients with suspected acute retroviral syndrome, check a viral load, as the EIA may not have had time to turn ⊕.

TREATMENT

- Begin antiretroviral therapy (ART) in all HIV-⊕ patients regardless of CD4 count. This includes asymptomatic patients and pregnant women.
- Counsel pregnant women with HIV to avoid breast-feeding to ↓ the risk of HIV transmission.
- Start ART in the setting of a needle stick involving blood from an HIV-⊕ patient.
- Regimens should include 2 nucleoside reverse transcriptase inhibitors (NRTIs) and a third drug from a **different category** (see Table 10-8).

TABLE 10-8. Categories of Antiretroviral Drugs

EXAMPLES	COMMON SIDE EFFECTS
NUCLEOSIDE REVERSE TRANSCRIPTASE INHIBITORS (NRTIs)	
Zidovudine (AZT)	Myopathy and bone marrow suppression.
Didanosine (ddI)	Pancreatitis.
Abacavir	Hypersensitivity reactions (eg, fever, chills, dyspnea).
Emtricitabine (FTC)	Diarrhea, nausea, and headache.
Lamivudine (3TC)	Same as those for emtricitabine.
Tenofovir (TNV)	Renal toxicity.
NON-NUCLEOSIDE REVERSE TRANSCRIPTASE INHIBITORS (NNRTIs)	
Efavirenz	CNS toxicity and teratogenicity.
Rilpivirine	Depression, headache, insomnia.
Nevirapine	Rash and hepatic failure.
PROTEASE INHIBITORS (PIs)[a]	
Atazanavir	Benign indirect hyperbilirubinemia.
Indinavir	Kidney stones.
Ritonavir	Potent P-450 inhibitor.
INTEGRASE STRAND TRANSFER INHIBITORS (INSTIs)	
Raltegravir (RAL)	Hypersensitivity reaction.
Dolutegravir (DTG)	Muscle weakness/rhabdomyolysis.

[a] All PIs can ↑ lipids, redistribute fat, and cause DM.

Q

A 37-year-old man with newly diagnosed HIV presents for routine care. His CD4 count is 35 and viral load 120,000 copies/mL. Which prophylaxis regimens should be started?

COMPLICATIONS

Complications are numerous and typically involve opportunistic infections and side effects from drugs. See Table 10-9 for prophylaxis indications.

Travel Medicine

FEVER IN THE RETURNED TRAVELER

Patients who present with a fever after international travel must be evaluated for tropical illnesses. Always consider common illnesses such as URI or UTI as causes of fever.

EXAM/DIAGNOSIS

- Obtain a thorough travel history, including location of travel, immunization status, food precautions taken (or not taken), and sexual exposures.
- Look for rashes, lymphadenopathy, hepatosplenomegaly, jaundice, and neurologic status on exam. Altered mental status after travel is considered a medical emergency.
- Initial evaluation should include a CBC with differential, a complete metabolic panel, blood cultures, thin and thick smears for malaria, and a UA and culture.
- See Table 10-10 for a list of possible causes, presentations, and treatment.

MALARIA PROPHYLAXIS

- Tailor prophylaxis to reflect the prevalence of resistant *Plasmodium falciparum* (high mortality) in the area of proposed travel. Most regimens start 1–2 weeks before travel and continue for 1 month after return.

TABLE 10-9. Prophylaxis in HIV

DISEASE	INDICATION	PROPHYLAXIS
PCP	CD4 < 200 or previous PCP or thrush.	TMP-SMX, dapsone, or atovaquone.
Mycobacterium avium complex (MAC)	CD4 < 50.	Azithromycin weekly.
Toxoplasma gondii	CD4 < 100 and *Toxoplasma* IgG ⊕.	TMP-SMX or dapsone + leucovorin + pyrimethamine.
TB	Recent contact or PPD > 5 mm.	INH for 9 months.
Pneumococcal pneumonia	All HIV-⊕ patients.	Vaccine. Repeat in 5 years.
Influenza	All HIV-⊕ patients.	Yearly vaccine.
Hepatitis B	All HIV-⊕ patients.	Hepatitis B vaccine.

A

The patient should be started on TMP-SMX for PCP and toxoplasmosis prophylaxis and should be given azithromycin for MAC prophylaxis. He should also be vaccinated against influenza (not the live vaccine), hepatitis B, and pneumococcus.

TABLE 10-10.   Causes, Diagnosis, and Management of Fever in the Returned Traveler

CAUSE	HIGH-RISK AREAS	METHOD OF TRANSMISSION	INCUBATION PERIOD	PRESENTATION	DIAGNOSIS	TREATMENT
Malaria	Africa, south-central and Southeast Asia, Western Pacific, Caribbean islands, Central America, South America	*Anopheles* mosquito bite	7–30 days	Malaise, headache, myalgias, jaundice, anemia, abnormal LFTs, thrombocytopenia, hypoglycemia	Serial thin and thick smears, at least × 3, looking for ring forms inside RBCs.	Antibiotic treatment varies depending on local resistance patterns. Blood products as needed for anemia.
Typhoid fever	South-central and Southeast Asia, southern Africa	Fecal-oral	5–21 days	Malaise, abdominal discomfort, diarrhea, hepato-splenomegaly, rose spots	Growth on blood, urine, or stool culture.	Fluoroquinolones.
Dengue fever	South-central and Southeast Asia, Western Pacific, Africa, Central America, South America, Caribbean islands	*Aedes* mosquito bite	3–10 days	Severe myalgias (also known as "breakbone fever" because of associated pain), headache, retroorbital pain, maculopapular rash, thrombocytopenia, hemorrhage	Primarily clinical; can check titers.	Supportive care/blood products as needed.

- Weekly chloroquine is the mainstay of therapy in chloroquine-sensitive areas.
- Mefloquine is active against chloroquine-resistant *P falciparum* and is also given weekly. Mefloquine resistance is present in Southeast Asia.
- Daily doxycycline or daily Malarone (atovaquone and proguanil) can be used in those who are unable to take mefloquine or who are traveling to chloroquine-resistant areas. Malarone can be used for short trips.
- **Precautions:**
  - Mefloquine has the potential for serious neuropsychiatric side effects and should not be prescribed to people with recent or active depression, psychosis, schizophrenia, or anxiety disorders.
  - Other effects of mefloquine include sinus bradycardia and QT-interval prolongation; avoid in patients on β-blockers or in those with known conduction disorders.

Infectious Diarrhea

- **Sx/Exam:** Diarrhea usually associated with abdominal pain +/– fever. Bloody diarrhea is typically due to enterohemorrhagic *E coli* (EHEC), *Campylobacter*, *Shigella*, and occasionally *Salmonella*.

- **DDx:** IBD, ischemic bowel, Whipple's disease, celiac disease, IBS, lactose intolerance, neuroendocrine disorders.
- **Dx:**
  - Diagnosis can frequently be made from symptoms alone. Because most cases of diarrhea are self-limited, studies are not usually warranted.
  - For patients with blood in the stool, fever, and severe abdominal pain, obtain a stool sample to examine for fecal leukocytes and send for culture.
  - Bloodwork may show leukocytosis, evidence of dehydration, hemolysis, or renal failure.
- **Tx:**
  - The most important treatment is fluid resuscitation; in children, use oral rehydration therapy. Avoid antimotility agents.
  - For travelers, consider an empiric fluoroquinolone or azithromycin if severe. Avoid antimicrobials in EHEC, as this could precipitate hemolytic-uremic syndrome. See Table 10-11 for guidelines on the treatment of specific organisms.

CLOSTRIDIUM DIFFICILE COLITIS

- Risk factors include recent antimicrobial use (other than metronidazole), recent hospitalization, and PPI use.
- **Sx/Exam:** Abdominal pain, diarrhea, nausea/vomiting (if ileus). Physical exam shows diffuse TTP.
- **Dx:**
  - Stool EIA for toxins A and B followed by confirmatory cell cytotoxic assay/oxygenic culture or PCR.
  - Also check KUB or CT of the abdomen and pelvis for toxic megacolon or associated ileus.
- **Tx:** Discontinue or minimize all antimicrobials. See Figure 10-15 for a treatment algorithm. Some patients may require fecal transplant or colectomy if symptoms do not resolve with antibiotics.

Tick-Borne Diseases

Lyme disease, Rocky Mountain spotted fever, human monocytic ehrlichiosis, human granulocytic anaplasmosis, and babesiosis are all transmitted to humans via tick bites. They are particularly prevalent in the Northeast, including Cape Cod, Martha's Vineyard, and Nantucket. See Table 10-12 for details.

Neutropenic Fever

Most often occurs after chemotherapy. Defined as a single temperature of > 38.3°C (101.3°F) or a sustained temperature of > 38°C (100.4°F) for > 1 hour in a neutropenic patient (ANC = PMNs + bands < 500).

Symptoms/Exam

- The skin should be examined for signs of erythema, rash, cellulitis, ulcers, or line infection.
- All indwelling lines should be carefully examined for subtle signs of infection, as erythema, tenderness, fluctuance, or exudate may be the only evidence of a serious "tunnel infection."
- Do not conduct a DRE unless perirectal abscess is suspected.

KEY FACT

Elderly patients or those on corticosteroids may not be able to mount a fever that meets the diagnostic criteria for neutropenic fever.

TABLE 10-11.   Common Pathogens Causing Diarrhea and Their Treatment

ORGANISM	RISK FACTORS	ANTIMICROBIAL TREATMENT
Salmonella spp.	Raw meat or improperly handled food; reptile exposure.	Fluoroquinolones if severe.
Shigella spp.	Child care workers.	Fluoroquinolones if severe.
Campylobacter jejuni	Raw/undercooked chicken, pork.	Azithromycin, fluoroquinolones if severe.
E coli	Contaminated food; undercooked beef (in particular *E coli* O157:H7).	Fluoroquinolones if severe. Do not use antimicrobials if *E coli* O157:H7 is implicated.
Vibrio spp.	Seafood.	Doxycycline if severe.
Yersinia enterocolitica	Raw/undercooked pork; unpasteurized milk.	Fluoroquinolones or TMP-SMX if severe.
S aureus	Inappropriately stored or handled food (eg, potato salad left out at room temperature, poor hand hygiene).	Not indicated.
Bacillus cereus	Reheated fried rice.	Not indicated.
Clostridium perfringens	Inappropriately stored or handled food.	Not indicated.
Giardia	Travelers, contaminated water, immune compromise.	Metronidazole, ART if HIV ⊕.
Cryptosporidium	Travelers, contaminated water, child care workers, immune compromise/HIV.	ART.
Cyclospora/Isospora	Travelers, contaminated water or produce, immune compromise/HIV.	TMP-SMX, ART.
Mycobacterium avium complex (MAC)	Immune compromise/HIV.	Clarithromycin + ethambutol, ART.
Microsporidium	Immune compromise/HIV.	Albendazole, ART.
C difficile	Antibiotic or health care facility exposure.	See Figure 10-15.
Norovirus/rotavirus/adenovirus	Child care workers, cruise ships.	Not indicated.
Hepatitis A	Travelers, contaminated water.	Not indicated.

DIAGNOSIS

- Obtain a CBC with differential, a complete metabolic panel, amylase, lipase, and a CXR.
- Obtain at least 2 sets of blood cultures and urine cultures. Consider sending stool and sputum cultures if clinically indicated. LP is warranted only if CNS symptoms are present.

TREATMENT

- Empiric antimicrobials should cover *Pseudomonas*. Use cefepime IV or a carbapenem IV.

Q

A 52-year-old man presents to the ED with altered mental status. He has a fever of 39°C (102.2°F), a heart rate of 130 bpm, and a BP of 100/60. His WBC count is 13,500 cells/mm³. What are the next most important steps in his management?

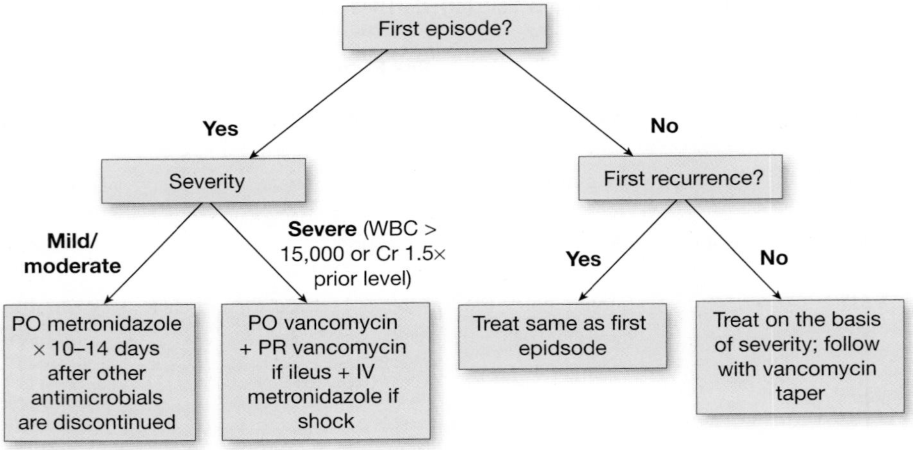

FIGURE 10-15. **Algorithm for the treatment of *Clostridium difficile* infection.**

- Consider vancomycin in patients with a history of MRSA infections, hypotension, persistent fever on empiric therapy, or skin or catheter site infections.
- Think about fungal infections (especially *Candida* and *Aspergillus*) in patients with 4–7 days of persistent fever, and begin amphotericin B, micafungin, or voriconazole.

Sepsis

Defined as 2 or more SIRS criteria **with evidence of infection.** Divided into 3 levels of severity (see Table 10-13). SIRS criteria are as follows:

- **Temperature:** $< 36°C$ ($< 96.8°F$) or $> 38°C$ ($> 100.4°F$).
- **Heart rate:** > 90 bpm.
- **Respiratory rate:** > 20 breaths/min or a P_{CO_2} of < 32 mm Hg.
- **Leukocytes:** $> 12,000$ cells/mm^3, < 4000 cells/mm^3, or $> 10\%$ bands on peripheral blood smear.

SYMPTOMS/EXAM

- Presents with nonspecific infectious symptoms such as fever, chills, and fatigue.
- Symptoms and signs suggestive of cellulitis, necrotizing fasciitis, meningitis, sinusitis, pneumonia, endocarditis, UTI, or GI infection are seen.
- Vital signs are abnormal (see the SIRS criteria above).
- Evidence of hypoperfusion includes cool, pale extremities, ↓ pulses, altered mental status, and ↓ urine output.

DIAGNOSIS

- Find the focus of infection on the basis of the history and physical exam.
- Always obtain blood cultures and sensitivities.
- Obtain a serum lactate to evaluate for end-organ hypoperfusion.

TREATMENT

- Early antimicrobial therapy and fluid resuscitation have been shown to ↓ mortality and are thus critical to the management of sepsis.
- The initial choice of antimicrobials should be based on the likely source or should be broad spectrum if the source is unclear. These should be tailored on the basis of culture data.

KEY FACT

Early initiation of appropriate antimicrobials is critical in the management of sepsis.

This patient is septic. Aggressive IV fluid resuscitation and broad-spectrum antibiotics should be initiated immediately to reduce mortality.

TABLE 10-12.   Clinical Features of Selected Tick-Borne Diseases

DISEASE	CAUSATIVE PATHOGEN	SYMPTOMS/EXAM	DIAGNOSIS	TREATMENT
Lyme disease	*Borrelia burgdorferi*; transmitted by *Ixodes* deer tick	**Early localized:** **Erythema migrans** (see Figure 10-16), fever, arthralgias, myalgias, lymphadenopathy. **Early disseminated:** Myocarditis +/− AV block, Bell's palsy, peripheral neuropathy, meningitis. **Late disseminated:** Arthritis, chronic neurologic symptoms.	ELISA as initial screen followed by Western blot or PCR as a confirmatory test.	Doxycycline or amoxicillin. **If cardiac or neurologic symptoms are present, treat with ceftriaxone.**
Rocky Mountain spotted fever	*Rickettsia rickettsii*; transmitted by a variety of ticks (different from those that transmit Lyme disease)	Fever, rash on palms and soles that spreads to the trunk, arthralgias, headache, thrombocytopenia, hyponatremia, ↑ transaminases.	Serum antibody titers.	Doxycycline.
Human monocytic ehrlichiosis, human granulocytic anaplasmosis	*Ehrlichia* spp., *Anaplasma phagocytophilum*; transmitted by several deer ticks; may be cotransmitted with Lyme disease	Nonspecific, such as fever, chills, malaise, headache, and myalgias with no physical exam findings. Patients often have **thrombocytopenia, leukopenia, and** ↑ **transaminases.**	Serology, PCR, or peripheral blood smear to look for intracytoplasmic inclusions (morulae).	Doxycycline.
Babesiosis	*Babesia* spp. (*Babesia* organisms infect RBCs)	Fever, chills, fatigue, myalgias. Bloodwork will reflect **hemolytic anemia.**	Peripheral blood smear looking for organisms inside RBCs (in **Maltese cross formation**) or PCR.	Clindamycin and quinine are preferred. Atovaquone and azithromycin are alternatives. Consider plasma exchange in those with severe infection (> 10% parasitemia, significant hemolytic anemia). If symptoms persist, consider coinfection with *Anaplasma/Ehrlichia* or Lyme disease.

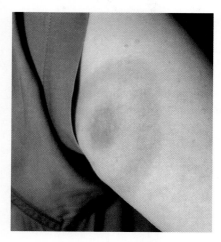

FIGURE 10-16.   Lyme disease. The classic "target" or "bull's-eye" lesion of erythema migrans is seen. (Used with permission of James Gathany, Public Health Image Library, Centers for Disease Control and Prevention, Atlanta, GA, as published in Papadakis MA et al. *Current Medical Diagnosis & Treatment 2015.* New York: McGraw-Hill, 2015, Figure 6-28.)

TABLE 10-13.   Severity of Sepsis

SEVERITY	CRITERIA
Sepsis	Meets at least 2 of the SIRS criteria with evidence of infection.
Severe sepsis	Meets the criteria for sepsis with evidence of end-organ damage.
Septic shock	Meets the criteria for sepsis with BP not responding to fluid resuscitation and necessitating the initiation of pressors and/or inotropes.

- Aggressive fluid resuscitation to maintain mean arterial pressure at > 65 mm Hg and urine output at > 0.5 mL/kg/hr should be initiated within the first 6 hours of the hospital course (including time in the ED).
- Consider central line access for cardiovascular and pulmonary monitoring as well as administration of high-volume fluid resuscitation, blood products, and/or pressors/inotropes.
- Consider an arterial line for continuous monitoring of BP.

COMPLICATIONS

Can lead to ARDS, DIC, multiorgan failure, and death.

Staphylococcal Toxic Shock Syndrome

A systemic response to staphylococcal infection, resulting in shock with multiorgan failure.

- Caused by toxic shock syndrome toxin-1 (TSST-1), a staphylococcal exotoxin that acts as a superantigen, activating multiple T cells at once and leading to massive cytokine release.
- Think of staphylococcal TSS in menstruating women (tampons can serve as a nidus for infection), in women with postpartum wounds, and in postsurgical patients with wounds that might serve as a source of infection.

SYMPTOMS

Fever, hypotension, a diffuse macular rash followed by desquamation (1–2 weeks later), and multiorgan failure (eg, diarrhea/vomiting, myalgias/rhabdomyolysis, renal failure, liver failure, thrombocytopenia, altered mental status).

DIAGNOSIS

Check blood, wound, and/or vaginal cultures for *Staphylococcus.*

TREATMENT

- Aggressive IV fluid resuscitation is essential owing to capillary leak caused by cytokine release.
- Any foreign bodies in the vaginal canal should be removed. If related to an infected wound, fluid collections should be drained.
- Antibiotic treatment should include a penicillinase-resistant penicillin for methicillin-susceptible *S aureus* or vancomycin for MRSA. All patients should be started on clindamycin to stop protein/toxin synthesis.

Fungal Infections

Typically affect immunocompromised patients and should always be considered in this population, but may also affect healthy adults. Fungus morphology may be as a yeast with spores, as a mold with hyphae, or both (see Table 10-14). Fungi that can present with both morphologies are referred to as dimorphic fungi and grow as a mold at room temperature and as a yeast at body temperature.

Antimicrobial Selection

When a pathogen has been definitively identified, it is important to choose an antimicrobial with narrow coverage. Table 10-15 illustrates common antimicrobials and their spectra of coverage. Table 10-16 reviews the mechanisms of action of the various antimicrobial classes and common adverse effects.

TABLE 10-14. Characteristics, Diagnosis, and Management of Fungal Infections

INFECTION	MORPHOLOGY	GEOGRAPHIC LOCATION/MODE OF TRANSMISSION	HISTORY/SYMPTOMS/EXAM	DIAGNOSIS	TREATMENT
Cryptococcosis	**Encapsulated yeast.**	Not localized to a particular region. Inhalation of pigeon droppings.	Self-limited pneumonia in healthy patients. Invasive with **meningo-encephalitis** if depressed T-cell function.	Antigen testing and culture of infected tissue (blood, sputum, CSF). May be seen with silver stain. **India ink test may show a halo 2° to capsule** (see Figure 10-17).	**Mild to moderate disease:** Fluconazole × 6–12 months. **Invasive disease or immuno-compromised hosts:** Amphotericin + flucytosine for 2 weeks followed by long-term fluconazole.
Histoplasmosis	Dimorphic fungus; narrow-based budding yeast on biopsy.	**Ohio/Mississippi River Valleys.** Inhalation of **bat guano or bird excrement, typically in caves or at construction sites.**	**Respiratory/flulike illness** in healthy host. Disseminated disease in immuno-compromised hosts, with **palatal ulcerations,** fever, weight loss, splenomegaly, and anemia/ **bone marrow suppression.**	Silver staining and culture of biopsied infected tissue +/− *Histoplasma* antigen tests of urine and serum.	**Mild to moderate disease without CNS involvement:** Itraconazole. **Severe/disseminated disease:** Amphotericin.

TABLE 10-14. **Characteristics, Diagnosis, and Management of Fungal Infections** *(continued)*

INFECTION	MORPHOLOGY	GEOGRAPHIC LOCATION/MODE OF TRANSMISSION	HISTORY/SYMPTOMS/ EXAM	DIAGNOSIS	TREATMENT
Coccidioido-mycosis	Dimorphic fungus; spherules with **endospores** on biopsy.	**Southwestern United States, particularly Arizona or the San Joaquin Valley in California.** Inhalation of spores from soil.	1° disease is usually a self-limited **pneumonia** with dry cough and fever. Disseminated disease affects the CNS (meningitis), skin **(erythema nodosum),** bones, and joints.	Silver stains of culture or biopsy, serologic studies, or antibody detection in CSF if meningitis is present.	Fluconazole or itraconazole. Amphotericin for severe pneumonia, disseminated infection (including CNS infection), and immuno-compromised patients.
Blastomycosis	Dimorphic fungus, **broad-based budding yeast** on biopsy.	Ohio/Mississippi River Valleys, states bordering the Great Lakes. Inhalation of spores from soil.	Most patients present with pneumonia. Up to 50% may have disseminated disease with a **verrucous-like rash**/subcutaneous nodules and/or **osteomyelitis.**	Direct visualization on wet prep and culture of infected tissues. With bone involvement, **lytic lesions may be seen on plain film.**	**Mild to moderate disease without CNS involvement:** Itraconazole. **Severe/disseminated disease:** Amphotericin.
Aspergillosis	Mold, **septated branched hyphae** on biopsy.	Not localized to a specific region. Inhalation of mold, which is abundant in nature.	Invasive aspergillosis may present with the classic triad of fever, pleuritic chest pain, and **hemoptysis.** Chronic pulmonary infection with **aspergilloma (fungus ball),** nodules, or **cavitary lesions.**	Direct visualization and culture of infected tissues, detection of anti-aspergillus IgG, +/− serum galacto-mannan antigen detection. May present with cavitary lesions or nodules with surrounding ground-glass infiltrates representing hemorrhage in invasive aspergillosis. Chronic infection can present with nodules or aspergilloma (fungus ball).	Voriconazole +/− surgical resection or embolization if uncontrolled hemoptysis.

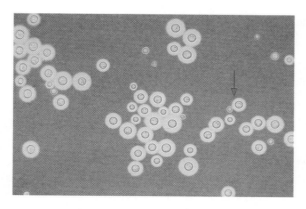

FIGURE 10-17. ***Cryptococcus neoformans.*** India ink preparation demonstrating budding yeast (arrow) and thick, translucent polysaccharide capsules outlined by the dark India ink particles. (Used with permission of Dr. L. Haley, Public Health Image Library, Centers for Disease Control and Prevention, Atlanta, GA, as published in Levinson W. *Review of Medical Microbiology and Immunology,* 12th ed. New York: McGraw-Hill, 2012, Fig. 50-7.)

TABLE 10-15. **Common Antimicrobials and Their Coverage**

ANTIMICROBIAL GROUP	COMMON EXAMPLES	ORGANISMS COVERED
Natural penicillins	Penicillin G, penicillin V	*T pallidum, Enterococcus,* streptococci, and rare penicillin-sensitive staphylococci.
β-lactamase-resistant penicillins	Dicloxacillin, methicillin (no longer used clinically, but important because of methicillin-resistant staphylococci), nafcillin, oxacillin	Used primarily for methicillin-sensitive staphylococci, but do cover some streptococci.
Aminopenicillins	Amoxicillin, amoxicillin/clavulanic acid, ampicillin, ampicillin/sulbactam	Natural penicillin coverage and *E coli, Proteus, H influenzae,* and *Enterococcus.* β-lactamase inhibitors add coverage for enteric gram-⊖ organisms and anaerobes.
Extended-spectrum penicillins	Piperacillin/tazobactam, ticarcillin/clavulanic acid	Aminopenicillin/β-lactamase inhibitor coverage in addition to resistant gram-⊖ organisms, including *Pseudomonas.*
First-generation cephalosporins	Cefazolin, cephalexin	Staphylococci, streptococci, *Proteus, E coli,* and *Klebsiella* **(PEcK).** Cephalosporins do not cover any enterococci.
Second-generation cephalosporins	Cefaclor, cefuroxime	First-generation cephalosporin coverage and *H influenzae,* **E**nterobacteriaceae, *Neisseria* **(HEN PEcK).**
Cephamycins	Cefotetan, cefoxitin	Second-generation cephalosporin coverage and gram-⊕/gram-⊖ anaerobes.
Third-generation cephalosporins	Cefotaxime, ceftazidime, ceftriaxone	Most gram-⊖ aerobes and gram-⊕ anaerobes. Ceftriaxone adds streptococcal coverage and ceftazidime adds *Pseudomonas* coverage.
Fourth-generation cephalosporins	Cefepime	Gram-⊖ aerobes, streptococci, and *Pseudomonas.*
Second-generation quinolones	Ciprofloxacin	Gram-⊖ aerobes and atypicals such as *Legionella, Mycoplasma,* and *Chlamydia.* Best *Pseudomonas* coverage of all quinolones.

TABLE 10-15. **Common Antimicrobials and Their Coverage** *(continued)*

ANTIMICROBIAL GROUP	COMMON EXAMPLES	ORGANISMS COVERED
Third-generation quinolones	Levofloxacin	Gram-⊖ aerobes, streptococci, and atypicals.
Fourth-generation quinolones	Gatifloxacin, moxifloxacin	Gram-⊕ organisms, some anaerobes, weak gram-⊖ coverage, and atypicals.
Carbapenems	Ertapenem, imipenem, meropenem	Gram-⊕ organisms (except resistant *Staphylococcus* and *Enterococcus*); gram-⊖ organisms, including *Pseudomonas* and anaerobes. Ertapenem has no *Pseudomonas* or *Enterococcus* coverage.
Macrolides	Azithromycin, erythromycin, clarithromycin	Gram-⊕ organisms and atypicals. High *S pneumoniae* resistance.
Aminoglycosides	Gentamicin, tobramycin	Gram-⊖ aerobes, including *Pseudomonas*.
Others	Aztreonam	Gram-⊖ aerobes, including *Pseudomonas*.
	Clindamycin	Gram-⊕ anaerobes, MRSA.
	Dalfopristin/quinupristin	MRSA and vancomycin-resistant enterococci (VRE).
	Linezolid	MRSA; VRE.
	Metronidazole	Anaerobes *(C difficile)*.
	TMP-SMX	Gram-⊖ organisms, gram-⊕ organisms, PCP.
	Vancomycin	MRSA and *C difficile* (PO only).
	Tetracyclines (doxycycline, minocycline, tigecycline)	Tick-borne infections, atypical organisms, streptococcus, and MRSA.

TABLE 10-16. **Mechanisms of Action and Adverse Effects of Selected Antimicrobial Classes**

Antimicrobial Group	Mechanism of Action	Adverse Effects
Penicillins	Inhibit bacterial cell wall synthesis.	Hypersensitivity reaction.
Cephalosporins	Inhibit bacterial cell wall synthesis; less susceptible to β-lactamases.	Hypersensitivity reaction.
Quinolones	Inhibit DNA synthesis.	Tendinopathy, QTc prolongation, myasthenia gravis exacerbation.
Carbapenems	Inhibit bacterial cell wall synthesis; highly resistant to β-lactamases.	Anemia, transaminitis.
Macrolides	Inhibit bacterial protein synthesis.	QTc prolongation, cholestasis.
Aminoglycosides	Inhibit bacterial protein synthesis.	Hearing loss, renal dysfunction.
Tetracyclines	Inhibit bacterial protein synthesis.	Tooth discoloration, skin photosensitivity, drug-induced lupus, GI upset.
Aztreonam	Inhibits bacterial cell wall synthesis.	Transaminitis, GI upset, neutropenia.
Clindamycin	Inhibits bacterial protein synthesis.	GI upset, rash.
Linezolid	Inhibits protein synthesis.	Bone marrow suppression, peripheral neuropathy, lactic acidosis.
Metronidazole	Inhibits bacterial DNA synthesis.	GI upset, peripheral neuropathy, disulfiram-like reaction with EtOH.
TMP-SMX	Inhibits bacterial DNA synthesis.	Hyperkalemia, thrombocytopenia, ↓ creatinine clearance.
Vancomycin	Inhibits bacterial cell wall synthesis.	Red man syndrome, thrombocytopenia. Rarely renal toxicity.

NOTES

CHAPTER 11

MUSCULOSKELETAL

KEY FACT

Libman-Sacks endocarditis, also known as verrucous endocarditis, is characterized by noninfectious, granular, pea-sized masses near the edge of a valve or valve ring.

MNEMONIC

SLE criteria—

DOPAMINE RASH

Discoid rash
Oral ulcers
Photosensitive rash
Arthritis
Malar rash
Immunologic criteria (⊕ anti-dsDNA or ⊕ anti-Sm)
NEurologic or psychiatric symptoms
Renal disease
ANA ⊕
Serositis (pleural, peritoneal, or pericardial)
Hematologic disorders (thrombocytopenia, anemia, or leukopenia)

Systemic Lupus Erythematosus (SLE)

A multisystem, chronic inflammatory disease that may affect the skin, joints, kidneys, lungs, nervous system, and serous membranes. Patients may experience acute flare-ups of their symptoms. SLE is generally 1° but sometimes occurs 2° to drug use (eg, hydralazine, penicillamine, procainamide, TNF inhibitors, minocycline). 2° SLE is reversible.

SYMPTOMS/EXAM

Disproportionately affects young African American women; also common among Asians and Hispanics. Findings by organ system include:

- **Constitutional:** Fatigue, weight loss, fever.
- **Musculoskeletal:** Arthritis is usually migratory and symmetric, often involving the hands. Joint symptoms affect > 90% of patients.
- **Skin: Many characteristic skin findings are associated with SLE.** These include **malar rash** (a "butterfly rash" over the cheeks and nose; see Figure 11-1), **discoid rash** (erythematous plaques with central atrophy), painless **oral ulcers,** Raynaud's phenomenon, and a **photosensitive rash.**
- **Renal:** Nephritis and nephrosclerosis, which can lead to renal failure.
- **Pulmonary: Pleurisy,** pleural effusion, interstitial lung disease, pulmonary hypertension, pneumonitis, alveolar hemorrhage.
- **Cardiovascular: Pericarditis,** pericardial effusion, verrucous endocarditis, ↑ risk of CAD.
- **CNS:** Seizures, headache, peripheral neuropathies, thromboembolic disease.
- **Psychological:** Delirium, anxiety, depression, psychosis.
- **Hematologic:** Thrombocytopenia, hemolytic anemia, leukopenia, thrombophilia, lymphadenopathy, splenomegaly.
- **GI: Peritonitis.**

DIAGNOSIS

- The diagnostic criteria for SLE are summarized in the mnemonic **DOPAMINE RASH.** Diagnosis is clinical and requires at least 4 of the 11 criteria listed.

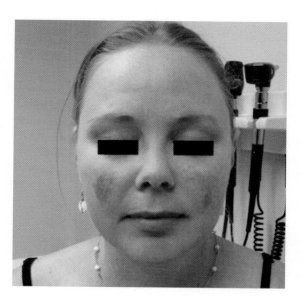

FIGURE 11-1. **Malar rash in a butterfly distribution.** (Reproduced with permission from Imboden JB et al. *Current Diagnosis & Treatment: Rheumatology,* 3rd ed. New York: McGraw-Hill, 2013, Plate 35.)

- The ANA test is the best screening measure for SLE. It is highly sensitive but nonspecific, whereas anti-dsDNA and anti-Sm antibodies are highly specific (sensitivity is much lower, at about 75% and 25%, respectively). Drug-induced lupus is associated with antihistone antibodies. ANA is ⊕ with significant titers (usually 1:160 or higher) in almost all cases.
- Active SLE (flare-up) presents with an ↑ in IgG and anti-dsDNA titers and a ↓ in complement levels (especially CH50, C3, and C4).
- Obtain anticardiolipin antibody and lupus anticoagulant assays to screen for antiphospholipid antibody syndrome. Most patients with antiphospholipid antibody syndrome do not have full-blown SLE.

TREATMENT

- Arthritis and mild serositis are treated with NSAIDs. Hydroxychloroquine is also routinely used.
- Steroids and immunosuppressants (cyclophosphamide, azathioprine), including biologic agents that target B cells (belimumab, rituximab), are used for refractory cases or in the presence of significant organ involvement.
- Active flare-ups are treated with steroids, which are tapered once remission has been induced.
- Patients with antiphospholipid antibody syndrome need lifelong anticoagulation with warfarin.
- Patient education should include protection from sunlight and other sources of UV light, maintenance of a balanced diet, smoking cessation, immunizations, and avoidance of pregnancy during active disease.

COMPLICATIONS

- SLE patients who become pregnant have a higher incidence of spontaneous abortion.
- Newborns who develop neonatal lupus can develop congenital complete heart block.
- Stroke etiologies in SLE include arterial and venous thrombosis, cardiogenic embolism, small vessel infarcts, and vasculitis.
- Antiphospholipid antibody syndrome predisposes patients to arterial and venous thrombosis.
- Mortality in SLE is frequently due to accelerated atherosclerosis, infections, malignancy, or renal disease.

Rheumatoid Arthritis (RA)

A symmetric, inflammatory, peripheral polyarthritis of unknown etiology with extra-articular manifestations that include pulmonary fibrosis, serositis, vasculitis, and rheumatoid nodules.

SYMPTOMS/EXAM

- Presents with insidious onset of a symmetrical arthritis. Polyarticular disease presents with a gradual onset and intermittent or migratory joint involvement.
- **Nonspecific** complaints include fever, fatigue, anorexia, and weight loss. Affected joints are swollen and tender (the MCP and PIP joints of the fingers, interphalangeal joints of the thumbs, wrists, and MTP joints of the toes are sites of arthritis early in the disease).
- Other findings include joint deformities (see Figure 11-2), atlantoaxial joint subluxation, carpal tunnel syndrome, and Baker's cyst.

Q   1

A 27-year-old woman presents with SLE, and you start her on hydroxychloroquine. What is a potential toxicity associated with the long-term use of this drug?

Q   2

A 58-year-old woman with warm and tender joints at her wrists and the bases of her fingers has failed methotrexate therapy for her RA and wants to try anti-TNF therapy. What should you remember to screen for before initiating this treatment?

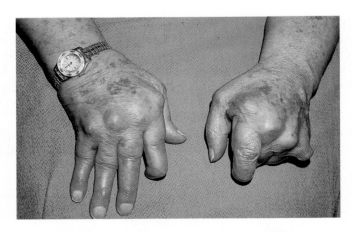

FIGURE 11-2.   Ulnar deviation of the MCP joints and swelling of the PIP joints in rheumatoid arthritis. Multiple subcutaneous rheumatoid nodules are also seen. (Reproduced with permission from Goldsmith LA et al. *Fitzpatrick's Dermatology in General Medicine,* 8th ed. New York: McGraw-Hill, 2012, Fig. 160-1A.)

KEY FACT

Atlantoaxial instability is a complication of RA that makes intubation riskier than normal.

- **Extra-articular features** may include anemia, fatigue, subcutaneous ("rheumatoid") nodules, neuropathy, episcleritis and scleritis, Sjögren's syndrome (dry eyes and mouth), pulmonary fibrosis, vasculitis, hepatosplenomegaly, pleuritis, lung nodules, pericarditis, and myocarditis.

DIAGNOSIS

- Diagnosed in the presence of 4 or more of the following criteria for 6 weeks:
    - Arthritis of 3 or more joint areas, most commonly the PIP, MCP, wrist, elbow, knee, or ankle (see Figure 11-3).
    - Arthritis of the hand joints (MCP, PIP, or wrists).

1   A

Retinal toxicity. Monitor the patient with baseline and follow-up ophthalmologic exams.

2   A

Screen for latent TB with a PPD test or QuantiFERON Gold, and test for hepatitis B and C antibodies.

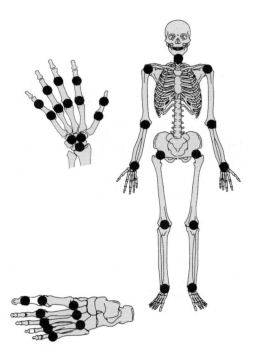

FIGURE 11-3.   Joint distribution in rheumatoid arthritis. RA involves almost all synovial joints in the body (vs osteoarthritis, which has a more limited distribution). (Reproduced with permission from Imboden JB et al. *Current Diagnosis & Treatment: Rheumatology,* 3rd ed. New York: McGraw-Hill, 2013, Fig. 15-1A.)

- Symmetric arthritis.
- Rheumatoid nodules (most commonly found at the elbow).
- ↑ CRP or ESR.
- Radiographic changes (obtain plain films of affected joints in all RA patients). Classic changes are symmetric joint space narrowing and periarticular osteopenia (see Figure 11-4).
- RF is nonspecific but is ⊕ in 75% of cases. **Anti–cyclic citrullinated peptide (anti-CCP)** antibody is much more specific for RA. Joint aspiration is inflammatory (see Table 11-1). Look for periarticular osteoporosis with erosions around the affected MCP and PIP joints on x-ray.

TREATMENT

- Start treatment with disease-modifying antirheumatic drugs (DMARDs) as soon as possible to prevent joint damage and long-term disability. Methotrexate is a first-line DMARD.
- In moderate to severe RA, initiate anti-inflammatory therapy with either an NSAID or a glucocorticoid, and start DMARD therapy.
- If methotrexate fails or is contraindicated, give anti-TNF treatment (etanercept, infliximab, adalimumab). Patients on TNF inhibitors are at ↑ risk for infections and possibly malignancies.
- Patients with acute exacerbations (ie, those who are febrile, toxic, or experiencing a rapid decline in function) are treated with a short course of prednisone.
- Other measures include weight loss, rest, smoking cessation, and physiotherapy. Screen for and treat osteoporosis resulting from steroid use.

Gout

A metabolic condition resulting from the intra-articular deposition of monosodium urate crystals and characterized by extracellular fluid urate saturation and hyperuricemia. Tissue deposition of urate crystals results in inflammatory changes and destructive consequences. Hyperuricemia results either from

KEY FACT

Clinical findings of RA hands:
- MCP and PIP involvement
- Sparing of the DIP joint
- Ulnar deviation
- Symmetric
- Swan-neck deformities
- Boutonnière deformities

KEY FACT

Methotrexate for RA is contraindicated in pregnant patients and in those with HIV, liver disease, renal failure, or bone marrow suppression.

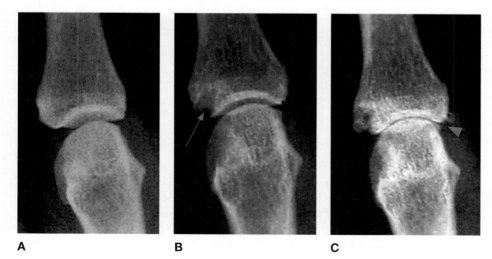

A   B   C

FIGURE 11-4.   Progression of radiographic findings in rheumatoid arthritis. (A) Normal MCP joint 1 year before the onset of RA. **(B)** Six months following disease onset, there is a bony erosion (arrow) adjacent to the joint along with joint space narrowing. **(C)** After 3 years of disease, diffuse loss of articular cartilage has led to marked joint space narrowing (arrowhead).
(Reproduced with permission from Imboden JB et al. *Current Rheumatology Diagnosis & Treatment*, 3rd ed. New York: McGraw-Hill, 2013, Fig. 15-3.)

Q

A 47-year-old man celebrates his birthday by going out for steak and beer. The following morning, his first MTP joint is red and painful even to light touch. He is on lovastatin, aspirin, hydrochlorothiazide, and niacin. Which of his medications likely contributed to his gout?

TABLE 11-1. Interpretation of Joint Aspiration

	NORMAL	NONINFLAMMATORY	INFLAMMATORY	INFECTIOUS	HEMORRHAGIC
Color	Clear	Xanthochromic	Yellow	Opaque	Bloody
Viscosity	High	High	Low	Low	Variable
WBCs/mm^3	< 200	200–3000	3000–50,000	> 50,000	Variable
% PMNs	< 25	< 25	> 50	> 75	Variable
Crystals	None	None	May be present	None	None
Differential	None	Osteoarthritis, SLE, trauma, aseptic, necrosis, scleroderma, Charcot's joint	Gout, pseudogout, RA, SLE, TB, scleroderma, ankylosing spondylitis, psoriatic arthritis	Bacterial, TB	Coagulopathy, trauma

KEY FACT

Monoarthritis? Think:
- Gout
- Septic arthritis
- Lyme disease
- Pseudogout
- Trauma

KEY FACT

Patients with gout should limit their intake of EtOH, as ethanol ↑ urate synthesis and ↓ uric acid excretion.

Hydrochlorothiazide and other thiazide diuretics interfere with the excretion of uric acid, thereby exacerbating gout.

excessive urate production or from ↓ renal uric acid excretion. Complications include nephrolithiasis and chronic urate nephropathy.

SYMPTOMS/EXAM

- Typically presents in **middle-aged, obese men** (90%). Those from the Pacific Islands are disproportionately affected. Incidence in women ↑ after menopause.
- Acute gout attacks often occur at night between periods of remission. The 3 stages are acute gouty arthritis, interval gout, and chronic recurrent and tophaceous gout.
- Patients initially present with severe pain, redness, and swelling in a single lower extremity joint (typically the first MTP joint); subsequent attacks may present in an additive fashion with multiple joints.
- Differentiate from pseudogout, in which symptoms may be severe and often affect the knee (> 50%) or shoulder. Involvement of the ankle, wrist, or olecranon bursa is more common in a recurrent episode of gouty arthritis.
- Common precipitants of attacks include a high-purine diet (eg, meats, alcohol), dehydration or diuretic use (thiazides), high-fructose corn syrup, stress, severe illness, trauma, and tumor lysis syndrome.
- Patients with long-standing disease may develop tophi that lead to joint deformation.

DIAGNOSIS

- Many patients with acute gouty arthritis have a history of years of asymptomatic hyperuricemia.
- The best initial test is arthrocentesis. Joint aspiration from warm, swollen joints helps distinguish inflammatory from noninflammatory disease as well as infectious from hemorrhagic processes (see Table 11-1). In gout, joint aspirate is inflammatory with needle-shaped, negatively birefringent (yeLLow when paraLLel to the condenser) crystals (see Figure 11-5 and Tables 11-1 and 11-2).
- Radiographs are normal in early gout. Characteristic punched-out erosions with overhanging cortical bone ("rat bites") are seen in advanced disease (see Figure 11-6).

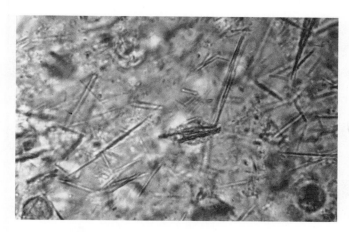

FIGURE 11-5. **Gout crystals.** Note the needle-shaped, negatively birefringent crystals. (Reproduced with permission from Longo DL et al. *Harrison's Principles of Internal Medicine,* 18th ed. New York: McGraw-Hill, 2012, Fig. 333-1.)

- Most patients have ↑ serum uric acid (which is neither sensitive nor specific). Thirty percent of patients have at least 1 normal uric acid level. Roughly 90% are underexcretors of uric acid, and the remainder are overproducers. Uric acid levels can be normal during a flare.

TREATMENT

- For acute attacks, administer high-dose NSAIDs (eg, indomethacin).
- Colchicine is useful if started within the first 24 hours of an attack or when there is a contraindication to the use of NSAIDs. Side effects include diarrhea, nausea, and bone marrow suppression.
- Use oral or intra-articular steroids when first-line therapy fails or is contraindicated.
- Once the acute attack resolves, begin maintenance therapy to ↓ serum uric acid levels (≤ 6 mg/dL). Allopurinol can be used in either overproducers or underexcretors; underexcretors should receive probenecid.
- Before starting probenecid, collect a 24-hour urine sample for uric acid while the patient is **off** hyperuricemia-inducing medications (eg, diuretics, alcohol, cyclosporine) to determine whether the hyperuricemia is due to undersecretion or overproduction of urate (see Table 11-3).
- Encourage a low-purine diet (eggs, cheese, fruit, and vegetables). Weight loss and BP control can also prevent flares.
- Renal complications of chronic hyperuricemia include nephrolithiasis and chronic urate nephropathy.

KEY FACT

Remember to **A**void **A**llopurinol in **A**cute gout **A**ttacks.

TABLE 11-2. **Differential Diagnosis of Gout and Pseudogout**

	GOUT CRYSTALS	**PSEUDOGOUT CRYSTALS**
Composition	Urate	Calcium pyrophosphate dihydrate
Shape	Needle shaped	Rhomboid shaped
Refringence	Negatively birefringent	Strongly positively birefringent
Red compensator	YeLLow when paraLLel	Blue when parallel
Response to colchicine	Good	Weak

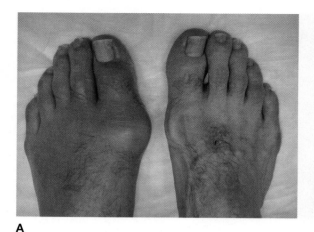
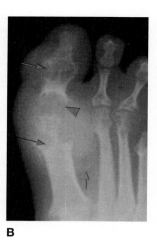

A **B**

FIGURE 11-6. Gout. (A) A swollen left first MTP joint with overlying erythema and warmth, characteristic of an acute gout attack (podagra). **(B)** AP radiograph of the right foot in a different patient showing the severe consequences of long-standing gout, including large, nonmarginal erosions with overhanging edges of bone (red arrows), soft tissue swelling, and destruction of the first MTP joint (arrowhead). Note the subtle calcification of a gouty tophus (orange arrow). (Image A reproduced with permission from LeBlond RF et al. *DeGowin's Diagnostic Examination*, 9th ed. New York: McGraw-Hill, 2009, Plate 30. Image B reproduced with permission from USMLE-Rx.com.)

Osteoarthritis (OA)

A chronic, noninflammatory joint disease characterized by degeneration of the articular cartilage, hypertrophy of the bone margins, and synovial membrane changes. OA can be 1° or 2° to trauma, chronic arthritis, or a systemic metabolic disorder (hevmochromatosis, Wilson's disease).

SYMPTOMS/EXAM

- Marked by insidious onset of joint pain without inflammatory signs (swelling, warmth, and redness).
- In contrast to the "morning stiffness" of inflammatory arthritis, OA worsens with activity during the day and improves with rest. Morning stiffness has a duration of < 30 minutes.
- 1° OA usually involves the following joints:
  - **Hands: DIP,** PIP, and first carpometacarpal joints. Classic DIP deformities are known as Heberden's nodes (see Figure 11-7). Contrast this with the classic MCP lesions of RA (see Figure 11-8).
  - **Feet:** First MTP joint.

TABLE 11-3. Causes of Hyperuricemia

	OVERPRODUCTION OF URIC ACID	UNDERSECRETION OF URIC ACID
24-hour urine collection for uric acid	> 800 mg/day	< 800 mg/day
Etiology	Idiopathic (1°), inherited enzyme defect, myeloproliferative disorders, lymphoproliferative disorders, tumor lysis syndrome, psoriasis	Chronic kidney disease, aspirin, diuretics

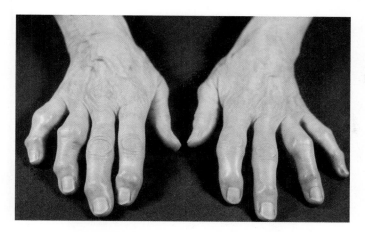

FIGURE 11-7.   Osteoarthritis. Severe osteoarthritis of the hands affecting the DIP joints (Heberden's nodes) and the PIP joints (Bouchard's nodes). (Reproduced with permission from Longo DL et al. *Harrison's Principles of Internal Medicine*, 18th ed. New York: McGraw-Hill, 2012, Fig. 332-2.)

■ **Knees, hips.**
■ **Spine:** C5, T9, and L3 are the most common spinal levels.

DIAGNOSIS

■ Diagnosed clinically in combination with radiographic findings showing joint space narrowing that is frequently asymmetric (see Figure 11-9), subchondral sclerosis, and osteophytes.
■ ANA, ESR, RF, and anti-CCP are normal. Joint fluid has a leukocyte count of < 2000.

TREATMENT

■ 1° treatment consists of weight loss, physiotherapy, and low-impact exercise.

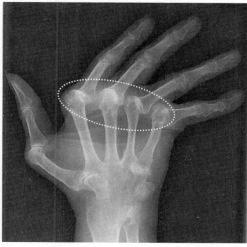

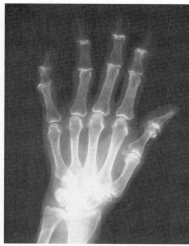

A   B

FIGURE 11-8.   Rheumatoid arthritis vs osteoarthritis. (A) Classic changes of RA include ulnar deviation at the MCP joints, destruction of carpal bones, and destruction of the radiocarpal and ulnocarpal joints. **(B)** OA changes include severe joint space narrowing at all DIP and PIP joints. Joint space narrowing at the carpometacarpal joint of the first digit is also seen. (Image A reproduced with permission from Brunicardi FC et al. *Schwartz's Principles of Surgery*, 9th ed. New York: McGraw-Hill, 2010, Fig. 44-18B. Image B reproduced with permission from Imboden JB et al. *Current Diagnosis & Treatment: Rheumatology*, 3rd ed. New York: McGraw-Hill, 2013, Fig. 43-1.)

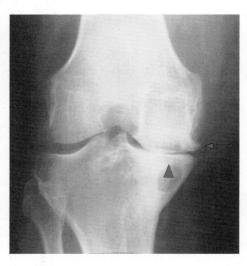

FIGURE 11-9. **Radiographic changes in knee osteoarthritis.** AP knee radiograph shows a narrowed joint space on the medial side of the joint only; subchondral sclerosis (arrowhead) and a cyst (lucency below the arrowhead); and osteophytes (arrow). (Reproduced with permission from Chen MY et al. *Basic Radiology*. New York: McGraw-Hill, 2004, Fig. 7-40.)

- For mild symptoms, use acetaminophen or NSAIDs. Intra-articular corticosteroid injections may be added for further pain control.
- Joint replacement is used for severe OA in patients who fail medical management and have marked limitation of their daily activities.

Low Back Pain (LBP)

LBP is the leading cause of missed workdays in the United States. Table 11-4 outlines common causes.

DIAGNOSIS

- Conduct a neurologic exam to determine if the spinal nerves are affected (see Table 11-5).
- Suspect spinal cord involvement if the Babinski reflex is upgoing or if there is sphincter laxity. An **UP**going toe is an **UP**per motor neuron sign.
- A ⊕ **straight leg raise test** (in which a supine patient experiences leg, buttock, or back pain in the affected leg at < 30° of elevation of the affected leg) is sensitive for spinal nerve irritation or radiculopathy. A ⊕ **crossed straight leg raise test** (in which a supine patient experiences leg, buttock, or back pain in the affected leg at < 30° of elevation of the **unaffected** leg) is specific for spinal nerve irritation.
- Order a **lumbar spine x-ray** for patients in whom osteomyelitis, cancer, fractures, or ankylosing spondylitis is suspected or for those who fail to improve after 2–4 weeks of conservative therapy. Consider screening for osteoporosis if fractures are seen on x-ray.
- An MRI should be ordered if cauda equina syndrome is suspected or if the patient has neurologic deficits for which surgery is being considered.

TREATMENT

- Patients with cauda equina syndrome or spinal nerve involvement require surgical evaluation. Degenerative LBP is treated with NSAIDs and physiotherapy. Ankylosing spondylitis is treated with TNF inhibitors and physiotherapy (see below).

KEY FACT

Order x-rays in geriatric patients with new-onset back pain or if the history and physical are suggestive of malignancy, infection, or inflammatory arthropathy.

TABLE 11-4.   Causes of Low Back Pain

	SYMPTOMS/EXAM	DIAGNOSIS
Cauda equina syndrome	Bowel and bladder incontinence or retention, saddle anesthesia. **A medical emergency.**	Order a stat MRI if cauda equina is suspected.
Degenerative processes	Chronic and progressive. **Degeneration of disks** leads to localized pain that can refer to adjacent spinal nerves (eg, pain that radiates down the thigh). Severe disk disease can lead to **spinal stenosis,** in which LBP worsens with standing and walking but improves with sitting or stooping forward (patients typically find it easier to walk uphill than downhill).	Order a lumbar spine x-ray to rule out other causes of LBP.
Neoplastic	1° or metastatic to bone. Suspect in elderly patients with unintentional weight loss or a history of cancer.	A tumor mass may be seen on lumbar spine x-ray. Bone scan or MRI can detect disease not seen on plain film.
Traumatic	Acute onset of LBP is temporally associated with a traumatic event. Look for local spinal tenderness 2° to a **fracture** or a **herniated disk** (pain worsens with cough; L4 or L5 nerve root compression). Paraspinal tenderness indicates **myofascial strain.**	CT may be necessary to confirm a fracture and to assess the spinal column for stability. Myofascial strain and disk herniations cannot be seen.
Osteomyelitis	Fever, chills, or IV drug use. **ESR** is often ↑↑.	X-ray may show disk narrowing and endplate destruction. MRI may be needed to aid in diagnosis and to assess for epidural abscess.
Ankylosing spondylitis	The typical patient is a young adult male presenting with chronic LBP that is worse in the morning and accompanied by sacroiliitis/arthritis of the hip, knee, or shoulder. Look for acute anterior uveitis, restriction of chest wall expansion, dactylitis, Achilles tendinitis, and plantar fasciitis. ↓ spinal mobility.	AP pelvic x-ray shows pseudo-widening, erosions, and sclerosis of the sacroiliac joint. The classic "bamboo spine" on lumbar x-ray is from ossification of spinal ligaments. HLA-B27 is 90% sensitive in Caucasians.
Referred	Can be 2° to disease from the aorta, kidneys, ureter, or pancreas.	Conduct a thorough abdominal exam.

- Most LBP from disk herniation will improve within 6 weeks; surgery should be considered in cases of progressive neurologic deficits.

Spondyloarthropathies

The family of spondyloarthropathies encompasses a group of inflammatory arthritides that sometimes overlap. These include:

- Ankylosing spondylitis
- Reactive arthritis (formerly known as Reiter's syndrome)

Q

A 69-year-old man presents with back pain of more than a year's duration that radiates down his legs. He reports that the pain worsens when he walks downhill but is relieved when he pushes his granddaughter's stroller. You diagnose presumed spinal stenosis and order an MRI. You should ask about changes in bowel and bladder function to rule out what complication?

TABLE 11-5.   Spinal Nerve Damage and Associated Sensorimotor Deficits

Nerve	Motor Deficits	Sensory Deficit	Reflexes
L3, L4	Problems in rising from a chair and heel walking.	Over the anterior knee or the medial calf.	↓ knee jerk.
L5	Problems with heel walking, extending the big toe, or dorsiflexing the ankle.	Over the medial aspect of the foot.	
S1	Problems with toe walking or plantar flexing the ankle.	Over the lateral aspect of the foot.	↓ ankle jerk.

- Psoriatic arthritis
- Spondyloarthritis associated with Crohn's disease and ulcerative colitis
- Juvenile-onset spondyloarthritis (including juvenile RA)

ANKYLOSING SPONDYLITIS

- A chronic inflammatory disease of the axial skeleton that presents with progressive stiffness of the spine that can lead to kyphosis, hip and shoulder pain, enthesitis, and ↓ chest expansion. Associated with HLA-B27 (see Table 11-4).
- Extra-articular involvement includes uveitis, aortitis, and IBD.
- **Dx:** X-ray of the lumbar spine shows the characteristic "bamboo spine."
- **Tx:** NSAIDs, exercise. In patients who do not respond to NSAIDs, consider a biological agent such as a TNF inhibitor.

REACTIVE ARTHRITIS

- An inflammatory arthritis, typically of the GI or GU tract, with pathogens such as *Campylobacter, Yersinia, Salmonella, Shigella, Chlamydia trachomatis,* and possibly *C difficile* and *Chlamydia pneumoniae.* Onset occurs days to weeks after infection. Formerly known as Reiter's syndrome.
- **Sx/Exam:** Usually affects the lower extremities asymmetrically, presenting as a mono- or oligoarthritis. Extra-articular symptoms include conjunctivitis, uveitis, and urethritis.
- **Tx:** NSAIDs are first line; intra-articular glucocorticoid injections for patients who are unresponsive to NSAIDs alone. DMARDs if refractory.

PSORIATIC ARTHRITIS

A

Cauda equina syndrome, which is a medical emergency and must therefore be ruled out.

- An inflammatory arthritis associated with psoriasis.
- **Sx/Exam:** Presents with pain and stiffness in the affected joint, joint line tenderness (enthesitis), nail pitting, asymmetric oligoarthritis, symmetric polyarthritis (similar to RA), and spondyloarthritis, including both sacroiliitis and spondylitis.
- **Tx:** Treatment usually begins with NSAIDs; if the arthritis remains active despite NSAIDs, consider methotrexate or a TNF inhibitor (infliximab, adalimumab, etanercept).

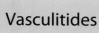

Vasculitides

Defined by the presence of inflammatory leukocytes in vessel walls **with subsequent tissue ischemia or hemorrhage. Vasculitis may occur as a 1° disease or 2° to another underlying pathology.** Treatment focuses on management of the underlying disease. Categorized on the basis of vessel size:

- **Large-vessel vasculitis:** Takayasu's arteritis, temporal arteritis.
- **Medium-vessel vasculitis:** Kawasaki disease, polyarteritis nodosa.
- **Small-vessel vasculitis:** Eosinophilic granulomatosis with polyangiitis (Churg-Strauss syndrome), granulomatosis with polyangiitis (Wegener's), Henoch-Schönlein purpura, cryoglobulinemic vasculitis.

TEMPORAL ARTERITIS (GIANT CELL ARTERITIS)

Affects older women more often than men by a ratio of 2:1. Can cause **blindness** 2° to occlusion of the **central retinal artery** (a branch of the internal carotid artery). Half of patients also have polymyalgia rheumatica.

SYMPTOMS/EXAM

- Classic symptoms consist of a new headache and scalp tenderness (eg, pain combing the hair) along with **temporal tenderness, jaw claudication,** and visual symptoms such as **monocular blindness.**
- Also associated with weight loss, myalgias/arthralgias, and fever.

DIAGNOSIS

Obtain an **ESR** (often > 100 mm/hr), a prompt ophthalmologic evaluation, and a **temporal artery biopsy.** Biopsy will reveal thrombosis; necrosis of the media; and lymphocytes, plasma cells, and giant cells.

TREATMENT

- Treat immediately with **high-dose prednisone** (40–60 mg/day) and continue for 1–2 months before tapering. Do not delay treatment, as blindness is permanent.
- Conduct serial eye exams for improvements or changes. Other complications include angina, stroke, and aortic aneurysm.

POLYARTERITIS NODOSA (PAN)

A systemic necrotizing vasculitis that involves medium-size muscular arteries. Most commonly affects middle-aged men. Not associated with the presence of ANCA.

SYMPTOMS

- Patients present with systemic symptoms (fatigue, weight loss, fever, arthralgias). Commonly affects the GI tract, skin, joints, nerves, and kidneys (multisystem involvement).
- Frequently presents with mononeuritis multiplex.

DIAGNOSIS

- Diagnosis is mostly clinical; common laboratory features include ↑ ESR, leukocytosis, thrombocytosis, and anemia.
- Tissue biopsy from muscle and skin (the most accurate test) reveals vasculitis.

KEY FACT

Treatment of temporal arteritis should not be delayed while awaiting biopsy results, as a biopsy may still be ⊕ even after 2 weeks of corticosteroid therapy.

Q

A 73-year-old woman comes to your office complaining of a headache that has developed over the past month along with pain when combing her hair. She has a palpable tender cord on her right temple, and you strongly suspect temporal arteritis. Should you wait to start systemic corticosteroids until she can get a temporal artery biopsy?

TREATMENT

Oral glucocorticoid monotherapy is first-line treatment; in patients whose glucocorticoid dose cannot be tapered, consider immunosuppressive medications (eg, cyclophosphamide).

Polymyalgia Rheumatica (PMR)

An inflammatory disease that causes severe pain and stiffness in proximal muscle groups without weakness or atrophy. Risk factors include female gender and age > 50. PMR is associated with giant cell arteritis, which may precede, coincide with, or follow polymyalgia symptoms. The average age at diagnosis is > 70 years.

SYMPTOMS/EXAM

- Typical symptoms include bilateral aching and morning stiffness lasting ≥ 30 minutes for at least 2 weeks.
- Patients present with pain and **stiffness of the shoulder and pelvic girdle** along with **fever,** malaise, weight loss, and minimal joint swelling.
- Patients classically have difficulty getting out of a chair or lifting their arms above their heads but have **no objective weakness.**

DIAGNOSIS

Look for concurrent **anemia** and an ↑↑ **ESR** that occasionally exceeds 100 mm/hr.

TREATMENT

Treat with **low-dose prednisone** (20 mg/day) followed by a long taper. Pain due to PMR responds rapidly to corticosteroids (in 2–4 days). The principal goal of treatment is symptom relief.

Fibromyalgia

A chronic pain disorder characterized by soft tissue and axial skeletal pain in the absence of joint pain or inflammation. It is typically a diagnosis of exclusion and can be frustrating to manage. Affects women more often than men, and prevalence ↑ with age.

SYMPTOMS/EXAM

- Presents as a syndrome of myalgias, insomnia, weakness, and fatigue in the absence of inflammation. Patients complain of muscle aches and stiffness with trigger points.
- Associated with depression, anxiety, and IBS.

DIAGNOSIS

- Lab testing is ⊖.
- The research criteria used for diagnosis require 11 of 18 tender **trigger points** (see Figure 11-10) that reproduce pain with palpation.

TREATMENT

- Treatment includes pregabalin, progressive physical reconditioning, improvement of restorative sleep, and supportive measures such as heat application.

KEY FACT

Polymyalgia causes **P**ain but not weakness.

KEY FACT

Long-term steroid use can cause osteoporosis. Screen with DEXA scans, and prevent and treat with calcium, vitamin D, weight-bearing exercise, and, when necessary, bisphosphonates.

No. It may be possible to get an accurate diagnostic biopsy weeks to months after starting treatment, but blindness resulting from temporal arteritis is permanent.

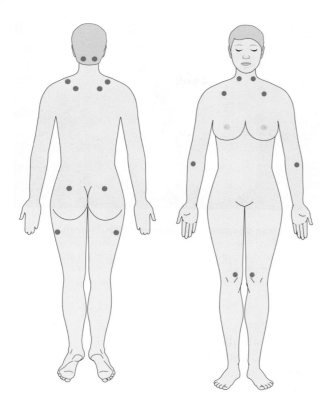

FIGURE 11-10.   Trigger points in fibromyalgia. (Reproduced with permission from Le T et al. *First Aid for the USMLE Step 2 CK,* 7th ed. New York: McGraw-Hill, 2010: 265.)

- Consider hydrotherapy, transcutaneous electrical nerve stimulation (TENS), stress reduction, psychotherapy, or low-dose antidepressants.

Polymyositis and Dermatomyositis

Polymyositis is a progressive systemic connective tissue disease characterized by muscle inflammation, muscle fiber necrosis, degeneration, and inflammatory cell infiltration. **Dermatomyositis** is characterized by similar muscle weakness, but with coexisting cutaneous involvement. Systemic manifestations include myocarditis, pulmonary fibrosis, and cardiac conduction deficits. More commonly seen in **older women** (50–70 years of age).

SYMPTOMS/EXAM

- **Polymyositis:** Presents with **symmetric,** progressive proximal muscle weakness that is sometimes accompanied by pain, resulting in the classic complaint of difficulty rising from a chair. Patients may have trouble swallowing and speaking and may eventually have difficulty breathing. Dyspnea may be a sign of pulmonary fibrosis.
- **Dermatomyositis:** May present with a **heliotrope rash** (a violaceous periorbital rash) and **Gottron's papules** (papules located on the dorsum of the hands over bony prominences; see Figure 11-11). New-onset dermatomyositis requires age-appropriate cancer screening because of its high association with internal malignancy.
- Table 11-6 compares the epidemiology and disease associations of polymyositis and dermatomyositis with those of inclusion body myositis.

Q

A 64-year-old woman with diffuse scleroderma and stable angina underwent an echocardiogram and was found to have pulmonary hypertension. What medication, although typically prescribed for other purposes, is a possible treatment for pulmonary hypertension?

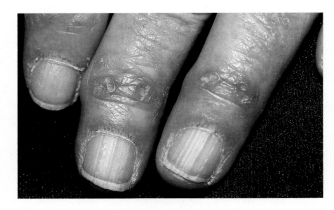

FIGURE 11-11.   Gottron's papules in dermatomyositis. Note the Gottron's papules over the DIP joints, a hallmark cutaneous feature of dermatomyositis, along with the prominent nail-fold telangiectasias and dystrophic cuticles. The combination of Gottron's papules and nail-fold changes is pathognomonic for dermatomyositis. (Reproduced with permission from Goldsmith LA et al. *Fitzpatrick's Dermatology in General Medicine,* 8th ed. New York: McGraw-Hill, 2012, Fig. 156-4.)

DIAGNOSIS

- Look for ↑ CK and **aldolase.**
- EMG demonstrates fibrillations. Muscle biopsy, which is necessary for definitive diagnosis, shows inflammatory cells and muscle degeneration.

TABLE 11-6.   Polymyositis, Dermatomyositis, and Inclusion Body Myositis

	POLYMYOSITIS	DERMATOMYOSITIS	INCLUSION BODY MYOSITIS
EPIDEMIOLOGY			
Age at onset	> 18 years.	Adulthood and childhood.	> 50 years.
Familial association	No.	No.	In some cases.
ASSOCIATED CONDITIONS			
Connective tissue diseases	Yes.[a]	Scleroderma and mixed connective tissue disease (overlap syndromes).	Yes, in up to 20% of cases.[a]
Systemic autoimmune diseases	Frequent.	Infrequent.	Infrequent.
Malignancy	No.	Yes, in up to 15% of cases.	No.

[a] SLE, RA, Sjögren's syndrome, systemic sclerosis, mixed connective tissue disease.

Adapted with permission from Longo DL et al. *Harrison's Principles of Internal Medicine,* 18th ed. New York: McGraw-Hill, 2012, Table 388-1.

A

Sildenafil. Remember that nitrates such as sublingual nitroglycerin are strongly contraindicated for 24 hours after the use of sildenafil or other PDE-5 inhibitors.

TREATMENT

■ High-dose **corticosteroids** generally result in improved muscle strength in 4–6 weeks and are then slowly tapered to the lowest effective dose for maintenance.

■ Methotrexate may be used as steroid-sparing therapy or for refractory symptoms.

Systemic Sclerosis (Scleroderma)

A multisystem disease with **symmetric thickening** of the skin on the face and extremities. It typically affects **women** 30–65 years of age. Diagnosis is clinical and is supported by biopsy. There are 2 subtypes: limited and systemic (see Table 11-7).

SYMPTOMS

■ Presents with prominent symmetrical skin thickening; loss of normal skin that gives the appearance of a tight face; and telangiectasias of the fingers, face, and lips.

■ Raynaud's phenomenon is an exaggerated vasoconstrictive response to stimuli such as cold temperature and emotional stress; digital ulceration may occur.

■ Systemic involvement of diffuse scleroderma includes GI (esophageal hypomotility leading to Barrett's esophagus and reflux), pulmonary (interstitial lung disease, fibrosis), and renal disease (scleroderma renal crisis).

DIAGNOSIS

■ In the presence of characteristic clinical findings, consider ANA as a screening test. Other tests include anti-topoisomerase I antibody (anti-Scl-70), which is highly specific but is present in only 30% of scleroderma patients.

■ Skin biopsy is generally not essential for confirmation of the diagnosis.

MNEMONIC

CREST syndrome

Calcinosis
Raynaud's phenomenon
Esophageal dysmotility
Sclerodactyly
Telangiectasias

TABLE 11-7.   **Limited vs Diffuse Scleroderma**

	LIMITED (CREST)	DIFFUSE
Skin involvement	Distal, face only	Generalized
Progression	Slow	Rapid
Immunologic finding	Anticentromere antibody	Anti-Scl-70 antibody
Prognosis	Fair	Poor
Calcinosis	+++	+
Telangiectasias	+++	+
Renal failure	None	++
Pulmonary interstitial fibrosis	+	+++

NOTES

NEPHROLOGY

Renal Basics

GLOMERULAR FILTRATION RATE (GFR) AND SURROGATES

- GFR is a marker of renal function defined by the amount of fluid entering Bowman's space from the glomeruli per minute. It cannot be directly measured but is approximated using creatinine clearance (CrCl).
- CrCl is estimated by the Cockcroft-Gault equation (based on age/sex/weight), whereas GFR is estimated by the Modification of Diet in Renal Disease (MDRD) equation (based on age/sex/race). CrCl generally overestimates GFR as creatinine is secreted into the tubule. Normal values are 100–130 mL/min/1.73 m^2.
- Oliguria is generally defined as a urine volume of < 500 mL/day, or approximately < 20 mL/hr.

INTERPRETING A URINALYSIS (UA)

Tables 12-1 and 12-2 offer guidelines for interpreting a UA.

TABLE 12-1.   Interpretation of UAs

TEST	INTERPRETATION
Proteinuria	A spot urine dip generally requires 100–150 mg/dL of protein to be ⊕; many dip tests can detect only albumin (not globulins or Bence Jones proteins). A full UA can detect both albumin and nonalbumin proteins, but there must be at least 1–10 mg of protein/dL for the UA to be ⊕.
Glucosuria	May indicate hyperglycemia; consider diabetes. May also indicate proximal tubule dysfunction, as in Fanconi's syndrome.
Ketonuria	Occurs with starvation, poorly controlled diabetes (eg, DKA), and alcohol intoxication. Urine ketones can also be ↑ following recent exercise and during pregnancy.
Hematuria/blood	A ⊕ value indicates myoglobin, hemoglobin, or RBCs in the urine.
Nitrite	Can become ⊕ with gram-⊖ bacteriuria.
Leukocyte esterase	Produced by WBCs; abnormal in urine; suggests a UTI.
pH	Alkalosis is most commonly associated with *Proteus* UTIs but may also be seen with some strains of *Klebsiella*, *Pseudomonas, Providencia,* and *Staphylococcus.* Acidosis with nephrolithiasis suggests uric acid or cystine stones. A pH of > 5.5 in the setting of metabolic acidosis suggests distal renal tubular acidosis (RTA).
Specific gravity	A rough estimate of urine osmolarity (U_{osm}).
Urobilinogen	Low sensitivity. ↑ urobilinogen occurs in hemolysis or hepatocellular disease; ↓ urobilinogen may suggest biliary obstruction.
Bilirubin	Bilirubin in the urine suggests a conjugated hyperbilirubinemia.
Epithelial cells	An excessive number of epithelial cells in the urine suggests a urine sample contaminated by surrounding skin.

TABLE 12-2. Urine Sediment Analysis

FINDING	ASSOCIATION
Hyaline casts	A normal finding, but an ↑ amount, while nonspecific, suggests a prerenal condition.
RBC casts, dysmorphic RBCs	Glomerulonephritis.
Waxy casts	Chronic kidney disease (CKD).
WBC casts	Pyelonephritis or interstitial nephritis.
Eosinophils	Allergic interstitial nephritis.
Coarse, granular, "muddy brown" casts	Acute tubular necrosis (ATN).
RBCs	Indicates hematuria. The absence of RBCs when the dipstick is ⊕ for blood suggests hemoglobinuria from hemolysis or myoglobinuria from rhabdomyolysis.
WBCs	A finding of more than a few WBCs is always abnormal except when the sample is contaminated (eg, with epithelial cells). Causes include infection, nephrolithiasis, neoplasm, acute interstitial cystitis, prostatitis, acute interstitial nephritis, strictures, and glomerulonephropathy.
Crystals	See the discussion of nephrolithiasis.
Yeast, bacteria	Indicate infection if the sample is not contaminated (eg, with epithelial cells).

FRACTIONAL EXCRETION OF SODIUM (Fe_{Na})

- Fe_{Na} is calculated using measured plasma and urine levels of sodium and creatinine. The acronym "**UP/UP**" can be used to remember the Fe_{Na} equation:

$$Fe_{Na} = (U_{Na} \times P_{Cr})/(U_{Cr} \times P_{Na})$$

  - A Fe_{Na} of < 1% suggests a **prerenal** state such as cardiorenal syndrome, dehydration, hepatorenal syndrome, or drug effects (eg, NSAIDs, ACEIs).
  - A Fe_{Na} of > 2% suggests **intrinsic** renal disease such as ATN, acute interstitial nephritis, vasculitis, or anything causing renal ischemia.
- Note that Fe_{Na} should be used only in patients with oliguria (< 500 mL of urine per day). Additionally, Fe_{Na} will be inaccurate in patients on diuretics and in those with CKD. In these instances, use the fractional excretion of urea (Fe_{urea}) to help determine the etiology of the renal injury (where U_{urea} = urine levels of urea and P_{urea} = plasma levels of urea):

$$Fe_{urea} = (U_{urea} \times P_{Cr})/(U_{Cr} \times P_{urea})$$

  - A Fe_{urea} of < 35% suggests a **prerenal** state.
  - A Fe_{urea} of > 50% suggests **intrinsic** renal disease.

Causes of anion gap metabolic acidosis—

MUDPILERS

Methanol
Uremia
Diabetic ketoacidosis
Paraldehyde
INH, **I**ron toxicity
Lactic acidosis
Ethylene glycol
Rhabdomyolysis
Salicylates

KEY FACT

Isopropyl alcohol ingestion causes an osmolal gap but does not cause an AG acidosis. Thus, it is important to calculate osmolal gap in all patients with suspected substance ingestion.

KEY FACT

Look for cherry-red maculae on funduscopic exam in patients with methanol intoxication.

KEY FACT

ACEIs prevent the normal degradation of bradykinin, which can cause a dry cough as a result of bronchoconstriction.

KEY FACT

In hypovolemia, look for hypokalemia and metabolic alkalosis due to activation of the RAA system. This is commonly referred to as "cohtraction alkalosis."

ACID-BASE DISORDERS

The algorithm for acid-base disorders is as follows:

1. **Identify the 1° disorder:**
   - **Respiratory alkalosis:** pH > 7.40, Pco_2 < 40.
   - **Respiratory acidosis:** pH < 7.40, Pco_2 > 40.
   - **Metabolic alkalosis:** pH > 7.40, HCO_3 > 24.
   - **Metabolic acidosis:** pH < 7.40, HCO_3 < 24.
2. Consider compensation, both metabolic and respiratory, and both acute and chronic. If different from that expected, consider a mixed picture.
   - **Expected compensation in metabolic acidosis:** $Paco_2 = 1.5 \times [HCO_3] + 8 +/- 2$ mm Hg.
     - If $Paco_2$ is less than expected, it suggests concurrent respiratory alkalosis.
     - If $Paco_2$ is more than expected, it suggests concurrent respiratory acidosis.
   - **Expected compensation in acute respiratory acidosis:** An ↑ of 1 mmol/L in HCO_3 for every 10-mm Hg ↑ in $Paco_2$ above 40 mm Hg. If the change in HCO_3 is less than this, it suggests concurrent metabolic acidosis.
   - **Expected compensation in chronic respiratory acidosis:** An ↑ of 4–5 mmol/L in HCO_3 for every 10-mm Hg ↑ in $Paco_2$ above 40 mm Hg. If the change in HCO_3 is more than this, it suggests concurrent metabolic alkalosis.
3. If the patient has metabolic acidosis, determine the anion gap, or AG (Na − [HCO_3 + Cl]). If the AG is ≥ 14, an AG metabolic acidosis exists. A normal AG is 12.
4. If the patient has an AG metabolic acidosis, determine the osmolal gap (measured serum osmolality − expected serum osmolality). Expected serum osmolality = (2 × Na) + (glucose/18) + (BUN/2.8). If the osmolal gap is > 10, suspect ingestion of a substance with high osmoles, such as ethylene or propylene glycol, methanol, or isopropyl alcohol.
5. If there is metabolic acidosis, determine the delta-delta (change in AG ÷ change in HCO_3). If the delta-delta is < 1, there is both an AG acidosis and a non-AG acidosis. If the delta-delta is > 2, there is both an AG metabolic acidosis and a metabolic alkalosis.

Figure 12-1 demonstrates a flow chart for evaluating acid-base disorders.

RENIN-ANGIOTENSIN-ALDOSTERONE (RAA) SYSTEM

- Renin is released by the juxtamedullary apparatus in response to ↓ renal blood flow.
- Renin converts angiotensinogen to angiotensin I, which is converted to angiotensin II by angiotensin-converting enzyme (ACE) in the lung and kidneys.
- ACE also degrades bradykinin, which acts as a vasodilator and a bronchoconstrictor.
- Angiotensin II causes direct arteriolar vasoconstriction, leading to ↑ total peripheral resistance and therefore ↑ BP. This especially affects the efferent arterioles of the glomerulus, leading to ↑ GFR.
- Angiotensin II stimulates aldosterone synthesis by the adrenal glands.
- Aldosterone ↑ sodium reabsorption and K^+ and H^+ excretion in the collecting duct.

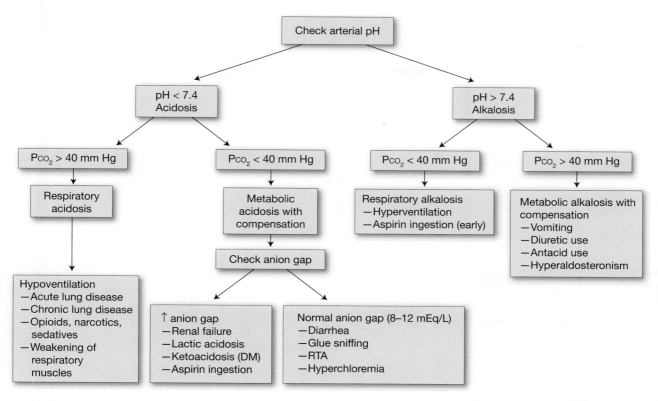

FIGURE 12-1. Acid-base disorders.

Electrolytes

SODIUM

Hyponatremia

Defined as a serum sodium level of < 135 mEq/L. This level may be falsely ↓ in hyperlipidemia, hyperglycemia, or hyperproteinemia and requires correction.

SYMPTOMS

- Often asymptomatic, but may present with **confusion, lethargy,** muscle cramps, and nausea.
- When serum sodium is low or rapidly decreasing, hyponatremia may lead to cerebral edema, which may result in seizures, status epilepticus, coma, or even death.

DIAGNOSIS

Assess volume status and check serum osmolality, urine osmolality, and urine sodium (see Figure 12-2).

TREATMENT

Treatment varies depending on whether the patient is symptomatic. "Symptomatic" refers to patients who have seizures/status epilepticus or altered mental status. See Figure 12-3.

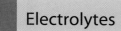

MNEMONIC

Causes of SIADH—

BCDE

Breathing (pulmonary): Small cell carcinoma, TB, pneumonia, pulmonary abscess
CNS: Meningitis, brain abscess, head trauma
Drugs: Clofibrate, phenothiazine, carbamazepine
Ectopic: Lymphoma, sarcoma, duodenal/pancreatic cancer

KEY FACT

ADH secretion is normally stimulated by ↑ plasma osmolarity. It acts on V2 receptors in the collecting duct to ↑ H_2O permeability, leading to free water reabsorption from the urine.

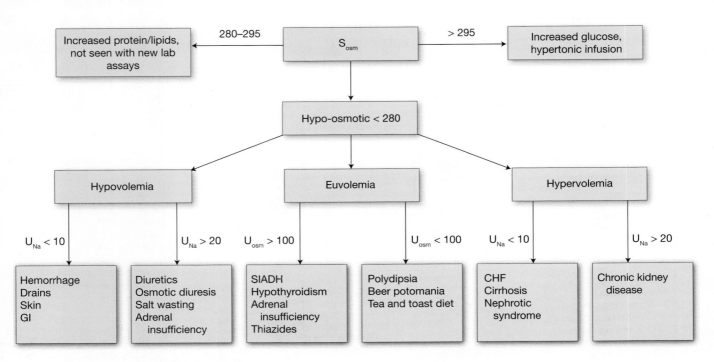

FIGURE 12-2.   Evaluation of hyponatremia.

KEY FACT

SIADH cannot be diagnosed in a hypovolemic patient regardless of plasma or urine osmolalities.

KEY FACT

The correction rate of sodium should not exceed 8–10 mEq/L/day. More rapid correction can result in osmotic demyelination syndrome, manifested by flaccid paralysis, dysarthria, dysphagia, and gait abnormalities.

Hypernatremia

Defined as a serum sodium level of > 147 mEq/L.

SYMPTOMS

Hyperpnea, weakness, restlessness, insomnia, altered mental status, coma.

DIAGNOSIS

- Assess volume status, urine output, U_{osm}, and U_{Na}.
- Hypernatremia from **dehydration** is usually due to ↑ insensible losses

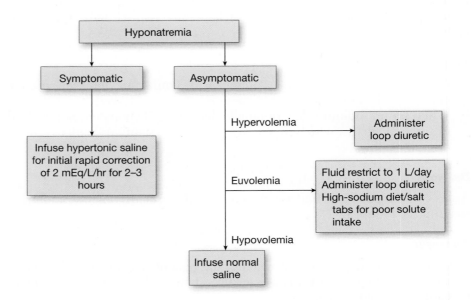

FIGURE 12-3.   Treatment of hyponatremia.

(burns, sweating, endotracheal intubation) or to diarrhea when the patient has **limited access to free water.** U_{osm} is usually > 700 mOsm/kg.

- Hypernatremia from ↑ **total body sodium** generally does **not** present with hypovolemia. Causes include excessive hydration with hypertonic fluids, dysfunction of central regulation, and mineralocorticoid excess (consider if the patient has hypokalemia and hypertension).
- Hypernatremia from **renal losses** (see Table 12-3) usually results in hypovolemia with U_{osm} < 700 mOsm/kg. Consider the clinical context in the setting of the U_{osm}/P_{osm} ratio to help determine the cause.

TREATMENT

- Always treat underlying causes (eg, DDAVP for central diabetes insipidus [DI]; a low-salt diet and thiazides for nephrogenic DI).
- Correct the free-water deficit with hypotonic saline, D_5W, or oral water.
- To prevent cerebral edema, do not correct hypernatremia at a rate of > 12 mEq/L/day.

POTASSIUM

Hypokalemia

Defined as a serum potassium level of < 3.5 mEq/L.

SYMPTOMS

- May be asymptomatic or present with fatigue, muscle weakness or cramps, ileus, hyporeflexia, paresthesias, and flaccid paralysis if severe.
- ECG may show T-wave flattening, U waves (an additional wave after the T wave), ST-segment depression, and QT prolongation followed by AV block and subsequent cardiac arrest.

DIAGNOSIS

- Order an ECG and check urine potassium.
- **Urine potassium > 20 mEq/L:** Usually indicates that the kidneys are wasting potassium. Acid-base status must be examined to further stratify the etiology.

TABLE 12-3.   Causes of Hypernatremia 2° to Renal Losses

	ETIOLOGY	COMMENTS
Osmotic diuresis	**Causes:** Mannitol, hyperglycemia, high-protein feeds, postobstructive diuresis.	U_{osm}/P_{osm} > 0.7.
Central DI	The pituitary does not make ADH. **Causes:** Tumor, trauma, neurosurgery, infection.	U_{osm}/P_{osm} < 0.7. U_{osm} should ↑ by 50% in response to DDAVP.
Nephrogenic DI	The kidneys are unresponsive to ADH. **Causes:** Renal failure, hypercalcemia, demeclocycline, lithium, sickle cell anemia.	U_{osm}/P_{osm} < 0.7. U_{osm} should not respond to DDAVP challenge.

KEY FACT

Hypernatremia often occurs with dehydration when a patient has no access to free water. Envision a salty desert.

KEY FACT

The main determinant of urinary potassium wasting is urinary flow rate. The greater the urine volume production, the more potassium is wasted.

Q 1

A 39-year-old man with a history of major depressive disorder is admitted for altered mental status. His initial labs show a serum HCO_3 of 14 mEq/L and an anion gap of 22. ABG shows a pH of 7.30, a $Paco_2$ of 20 mm Hg, and a Pao_2 of 150 mm Hg. On the basis of his acid-base status, what ingestion should you suspect?

Q 2

A 65-year-old man with a history of CAD and smoking is brought to the ED for gait impairment and confusion. A BMP shows a serum sodium level of 115 mEq/L. He is euvolemic on exam, and his urine osmolality is 295 mOsm/kg. What is the next best step in treatment?

KEY FACT

Replace **magnesium,** as deficiency leads to an ↑ in urinary potassium wasting, making potassium repletion more difficult.

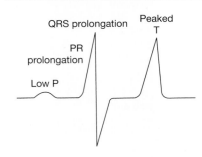

FIGURE 12-4. **Effects of hyperkalemia as seen on ECG.**

MNEMONIC

Treatment of hyperkalemia—

C BIG K Drop

Calcium gluconate
Bicarbonate/**B**eta agonist (albuterol)
Insulin
Glucose
Kayexalate
Diuretic/**D**ialysis

---

1   **A**

The patient has a mixed metabolic acidosis and respiratory alkalosis. His pH is < 7.40, indicating that he has a 1° metabolic acidosis. The expected compensation is a drop in his Pa_{CO_2} of $1.2 \times [24 - HCO_3] = 12$, or a Pa_{CO_2} of 28 mm Hg. However, his actual Pa_{CO_2} is lower than this, indicating that he has a 1° respiratory alkalosis as well. This is commonly seen in salicylate poisoning.

2   **A**

This patient's euvolemia and high urine osmolality suggest SIADH. You should restrict his free water intake and monitor his sodium closely to ensure a rise of no more than 0.5 mEq/L/hr to prevent osmotic demyelination syndrome.

- **Metabolic acidosis:** Type I RTA, lactic acidosis, or ketoacidosis.
- **Metabolic alkalosis:** 1° or 2° hyperaldosteronism (check plasma renin activity and plasma aldosterone concentration), Cushing's syndrome (check 24-hour urine cortisol), diuretics (loop or thiazide).
- **Variable pH:** Gentamicin, platinum-containing chemotherapeutic agents, hypomagnesemia.
- **Urine potassium < 20 mEq/L:** Usually indicates a nonrenal source of hypokalemia. This could be from **transcellular shift** (eg, insulin, β_2-agonists, alkalosis, periodic paralysis) or from **GI losses** (eg, diarrhea, chronic laxative abuse, vomiting, NG suction).

TREATMENT

- Treat the underlying disorder.
- Provide oral and/or IV **potassium repletion.** Replace cautiously in patients with renal insufficiency.

Hyperkalemia

Defined as a serum potassium level of ≥ 5 mEq/L.

SYMPTOMS

- Usually asymptomatic, but may present with muscle weakness and abdominal distention.
- ECG may show tall, peaked T waves and PR prolongation followed by loss of P waves and QRS widening that progresses to sine waves, ventricular fibrillation, and cardiac arrest (see Figure 12-4).

DIAGNOSIS

- Order a repeat blood draw unless suspicion is high, as hemolysis can result in an artificially high serum potassium level.
- Obtain an ECG.
- Urine potassium levels can help determine the etiology of the hyperkalemia.
  - **Urine potassium < 40 mEq/L:** Usually indicates that the hyperkalemia is caused by ↓ potassium excretion by the kidneys. Causes include renal insufficiency, drugs (eg, spironolactone, triamterene, amiloride, ACEIs, TMP, NSAIDs), and mineralocorticoid deficiency (type IV RTA). A plasma renin activity and plasma aldosterone concentration should be ordered if a mineralocorticoid deficiency is suspected.
  - **Urine potassium > 40 mEq/L:** Usually points to a nonrenal etiology. Causes include **cellular shifts** resulting from tissue injury, tumor lysis, insulin deficiency, acidosis, retroperitoneal hemorrhage, drugs (eg, succinylcholine, digitalis, arginine, α-blockers), and **iatrogenic** factors such as excessive potassium repletion.

TREATMENT

- Values > 6.5 mEq/L or ECG changes (especially PR prolongation or wide QRS) require emergent treatment (see the mnemonic **C BIG K Drop**).
- **Calcium gluconate** (for cardiac cell membrane stabilization) should be given immediately to prevent arrhythmias.
- Temporary treatment includes β_2-agonists, insulin and glucose, and sodium bicarbonate.
- Long-lasting elimination requires Kayexalate and a loop diuretic.
- **Restrict dietary potassium** and discontinue any medications that may be contributing to the hyperkalemia.
- Patients with severe or symptomatic hyperkalemia, with hyperkalemia refractory to the above management, or on **chronic** hemodialysis may require acute **hemodialysis.**

CALCIUM

Hypocalcemia

Defined as a serum calcium level of < 8.4 mg/dL. Etiologies include ↓ GI absorption (as found in hypoparathyroidism, pseudohypoparathyroidism, vitamin D deficiency, malabsorption, renal failure, critical illness, and hypomagnesemia), acute pancreatitis, rhabdomyolysis, tumor lysis, and diuretics. Don't forget to check a calcium level after a total thyroidectomy.

SYMPTOMS

Paresthesias, circumoral numbness, tetany, lethargy, confusion, seizures, Trousseau's sign, Chvostek's sign, QT prolongation.

TREATMENT

- Replace with oral calcium carbonate or IV calcium gluconate.
- **Correct for hypoalbuminemia.** For every 1-mg/dL ↓ in albumin, ↑ the calcium level by 0.8 mg/dL. Alkalosis ↑ calcium binding to albumin.

Hypercalcemia

Defined as a serum calcium level of > 10.2 mg/dL. Etiologies are outlined in the mnemonic **CHIMPANZEES**.

SYMPTOMS

May present with **stones** (kidney stones), **bones** (fractures), abdominal **groans** (anorexia, nausea, constipation), and **psychiatric overtones** (weakness, fatigue, altered mental status). Consider in patients with pancreatitis, refractory PUD, a personal or family history of kidney stones, or bone pain.

DIAGNOSIS

- Inquire about diet and vitamin supplementation.
- Check calcium, phosphate, albumin, ionized calcium, and alkaline phosphatase. Also consider vitamin D levels, SPEP, TSH, and imaging. Check an ECG, which may show a short QT interval.
- Hyperparathyroidism is a common cause of hypercalcemia, so check PTH and parathyroid hormone–related peptide (PTHrP) levels.
- **Elevated or inappropriately normal PTH** (which should be suppressed in the setting of hypercalcemia): Points to 1° hyperparathyroidism (eg, from adenoma, hyperplasia, carcinoma, or MEN 1/2) as the likely cause (see Chapter 5 for more details). Consider an ectopic PTH-producing tumor as well.
- **Low PTH:**
  - Indicates that the cause could be excessive calcium or vitamin D intake, granulomatous disease, sarcoidosis, malignancy (eg, hematologic, lymphoproliferative, multiple myeloma, bone metastases), milk-alkali syndrome, or Paget's disease.
  - PTHrP secretion from cancer cells (often squamous cell carcinoma) can cause a paraneoplastic hypercalcemia. The ↑ calcium suppresses the normal parathyroid gland, resulting in low PTH levels.
  - Testing options include phosphate, vitamin D, TSH, serum immunoelectrophoresis (for MGUS or myeloma), alkaline phosphatase (for Paget's), GGT (to determine the origin of the ↑ alkaline phosphatase), spot urine calcium, spot urine creatinine, BUN/creatinine, and x-rays/bone scan (to look for lytic lesions).

MNEMONIC

Causes of hypocalcemia—

HIPOCAL

Hypoparathyroidism/hypomagnesemia
Infection
Pancreatitis
Overload (rapid volume expansion)
Chronic kidney disease
Absorption abnormalities
Loop diuretics

KEY FACT

In patients with hypocalcemia, look for **Trousseau's and Chvostek's signs,** which are due to ↑ neuromuscular irritability.

- **Trousseau's sign:** Elicited by inflating a BP cuff to greater than the patient's SBP for 3 minutes, leading to carpopedal spasm.
- **Chvostek's sign:** Elicited by tapping on the patient's jaw over the course of the facial nerve, leading to spasms of the facial muscles.

MNEMONIC

Causes of hypercalcemia—

CHIMPANZEES

Calcium supplementation
Hyperparathyroidism
Iatrogenic/**I**mmobility
Milk-alkali syndrome
Paget's disease
Addison's disease/**A**cromegaly
Neoplasm
Zollinger-Ellison syndrome
Excess vitamin A
Excess vitamin D
Sarcoidosis

KEY FACT

Distinguish hyperparathyroidism from excess vitamin D by checking phosphate levels. PTH → ↓ phosphate reabsorption in the kidney. Vitamin D → ↑ phosphate reabsorption in the GI tract.

- ↑ **Ca,** ↑ **phosphate:** Think of excess vitamin D.
- ↑ **Ca,** ↓ **phosphate:** Think hyperparathyroidism.

TREATMENT

- The first step in treatment is to **hydrate** the patient with IV fluids. Furosemide should be given only if you are certain that the patient is adequately volume resuscitated.
- Identify and treat the underlying cause.
- Discontinue all drugs that can cause hypercalcemia (eg, thiazides).
- Patients with symptomatic hypercalcemia or a serum calcium level of > 14 mg/dL require **IV bisphosphonates** (eg, pamidronate) or **calcitonin.** However, each takes 12–24 hours to have an effect, and the therapeutic benefits of both may be short-lived.
- Place the patient on a low-calcium diet.
- For 1° hyperparathyroidism, parathyroidectomy is needed.
- **Hemodialysis** is a last resort.

Diuretics

Table 12-4 lists commonly used diuretics, their mechanism of action, and their adverse effects. See Figure 12-5 for a depiction of diuretics and their underlying mechanisms.

TABLE 12-4. **Mechanism of Action and Adverse Effects of Selected Diuretics**

DIURETIC CLASS	EXAMPLES	MECHANISM OF ACTION	ADVERSE EFFECTS
Thiazides	HCTZ, chlorthalidone	Inhibition of the Na-Cl channel in the distal convoluted tubule.	▪ **Hyper**calcemia ▪ Hyponatremia ▪ Hypokalemia ▪ Hyperuricemia ▪ Hyperglycemia ▪ Hyperlipidemia ▪ Hypomagnesemia
Loop diuretics	Furosemide, bumetanide, torsemide, ethacrynic acid	Inhibition of the Na-K-2Cl channel in the thick ascending limb of the loop of Henle.	▪ **Hypo**calcemia ▪ Hypokalemia ▪ Hyperuricemia ▪ Ototoxicity
Carbonic anhydrase inhibitors	Acetazolamide	Inhibition of carbonic anhydrase in the proximal tubule, leading to NaCl and $NaHCO_3$ loss.	▪ **Hypo**kalemia ▪ Fatigue ▪ Diarrhea
Potassium-sparing diuretics	Eplerenone, spironolactone, triamterene, amiloride	Inhibition of the sodium channel in the cortical collecting duct; eplerenone and spironolactone also antagonize aldosterone receptor, which prevents potassium loss into urine.	▪ **Hyper**kalemia ▪ Gynecomastia (spironolactone only; due to cross-reactivity and blockade of androgen receptor) ▪ Hypertriglyceridemia

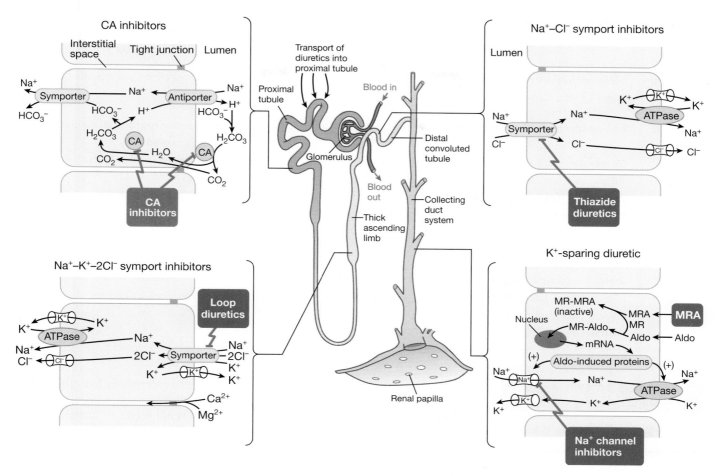

FIGURE 12-5. **Site and mechanism of action of diuretics.** Diuretics target and block the action of epithelial proteins involved in solute transport. The site and mechanism of action of a given class of diuretics are determined by the specific protein inhibited by the diuretic. CA = carbonic anhydrase; MR = mineralocorticoid receptor; MRA = mineralocorticoid receptor antagonist; Aldo = aldosterone. (Reproduced with permission from Brunton LL et al. *Goodman & Gilman's The Pharmacological Basis of Therapeutics*, 12th ed. New York: McGraw-Hill, 2011, Figure 25-13.)

Acute Kidney Injury (AKI)

An ↑ in serum creatinine of ≥ 0.3 mg/dL within 48 hours; an ↑ in serum creatinine ≥ 1.5 times the baseline within the past 7 days; or a urine volume of < 0.5 mL/kg/hr for 6 hours.

SYMPTOMS/EXAM

- Patients are often asymptomatic but may present with dyspnea, edema/anasarca, **uremic symptoms** (eg, anorexia, nausea, malaise, hyperpigmented skin, asterixis, pericarditis [listen for a friction rub]), and anemia.
- Exam should include checking BP, daily weights, and assessment of volume status. Other findings are specific to the etiology of the renal failure.

DIAGNOSIS

- AKI is categorized as prerenal, intrinsic, or postrenal (see Table 12-5).
- To determine the etiology, order urine sodium (or urea if the patient is on diuretics or has CKD), urine creatinine, and a UA with micro and urine eosinophils. Calculate the Fe_{Na} (see the discussion of renal basics) and look at the urine sediment under the microscope. Order a renal ultra-

Q **1**

A 55-year-old hospitalized woman with a history of CKD is receiving IV antibiotics for pyelonephritis. On hospital day 2, her serum potassium level is 5.8 mEq/L; the specimen was not hemolyzed. What do you do next?

Q **2**

A 65-year-old man presents to the ED from clinic after routine labs show a serum creatinine level of 3.8 mg/dL, up from 1.1 mg/dL 3 months ago. He states that his urine "mostly dribbles out." On exam, you feel a suprapubic mass. What should you do next?

TABLE 12-5.   Laboratory Findings Associated with Acute Kidney Injury

Class	Cause	Fe$_{Na}$	UA
Prerenal	Dehydration (anorexia, burns, GI losses), ACEIs, NSAIDs, renal artery stenosis, shock, cardiorenal syndrome, hepatorenal syndrome.	< 1%	Bland, or may see hyaline casts.
Intrinsic	**Interstitial:** Acute interstitial nephritis (eg, due to antibiotics, systemic infection), multiple myeloma. **Glomerular:** Nephritic syndrome, multiple myeloma. **Tubular:** ATN (see Table 12-6 for a list of causes), multiple myeloma. **Vascular:** Emboli, vasculitis, thrombotic microvascular angiopathy (usually due to antiphospholipid antibody syndrome), renal vein thrombosis.	> 1%	**Glomerulonephritis:** RBCs and RBC casts, protein. **Acute interstitial nephritis:** Eosinophils, WBCs and WBC casts. **ATN:** Pigmented granular ("muddy brown") casts. **Multiple myeloma:** Bence Jones protein, RBCs and RBC casts.
Postrenal	**Ureteral stenosis:** Papillary necrosis (usually due to overuse of NSAIDs), blood clot, retroperitoneal fibrosis, malignancy. **Bladder neck:** Anticholinergics, malignancy. **Prostate:** BPH, cancer, prostatitis.	Variable	Variable—bland or RBCs.

KEY FACT

A Fe$_{Na}$ < 1% suggests prerenal failure.

---

1   **A**

Get an ECG, which may show serious signs of hyperkalemia. Next, follow the mnemonic **C BIG K Drop.** Administer calcium to stabilize the heart; then give bicarbonate, albuterol, insulin, and glucose for a fast-acting but short-lived response. Kayexalate and furosemide can then be given to dispose of excess potassium.

2   **A**

The mass is likely a full bladder resulting from urinary retention 2° to BPH, a common cause of renal failure among elderly men. After asking the patient to void, place a Foley catheter. If he has a large postvoid residual, keep his Foley in place and start α-blockers and 5α-reductase inhibitors for BPH.

---

sound +/– Dopplers (if renal artery stenosis is suspected) to look for hydronephrosis suggestive of urinary tract obstruction.

- Listen for a renal artery bruit characteristic of renal artery stenosis.
- Suspect a vascular cause in predisposed patients (eg, those with a hypercoagulable state) presenting with abdominal pain.
- Order a serum and urine protein electrophoresis (SPEP/UPEP) if multiple myeloma is suspected.
- Men should have a prostate exam in cases of postrenal failure.

TREATMENT

- **Prerenal etiologies:** Treat with IV fluids unless cardiorenal syndrome is suspected, in which case treat with diuresis.
- **Intrinsic disease:** Treat the underlying cause or remove the offending agent.
- **Postrenal etiologies:** Alleviate the obstruction with Foley catheter placement or urologic intervention if needed.
- In addition to the above, protect the kidneys with the interventions that follow.

TABLE 12-6.   Causes of Acute Tubular Necrosis

Cause	Examples
Exogenous nephrotoxins	Chemotherapeutic agents (cisplatin, methotrexate) and other immunosuppressants (cyclosporine, tacrolimus), aminoglycosides, amphotericin B, cephalosporins, heavy metals, and radiocontrast dyes (effects can be minimized by hydration and oral *N*-acetylcysteine).
Endogenous nephrotoxins	Hyperuricemia, rhabdomyolysis, massive intravascular hemolysis, Bence Jones proteins (from multiple myeloma).
Ischemic	All causes of shock, including a prolonged prerenal state.

- Discontinue nephrotoxic medications and ↓ any renally excreted medications in proportion to the GFR.
- Avoid contrast studies unless they are essential.
- Keep total body balance even unless there is rhabdomyolysis, in which case treat with aggressive fluid resuscitation to keep urine output > 300 mL/hr.
- Initiate a low-potassium and low-phosphate diet.
- Monitor for hyperkalemia, hypocalcemia, and hyperphosphatemia. Start a phosphate binder if phosphate is ↑.
- If the pH is < 7.2, bicarbonate may be used to treat a non-AG acidosis or to temporize an AG metabolic acidosis (until dialysis or renal recovery).
- Dialyze if indicated (see the mnemonic **AEIOU**).

Contrast Nephropathy

- Characterized by an acute decline in GFR that occurs 24–48 hours after a patient receives IV radiocontrast.
- Risk factors include preexisting renal insufficiency, diabetes, ↓ effective arterial volume, a high volume of contrast, and concomitant nephrotoxic medications.
- Patients with an ↑ risk of developing contrast nephropathy should receive prophylaxis with infusion of normal saline or sodium bicarbonate and oral acetylcysteine.
- **Tx:** Treatment is supportive. The renal injury usually resolves in 1 week.

Hematuria

Defined as 3 or more RBCs/hpf on urine microscopy. Gross hematuria is present when blood is visible to the naked eye.

DIFFERENTIAL

Pseudohematuria is defined as urine that gives the false impression of hematuria either grossly or by laboratory testing. It may result from certain drugs, foods, or dyes that cause myoglobinuria, hemoglobinuria, or simple discoloration of urine.

DIAGNOSIS

- See Figure 12-6 for a diagnostic algorithm.
- Urine cytology is no longer routinely recommended as part of the hematuria workup.
- If the workup is still ⊖ and suspicion is high, a **renal angiogram** may be ordered to look for vascular causes (eg, renal vein thrombosis, varices, aneurysms, AVMs).
- Patients on anticoagulants with hematuria should still receive a full workup.

Proteinuria

Urinary protein excretion of > 150 mg/24 hrs. **Nephrotic syndrome** consists of severe proteinuria that is defined as a daily urinary protein excretion of > 3.5 g (see the following section). Moderately ↑ albuminuria is defined as a **persistent** daily urinary protein excretion of 30–300 mg. Transient proteinuria can occur with infection, stress, and illness.

KEY FACT

Prostaglandins cause dilation of afferent arterioles in the nephron, leading to ↑ renal blood flow and GFR. NSAIDs block prostaglandin synthesis, leading to a prerenal state.

MNEMONIC

Indications for emergent dialysis—

AEIOU

Acidosis
Electrolytes (hyperkalemia)
Ingestion (of toxins)
Overload (volume)
Uremic symptoms (encephalopathy, pericarditis)

KEY FACT

Remember—true hematuria must have RBCs.

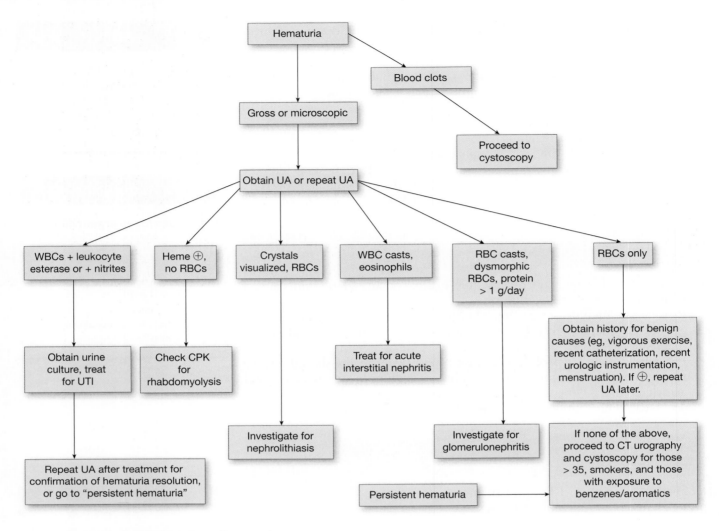

FIGURE 12-6. **Diagnostic workup of hematuria.**

SYMPTOMS/EXAM

Presentation is generally unremarkable unless the patient has nephrotic-range proteinuria. In such instances, patients usually present with generalized edema and/or frothy urine.

DIAGNOSIS

To ascertain the cause of proteinuria, it is important to know the quantity and type of protein involved. To determine this, proceed as follows (see also Table 12-7):

- Obtain a 24-hour urine collection to quantify daily urinary protein excretion. If this is not possible, check a spot urine protein/creatinine ratio (normal is < 0.2; nephrotic syndrome is > 3.0).
- Check a UA, electrolytes, BUN/creatinine, UPEP, and serum total protein.
- Examine urine sediment. A benign appearance suggests benign causes, whereas RBCs and RBC casts suggest acute nephritic syndrome and fat bodies point to nephrotic syndrome. (See below for the differences between nephritic and nephrotic syndromes.)
- A UA significant only for protein in the absence of other signs of renal disease suggests **benign proteinuria**. Causes include pulmonary edema, CHF, fever, exercise, head injury, CVA, stress, orthostatic proteinuria, and idiopathic factors.

TABLE 12-7. **Location of Renal Disease in Proteinuria**

LOCATION	URINE PROTEIN	LAB FINDINGS	ETIOLOGIES
Interstitial nephritis	< 2 g/24 hrs	Routine UA shows WBCs, WBC casts, and eosinophils.	Infection, medications (NSAIDs, quinolones, sulfonamides, rifampin), connective tissue diseases (SLE, sarcoidosis, Sjögren's syndrome).
Glomerular disease	> 2 g/24 hrs	Routine UA shows RBCs or RBC casts.	See the discussion of nephritic and nephrotic syndromes.
Overflow proteinuria	< 2 g/24 hrs; mostly light-chain or low-molecular-weight proteins	↑ serum protein.	Amyloid, multiple myeloma (may also present with massive proteinuria), lymphoproliferative disease, hemoglobin, myoglobin.

TREATMENT

- Treat any underlying causes.
- Treat hyponatremia with free water restriction and peripheral edema with a loop diuretic.
- Diabetics with proteinuria should be started on an ACEI.
- Proteinuria itself does not require treatment. Patients in whom proteinuria persists for many years are at ↑ risk for renal failure. In these cases, consider a low-salt and low-protein diet with < 0.8 g protein/kg per day.

Nephritic and Nephrotic Syndromes

Nephritic and nephrotic syndromes are disorders of the glomerulus.

- **Nephrotic syndrome:** Due to loss of glomerular basement membrane function 2° to fusion of podocytes. This results in loss of large plasma proteins into the urine, which is responsible for many of the manifestations associated with the syndrome.
- **Nephritic syndrome:** Due to inflammation of the glomerulus 2° to neutrophilic infiltration.

See Table 12-8 for a comparison of nephritic and nephrotic syndromes and Tables 12-9 to 12-11 for the causes of each.

Chronic Kidney Disease (CKD)

An irreversible or only partially reversible state in which the kidneys have lost the ability to regulate some combination of the body's fluid state, electrolyte levels, and acid-base status. Erythropoiesis and vitamin D metabolism are often compromised as well.

SYMPTOMS/EXAM

- May be asymptomatic or present with a clinical picture that appears inconsistent with the severity of the disease. If mild or gradual, other organ systems may compensate (eg, hyperventilation to blow off CO_2).
- As CKD worsens—ie, as GFR approaches zero—uremic and anemic symptoms worsen, and patients appear progressively more ill.
- Urine volume may remain normal despite marked changes in serum (ele-

Q

A mother brings her 2-year-old boy to the clinic because his face seems swollen and he feels heavier. The child recently had a URI, and though his upper respiratory symptoms have improved, he has grown more fatigued. You note dependent edema. UA reveals 3+ protein, light microscopy shows normal-appearing glomeruli, and biopsy reveals podocyte effacement. What is your diagnosis?

TABLE 12-8.   **Nephritic and Nephrotic Syndromes**

	NEPHRITIC SYNDROME	NEPHROTIC SYNDROME
Defining features	Proteinuria (usually < 3.5 g/day). Edema. Oliguria, hematuria, hypertension.	Proteinuria > 3.5 g/day. Edema. Hypoalbuminemia, hyperlipidemia. Hypercoagulability (due to loss of protein C and S and antithrombin III). Immunodeficiency (due to loss of immunoglobulins/complement protein).
UA findings	**Dysmorphic RBCs,** RBC casts.	Bland, RBCs, or fatty vacuoles in a **Maltese cross pattern.**
Diagnosis	Check complement levels, ANCA, ANA, anti-dsDNA, cryoglobulin, a hepatitis panel, anti-GBM antibodies, antistreptolysin antibody, and blood cultures. A renal biopsy is the gold standard of diagnosis.	Evaluate for nonrenal causes with ANA, a hepatitis panel, RPR, a fasting glucose or HbA$_{1c}$, a pregnancy test, and HIV ELISA. A biopsy may be needed for definitive diagnosis.
Treatment	Treat inflammatory disorders with steroids and cytotoxic agents. In cases 2° to systemic disease, treat the underlying disorder.	Treat as per proteinuria. Patients with hyperlipidemia should be started on a statin. Patients who develop thrombosis require anticoagulation. Pneumovax is recommended.

KEY FACT

Urine volume may be completely normal in acute and chronic renal failure.

Minimal change disease, a common cause of nephrotic syndrome in children that results from effacement of glomerular epithelial foot processes. It is treated with steroids and has an excellent prognosis.

vation) or urine (reduction) electrolytes, urea nitrogen levels, and creatinine. Urine output will ↓ as CKD reaches a terminal stage.

DIAGNOSIS

- A serum creatinine that is > 1.4 mg/dL for > 3 months is generally considered diagnostic. Lower cutoffs are applied to patients with less muscle mass (often shorter or older patients), particularly women, and higher cutoffs to large, muscular patients (remember to examine the labs **and** the patient).
- Note that high-protein diets, rhabdomyolysis, and certain medications (eg, cimetidine, TMP) can ↓ creatinine excretion, in which case serum creatinine may be high without renal impairment.

TREATMENT

- Appropriate identification and treatment of the cause is critical to preventing disease progression. Most causes are similar to those of AKI.
- Follow the indications for dialysis as laid out in the discussion of AKI.
- For intrinsic renal disease, it is important to optimize the kidney in other respects—ie, to control hypertension, avoid nephrotoxic drugs, control blood glucose level, restrict protein intake, and control lipids. Patients should be placed on a renal diet to prevent a high potassium load.
- Long-term treatment often involves erythropoietin (if the patient is ane-

TABLE 12-9. 1° Renal Causes of Nephrotic Syndrome

PATHOLOGY	DESCRIPTION	HISTORY/PE	LABS	TREATMENT/PROGNOSIS
Minimal change disease	Effacement of glomerular basement membrane podocytes.	Patients are prone to infections and thrombotic events. Common in children; idiopathic.	Light microscopy appears **normal.** Electron microscopy shows **effacement of epithelial foot processes** with lipid-laden renal cortices.	Steroids; excellent prognosis.
Focal segmental glomerulosclerosis	Glomerular sclerosis. Not all glomeruli are affected.	The typical patient is a young African American male with uncontrolled hypertension. Associated with HIV infection and IV drug use, but may be idiopathic.	Microscopic hematuria; biopsy shows sclerosis in capillary tufts.	Prednisone, cytotoxic therapy.
Membranous nephropathy	**The most common nephropathy in adult Caucasians;** an immune complex disease.	Associated with HBV, syphilis, **malaria,** and gold.	**"Spike and dome"** appearance due to granular deposits of IgG and C3 at the basement membrane.	Prednisone and cytotoxic therapy for severe disease.
Membranoproliferative glomerulonephritis (MPGN)	Can also be nephritic syndrome. Can be immune complex or complement mediated.	Slow progression to renal failure. Type I is associated with HCV, cryoglobulinemia, SLE, and subacute bacterial endocarditis.	**"Tram-track"** double-layered basement membrane. Type I has subendothelial deposits; type II involves a C3 nephritic factor; both types have $\downarrow$ C3.	Steroids and cytotoxic agents may help.

Adapted with permission from Le T et al. *First Aid for the USMLE Step 2 CK,* 7th ed. New York: McGraw-Hill, 2010: 487–488.

mic), vitamin D, phosphate binders, and calcium. Bicarbonate may be used for severe acidosis.

- Prepare the patient for dialysis. Avoid IVs in the arm that will be used for AV shunts.
- The only definitive treatment for irreversible end-stage renal disease is transplantation.

Renal Tubular Acidosis (RTA)

May occur 2° to renal or adrenal disease, or may be a 1° disease. Due to a net $\downarrow$ in either tubular hydrogen (H^+) secretion or bicarbonate reabsorption that leads to a **non-anion-gap metabolic acidosis.** There are 4 types of RTA (see Table 12-12), but only 3 are clinically important. **Type IV (distal)** is the most common; type III is uncommon and is seen only in children.

DIAGNOSIS

Usually asymptomatic. See Figure 12-7 for a diagnostic algorithm.

TABLE 12-10.   **2° Causes of Nephrotic Syndrome**

PATHOLOGY	DESCRIPTION	HISTORY/PE	LABS	TREATMENT/PROGNOSIS
Diabetic nephropathy	Has 2 characteristic forms: diffuse hyalinization and nodular glomerulosclerosis **(Kimmelstiel-Wilson lesions).**	Patients generally have long-standing, poorly controlled diabetes mellitus (DM).	Thickened GBM; ↑ **mesangial matrix.**	Tight control of blood sugar; ACEIs.
Lupus nephritis	Both nephrotic and nephritic. The severity of renal disease often determines overall prognosis.	Proteinuria or RBCs on UA may be found during evaluation of SLE patients.	Mesangial proliferation; subendothelial immune complex deposition leading to ↓ C3 and C4.	Prednisone and cytotoxic therapy may reduce disease progression.
Renal amyloidosis	Both nephritic and nephrotic. Due to deposition of proteins in **beta-pleated sheet** configuration or light chains. 1° (plasma cell dyscrasia) and 2° (infectious or inflammatory) are the most common.	Patients may have a plasma cell dyscrasia (eg, multiple myeloma) or a chronic inflammatory disease (eg, RA, TB). The β_2-microglobulin subtype is associated with long-term hemodialysis.	Abdominal fat biopsy; seen with **Congo red stain; apple-green birefringence** under polarized light.	Prednisone and melphalan. Bone marrow transplantation may be used if 2° to a plasma cell dyscrasia.

Adapted with permission from Le T et al. *First Aid for the USMLE Step 2 CK,* 7th ed. New York: McGraw-Hill, 2010: 487–488.

TABLE 12-11.   **Causes of Nephritic Syndrome**

PATHOLOGY	DESCRIPTION	HISTORY/PE	LABS	TREATMENT/PROGNOSIS
PAUCI-IMMUNE/ANCA ⊕				
Microscopic polyangiitis	Necrotizing vasculitis without granuloma formation.	Pulmonary nodules/ hemoptysis, purpura.	⊕ p-ANCA, normal complement levels.	Steroids and immunosuppressants (cyclophosphamide or rituximab) +/− plasmapheresis.
Granulomatosis with polyangiitis (formerly Wegener's)	Necrotizing vasculitis with granuloma formation.	Oral ulcers, sinusitis, pulmonary nodules/ cavities with hemoptysis.	⊕ c-ANCA, normal complement levels.	Same as above.
Eosinophilic granulomatosis with polyangiitis (formerly Churg-Strauss)	Necrotizing vasculitis with granuloma formation, with associated eosinophilia.	Asthma, allergic rhinitis, peripheral neuropathy.	⊕ p-ANCA, normal complement levels.	Same as above.

TABLE 12-11. **Causes of Nephritic Syndrome** *(continued)*

PATHOLOGY	DESCRIPTION	HISTORY/PE	LABS	TREATMENT/PROGNOSIS
		ANTI-GBM ⊕		
Goodpasture's syndrome	Linear deposits of IgG directed primarily against type IV collagen, type II hypersensitivity reaction.	Pulmonary hemorrhage with renal disease.	⊕ anti-GBM, normal complement levels.	Steroids and immunosuppressants (cyclophosphamide or rituximab) +/− plasmapheresis.
Anti-GBM disease	Linear deposits of IgG directed primarily against type IV collagen, type II hypersensitivity reaction.	Isolated renal disease.	⊕ anti-GBM, normal complement levels.	Same as above.
		IMMUNE COMPLEX MEDIATED		
Poststreptococcal glomerulonephritis	Subepithelial humps and subendothelial immune complex deposition (**"lumpy-bumpy"** appearance).	Recent group A streptococcal infection.	⊕ antistreptolysin O antibody, ↓ C3.	Treat the underlying infection.
Cryoglobulinemia	Subendothelial deposits of cryoglobulins (immune complexes and complements that precipitate when refrigerated).	HCV infection.	⊕ cryocrit, ↓ C3 and C4.	Same as above.
Endocarditis	Subendothelial and subepithelial immune complex deposition.	Cardiac murmur, splinter hemorrhages, Janeway lesions, Osler's nodes.	⊕ blood cultures, ↓ C3.	Same as above.
IgA nephropathy/ Henoch-Schönlein purpura (HSP)	Mesangial IgA immune complex deposition, common in children.	Hematuria 24–48 hours after upper respiratory or GI tract infection. HSP presents with palpable purpura, joint pain, abdominal pain, and hematuria.	Normal complement levels.	ACEIs if proteinuria. Steroids +/− cyclophosphamide.
Alport syndrome	X-linked recessive genetic mutation of type IV collagen, **foam** (lipid-laden) **cells** in glomerular interstitium.	Sensorineural hearing loss, ocular defects.	Normal complement levels.	ACEIs if proteinuria.
Lupus nephritis	See Table 12-10.			
MPGN	See Table 12-9.			

TABLE 12-12.   Types of Renal Tubular Acidosis

	TYPE I (DISTAL)	TYPE II (PROXIMAL)	TYPE IV (DISTAL)
Defect	H^+ secretion.	HCO_3^- reabsorption.	Aldosterone deficiency or resistance leads to defects in Na^+ reabsorption, H^+ and K^+ excretion, and ↓ ammoniagenesis.
Etiologies (most common)	Hereditary, amphotericin, collagen vascular disease (eg, scleroderma), cirrhosis, nephrocalcinosis.	Hereditary, carbonic anhydrase inhibitors, Fanconi's syndrome, tenofovir.	Hyporeninemic hypoaldosteronism with DM; hypertension, chronic interstitial nephritis.
Treatment	Potassium citrate or sodium bicarbonate.	Potassium citrate.	Furosemide, Kayexalate.
Complications	Nephrolithiasis.	Rickets, osteomalacia.	Hyperkalemia.

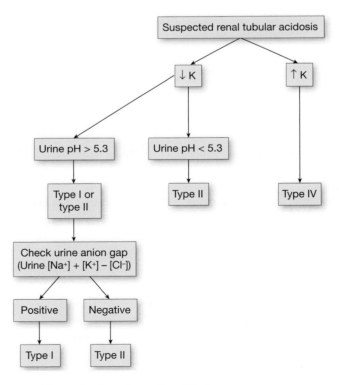

FIGURE 12-7.   Diagnosis of renal tubular acidosis.

TABLE 12-13. **Types of Nephrolithiasis**

TYPE	FREQUENCY	ETIOLOGY AND CHARACTERISTICS	TREATMENT
Calcium oxalate/ calcium phosphate	83%	The most common causes are **idiopathic hypercalciuria**, ↑ urine uric acid 2° to diet, IBD, and 1° hyperparathyroidism. Alkaline urine; octahedron crystals. Radiopaque.	Hydration, surgical removal. Thiazide diuretics in the setting of hypercalciuria to reabsorb calcium and prevent further stones.
Struvite (Mg-NH$_4$-PO$_4$)	9%	"Triple phosphate" stones. Associated with urease-producing organisms (eg, *Proteus*). Form staghorn calculi. Alkaline urine; rectangular, "coffin lid" crystals. Radiopaque.	Hydration, treat UTI if present, surgical removal.
Uric acid	7%	Associated with gout and high purine turnover states. Acidic urine (pH < 5.5). Diamond or rhomboid crystals. **Radiolucent on KUB, but seen on CT.**	Hydration, alkalinize urine with citrate or carbonic anhydrase inhibitor, surgical removal. Allopurinol to prevent further stones.
Cystine	1%	Due to a defect in renal transport of certain amino acids (**COLA—C**ystine, **O**rnithine, **L**ysine, and **A**rginine). **Hexagonal crystals.** Radiopaque.	Hydration, alkalinize urine, penicillamine, surgical removal.
Indinavir	Rare	Patients will be on protease inhibitors for HIV. Stones consist of precipitated indinavir. **Radiolucent on KUB and CT.**	Hydration, surgical removal.

Adapted with permission from Le T et al. *First Aid for the USMLE Step 2 CK,* 7th ed. New York: McGraw-Hill, 2010: 489.

Nephrolithiasis

Stones most commonly occur in males in the third and fourth decades of life. Risk factors include a ⊕ family history, **low fluid intake,** gout, status post-colectomy/ileostomy, chronic diarrhea, sarcoid, specific enzyme disorders, RTA, and hyperparathyroidism. Stones are most commonly composed of calcium oxalate but may also be calcium phosphate, struvite, uric acid, or cystine (see Table 12-13).

SYMPTOMS/EXAM

Presents with **acute onset of severe, colicky flank pain** that may **radiate to the testes or vulva** and may be associated with nausea and vomiting. Patients are unable to get comfortable and shift position frequently (vs those with peritonitis, who remain still).

DIAGNOSIS

- Labs, examination, and imaging together make the diagnosis.
- Gross or **microscopic hematuria** and an **altered urine pH** may be noted on UA. Check serum calcium, a CBC, and serum creatinine, and look for signs of UTI (which may be the cause of infection leading to struvite stones or 2° to obstruction from other stones).
- Tenderness may be present in the costovertebral areas or in either abdomi-

Q

A 38-year-old HIV-⊕ woman on antiretrovirals has a 2-day history of fevers and right flank pain. Exam reveals right CVA tenderness. UA shows 20–50 RBCs/hpf and 20–50 WBCs/hpf. CT reveals moderate right-sided hydronephrosis along with perinephric and periureteral stranding. Two hours after presentation, her BP goes from 120/75 to 82/50. She is also tachycardic to the 150s, and her temperature is 40.1°C (104.2°F). What do you do?

nal lower quadrant. It may be difficult to distinguish pain associated with nephrolithiasis from that originating in the ovaries, fallopian tubes, intestines, or gallbladder.

- Imaging is critical. A noncontrast renal-protocol abdominal CT scan is the principal means of diagnosis and can visualize all stones except indinavir. A **KUB** can often detect radiopaque stones, and **IVP** can detect stones that are radiolucent on KUB. These modalities are rarely used for the 1° diagnosis of nephrolithiasis, but a KUB is often used to follow known radiopaque stones (see Figure 12-8).
- All urine should be strained, and if a stone is passed, it should be recovered and sent to the lab for analysis.

TREATMENT

- **Hydration and analgesia** are the initial treatment; additional treatment is based on the size of the stone.
- Stones < 5 mm in diameter almost always pass without surgical intervention. Typically a 4- to 6-week course of medical expulsion therapy is first attempted, consisting of α-blockers (for both male and female patients), pain control, and time.
- Stones up to 3 cm in diameter can be treated with **extracorporeal shockwave lithotripsy** (ESWL) or percutaneous nephrolithotomy. Stones may also be treated with ureteroscopy and percutaneous nephrolithotomy.
- In cases where stones are 2° to hypercalciuria, thiazide therapy should be initiated.
- Patients who present with fever and an obstructing stone require immediate drainage of the kidney by way of ureteral stenting or nephrostomy tubes. Failure to treat in a timely fashion will result in urosepsis and possibly death.
- Preventive measures include hydration and a diet low in salt and animal protein. Additional prophylactic measures depend on stone composition and urine electrolyte profile.

KEY FACT

The recommended diet for a patient with a calcium stone is a normal-calcium diet. Low-calcium and high-calcium diets can both exacerbate the problem! A diet low in animal protein is recommended for **all** kinds of stones.

The patient likely has sepsis 2° to UTI. She requires aggressive fluid resuscitation and empiric antibiotics after urine and blood cultures. Call urology for a presumed indinavir stone despite lack of visualization on CT.

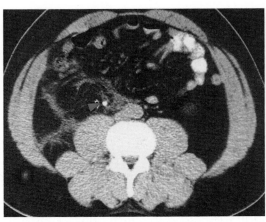
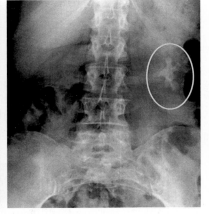

A   B

FIGURE 12-8.   Nephrolithiasis. (A) Transaxial CT without IV contrast shows a right ureteral calculus (arrowhead) with surrounding inflammatory changes of retroperitoneal fat. **(B)** AXR shows a left staghorn or struvite ($Mg\text{-}NH_4\text{-}PO_4$) stone filling the collecting system of the right kidney. (Image A reproduced with permission from Chen MY et al. *Basic Radiology*. New York: McGraw-Hill, 2004, Fig. 9-31. Image B reproduced with permission from USMLE-Rx.com.)

NEUROLOGY

Localization

Localization can be determined by the history and physical exam and is facilitated by dividing findings into peripheral vs central lesions (see Table 13-1) and upper motor neuron (UMN) vs lower motor neuron (LMN) lesions (see Table 13-2 and Figure 13-1).

- **Peripheral lesions:** Involve segmental loss; symptoms are ipsilateral to the lesion.
- **Central lesions:** Sensation below the level of the lesion is contralateral for crude touch, pain, and temperature and ipsilateral for fine touch and proprioception (for spinal cord lesions).

Stroke

Can be ischemic or hemorrhagic. Table 13-3 describes the causes, risk factors, and presentation of both; Table 13-4 and Figure 13-2 outline affected vessels and their associated deficits.

TABLE 13-1.   Lesion Location and Associated Symptoms

LOCATION	SYMPTOMS	EXAMPLES
PERIPHERAL LESIONS		
Neuromuscular junction	Fatigable weakness, symmetric pattern, no sensory loss; the face and proximal limbs are most often affected.	Myasthenia gravis.
Peripheral nerve	Distal asymmetric or symmetric pattern; ↓ sensation in a patch innervated by nerve; LMN signs.	Diabetic neuropathy; axonal injury/demyelination.
Nerve root	Shooting pain; weakness and reflex loss in movement corresponding to the root; dermatomal sensory change; LMN signs.	Prolapsed disk; herpes zoster.
CENTRAL LESIONS		
Spinal cord	"Band" with ↓ sensation and UMN signs below the level of the lesion; bladder/bowel dysfunction.	Cord compression.
Brainstem	Cranial nerve deficits, possible stupor/coma, hemibody UMN signs and sensory changes.	Stroke.
Cerebellum	Ipsilateral ataxia, nystagmus, dysmetria, breakdown of rapid alternating movements.	Hemisphere lesions (ipsilateral clumsiness of distal limbs). Vermis lesions (truncal ataxia).
Basal ganglia	Extrapyramidal signs (rigidity, bradykinesia, tremor), visual field cuts.	Parkinson's disease.
Cortical brain	Cortical signs (aphasia → left hemisphere; neglect → right hemisphere, gaze deviation); UMN weakness that is not fully hemibody (eg, face and arm > leg); sensory changes that are not fully hemibody.	Unilateral occipital lobe lesion (contralateral homonymous hemianopia).

TABLE 13-2.   UMN vs LMN Lesions

	UMN LESIONS	LMN LESIONS
Anatomy	Motor cortex → internal capsule → pons → medulla (pyramidal decussation) → corticospinal tract ("CNS lesions").	Anterior horn cell → ventral root → plexus → peripheral nerve ("PNS lesions").
Paresis (muscle weakness)	Affect the upper extremity extensors more than the flexors and the lower extremity flexors more than the extensors.	Affect the distribution of the anterior horn cell, plexus, or peripheral nerve involved.
Tone	Spasticity.	Flaccidity.
Wasting	Absent.	Present.
DTRs	Hyperactive.	Hypoactive or absent.
Plantar reflexes	Upgoing (⊕ Babinski's).	Downgoing (normal).
Fasciculations	Absent.	Present.
Examples	Strokes, TIA, brain tumors, head trauma, MS, epidural abscess.	Guillain-Barré syndrome, neuropathies, **Bell's palsy,** herpes zoster, Lyme disease, cauda equina syndrome.

DIAGNOSIS

- Check airway, breathing, and circulation; order a stat glucose. Keep NPO until intracranial hemorrhage has been ruled out and the patient has been assessed for dysphagia (aspiration risk).
- Order a **head CT without contrast** to rule out bleed.
  - **Hypodense** = ischemic stroke.
  - **Hyperdense** = hemorrhagic stroke.
- Further evaluation includes:
  - **MRA or CT angiography:** To evaluate vessels, including the carotids and circle of Willis.
  - **Transesophageal echocardiography:** To evaluate for cardiac origins of emboli and patent foramen ovale.
  - **Labs:** CBC, electrolytes, coagulation studies, HbA_{1c}, fasting lipids.
  - **Telemetry or ECG:** To evaluate for atrial fibrillation (AF).

TREATMENT

- Ischemic stroke:
  - **Candidates for IV recombinant tPA:** Keep BP < 185/110.
    - Candidates include those who have a symptom duration of < 4.5 hours, are > 18 years of age, and have a CT without hemorrhage and a measurable neurologic deficit.
    - Do **not** give tPA if stroke/head trauma occurred in the past 3 months; if the patient is pregnant/lactating; or if there is a history of intracerebral hemorrhage (ICH) or major surgery in the last 2 weeks, acute MI in the last 3 months, LP in the last 7 days, or uncontrolled hypertension requiring aggressive therapy.
  - **Patients who are not tPA candidates:** Allow permissive hypertension (> 160/> 80 and < 210/< 110) for 24 hours.
  - **Antiplatelet agents:** Aspirin ↓ the incidence of a second event. Patients already on aspirin may be given clopidogrel, ticlopidine, or dipyridamole.

Q 1

A 32-year-old woman in her third trimester of pregnancy develops sudden onset of hemifacial weakness, diminished taste, hyperacusis, and difficulty closing the eye. What is the diagnosis?

Q 2

An 81-year-old woman with a history of hypertension presents with sudden onset of left-sided weakness. She displays left-sided neglect and left facial and arm paralysis with relative sparing of the left leg. Which vessel territory is affected?

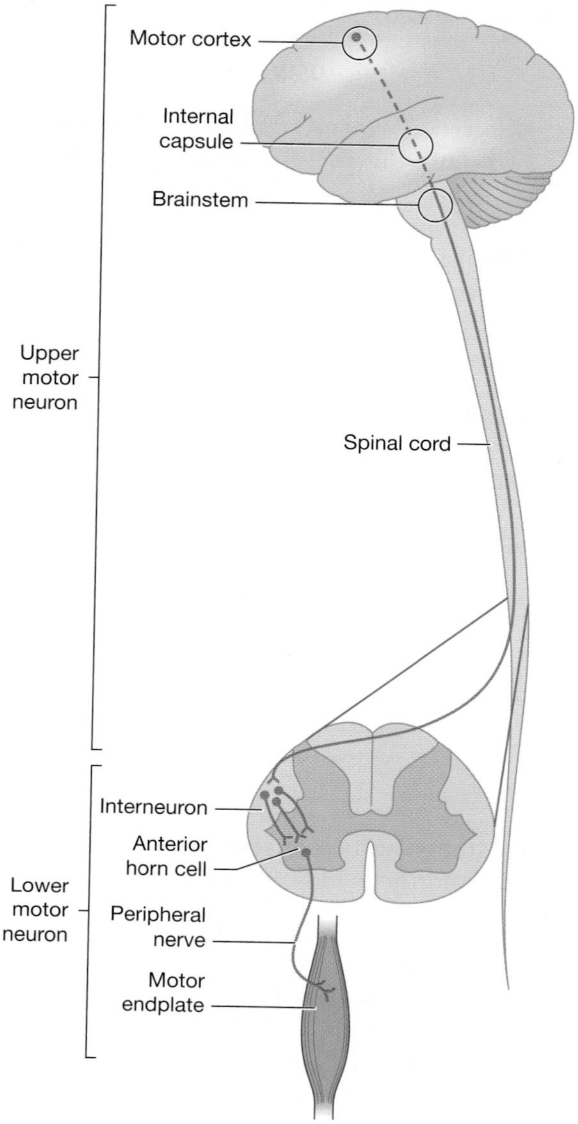

FIGURE 13-1.   Anatomic basis of UMN and LMN function. (Reproduced with permission from Greenberg DA et al. *Clinical Neurology*, 8th ed. New York: McGraw-Hill, 2012, Fig. 9-1.)

- **Hemorrhagic stroke:** Lower systolic BP to < 160 unless intracranial pressure is very high; **obtain an urgent neurosurgical evaluation** for possible posterior craniotomy for cerebellar ICHs > 3 cm or aneurysm clipping/coiling in subarachnoid hemorrhage (SAH). Treat coagulopathies.

PREVENTION

2° stroke prevention measures include:

- **Antiplatelet therapy:** Aspirin, aspirin/dipyridamole (Aggrenox), or clopidogrel (Plavix).
- **BP goals:** < 140/90.
- **Lipid goals:** LDL of < 70 mg/dL.
- Discontinuation of smoking.
- If > 50% carotid stenosis is seen on angiography, refer for observation and evaluation for carotid endarterectomy.
- If AF is present or if LVEF is ≤ 25%, consider warfarin.

---

1   **A**

Bell's palsy. The facial nerve (CN VII) consists of branches to the muscles of facial expression as well as to the sensory (taste to the anterior two-thirds of the tongue) and parasympathetic (glands of the head and neck) branches.

2   **A**

Stroke involving the right MCA territory. This is supported by the neglect (a cortical sign) and sparing of the left leg, indicating preservation of the ACA territory. The MCA supplies the lateral frontal, parietal, and temporal cortex; the ACA supplies the territory for motor control of the left leg.

TABLE 13-3. Ischemic vs Hemorrhagic Stroke

	Ischemic	Hemorrhagic
Definition	Infarction of CNS tissue; 85% of all strokes (see Figure 13-3). **Transient ischemic attack (TIA):** Episode of neurologic dysfunction caused by focal brain, spinal cord, or retinal ischemia without acute infarction. Absence of findings on imaging; typically lasts 10–60 minutes.	**ICH:** Focal bleeding from a blood vessel in brain parenchyma (see Figure 13-4). **SAH:** Sudden bleeding in the subarachnoid space.
Cause	Cerebral artery thrombosis or embolism (from heart or neck vessels) causing vessel obstruction.	**ICH:** Usually results from a ruptured small atherosclerotic artery weakened by chronic hypertension. **SAH:** The most common cause is head trauma, but spontaneous bleeding results from a ruptured aneurysm.
Risk factors	Untreated hypertension, AF, diabetes, cigarette smoking, recent MI, valvular heart disease, carotid artery disease, TIA, hyperlipidemia, OCP use, illicit drug use (cocaine, amphetamines).	High blood pressure, cigarette smoking, OCP use, excessive alcohol consumption, illicit drug use.
Symptoms/exam	Abrupt, dramatic onset of focal neurologic symptoms.	Headache, vomiting, hypertension, and impaired consciousness.

TABLE 13-4. Vessels Affected in Stroke and Associated Symptoms

Vessel Affected	Deficit
MCA stroke	Contralateral hemiparesis of the face, hand, and arm; contralateral hemisensory deficit in the same distribution; ipsilateral gaze preference; facial droop (UMN pattern). Contralateral homonymous hemianopia; neglect of contralateral limbs; apraxia. **Broca's (expressive) aphasia:** Nonfluent speech; poor repetition and naming but good auditory comprehension (usually associated with left hemispheric stroke). **Wernicke's (receptive) aphasia:** Poor auditory comprehension, repetition, and naming but fluent speech (usually associated with left hemispheric stroke).
ACA stroke	Leg paresis.
PCA stroke	Homonymous hemianopia with macular sparing; prosopagnosia (affects occipital lobe).
Basilar artery stroke	Coma, cranial nerve palsies, "locked-in" syndrome (affects the brainstem).
Lacunar stroke	Pure motor or sensory deficit; dysarthria; hemiparesis of the face, arm, and leg (affects the thalamus, internal capsule, and midbrain).

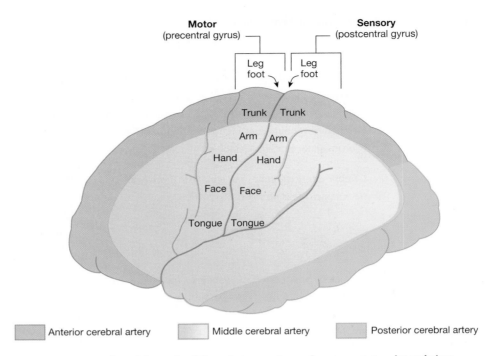

Motor
(precentral gyrus)

Sensory
(postcentral gyrus)

Leg
foot

Leg
foot

Trunk / Trunk

Arm / Arm

Hand / Hand

Face / Face

Tongue / Tongue

☐ Anterior cerebral artery   ☐ Middle cerebral artery   ☐ Posterior cerebral artery

FIGURE 13-2.   **Arterial supply of the primary motor and sensory cortex, lateral view.**
(Adapted with permission from Aminoff M, Greemberg D, Simon R: *Clinical Neurology*, 9th edition. New York, NY: McGraw-Hill Education; 2015.)

Seizures

May be partial or generalized (see Table 13-5).

- **Partial:** Involve only 1 part of the brain; can progress to generalized.
- **Generalized:** Arise from both cerebral hemispheres.

Status epilepticus is defined as continuous seizures or repetitive, discrete seizures with impaired consciousness in the interictal period. It is a medical emergency with up to a 20% mortality rate.

KEY FACT

Jacksonian march seizure activity presents as progressive jerking that spreads from one limb to the next on the ipsilateral side.

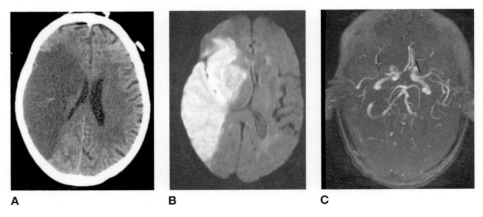

A   B   C

FIGURE 13-3.   **Acute ischemic stroke.** Acute left hemiparesis in a 62-year-old woman. **(A)** Noncontrast transaxial head CT with loss of gray and white matter differentiation and asymmetrically decreased size of the right lateral ventricle in a right MCA distribution (indicating mass effect). **(B)** Transaxial diffusion-weighted MRI with reduced diffusion in the same distribution, consistent with an acute infarct. **(C)** Maximum-intensity projection of a transaxial time-of-flight MRA shows the cause: an abrupt occlusion of the proximal right MCA (arrow). Compare with the normal left MCA (arrowhead). (Reproduced with permission from USMLE-Rx.com.)

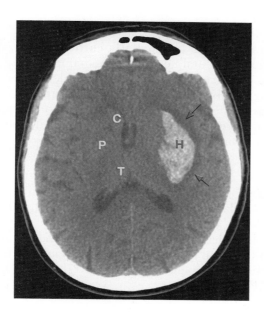

FIGURE 13-4. **Intracerebral hemorrhage.** Transaxial image from a noncontrast head CT shows an intraparenchymal hemorrhage (H) and surrounding edema (arrows) centered in the left putamen, a common location for hypertensive hemorrhage. C, P, and T denote the normal contralateral caudate, putamen, and thalamus. (Reproduced with permission from Fauci AS et al. *Harrison's Principles of Internal Medicine,* 17th ed. New York: McGraw-Hill, 2008, Fig. 364-17.)

EXAM

- **Fever** suggests CNS infection.
- Look for **tongue biting, urinary incontinence,** and **meningeal signs** (nuchal rigidity, ⊕ Brudzinski's, ⊕ Kernig's).

KEY FACT

Postictally, seizure patients may have a focal neurologic deficit that mimics a stroke (eg, Todd's paralysis) and resolves within minutes to days.

TABLE 13-5. **Partial vs Generalized Seizures**

SUBTYPE	PRESENTATION
PARTIAL SEIZURES	
Simple	Acute onset of motor, sensory, autonomic, or psychiatric symptoms; **no alteration of consciousness.**
Complex	Same symptoms as simple partial seizures, but with **transient alteration of consciousness** (may begin with aura).
GENERALIZED SEIZURES	
Tonic-clonic ("grand mal")	Acute loss of consciousness; tonic phase (stiffening of body) followed by clonic phase (jerking of body). Postictal period (deep sleep) presents with incontinence, confusion, low serum HCO_3, and ↑ serum CK and prolactin.
Absence ("petit mal")	Acute brief lapses of consciousness; no loss of postural control; begin in childhood (ages 4–8). No postictal period.
Atonic	Acute brief loss of postural control and consciousness (1–2 seconds).
Myoclonic	Acute shocklike contraction of muscle groups (jerks).

Q

A 27-year-old woman with a history of epilepsy is planning her first pregnancy. What should you recommend for her prenatal care?

DIFFERENTIAL

- ICH, acute or **old stroke (particularly cortical),** SAH, meningitis, head injury, subdural or epidural hematoma, migraines.
- **Hyponatremia** (or changes in magnesium, calcium, or glucose), **EtOH withdrawal,** cocaine or amphetamine intoxication.
- Medications associated with seizures include imipramine, meperidine, INH, imipenem, bupropion, **fluoroquinolones,** and metronidazole.
- 1° **CNS tumor** or brain metastases.

DIAGNOSIS

- **Labs:** Order a CBC, electrolytes, glucose, magnesium, calcium, ammonia, an EtOH level, a toxicology screen, and an antiepileptic drug level if appropriate.
- **EEG:** To establish a baseline, localize the focus, and confirm the diagnosis.
- **CT** or **MRI** of the brain is indicated in any new adult-onset seizure.
- If **CNS infection is suspected, get an LP**—but only if there is **no evidence of** ↑ **ICP.**

TREATMENT

- **Acute:**
  - Check **ABCs; intubation may be required to protect the airway.**
  - Gently turn the patient onto his left side to prevent aspiration. Unless the patient is being intubated, do not put anything into his mouth (eg, tongue blade, fingers)!
  - Always check a **glucose level,** as hypoglycemia is a common cause of convulsions. If the patient is hypoglycemic, give IV thiamine and then glucose. If the glucose level is normal, give lorazepam 0.1 mg/kg in 2-mg increments each over 2–3 minutes up to 8 mg.
  - If the seizure continues, give fosphenytoin 15–20 mg/kg at a rate no faster than 150 mg/min. If the seizure persists, consider induction of coma with anesthetic (propofol, midazolam, phenobarbital).
- **Chronic:** Table 13-6 outlines pharmacotherapeutic options for the long-term prevention of seizures.

Brain Death

A state characterized by the absence of cerebral and brainstem function with maintenance of other organs through artificial means. Distinguish between vegetative state and coma as follows:

- **Vegetative state:** The patient is awake but unaware (may move eyes, but no responsive behavior).
- **Coma:** The patient is unconscious and unarousable.

KEY FACT

Signs and symptoms of ↑ ICP include headache on awakening, nausea/vomiting, drowsiness, diplopia, blurry vision, papilledema, and CN VI palsies.

KEY FACT

Most antiepileptic drugs are teratogenic. Rule out pregnancy before starting treatment.

KEY FACT

Carbamazepine, an antiepileptic drug, is used as therapy for trigeminal neuralgia.

Epilepsy is a brain disorder characterized by recurrent seizures. Do not take a pregnant woman off her antiepileptic drugs. Valproate is the most teratogenic, so switching to another drug (eg, carbamazepine) is recommended before pregnancy. Taking 400 μg of folic acid daily is also recommended, as are regular checks of serum drug levels.

TABLE 13-6.　First-Line Drugs for the Prevention of Seizure

PARTIAL ONSET[a]	1° GENERALIZED	ABSENCE	MYOCLONIC, ATONIC
Carbamazepine	Valproate	Ethosuximide	Valproate
Lamotrigine	Lamotrigine	Valproate	
Phenytoin			
Valproate			

[a] Includes simple partial, complex partial, and secondarily generalized seizures.

DIAGNOSIS

- Exclude sedative medications, hypothermia, hypotension, or metabolic derangements.
- Examine for absent brainstem functions. A comatose state (injury to the reticular activating system) would present with unresponsiveness to verbal, tactile, or painful stimuli.
- Examine for absent brainstem reflexes (see Table 13-7).
- Complete apnea is denoted by no respirations at a $Paco_2$ of 60 mm Hg, or 20 mm Hg above normal values (apnea test).
- **Confirmatory testing:** A clinical diagnosis can be made on the basis of an apnea test and the absence of brainstem reflexes. If these are not conclusive, the following confirmatory tests may be conducted:
  - **Angiography** (conventional, MRI, or radionuclide): Brain death is demonstrated by the absence of vessel filling at the carotid bifurcation/circle of Willis.
  - **EEG.**
  - **Transcranial Doppler ultrasonography:** Look for small systolic peaks without diastolic flow.

Epidural Hematoma

- An accumulation of blood between the skull and the dura. Typically results from tearing of the **middle meningeal artery** 2° to head trauma. A **neurologic emergency.**
- **Sx/Exam:** The patient is initially unconscious from concussion, followed by a "lucid interval" during which the hematoma subclinically expands. Lethargy and rapid neurologic deterioration follow with signs of herniation (eg, fixed, dilated pupil).
- **Dx:** Head CT without contrast shows a **biconvex, lens-shaped hyperdensity** that respects cranial suture lines (see Figure 13-5A).
- **Tx:** Open craniotomy and evacuation of blood if > 30 cm³ of hematoma. If the hematoma is < 30 cm³ and < 15 mm thick with < 5 mm midline shift and a GCS > 8 with no focal deficit, you may observe.

Subdural Hematoma

- An accumulation of blood between the arachnoid membrane and the dura. Typically results from blunt head trauma (commonly a fall) that

TABLE 13-7. **Evaluation for Absent Brainstem Functions**

ABSENT REFLEX	DEFINITION	NERVES INVOLVED
Pupillary light	No change in pupil size in response to bright light.	CN II, III
Corneal	No blinking when the cornea is touched.	CN V, VII
Oculovestibular	No deviation of eyes to stabilize images on retina during head movement/simulated head movement.	CN III, IV, VI, VIII
Gag	No response when the posterior pharynx is stimulated.	CN IX, X

KEY FACT

Common causes of coma include ischemic brain injury, traumatic brain injury, and metabolic derangements (eg, profound hypoglycemia).

KEY FACT

For comatose patients, evaluate for nonconvulsive status epilepticus with an EEG.

Q

A 23-year-old man presents after a motor vehicle accident. He opens his eyes when asked, is disoriented and confused, and is able to pinpoint the locations of his pain. What is his score on the Glasgow Coma Scale?

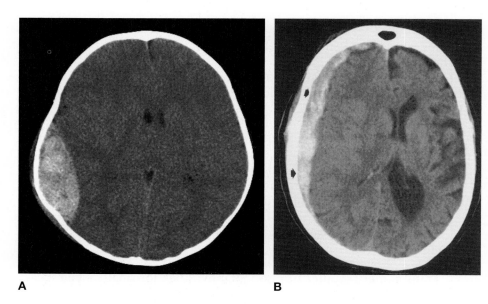

F I G U R E 1 3 - 5 .   **Acute epidural and subdural hematoma. (A)** Noncontrast transaxial CT showing a right temporal acute epidural hematoma. Note the characteristic biconvex shape. **(B)** Noncontrast transaxial CT demonstrating a right acute holohemispheric subdural hematoma. Note the characteristic crescentic shape. (Image A reproduced with permission from Doherty GM. *Current Diagnosis & Treatment: Surgery*, 13th ed. New York: McGraw-Hill, 2010, Fig. 36-8. Image B reproduced with permission from Chen MY et al. *Basic Radiology*. New York: McGraw-Hill, 2004, Fig. 12-32.)

leads to rupture of the **bridging veins** (common in the **elderly** and in **alcoholics**).

- **Sx/Exam:** Presents with headache, altered mental status, and possible hemiparesis.
- **Dx:** Head CT shows a **crescent-shaped,** concave hyperdensity that may have a less distinct border and does not cross the midline (see Figure 13-5B).
- **Tx: Surgical evacuation** of blood if symptoms are present or if the lesion is increasing in size.

Spinal Cord Compression

A neurologic emergency! Evaluate for trauma (immobilize the neck if necessary), localize the lesion, image the spine, and call neurosurgery (see Figure 13-6).

SYMPTOMS/EXAM

- Presents with back pain, paresthesias, weakness, and bladder/bowel incontinence or retention.
- Exam reveals bilateral weakness, a sensory level (by pinprick), hyperreflexia below the sensory level, saddle anesthesia, and loss of anal wink. The last 2 findings are common with conus medullaris and cauda equina involvement.
- Complete cord transection initially presents with spastic paralysis followed by flaccid paralysis (because of loss of UMN inhibition that causes initial spasticity).

KEY FACT

Loss of anal reflex ("anal wink") indicates a lesion at S2–S4.

The patient's score is 12. A GCS score of 13–15 is considered mild disability, 9–12 is considered moderate, and < 8 is considered severe.

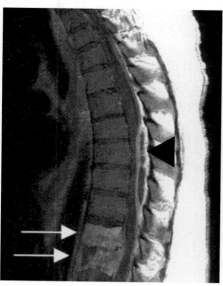
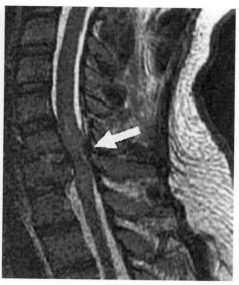

A   **B**

FIGURE 13-6.   Spinal cord compression. (A) Sagittal postcontrast MRI shows diskitis/ osteomyelitis (arrows) and a rim-enhancing epidural abscess (arrowhead) compressing the spinal cord. **(B)** Sagittal T2-weighted MRI in another patient shows a traumatic fracture at C6–C7 compressing the spinal cord. Note the abnormally high signal within the spinal cord (arrow).
(Image A reproduced with permission from Tintinalli JE et al. *Tintinalli's Emergency Medicine: A Comprehensive Study Guide*, 6th ed. New York: McGraw-Hill, 2004, Fig. 305-5. Image B reproduced with permission from Doherty GM. *Current Diagnosis & Treatment: Surgery*, 13th ed. New York: McGraw-Hill, 2010, Fig. 36-12.)

DIFFERENTIAL

The etiologies of spinal cord compression include:

- **Trauma:** Motor vehicle accidents; sports-related injuries.
- **Infection:** Epidural abscess in IV drug users; spinal TB (Pott's disease) in immunocompromised patients; vertebral osteomyelitis.
- **Neoplasms:** Metastases are most common.
- **Degenerative disease:** Cervical and lumbar disk herniations.
- **Vascular:** Infarction, epidural and subdural hematomas, and AVMs are rare.

DIAGNOSIS

Spinal MRI; CT or CT myelography for patients in whom MRI is contraindicated (eg, those with pacemakers).

TREATMENT

- Administer steroids within 8 hours of symptom onset (controversial).
  - **Acute spinal cord injury:** Methylprednisolone bolus. Wait 45 minutes; then give a continuous infusion of methylprednisolone over the next 24 hours.
  - **Spinal tumor:** Dexamethasone 100 mg IV bolus.
- **Fractures, subluxations, and dislocations:** Surgical reduction.
- **Epidural abscess:** Neurosurgical drainage and broad-spectrum antibiotics (a third-generation cephalosporin, vancomycin, and metronidazole).

Headache

Table 13-8 outlines the differential for headache.

KEY FACT

Trauma to the neck should be suspected if there is trauma to the face and body.

KEY FACT

Always look for a sensory level when considering a spinal cord process. The pinprick test is precise and reproducible.

Q

A 58-year-old woman who is being treated with estrogen presents with an inability to walk or to urinate. Exam shows a distended bladder, ↓ rectal tone, spastic weakness in the bilateral lower extremities, and bilateral ankle clonus. Where is the lesion, and what are the most likely etiologies?

TABLE 13-8.   **Presentation, Diagnosis, and Treatment of Headache**

Type	Symptoms	Exam/Diagnosis	Treatment
Tension	Tight, bandlike pain bilaterally.	Exam is usually normal. A clinical diagnosis.	NSAIDs/acetaminophen; relaxation techniques.
Migraine	Episodic and severe with sensitivity to light, sound, and movement; may be accompanied by nausea, vomiting, photophobia, and phonophobia. **Common migraine:** Without aura. **Classic migraine:** With aura (eg, visual disturbances and paresthesias preceding headache).	Exam is usually normal. A clinical diagnosis that has a familial predisposition; more common in women.	Eliminate triggers. **Mild:** NSAIDs + antiemetic (eg, metoclopramide). **Moderate:** Triptans. **Severe:** IV hydration, antiemetics, dexamethasone, prochlorperazine, or ergotamine. **Prevention:** TCAs, valproate, β-blockers.
Cluster	Brief, severe, unilateral, **periorbital** headache; attacks occur at the same hour each day.	Exam reveals ipsilateral lacrimation, conjunctival injection, Horner's syndrome, and nasal congestion; more common in men.	100% O$_2$ or low-dose prednisone.

KEY FACT

Horner's syndrome presents with ipsilateral miosis (pupillary constriction), ipsilateral ptosis (eyelid droop), and ipsilateral anhidrosis (lack of sweating) of the face.

KEY FACT

Severe, sudden-onset headache should raise concern for a subarachnoid/aneurysm rupture.

The lesion is likely in the spinal cord at the lumbar level or higher. The most likely etiologies are neoplastic, infectious, inflammatory, vascular, or structural processes (disk herniation). In rare cases, the etiology may be a metastatic lesion at the thoracic level from a 1° breast cancer 2° to estrogen treatment.

DIAGNOSIS

Obtain a CT scan with:

- A headache that is acute and extremely severe ("**thunderclap headache**").
- A headache that is progressive over days to weeks, particularly if it is not similar to previous headaches.
- Focal neurologic signs.
- Papilledema.
- A headache in an immunocompromised patient (eg, HIV).

Guillain-Barré Syndrome (GBS)

An **acute polyradiculoneuropathy** (root and peripheral nerve process) that usually has an **autoimmune** basis. It typically presents as an **ascending** motor paralysis with **areflexia**, autonomic involvement (eg, postural hypotension), and possible sensory symptoms. Seventy percent of patients have a recent history of respiratory or GI **infection** (particularly *Campylobacter jejuni*).

SYMPTOMS/EXAM

Exam shows leg > arm weakness, facial weakness with difficulty handling secretions, **absent reflexes**, proprioception > pain/temperature sensation, postural hypotension, and respiratory failure.

DIAGNOSIS

- A clinical diagnosis supported by ancillary tests that are most effective at excluding mimics (eg, acute myelopathies, botulism, diphtheria, Lyme disease).
- **LP:** Typically shows ↑ protein with normal WBC levels ("**albuminocytologic dissociation**"), but often normal in the first 48 hours.
- **CBC:** May show an ↑ WBC count. Obtain an ESR and a Lyme titer.
- **Nerve conduction study:** May show evidence of demyelination.

TREATMENT

- Give **IVIG** or **plasmapheresis** as soon as possible.
- Measure **vital capacity** and **maximum inspiratory force** to monitor for respiratory compromise.
- Watch for **autonomic instability,** including hypotension, temperature dysregulation, and cardiac arrhythmias.

Myasthenia Gravis (MG)

An autoimmune disorder in which antibodies attack the acetylcholine (ACh) receptors at the neuromuscular junction. Has a bimodal age distribution with an earlier peak in the 30s–40s (women) and a late peak in the 70s–90s (men).

SYMPTOMS/EXAM

The main features of MG are **weakness** and **fatigability** of the skeletal muscles. The weakness may be worse at the end of the day or after exercise and may improve with rest. There is an ↑ in weakness with repeated use of the skeletal muscles (fatigability). Categorized as follows:

- **Ocular MG:** Muscle weakness limited to the eyelids and extraocular muscles, with ptosis and/or diplopia. Fifty percent of patients go on to develop generalized MG.
- **Generalized MG:** Weakness may be seen in ocular, bulbar (dysarthria, dysphagia, fatigable chewing), facial (expressionless), limb, and respiratory muscles. Worsening respiratory muscle strength can lead to respiratory failure, or a **"myasthenic crisis."**

DIFFERENTIAL

Lambert-Eaton myasthenic syndrome (antibodies attack presynaptic voltage-gated calcium channels), botulism, drug-induced myasthenia, motor neuron diseases (eg, ALS), generalized fatigue, intracranial mass, hyperthyroidism.

DIAGNOSIS

- **Edrophonium chloride (Tensilon)** is an acetylcholinesterase inhibitor that prolongs the presence of ACh at the neuromuscular junction. A ⊕ test results in an immediate ↑ in the strength of affected muscles.
- Immunologic assays for **ACh receptor antibody;** if seronegative, **muscle-specific kinase (MuSK) antibodies.**
- **Repetitive nerve stimulation:** The nerve is stimulated and action potentials are measured in muscles. In MG, there is a rapid ↓ in the amplitude of action potentials.
- **Single-fiber electromyography:** Measures single-muscle-fiber discharges. The most sensitive diagnostic test for MG.

TREATMENT

- **Symptomatic treatment:** First-line treatment is an acetylcholinesterase inhibitor (pyridostigmine).
- **Chronic immunomodulating agents:** Corticosteroids, azathioprine, cyclosporine, mycophenolate mofetil.
- **For myasthenic crisis:** Plasmapheresis and/or IVIG.
- **Surgery:** Thymectomy (to remove the source of antibodies).

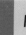

KEY FACT

Even if the head CT is ⊖, get an LP when there is high suspicion for SAH. Fifteen percent of patients with an aneurysmal SAH have a ⊖ CT. LP will show high RBCs in all tubes and xanthochromia (yellow CSF).

KEY FACT

Neuromuscular blocking agents used during anesthesia can unmask or worsen MG, leading to prolonged postoperative weakness and ventilator dependence.

Q   **1**

A 33-year-old man who is recovering from a recent infection presents with an inability to stand up from a sitting position. Exam shows an absence of reflexes. What is his diagnosis?

Q   **2**

A 31-year-old man complains that when he looks up to catch a baseball, he sees 2 balls and cannot make the catch. Exam shows ptosis and weakness in all extraocular muscles. He also complains of generalized fatigue. What is the likely diagnosis?

Vertigo

An illusion of movement of either the patient or his/her surroundings. Non-vestibular causes of dizziness include orthostatic hypotension, cardiac arrhythmia, and presyncope/syncope. Once a diagnosis of vertigo has been established, one must determine whether it is peripheral or central (see Table 13-9).

Multiple Sclerosis (MS)

A disorder involving inflammation and destruction of CNS myelin, likely from an autoimmune process. **Young women** are at higher risk, as are those who reside in **northern latitudes.**

SYMPTOMS

- The most common symptoms are sensory loss, optic neuritis, weakness, paresthesias, diplopia, and ataxia.
- The 4 clinical courses of MS are relapsing-remitting, 2° progressive, 1° progressive, and progressive/relapsing.

EXAM

Classic findings include:

- Hyperreflexia, **weakness,** and ataxia.
- **Lhermitte's sign:** Radiating/shooting pain up or down the spine on flexion or extension.
- **Optic neuritis:** ↓ visual acuity; pain with eye movements; central scotoma; red desaturation.

TABLE 13-9.   Peripheral vs Central Vertigo

	PERIPHERAL	CENTRAL
Pathology	Lesion of the vestibular apparatus of the inner ear or CN VIII.	Lesion of brainstem vestibular nuclei or their connections.
Symptoms	Intermittent, **positional** vertigo; may be associated with tinnitus, hearing loss, and postural unsteadiness. Nystagmus is rotary, unidirectional, and fatigable. Fixation of gaze stops vertigo.	Vertigo is **not positional** and may have accompanying cranial nerve injuries (facial droops, dysarthria, absent corneal reflexes). Nystagmus changes direction with gaze; vertical nystagmus is highly specific for central vertigo. Visual fixation does not stop vertigo.
Diagnosis	See Figure 13-7.	See Figure 13-7.
Treatment	Canalith repositioning (Epley maneuver) for BPPV; physical therapy, antihistamines/benzodiazepines/scopolamine.	Treat the underlying cause.

1   **A**

Guillain-Barré syndrome. This patient demonstrates the classic ascending motor paralysis that follows his recent history of infection.

2   **A**

Myasthenia gravis. The lesion is in the neuromuscular junction isolated to the eyes. These symptoms can also occur in MS, but the latter is accompanied by other symptoms, such as paresthesias.

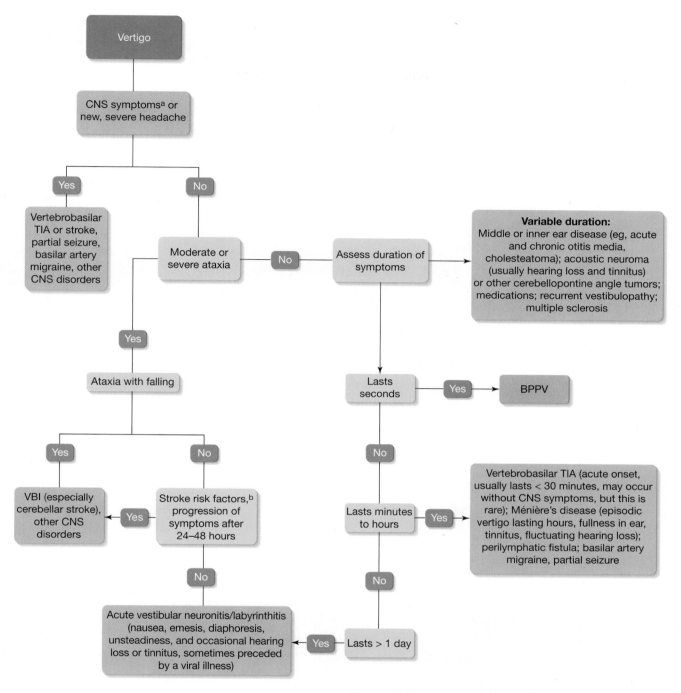

FIGURE 13-7. **Diagnostic approach to vertigo.** (Reproduced with permission from Henderson MC et al. *The Patient History: An Evidence-Based Approach to Differential Diagnosis,* 2nd ed. New York: McGraw-Hill, 2012, Fig. 6-2.)

[a] CNS symptoms = focal or sensory or motor deficits, brainstem findings (eg, dysarthria, diplopia, dysphagia).
[b] Stroke risk factors = advanced age, smoking, dyslipidemia, family history, DM, hypertension, AF, CAD, CHF, peripheral vascular disease.

- **Afferent pupillary defect (Marcus Gunn pupil):** The pupil paradoxically dilates to a light stimulus as a result of delayed conduction.
- **Internuclear ophthalmoplegia (MLF syndrome):** The classic finding is weakness on adduction of the ipsilateral eye with nystagmus on abduction of the contralateral eye, together with incomplete or slow abduction of the ipsilateral eye on lateral gaze with complete preservation of convergence.

DIAGNOSIS

- **Brain MRI with gadolinium:** Reveals multiple focal **periventricular areas of** ↑ **signal,** called **Dawson's fingers** (see Figure 13-8).
- **CSF:** Shows ↑ protein (myelin basic protein, **oligoclonal bands**).
- **Visual evoked potentials:** Demonstrate delayed conduction.

TREATMENT

- Treat acute exacerbations with methylprednisolone/prednisone.
- Manage relapsing-remitting disease with prophylactic agents such as **interferon-β$_{1a/1b}$** or glatiramer acetate.
- If there is poor response or intolerance to prophylactic agents, use natalizumab.
- Baclofen may be given for spasticity.

Muscular Dystrophy

A group of hereditary progressive muscle-based diseases. The most common form is **Duchenne's muscular dystrophy,** which is **X-linked** and caused by a defect in the gene encoding the dystrophin protein.

SYMPTOMS/EXAM

- Presents between ages 3 and 5; patients progress to being wheelchair bound in childhood. Death is due to pulmonary complications in adolescence.
- Presents with **toe walking,** waddling gait, and inability to run or climb stairs.
- In attempting to rise to a standing from a supine position, patients use their arms to climb up their bodies (**Gowers' sign**).
- Proximal and girdle muscle **weakness** and **pseudohypertrophy** of the calves are apparent on exam.

DIAGNOSIS

- **Serum CK** levels are ↑ to 20–100 times normal.
- Genetic testing for the **dystrophin gene mutation;** muscle biopsy with immunohistochemistry.

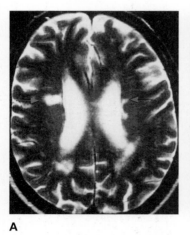
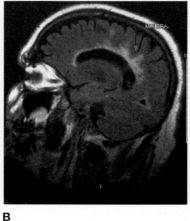
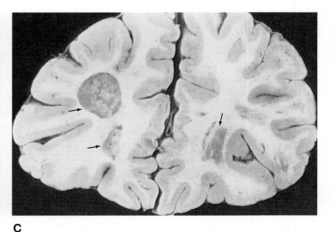

A   **B**   **C**

FIGURE 13-8.   Multiple sclerosis. Transaxial T2-weighted MRI (**A**) and sagittal FLAIR image (**B**) showing multiple MS plaques (arrows) in the periventricular matter oriented radially from the corpus callosum ("Dawson's fingers"). (**C**) Areas of demyelination of the white matter (arrows) in the frontal lobe of a patient with multiple sclerosis. (Images A and B reproduced with permission from Ropper AH, Samuels MA. *Adams & Victor's Principles of Neurology,* 9th ed. New York: McGraw-Hill, 2009, Fig. 36-1. Image C reproduced with permission from Waxman SG. *Clinical Neuroanatomy,* 27th ed. New York: McGraw-Hill, 2013, Fig. 25-9.)

TREATMENT

Prednisone slows disease progression by up to 3 years.

Parkinson's Disease (PD)

A neurodegenerative disease clinically diagnosed by at least 2 out of 4 cardinal features: resting tremor, bradykinesia, muscular rigidity, and postural instability. It is due to ↓ dopaminergic transmission in the basal ganglia resulting from neuronal degeneration in the **substantia nigra**.

SYMPTOMS

- The peak age of onset is in the early 60s.
- **Motor symptoms:** Progressive slowness in dressing, walking, feeding, or writing; difficulty rising from a chair; hesitancy in initiating gait; frequent falls and loss of balance; loss of facial expression; smaller handwriting (micrographia).
- **Nonmotor symptoms:** Sleep disorders (restless legs and REM sleep behavior disorder); sensory abnormalities and pain; autonomic dysfunction.
- **Neuropsychiatric symptoms:** Depression, anxiety, cognitive impairment (including psychosis).

EXAM

Exam reveals the following:

- **Resting tremor:** A 4- to 6-Hz tremor that is initially unilateral, with distal prominence and pill rolling.
- **Bradykinesia:** Slowness and paucity of movement with ↓ amplitudes. Patients have a slow blink rate and few facial expressions (masked facies).
- **Rigidity:** ↑ muscle tone that is present in all directions of movement may be **cogwheel rigidity.**
- **Loss of postural reflexes:** Patients cannot remain balanced if pushed from the front or from behind.

TREATMENT

- **Carbidopa/levodopa:** Most effective. Carbidopa blocks the metabolism of levodopa in the periphery. Levodopa is an amino acid precursor to dopamine that crosses the blood-brain barrier. First-line treatment for patients > 70 years of age.
- **Dopamine agonists:** Direct agonists of the dopamine receptor; effective as monotherapy or as adjuncts to carbidopa/levodopa. They include nonergot alkaloids (pramipexole, ropinirole) and ergot alkaloids (bromocriptine). First-line treatment for patients < 50 years of age (eventually will require carbidopa/levodopa).
- **Adjunctive therapy:** MAO-B inhibitors (selegiline), COMT inhibitors (entacapone), amantidine, anticholinergics.
- **Surgical:** Deep brain stimulation in the subthalamus or pallidum; pallidotomy.

Huntington's Disease (HD)

An adult-onset neurodegenerative disease that is genetically inherited in an autosomal dominant pattern. It is caused by neuronal loss in the cerebral cortex and basal ganglia.

MNEMONIC

Key Parkinson's signs—

PARKINSON'S

Pill rolling
Akinesia/bradykinesia
Rigidity
Kyphosis
Instability
Neck/head tremor
Shuffling gait
Oculogyric crisis (fixation of the eyes in upward deviation)
"**N**ose tap" (tapping on the glabella, the area of the forehead above the nose)
Small writing (micrographia)

Q **1**

A 43-year-old woman complains of severe dizziness every time she turns her head abruptly. She states that the episodes make her feel as though the world is moving around her. She denies accompanying symptoms, takes no medications, and says that the episodes usually resolve on their own. What is her diagnosis?

Q **2**

A 65-year-old man presents with tremor of the right hand and a voice that has become softer over the years. Exam shows hypophonia, a 4-Hz resting tremor, mild right-sided rigidity, and micrographia. What is the diagnosis?

SYMPTOMS/EXAM

- Choreiform (dancelike) movements.
- Gradual dystonia, bradykinesia, rigidity, dysarthria, and dysphagia (parkinsonian symptoms).
- Cognitive decline, dementia, and depression/anxiety/psychosis may be present.

DIAGNOSIS

- Diagnosed by clinical exam and family history.
- Genetic tests (mandatory only with no family history) reveal expansion of CAG repeats in the huntingtin gene.
- HD can have genetic anticipation; disease severity ↑ and age of onset ↓ with each successive generation (due to ↑ expansion of CAG repeats).

TREATMENT

Treatment is symptomatic and careful follow-up is necessary, as some treatments may worsen symptoms.

- **Chorea:** Benzodiazepines, valproate, or dopamine-depleting agents such as tetrabenazine.
- **Parkinsonian features:** Carbidopa/levodopa or dopamine agonists.
- **Depression:** SSRIs.
- **Psychosis:** Atypical (second-generation) antipsychotics are preferred to minimize extrapyramidal side effects.

Amyotrophic Lateral Sclerosis (ALS)

A neurodegenerative, progressive motor neuron disease. Involves both LMNs and UMNs in a pure motor disorder (sensations are intact). Roughly 5–10% of cases are familial. Peak occurrence is at 55–75 years of age; has a 2:1 male-to-female ratio.

SYMPTOMS/EXAM

- Patients have progressive muscular weakness, muscle wasting, spasticity, respiratory insufficiency, and possible dementia.
- Exam reveals **UMN signs** (spasticity, weakness, ⊕ Babinski's), **LMN signs** (muscle atrophy, fasciculations), and **bulbar signs** (dysarthria, dysphagia, tongue fasciculations).

DIAGNOSIS

EMG shows widespread denervation. Muscle biopsy reveals neurogenic atrophy.

TREATMENT

ALS is an incurable, progressive disease. Treatment with BiPAP and **riluzole,** which inhibits glutamate release, has been associated with modest improvement.

Dementia

Progressive cognitive decline that interferes with the performance of the activities of daily living. Differs from mild cognitive impairment (MCI) in that

---

KEY FACT

Look for UMN **and** LMN signs with ALS.

---

1   **A**

Benign paroxysmal positional vertigo. The woman's symptoms are caused by free-moving canaliths in the vestibular canals.

---

2   **A**

Parkinson's disease. The lesion is in the left basal ganglia, specifically the substantia nigra, which will show neuronal degeneration and Lewy bodies at autopsy.

MCI symptoms are less severe, presenting with memory loss and attention deficits that exceed those of normal aging but do not interfere with activities of daily living.

SYMPTOMS

- **Impairment of recent memory** is typically the first sign.
- Subsequent manifestations include deficits in visuospatial ability (depth perception), language (speech or naming), calculation, or problem solving; behavioral and personality changes; and depression.

EXAM

Exam reveals cortical signs specific to each region:

- **Frontal:** Executive function breakdown, primitive reflexes, gait instability, personality changes.
- **Temporal:** Aphasia, memory loss, behavioral changes.
- **Parietal:** Calculation difficulties, left/right confusion, writing problems, inability to recognize fingers.
- **Occipital:** Simultagnosia (inability to synthesize full visual scenes), visual delusions.

DIFFERENTIAL

- **Reversible causes that mimic dementia:** Alcoholism, thyroid disease, vitamin deficiencies (B_{12}), drug and medication intoxication, chronic infections (HIV, neurosyphilis), depression ("pseudodementia"), subdural hematoma, delirium, and normal pressure hydrocephalus.
- **Nonreversible causes** (neurodegenerative diseases):
  - **Alzheimer's disease:** Memory loss.
  - **Frontotemporal dementia:** Apathy, poor judgment, language changes.
  - **Diffuse Lewy body dementia:** Visual hallucinations, fluctuations in baseline cognition, REM sleep disorders, parkinsonism.
  - **Creutzfeldt-Jakob disease:** Myoclonus, ataxia, personality changes.
  - **Vascular (multi-infarct) dementia:** Falls, apathy, weakness. May be sudden and stepwise in onset.

DIAGNOSIS

- Conduct a complete history and exam, a mini-mental status exam, and neuropsychological testing.
- Review medications.
- Check a CBC, electrolytes, B_{12}, TSH, VDRL, HIV, and a urine toxicology screen.
- Obtain a CT and possibly an MRI of the brain.

TREATMENT

- Treat reversible conditions that mimic dementia.
- Alzheimer's disease:
  - **Acetylcholinesterase inhibitors:** Include donepezil (Aricept), rivastigmine (Exelon), and galantamine (Reminyl). Use early in the course of disease.
  - **NMDA glutamate receptor antagonists:** Memantine (Namenda) for more advanced disease.
- Offer social support and assisted-living interventions.

Q

A 58-year-old inebriated man presents to the ED. He is uncoordinated, and review of his medical chart shows that he has a significant history of alcoholism. What treatment should the patient be given?

Wernicke-Korsakoff Syndrome

A nutritional disorder of the nervous system caused by a deficiency in thiamine (vitamin B$_1$), resulting in symmetrical lesions in the mammillary bodies. It is a syndrome complex consisting of **Wernicke's encephalopathy** and **Korsakoff's amnesia,** which may be seen separately.

SYMPTOMS/EXAM

- **Wernicke's encephalopathy:** Characterized by the triad of **ataxia, ophthalmoplegia,** and **confusion.**
- **Korsakoff's psychosis (amnesia):** Characterized by **impaired short-term memory. Confabulation** may be an accompanying symptom.

DIAGNOSIS

A clinical diagnosis. MRI may be used to rule out structural lesions.

TREATMENT

A **medical emergency.** Treat with high-dose thiamine (up to 500 mg). **Give thiamine before glucose,** as administering glucose in the absence of thiamine may precipitate neuronal death.

A

IV electrolytes and thiamine. He should also be put on watch for signs of alcohol withdrawal. Chronic alcoholics are malnourished and lack many vitamins, including thiamine, which can subsequently cause Wernicke-Korsakoff syndrome.

CHAPTER 14

OBSTETRICS

Determination of Gravidity and Parity

The mnemonic **G TPAL** provides a useful way to obtain an overview of a patient's obstetric history:

- **G** = Total number of pregnancies a patient has ever had, including miscarriages, abortions, and live births.
- **T** = Number of **term** deliveries > 37 weeks.
- **P** = Number of **preterm** deliveries between 20 and 36 weeks.
- **A** = Number of **abortions** or miscarriages of a pregnancy < 20 weeks.
- **L** = Number of **living** children a patient has.

Hence, a woman who is a G3P2012 has had 3 total pregnancies, 2 full-term deliveries, 1 miscarriage or abortion, and 2 living children.

Prenatal Care and Nutrition

All prenatal visits should document weight, BP, extremity edema, urine protein and glucose, fundal height (> 20 weeks), and fetal heart rate. Further recommendations are as follows:

- **Weight gain:** Women with a normal prepregnancy BMI should gain a total of 25–35 lbs during the pregnancy; obese women should gain less (11–20 lbs) and underweight women more.
- **Nutrition:** Requirements for total calories, protein, iron, folate, calcium, and zinc should ↑. All patients should take prenatal vitamins.
- **Caloric intake:** An additional 300 kcal/day is needed during pregnancy and 500 kcal/day during breast-feeding.
- **Folate:** Supplement with 400 µg/day to ↓ the risk of neural tube defects (NTDs). **Women with twin gestations or a prior history of a fetus with NTDs should receive 4 mg/day.**
- **Iron:** Supplement in the latter half of pregnancy to prevent anemia.
- **Calcium:** Supplement in the later months of pregnancy and during breast-feeding.
- **Smoking and alcohol cessation.**
- **Screening for domestic violence.**
- **Prenatal labs:** See Table 14-1 for lab work that should be scheduled during pregnancy.

Aneuploidy Screening and Diagnostic Testing

PRENATAL ANEUPLOIDY SCREENING

All 3 of the following screenings are done separately in the pregnancy and together comprise the **integrated screen:**

1. **First-trimester serum markers** (10–14 weeks): Maternal serum β-hCG and pregnancy-associated plasma protein-A (PAPP-A).
2. **Nuchal translucency ultrasound** (10–14 weeks): Measures the thickness between the skin and cervical spine to stratify the fetal risk of having trisomy 21.

TABLE 14-1. **Prenatal Labs During Pregnancy**

GESTATIONAL AGE (GA)	LABS TO BE OBTAINED
Initial visit	CBC, blood type, Rh antibody screen, UA with culture, Pap smear, cervical gonorrhea and chlamydia cultures, rubella antibody titer, hepatitis B surface antigen, syphilis screen, PPD, HIV. Toxoplasmosis and sickle cell screening for at-risk patients. Women with risk factors for gestational diabetes (ie, prior gestational diabetes or a family history in a first-degree relative) should get early glucose testing and an HbA_{1c}.
6–11 weeks	**Ultrasound** to determine GA (more accurate than later scans).
10–14 weeks	**Ultrasound** to determine **nuchal translucency** for all patients. **First-trimester serum aneuploidy screening** for all patients. Offer **chorionic villus sampling** to high-risk patients.
15–19 weeks	**Quad screen (ie, second-trimester aneuploidy screening).** Offer **amniocentesis** to patients with abnormal screening.
18–21 weeks	**Screening ultrasound** to survey fetal anatomy, placental location, and amniotic fluid.
24–28 weeks	**One-hour glucose challenge test.** If ≥ 140 mg/dL, follow with a 3-hour glucose tolerance test. Repeat hemoglobin/hematocrit.
28 weeks	**RhoGAM** injection for Rh-⊖ patients. Start fetal kick counting (the patient should count 10 fetal movements in 2 hours).
35–37 weeks	Screen for **group B streptococcus** (GBS) with a rectovaginal swab. Repeat hemoglobin/hematocrit. Cervical gonorrhea and chlamydia cultures, RPR, and HIV (in at-risk patients). Assess fetal position with Leopold maneuvers and ultrasound.

3. **Second-trimester serum markers (aka the "quad screen") (15–19 weeks):** Maternal serum α-fetoprotein (MSAFP), unconjugated estriol, hCG, and inhibin A (see Table 14-2).

Any MSAFP result that is > 2.5 multiples of the mean (MoM) can signify an open NTD, an abdominal wall defect, multiple gestation, incorrect dating, fetal death, or placental abnormalities.

TABLE 14-2. **Detection of Genetic Abnormalities with Quad Screening**

	NEURAL TUBE DEFECT	TRISOMY 18	TRISOMY 21
MSAFP	↑	↓	↓
Estriol	Not used	↓	↓
Inhibin A	Not used	↔	↑

Q

A 39-year-old G2P0010 woman at 10 weeks' gestation has a history of a second-trimester pregnancy loss from trisomy 21. What is the next step?

Prenatal Diagnostic Testing

CHORIONIC VILLUS SAMPLING

- Performed to evaluate possible genetic diseases at an earlier time than is possible with amniocentesis, with comparable diagnostic accuracy.
- The preferred test for woman at baseline ↑ risk of having a child with aneuploidy—ie, a history of affected children or advanced maternal age.
- Done at **10–12 weeks' gestation via transabdominal or transvaginal** aspiration of chorionic villus tissue (a precursor of the placenta). Risks include fetal loss (1–5%) and an association with distal limb defects.

AMNIOCENTESIS

- Amniocentesis can be done for genetic testing, typically between 15 and 20 weeks' gestation, to detect genetic diseases or congenital malformations as described above. It is usually done to confirm the diagnosis if the integrated screen is abnormal.
- Amniocentesis can also be used for nongenetic evaluation:
    - In **Rh-sensitized pregnancy** to ascertain fetal blood type or to detect fetal hemolysis.
    - To detect infection in a woman suspected of having chorioamnionitis before the rupture of membranes (ROM).
    - For the evaluation of **fetal lung maturity** in the third trimester.
- Risks include fetal-maternal hemorrhage (1–2%) and fetal loss (0.5%).

Tests of Fetal Well-Being

NONSTRESS TEST (NST)

- Fetal heart rate is monitored externally by Doppler. A normal baseline fetal heart rate is 110–160 bpm.
- **Variability** is defined as the beat-to-beat changes from the baseline. It is a marker of normal neurologic function and fetal pH.
    - **Absent:** No change from baseline (abnormal).
    - **Minimal:** Change from 1 to 5 bpm from baseline (can be normal or abnormal).
    - **Moderate:** Change from 6 to 25 bpm from baseline (most reassuring pattern).
    - **Marked:** Change from ≥ 26 bpm (significance is unclear).
- A **normal response** after 32 weeks' gestation is an acceleration of ≥ 15 bpm above baseline lasting ≥ 15 seconds.
- A "reactive" NST includes **2 accelerations** in a **20-minute** period (see Figure 14-1).
- A "nonreactive" NST has < 2 accelerations in a 20-minute period and warrants a biophysical profile or a contraction stress test (see below).
- A nonreactive NST can be due to fetal sleep cycle, a fetal CNS anomaly, or maternal sedative or narcotic use.

This woman's baseline risk is higher for aneuploidy given her history of an affected pregnancy and her advanced maternal age. Therefore, a chorionic villus sampling could be done early in the pregnancy and would be confirmatory.

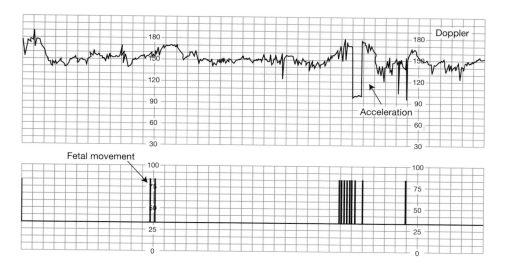

FIGURE 14-1. **Reactive nonstress test.** (Adaped with permission from Cunningham FG et al. *Williams Obstetrics,* 23rd ed. New York: McGraw-Hil, 2010, Fig. 15-7.)

CONTRACTION STRESS TEST (CST)

- Used to assess uteroplacental dysfunction. Can help predict how a baby will tolerate labor.
- Fetal heart rate is monitored during spontaneous or induced (nipple stimulation or pitocin) contractions.
- A normal or "negative" CST has no late decelerations and is highly predictive of fetal well-being.
- An abnormal or "positive" CST is defined by late decelerations in conjunction with at least 50% of contractions. A minimum of 3 contractions within a 10-minute period must be present for an adequate CST.

BIOPHYSICAL PROFILE (BPP)

- Ultrasound is used to assess 5 parameters (see the mnemonic **Test the Baby, MAN**).
- A score of 2 (normal) or 0 (abnormal) is given to each of the parameters.
  - A normal or "negative" test (a score of 8–10) is reassuring for fetal well-being.
  - An abnormal or "positive" test (a score < 6) is worrisome for fetal compromise.

FETAL HEART RATE DECELERATIONS

Table 14-3 outlines different types of heart rate patterns seen in near-term and term fetuses.

Normal Labor and Delivery

DEFINITIONS

- **Preterm delivery:** Delivery at 20 to < 37 weeks.
- **Term delivery:** Delivery at 37 to < 42 weeks.
- **Postterm delivery:** Delivery at ≥ 42 weeks.

MNEMONIC

When performing a BPP, remember to—

Test the Baby, MAN!

Fetal **T**one
Fetal **B**reathing
Fetal **M**ovements
Amniotic fluid volume
Nonstress test

Q

A 28-year-old G4P2012 woman with 2 healthy children at 16 weeks' gestation has an abnormal integrated screen that raises concern for trisomy 21. What is the next step?

TABLE 14-3.   **Fetal Heart Rate Patterns**

TYPE OF DECELERATION	DESCRIPTION	SCHEMATIC	COMMON CAUSE
Variable	Variable onset of abrupt (< 30-sec) slowing of fetal heart rate. Can be, but is not necessarily, associated with contractions. The return is similarly abrupt in most situations.		Umbilical cord compression.
Early	Deceleration begins and ends at approximately the same time as maternal contractions.		Fetal head compression (**no fetal distress**).
Late	Decelerations begin after onset of maternal contractions and persist until after the contractions are finished. The time from baseline to nadir is > 30 sec.		Late decelerations indicate fetal hypoxia (**fetal distress**). If late decelerations are repetitive and severe, immediate delivery is necessary.

Images reproduced with permission from Cunningham FC et al. *Williams Obstetrics,* 24th ed. New York: McGraw-Hill, 2014, Figs. 24-14, 24-16, and 24-18.

A

This patient's baseline risk for aneuploidy is low, which is likely why she was not offered a chorionic villus sampling earlier in her pregnancy and instead proceeded with integrated screening. However, now that she has abnormal screening results, the next step depends on her desire to confirm the diagnosis. If she desires further testing, amniocentesis would be confirmatory.

- Labor is defined by painful contraction with cervical change. The cervix can be assessed using the Bishop score, which indicates the likelihood of a successful vaginal delivery:
  - **Position:** Posterior, midposition, or anterior (0–2 points).
  - **Centimeters dilated:** 0–10 cm (0–3 points).
  - **Consistency:** Firm, medium, soft (0–2 points).
  - **Effacement:** 0–100% effaced (0–3 points).
  - **Station:** −3 to +3 station (0–3 points).
- A Bishop score of > 8 predicts a high likelihood of successful vaginal delivery, whether spontaneous or induced.

TABLE 14-4.   **Pregestational vs Gestational Diabetes Mellitus**

	PREGESTATIONAL	GESTATIONAL
Definition	Diagnosed **before pregnancy.**	Diagnosed **during pregnancy.**
Risk factors	Family history, autoimmune disorders (type 1), obesity (type 2).	Obesity, family history (in a first-degree relative), prior history of DM in pregnancy.
Diagnosis	See above.	Diagnosed if the 1-hour glucose test is ≥ 140 mg/dL **and** the follow-up 3-hour glucose test has at least 2 ↑ levels.
Treatment	Strict control of blood glucose levels with diet, exercise, and glycemic agents or **insulin.** ▪ **Fasting morning:** < 95 mg/dL. ▪ **Two-hour postprandial:** < 120 mg/dL.	ADA diet and regular exercise. If blood sugars are ↑ after 1 week, glyburide can be added. If glyburide is not sufficient, initiate insulin therapy.
Labor	Fingersticks every 4 hours in early labor and every 1–2 hours while the patient is in active labor, with dextrose infusion +/− an insulin drip to maintain tight glycemic control.	**Diet controlled:** ▪ **A1:** Fingersticks on admission. ▪ **A2:** Same as pregestational.
Postpartum	Continue glucose monitoring. Does not need to be as tight as in labor, as the body's insulin requirements quickly ↓.	Resume normal diet; no insulin is required. Perform a 2-hour glucose tolerance test at the postpartum visit to ensure resolution of diabetes.
Complications		
Fetus	Congenital malformations, stillbirth, macrosomia, IUGR, hypoglycemia, shoulder dystocia, birth trauma.	Hypoglycemia from hyperinsulinemia; macrosomia; birth trauma.
Mother	Hypoglycemia, DKA, spontaneous abortion, polyhydramnios, preterm labor, worsening end-organ dysfunction, ↑ risk of preeclampsia.	Perineal trauma from macrosomic infant; ↑ lifetime risk of developing DM.

STAGES OF LABOR

- **First stage:** The time from the onset of labor to 10 cm of dilation.
  - **Early labor:** Can last up to 20 hours for nulliparous women and 14 hours for multiparous women.
  - **Active labor:** Starts at 6 cm of dilation.
- **Second stage:** The time from complete dilation to delivery of the baby.
- **Third stage:** The time from delivery of the baby to delivery of the placenta.

Medical Complications of Pregnancy

DIABETES MELLITUS (DM)

The **most common** medical complication of pregnancy. See Table 14-4 for a comparison of pregestational and gestational DM.

Q

A 36-year-old G3P2002 woman at 10 weeks' gestation presents for her first prenatal visit. She has a history of 2 previous pregnancies complicated by gestational diabetes. Her last delivery was complicated by shoulder dystocia. Which tests should you order for her?

TABLE 14-5. **Mild and Severe Preeclampsia vs Eclampsia**

	MILD PREECLAMPSIA	SEVERE PREECLAMPSIA	ECLAMPSIA
Symptoms/ exam	**SBP ≥ 140 or DBP ≥ 90** on 2 or more occasions 4 hours apart. **Proteinuria** (≥ 300 mg/24 hrs).	**SBP ≥ 160 or DBP ≥ 110** on > 2 occasions 4 hours apart. **Proteinuria** (≥ 5 g/24 hrs). HELLP syndrome (see mnemonic). Oliguria (< 500 mL/24 hrs). Pulmonary edema.	**Seizures with the diagnosis of preeclampsia.**
Treatment	Deliver at 37 weeks or if preeclampsia worsens. If far from term, observation and conservative management. Magnesium sulfate is no longer recommended for seizure prophylaxis.	Deliver at 34 weeks. Hydralazine, labetalol, or nifedipine for BP control. Magnesium sulfate for seizure prophylaxis. Continue magnesium sulfate postpartum for at least 12–24 hours after delivery. Watch for magnesium toxicity; treat toxicity with IV calcium gluconate.	**Magnesium sulfate to control seizures.** Monitor ABCs closely. When stable, deliver. Seizures may occur before delivery, during delivery, and up to 6 weeks postpartum.
Complications	Fetal distress, stillbirth, placental abruption, DIC, seizures, fetal/maternal death, cerebral hemorrhage.	Same as with mild preeclampsia.	Fetal/maternal death.

 MNEMONIC

HELLP syndrome:

Hemolysis (LDH, uric acid, Hb, Hct)
Elevated **L**iver enzymes (AST/ALT)
Low **P**latelets (< 150)

The patient is at high risk of developing gestational diabetes again in this pregnancy. It is important to offer an early 1-hour glucose challenge test and HbA₁c.

PREECLAMPSIA

Preeclampsia is defined as hypertension and proteinuria that develop after 20 weeks' gestation. It is thought to be due to ↓ organ perfusion 2° to vasospasm and endothelial activation. Risk factors include nulliparity, African American ethnicity, extremes of age (< 18 or > 40 years), multiple gestations (ie, twins), renal disease, SLE, antiphospholipid antibody syndrome, and chronic hypertension. Characterized as mild or severe:

- **Mild:** Systolic BP (SBP) ≥ 140, diastolic BP (DBP) ≥ 90, and ≥ 300 mg protein on 24-hour urine.
- **Severe:** SBP ≥ 160, DBP ≥ 110, ≥ 5 g protein on 24-hour urine, symptoms of preeclampsia (headache, blurry vision, RUQ/epigastric pain), or abnormal labs (↑ AST, ALT, creatinine, LDH, or uric acid or low platelets).

Eclampsia is defined as seizures in a patient with preeclampsia.

SYMPTOMS/EXAM

Table 14-5 details the differences in the presentation and treatment of mild preeclampsia, severe preeclampsia, and eclampsia.

DIAGNOSIS

- Check UA, 24-hour urine for protein and creatinine clearance, CBC, creatinine, uric acid, LDH, and AST/ALT.
- PT/PTT, INR, fibrinogen, and a toxicology screen to rule out other causes.
- Diagnosis is based on clinical findings as described in Table 14-5.

TREATMENT

Definitive treatment is **delivery.** Severe preeclamptics should receive magnesium sulfate for seizure prophylaxis. See Table 14-5 for management.

KEY FACT

The only cure for preeclampsia is delivery. However, patients are still at risk up to 6 weeks postpartum.

THYROID DISEASE IN PREGNANCY

- **Hypothyroidism in pregnancy:** The most common cause is autoimmune (Hashimoto's) thyroiditis.
  - Sequelae include an ↑ rate of spontaneous abortion, preterm delivery, hypertensive disorders, and placental abruption.
  - **Tx:** Levothyroxine can be used. Consider treating women with subclinical hypothyroidism.
- **Subclinical hyperthyroidism:** hCG and TSH have a common α subunit that can stimulate the production of T_3 and T_4. Therefore, transient subclinical hyperthyroidism can occur in the first trimester.
- **Hyperthyroidism in pregnancy:** Most commonly caused by Graves' disease and pregnancy hyperthyroidism.
  - Sequelae include spontaneous abortion, preterm labor, and intrauterine fetal demise. In the fetus, it can cause fetal tachycardia, fetal goiter, and advanced bone age. **Thyroid storm** can be caused by labor, infection, or preeclampsia.
  - **Tx:**
    - Radioiodine is contraindicated in pregnancy.
    - β-blockers (atenolol or propranolol) can be used for the management of symptomatic tachycardia.
    - Propylthiouracil (PTU) can be used in the first trimester but should be avoided in the second and third trimesters given the ↑ risk of PTU hepatotoxicity.
    - Methimazole should be avoided in the first trimester because of its teratogenic effects during organogenesis. In the second trimester, it is safer to use than PTU.

HYPEREMESIS GRAVIDARUM

- Refractory vomiting that leads to **weight loss,** poor weight gain, dehydration, ketosis from starvation, and metabolic alkalosis. Symptoms peak at 9 weeks but typically improve by 20 weeks.
- Risk factors include nulliparity, multiple gestation, and trophoblastic disease.
- **DDx:** Rule out molar pregnancy, hepatitis, gallbladder disease, reflux, and gastroenteritis.
- **Dx:** Labs show **hyponatremia** and a hypokalemic, hypochloremic **metabolic alkalosis.** Ketonuria on UA suggests starvation ketosis.
- **Tx:** If there is evidence of weight loss, dehydration, or altered electrolytes, **hospitalize** and give antihistamines, vitamin B_6, metoclopramide or ondansetron, IV hydration, and electrolyte replacement. Advance the diet slowly and avoid fatty foods.

Peripartum Complications

POSTPARTUM HEMORRHAGE

KEY FACT

If postpartum uterine bleeding persists after conventional therapy, lifesaving techniques include uterine/internal iliac artery ligation, uterine balloon tamponade, and hysterectomy.

- Defined as blood loss of > 500 mL during a vaginal delivery or > 1000 mL during a cesarean section occurring before, during, or after delivery of the placenta. Table 14-6 summarizes common causes.
- Complications include **Sheehan's syndrome** (see below) and DIC.

TABLE 14-6.   Common Causes of Postpartum Hemorrhage

	UTERINE ATONY	GENITAL TRACT TRAUMA	RETAINED PLACENTAL TISSUE
Cause	Uterine overdistention (multiple gestation, polyhydramnios), exhausted myometrium, uterine infection, grand multiparity.	Precipitous delivery, operative vaginal delivery, large infant, laceration.	Placenta accreta/increta/percreta, placenta previa, prior C-section, curettage, accessory placental lobe, retained membranes.
Diagnosis	Palpation of a soft, enlarged, "boggy" uterus.	Inspection of the cervix, vagina, and vulva for lacerations or hematoma.	Inspection of the placenta and uterine cavity. Ultrasound to look for retained placenta.
Treatment	Vigorous bimanual massage. Oxytocin infusion. Methylergonovine if not hypertensive; PGF$_{2a}$ if not asthmatic; misoprostol.	Surgical repair of the defect.	Removal of remaining placental tissue.

SHEEHAN'S SYNDROME (POSTPARTUM HYPOPITUITARISM)

- The most common cause of anterior pituitary insufficiency in adult females. It occurs 2° to **pituitary ischemia,** usually as a result of postpartum blood loss and hypotension.
- **Sx/Exam:**
    - The most common presenting symptom is **failure to lactate** as a result of ↓ prolactin levels.
    - Other symptoms include lethargy, anorexia, weight loss, amenorrhea, and loss of sexual hair, but these may not be recognized for many years.
- **Tx: Lifelong hormone replacement therapy** (corticosteroids, levothyroxine, estrogen and progesterone).

INTRAPARTUM AND POSTPARTUM FEVERS

Most commonly due to **infections** (see Table 14-7). Remember the mnemonic **the 7 W's** for the causes of postpartum fever.

MASTITIS

- Cellulitis of the periglandular tissue in breast-feeding mothers. Typically due to *S aureus;* occurs at about 2–4 weeks postpartum.
- **Sx/Exam:** Breast pain and redness along with a **high fever,** chills, and flu-like symptoms. Look for **focal** breast erythema, swelling, and tenderness. **Fluctuance** points to a breast abscess.
- **DDx:** Distinguish from simple breast engorgement, which can present as a swollen, firm, tender breast with low-grade fever. Do not treat simple breast engorgement with antibiotics.
- **Dx:** Diagnosis includes breast milk cultures and CBC.
- **Tx: Dicloxacillin** or **erythromycin.** Continue nursing or manually expressing milk to prevent milk stasis. If an abscess is present, treat with needle aspiration. Incision and drainage should be reserved for large or recurrent abscesses.

MNEMONIC

The 7 W's of postpartum fever:

Womb—endomyometritis
Wind—atelectasis, pneumonia
Water—UTI
Walk—DVT, pulmonary embolism
Wound—incision, lacerations
Weaning—breast engorgement, mastitis, breast abscess
Wonder drugs—drug fever

KEY FACT

The treatment of mastitis includes antibiotics and continued breast-feeding.

KEY FACT

Contraindications to breast-feeding include HIV infection and certain drugs (eg, tetracycline, chloramphenicol).

TABLE 14-7. **Common Infections During Labor and After Delivery**

	CHORIOAMNIONITIS	ENDOMETRITIS
Definition	Infection of the **chorion, amnion,** and **amniotic fluid,** diagnosed **during labor.**	Infection of the **uterus,** diagnosed **after delivery.**
Risk factors	**Prolonged ROM.**	**C-section,** prolonged ROM.
Symptoms/ exam	Fever with no other obvious source **and** 1 of the following: ▪ Fetal tachycardia ▪ Maternal tachycardia ▪ Fundal tenderness ▪ Foul-smelling amniotic fluid	Fever within 24 hours postpartum without an obvious source.
Diagnosis	Clinical; CBC with differential.	Pelvic exam to rule out hematoma or retained membranes. CBC with differential, UA and urine culture, and blood cultures as indicated.
Treatment	Delivery of the fetus (chorioamnionitis is **not** an indication for cesarean delivery). Postpartum treatment is controversial. Some clinicians treat with a single dose of antibiotics for 24 hours postpartum; others discontinue therapy after the baby is born.	Antibiotics until the patient is afebrile for 24 hours.

Postpartum Mental Health

- **Definitions:**
  - **"Postpartum blues":** Mild depressive symptoms that develop within a few days of delivery and resolve within 2 weeks.
  - **Postpartum depression:** Major depressive disorder occurring within 12 months of giving birth.
  - **Postpartum psychosis:** Psychotic symptoms that develop within 2 weeks of giving birth.
- Medications usually **avoided in pregnancy** are:
  - **Fluoxetine:** Has a longer half-life and is transferred in breast milk, with the potential to accumulate in higher levels in the baby.
  - **Paroxetine:** Associated with congenital cardiac defects in the newborn.

KEY FACT

In pregnant women with depression, sertraline and citalopram are safe, effective mediations for treatment.

Teratogens in Pregnancy

- **Radiation:** Diagnostic and nuclear medicine studies have not been shown to pose any risk of fetal teratogenicity if overall exposure during pregnancy is < 5000 mrads. If possible, however, imaging with contrast should be avoided during pregnancy. Table 14-8 outlines radiation exposure levels associated with imaging procedures.
- **Medications:** See Table 14-9 for safe and teratogenic medications during pregnancy.
- **FDA pregnancy risk factor categories** are as follows:
  - **Class A:** Safe in human studies.
  - **Class B:** Generally safe; no ↑ risk in animal studies, but no adequate studies in humans.

TABLE 14-8. **Radiation Exposure Resulting from Common Radiologic Procedures**

RADIOLOGIC FILM	EXPOSURE (mrad)
Abdominal x-ray (1 view)	100
Chest x-ray (2 views)	0.02–0.07
CT head/chest	< 1000
CT abdomen/ lumbar spine	3500
MRI	0
Ultrasound	0

TABLE 14-9.   Safe vs Teratogenic/Unsafe Medications During Pregnancy

INDICATION	SAFE FOR USE	CONTRAINDICATED
Acne	Benzoyl peroxide.	Vitamin A and derivatives (eg, isotretinoin, etretinate) → heart and great vessel defects, craniofacial dysmorphism, and deafness.
Antibiotics	Penicillins, cephalosporin, macrolides.	Tetracycline → discoloration of deciduous teeth. Quinolones → cartilage damage. Sulfonamides late in pregnancy → kernicterus. Streptomycin → CN VIII damage/ototoxicity.
Bipolar disorder	Assess the risks and benefits of medications.	Lithium → congenital heart disease and Ebstein's anomaly (also avoid if the mother is breast-feeding).
Cancer	Alkylating agents can be used in the second and third trimesters.	Folic acid antagonists → abnormalities of the neural tube and cranium.
Contrast solution	Indigo carmine.	Methylene blue → jejunal and ileal atresia.
Depression	Assess risks vs benefits; TCAs, SSRIs.	SSRIs may cause persistent pulmonary hypertension of the newborn, poor feeding, and/or jitteriness.
GERD	OTC antacids (calcium carbonate, milk of magnesia), ranitidine, cimetidine, omeprazole.	Alka-Seltzer (has aspirin).
Headache/migraine	Acetaminophen, codeine, caffeine.	Avoid aspirin in late pregnancy in light of the risk of bleeding to the mother. Ergotamines have abortifacient potential and a theoretical risk of fetal vasoconstriction.
Hypertension	Labetalol, hydralazine, nifedipine, methyldopa, clonidine.	ACEIs and ARBs → fetal renal damage and oligohydramnios.
Hyperthyroidism	PTU.	Methimazole → aplasia cutis.
Hypothyroidism	Levothyroxine.	—
Nausea/vomiting	Pyridoxine (B$_6$), doxylamine, prochlorperazine, metoclopramide, ondansetron, granisetron, promethazine.	—
Pain	Acetaminophen, menthol, topical patches, morphine, hydrocodone, propoxyphene, meperidine. These medications should not be used continuously.	Avoid NSAIDs in late pregnancy for > 48 hours. When used over a long period, will → premature closure of the ductus arteriosus.
Seizure	Use an anticonvulsant that works best to control maternal seizures. Monotherapy at the lowest dose is preferred. Folate supplementation should be started 3 months before conception.	Phenytoin → dysmorphic facies, microcephaly, mental retardation, hypoplasia of the nails and distal phalanges, and NTDs. Valproic acid → craniofacial defects and NTDs. Carbamazepine → craniofacial defects, mental retardation, and NTDs. Phenobarbital → **cleft palate and cardiac defects.** Trimethadione and paramethadione have strong teratogenic potential and → mental retardation, speech difficulty, and abnormal facies.

TABLE 14-9.   Safe vs Teratogenic/Unsafe Medications During Pregnancy *(continued)*

INDICATION	SAFE FOR USE	CONTRAINDICATED
Thromboembolic disease	Heparin, low-molecular-weight heparin. Warfarin must be used in cases of highly thrombogenic artificial heart valves.	Warfarin → fetal nasal hypoplasia and bony defects (chondrodysplasia).
URI	Guaifenesin, acetaminophen, diphenhydramine, loratadine.	Ibuprofen can be used judiciously before 30 weeks but is generally avoided in pregnancy, as it can cause premature closure of the ductus arteriosus.

- **Class C:** Avoid in the first trimester if possible; some harm in animals but no adequate human studies, or no human or animal data are available
- **Class D:** Likely associated with human risks based on studies, but the benefits may outweigh the risks (eg, phenytoin). Use cautiously.
- **Class X:** Teratogenic; risks outweigh benefits.

Obstetric Complications of Pregnancy

FIRST-TRIMESTER BLEEDING

The differential diagnosis includes:

- **Ectopic pregnancy:** Any woman with a ⊕ pregnancy test and vaginal bleeding should have a transvaginal ultrasound to confirm intrauterine pregnancy.
- **Miscarriage:**
  - **Threatened:** Closed cervix + fetal heart tones.
  - **Inevitable:** Dilated cervix with painful contractions.
  - **Missed:** Nonviable intrauterine pregnancy.
  - **Incomplete:** Nonviable pregnancy with some tissue still in the uterus.
  - **Complete:** Empty uterine cavity following spontaneous abortion.
- **Ectropion:** An endocervical canal that everts to face the vagina. Very friable; can often bleed after intercourse.
- **Subchorionic hemorrhage:** Can cause heavy, light, or no bleeding. Should be evaluated and followed by ultrasound.

INTRAUTERINE GROWTH RESTRICTION (IUGR)

- Defined as an estimated fetal weight at or below the 10th percentile for GA. See Table 14-10 for common causes of IUGR.
- **Sx/Exam:** Suspect IUGR clinically if the difference between fundal height and GA is > 2 cm in the second trimester or > 3 cm in the third trimester.
- **Tx: Focus on prevention**—eg, smoking cessation, BP control, and dietary changes. Order an ultrasound every 2–4 weeks to assess interval growth. Also check umbilical artery Dopplers to assess for fetoplacental dysfunction. Deliver once the pregnancy reaches term.

OLIGOHYDRAMNIOS AND POLYHYDRAMNIOS

Table 14-11 contrasts oligohydramnios with polyhydramnios.

TABLE 14-10.   Causes of Intrauterine Growth Restriction

FETAL	MATERNAL
Chromosomal abnormalities: Trisomy 21 is most common, followed by trisomies 18 and 13. **Infection: CMV is most common;** then toxoplasmosis. Placental abnormalities, uterine abnormalities, multiple gestations.	**Hypertension.** **Drugs: Cigarette** smoking is most common; also alcohol, heroin, methamphetamines, and cocaine. **SLE.** Maternal thrombophilia. Malnutrition, malabsorption (eg, CF). Ethnic/genetic variation.

RHESUS (Rh) ISOIMMUNIZATION

When fetal Rh-⊕ RBCs leak into Rh-⊖ maternal circulation, **maternal anti-Rh IgG antibodies** can form. These antibodies can cross the placenta and react with fetal Rh-⊕ RBCs, leading to fetal hemolysis (erythroblastosis fetalis) and hydrops fetalis.

TREATMENT

- **Give RhoGAM to Rh-⊖ women:**
    - With prior delivery of an Rh-⊕ baby.
    - If the father is Rh ⊕, Rh status is unknown, or paternity is uncertain.
    - If the baby is Rh ⊕ at delivery.
    - If the woman has had ectopic pregnancies, abortions, amniocentesis or other traumatic procedures during pregnancy, vaginal bleeding, blood transfusions, or placental abruption.
- Sensitized Rh-⊖ women with titers > 1:16 should be closely monitored for evidence of fetal hemolysis with serial ultrasound and middle cerebral artery Doppler velocimetry.
- In severe cases, intrauterine blood transfusion via the umbilical vein or preterm delivery is indicated.

TABLE 14-11.   Oligohydramnios vs Polyhydramnios

	OLIGOHYDRAMNIOS	POLYHYDRAMNIOS
Definition	Amniotic fluid index (AFI) ≤ 5 cm on ultrasound.	AFI ≥ 25 cm on ultrasound.
Causes	**Fetal urinary tract abnormalities** (renal agenesis, polycystic kidneys, GU obstruction). Chronic uteroplacental insufficiency, ROM.	Normal pregnancy, uncontrolled maternal DM, multiple gestations, pulmonary abnormalities, fetal anomalies (duodenal atresia, tracheoesophageal fistula).
Diagnosis	Ultrasound for anomalies. Rule out ROM with ferning test and Nitrazine paper.	Ultrasound for fetal anomalies; glucose testing for DM.
Treatment	Possible amnioinfusion during labor to prevent cord compression.	Depends on the cause; therapeutic amniocentesis.
Complications	**Cord compression** → fetal hypoxia. Musculoskeletal abnormalities (facial distortion, clubfoot). Pulmonary hypoplasia, IUGR.	Preterm labor, placental abruption, fetal malpresentation, cord prolapse.

TABLE 14-12.   **Common Causes of Third-Trimester Bleeding**

	PLACENTAL ABRUPTION	PLACENTA PREVIA	UTERINE RUPTURE
Pathophysiology	**Placental separation** from the site of uterine implantation before delivery of the fetus.	**Abnormal placental implantation** near or covering the os.	**A complete rupture disrupts the entire thickness of the uterine wall.**
Risk factors	**Hypertension,** abdominal/pelvic trauma, tobacco or **cocaine use,** uterine distention.	**Prior C-section,** grand multiparity, multiple gestations, prior placenta previa.	**Prior uterine scar,** uterine anomalies, grand multiparity.
Symptoms	Abdominal pain; vaginal bleeding that does not spontaneously cease. Prolonged tightening of the abdomen coupled with prolonged contraction. **Fetal distress.**	Painless vaginal bleeding that ceases spontaneously with or without uterine contractions. The first bleeding episode usually occurs in the second or third trimester. **Usually no fetal distress.**	Severe abdominal pain, usually during labor, typically at the scar site. Change in the shape of the abdomen. **Fetal distress.** Loss of fetal station.
Diagnosis	**Primarily clinical.** Ultrasound to look for retroplacental hemorrhage (low sensitivity).	**Ultrasound** for placental position.	**Primarily clinical; based on symptoms and fetal distress.**
Treatment	**Mild abruption or premature infant:** Hospitalization, fetal monitoring, type and cross, bed rest. **Moderate to severe abruption:** Stabilize, type and cross, immediate delivery.	**No cervical exams!** Stabilize patients with a premature fetus. Serial ultrasound to assess fetal growth and resolution of previa. C-section for total or partial previa or if the patient/infant is in distress.	**Immediate C-section** with delivery of the infant and repair of the rupture.
Complications	Hemorrhagic shock; DIC; fetal death with severe abruption.	↑ risk of placenta accreta. Persistent hemorrhage requiring hysterectomy.	Fetal and maternal death.

THIRD-TRIMESTER BLEEDING

May be benign or pathologic.

- Benign causes include bleeding from ectropion. Most commonly, bleeding in the third trimester results from cervical change once labor starts and bloody show.
- Pathologic causes include bloody show, preterm labor, vasa previa, genital tract lesions, and trauma (eg, intercourse); see Table 14-12.

Abnormal Labor and Delivery

PRETERM PREMATURE RUPTURE OF MEMBRANES (PPROM)

PPROM is defined as spontaneous ROM at < **37 weeks,** before the onset of labor. Distinguished from premature rupture of membranes (PROM), which

Q

A 32-year-old G1P0 at 34 weeks' gestation with a diagnosis of preeclampsia presents with a refractory headache and nausea. She is found to have a BP of 208/112 and 3+ protein on urine dipstick. Her labs are pending. What is the next step?

refers to loss of fluid at term that is **premature to labor,** or the onset of contractions. Risk factors include low socioeconomic status, young maternal age, smoking, and STDs.

Symptoms/Exam

- Patients may complain of feeling a "gush of fluid."
- Sterile speculum exam shows pooling of amniotic fluid in the posterior vaginal vault.
- Look for cervical dilation.

Diagnosis

- **Nitrazine paper test:** Paper turns blue in alkaline amniotic fluid.
- **Fern test:** A ferning pattern is seen under the microscope after amniotic fluid dries on glass slide.

Treatment

- Obtain cultures and/or wet mounts to look for infectious causes. If signs of infection are present, assume **amnionitis** (maternal fever, fetal tachycardia, foul-smelling amniotic fluid). Give antibiotics (ampicillin +/– gentamicin) and **induce labor** regardless of GA.
- If no signs of infection are present and GA is **24–33 + 6 weeks,** treat with **antibiotics (ampicillin and erythromycin)** to prolong pregnancy for 1 week and **steroids** for fetal lung maturation. Give magnesium sulfate for tocolysis for 48 hours until the steroid dose is complete.
- Deliver at 34 weeks regardless of whether there is evidence of infection.

PRETERM LABOR

Labor between 20 and < 37 weeks' gestation. **Labor** is defined as painful contractions with cervical change. If a patient is having only painful contractions without cervical dilation, these are called **preterm contractions.**

Symptoms/Exam

- Patients may complain of menstrual-like cramps, uterine contractions, low back pain, pelvic pressure, new vaginal discharge, or bleeding.
- If preterm labor leads to preterm delivery, it can result in fetal respiratory distress syndrome, intraventricular hemorrhage, retinopathy of prematurity, necrotizing enterocolitis, or fetal death.

Diagnosis

- Obtain an **ultrasound** to verify GA, fetal presentation, and AFI.
- Look for **regular** uterine contractions (6 contractions in 1 hour) coupled with a concurrent cervical change at < 37 weeks' gestation.

Treatment

- Begin with **hydration.**
- If gestational age is < 34 weeks, **administer steroids (to accelerate fetal lung maturity),** and give magnesium sulfate for tocolysis during the steroid dose.
- If gestational age is > 34 weeks, do not attempt tocolysis. Proceed with expectant management.
- Give **penicillin or ampicillin** for GBS prophylaxis if preterm delivery is likely.

KEY FACT

The 3 signs of ROM are pooling of fluid on speculum exam, a ⊕ Nitrazine test, and ferning on microscopy.

KEY FACT

Magnesium sulfate works as a tocolytic and also ↓ the risk of cerebral palsy when administered before 32 weeks. Once steroids have been administered, stop the magnesium sulfate to avoid masking signs of infection and labor.

KEY FACT

Steroids accelerate the development of type I pneumocytes, which help with gas exchange within the alveoli, and type II pneumocytes, which produce surfactant.

A

The patient is presenting with severe preeclampsia that raises concern for the development of eclampsia. You should administer antihypertensives and magnesium for seizure prophylaxis and prepare for emergent delivery.

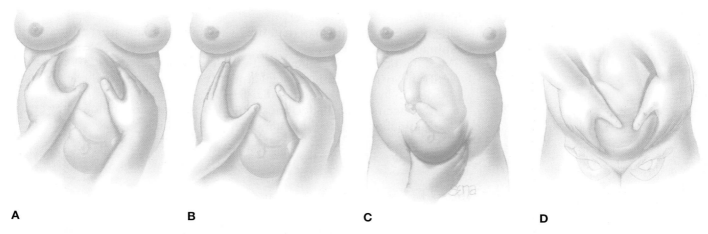

A   **B**   **C**   **D**

FIGURE 14-2. **Leopold maneuvers.** Maneuvers are performed with the fetus in a longitudinal lie in the left occiput anterior position. (Reproduced with permission from Cunningham FG et al. *Williams Obstetrics,* 23rd ed. New York: McGraw-Hill, 2010, Fig. 17-8.)

FETAL MALPRESENTATION

Defined as any presentation other than cephalic (head down). Breech presentation is the most common fetal malpresentation (affects 3% of all pregnancies).

DIAGNOSIS

- Perform Leopold maneuvers to identify fetal lie (see Figure 14-2).
  - Rock the thumb and index finger above the pubic symphysis to determine if there is a bony head presenting (vs soft tissue).
  - Palpate the remainder of the uterus for feet and the position of the back.
- Check with ultrasound if there is **any** doubt.

TREATMENT

- **Follow:** Up to 75% of cases spontaneously change to cephalic presentation by 38 weeks.
- **External cephalic version** can be attempted at 37 weeks in the setting of persistent malpresentation.
  - Involves pressure applied to the maternal abdomen to turn the infant.
  - Risks are placental abruption and cord compression; the infant **must** be monitored after the procedure, and consent must be obtained for emergent C-section.

SHOULDER DYSTOCIA

Defined as difficult delivery due to entrapment of the fetal shoulder at the level of the pubic bone. Risk factors include:

- A prior history of a shoulder dystocia
- Fetal macrosomia or inadequate pelvis

DIAGNOSIS

- A prolonged second stage of labor with retraction of the head ("turtle sign") back into the vaginal canal after pushing.
- After delivery of the head, there is difficulty delivering the anterior shoulder without performing additional maneuvers.

Q   **1**

A 27-year-old G1P1001 just delivered a healthy female infant weighing 9.5 lbs (4.3 kg). After delivery of the placenta, the patient was noted to have brisk vaginal bleeding with an estimated blood loss of 700 mL. What is the most likely cause of her hemorrhage?

Q   **2**

A 31-year-old healthy woman develops fevers (39.1°C/102.4°F) and severe uterine tenderness 8 hours after a C-section is performed for fetal malposition. The baby is doing well, and the amniotic fluid at C-section was clear. What is the likely source of infection?

Q   **3**

Two days after having an uncomplicated vaginal delivery, a 26-year-old G1P1 tells you that she has developed insomnia. Although she says that she is very happy with the baby, she complains of being anxious and irritable. What is her most likely diagnosis?

TREATMENT

- Flex and open the maternal hips (McRoberts maneuver) followed by suprapubic pressure.
- Most dystocias will be relieved with these 2 maneuvers:
  - Delivery of the posterior fetal arm or internal rotation of the fetal shoulders to lessen the shoulder diameter.
  - Replacement of the fetal head into the vaginal canal followed by cesarean section (Zavanelli maneuver).

INDICATIONS FOR CESAREAN SECTION

Table 14-13 outlines the indications for C-section.

Postdelivery Care

- Calculate the Apgar score. Each category can be scored 0, 1, or 2 points.
  - Strength and regularity of the heartbeat (HR > 100 or < 100)
  - Lung maturity (regular or irregular breathing)
  - Muscle tone and movement (active or limp)
  - Skin color (blue or pink)
  - Reflex responses to irritable stimuli (crying/whimpering/silence)
- Give topical erythromycin for chlamydial conjunctivitis and ophthalmia neonatorum (*Neisseria gonorrhoeae*).
- Administer vitamin K injection to prevent bleeding from vitamin K deficiency.

Spontaneous and Recurrent Abortion

SPONTANEOUS ABORTION (SAB)

Defined as **nonelective** termination of pregnancy at < 20 weeks' gestation. Also known as "miscarriage." Occurs in 10–15% of clinically recognizable pregnancies. Risk factors include advanced maternal age, a history of pregnancy loss, poorly controlled diabetes, antiphospholipid syndrome, thrombophilia, and structural uterine or cervical abnormalities.

SYMPTOMS/EXAM

Differentiate types of SABs on the basis of symptoms, cervical exam, and ultrasound (see Table 14-14).

1

The most common cause of postpartum hemorrhage is uterine atony. This patient's risk factor was having a baby large for gestational age, which caused uterine overdistention and inability to contract well postdelivery.

2

The uterus (endometritis). This is a rapid postoperative presentation, making the standard causes of postoperative fever less likely.

3

This patient most likely has "postpartum blues," which typically arises 2–3 days after delivery and resolves within 2 weeks. If her symptoms persist or worsen, she will need evaluation for postpartum depression.

TABLE 14-13. **Indications for Cesarean Section**

MATERNAL FACTORS	FETAL AND MATERNAL FACTORS	FETAL FACTORS
Prior C-section	Cephalopelvic disproportion	Fetal malposition
Active genital herpes infection	Placenta previa/placental abruption	Fetal distress
Cervical carcinoma	Labor dystocia, or abnormal progression of labor	Cord prolapse
Maternal trauma/demise		Erythroblastosis fetalis (Rh incompatibility)

TABLE 14-14.   Types of Spontaneous Abortions

TYPE	SYMPTOMS	CERVIX/ULTRASOUND	TREATMENT
Threatened abortion	Minimal bleeding +/− cramping. Most cases are thought to be due to implantation bleeding. **No products of conception (POC) are expelled.**	Closed os; ⊕ gestational sac.	Expectant management; consider pelvic rest for several weeks.
Inevitable abortion	Cramping with bleeding and cervical dilation. **No POC are expelled.**	Open os; normal ultrasound.	Expectant or D&C.
Missed abortion	Often no symptoms. **No POC are expelled.**	Closed os; no fetal cardiac activity; retained fetal tissue on ultrasound.	Can allow up to 2 weeks for POC to pass; offer medical management with misoprostol or D&C.
Incomplete abortion	Cramping with bleeding. **Some POC are expelled.**	Open os; normal ultrasound.	Expectant, medical management with misoprostol or D&C.
Complete abortion	Slight bleeding; pain has usually ceased. **All POC are expelled.**	Closed os; empty uterus on ultrasound.	None.
Septic abortion	Constitutional symptoms; malodorous discharge. Patients often have a recent history of therapeutic abortion; maternal mortality is 10–50%.	Cervical motion tenderness.	**Monitor** ABCs; D&C, IV antibiotics, supportive care.

TREATMENT

- Hemodynamic monitoring for significant bleeding.
- Check β-hCG to confirm pregnancy and transvaginal ultrasound to establish GA and rule out ectopic pregnancies; assess fetal viability or check for remaining tissue in the setting of a completed abortion.
- Check blood type and antibody screen; give RhoGAM if appropriate.

> **KEY FACT**
>
> All women with potential SABs should receive RhoGAM if the mother is Rh ⊖.

RECURRENT ABORTION

- Defined as 3 or more consecutive pregnancy losses before 20 weeks' gestation.
- Usually due to **chromosomal** or **uterine abnormalities,** but can also result from hormonal abnormalities, infection, or systemic disease.
- **Dx:** Based on clinical and lab findings.
  - Perform a pelvic exam (to look for anatomic abnormalities).
  - Check cervical cultures for chlamydia and gonorrhea.
  - Perform a maternal and paternal genetic analysis.
  - Obtain a hysterosalpingogram to look for uterine abnormalities.
  - Order TFTs, progesterone, lupus anticoagulant, and anticardiolipin antibody.
- **Tx:** Treatment is based on the diagnosis.

NOTES

GYNECOLOGY

Review of the Menstrual Cycle

- A normal menstrual cycle is 28 days with bleeding for 2–6 days.
  - The first day of bleeding = day 1 of the cycle.
  - Ovulation typically occurs at day 10–14.
  - Menstrual cycles are most irregular in the 2 years following menarche and 3 years preceding menopause.
  - Menopause is characterized by rises in FSH and LH.
- Table 15-1 and Figure 15-1 offer an overview of the physiologic changes involved in the menstrual cycle.

Abnormal Uterine Bleeding

Abnormalities in the frequency, duration, volume, and/or timing of menstrual bleeding. A useful mnemonic for categorizing its causes is **PALM-COEIN** (see Table 15-2).

EXAM

- Take a thorough menstrual history to determine the onset of abnormal bleeding, quantity, and how often bleeding occurs.
- Perform a speculum exam to assess for any vaginal or cervical lesions that may be causing the bleeding (eg, cervical polyps). Conduct a bimanual exam to assess the size, shape, and contour of the uterus and ovaries.

DIAGNOSIS

- Initial lab work includes β-hCG (always rule out pregnancy!), CBC, TSH, and prolactin.
- Pelvic ultrasound to look for structural causes.
- Other testing includes:
  - Saline infusion sonohysterography to look for polyps in the cavity.
  - Endometrial biopsy (for women ≥ 45 years of age or younger women with risk factors for endometrial hyperplasia/malignancy).
  - Hysteroscopy for direct visualization of the endometrial cavity.
- In older women, consider FSH/LH. An ↑ in both FSH and LH is suggestive of menopause, as the ovaries can no longer respond to hormonal signals by producing estrogen and progesterone.

KEY FACT

Women ≥ 45 years of age with abnormal uterine bleeding should have an endometrial biopsy to rule out malignancy.

TABLE 15-1.   Overview of the Normal Menstrual Cycle

ORGAN	PHASE
Ovary	**Follicular phase:** The ovary prepares the follicle for ovulation after stimulation by FSH from the pituitary gland.
	Luteal phase: After the LH surge, the egg is released from the ovary.
Uterus	**Proliferative phase:** The endometrium thickens.
	Secretory phase: The corpus luteum makes estrogen and progesterone to prepare the endometrium for implantation. If no implantation occurs, the drop in estrogen and progesterone results in shedding of the endometrium (ie, menses).

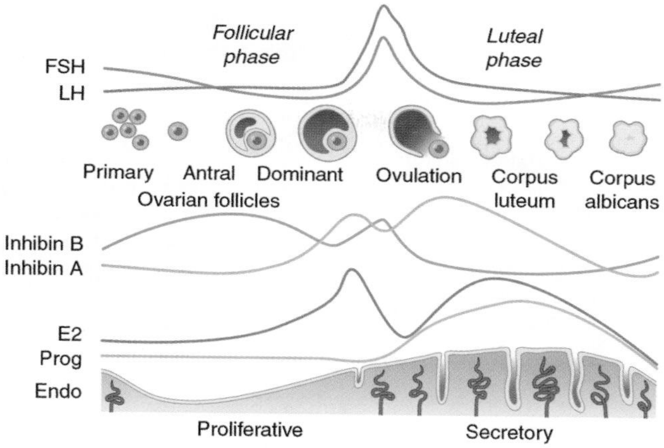

FIGURE 15-1. **The normal menstrual cycle.** (Reproduced with permission from Fauci AS et al. *Harrison's Principles of Internal Medicine,* 17th ed. New York: McGraw-Hill, 2008, Fig. 347-8.)

TREATMENT

- Treat the underlying cause.
- Acute, profuse bleeding can be treated with high-dose oral progesterone, high-dose combined OCPs, high-dose IV estrogen, D&C, uterine artery embolization, uterine balloon tamponade, or hysterectomy.

Amenorrhea

Defined as either 1° or 2° amenorrhea.

- **1° amenorrhea:** Absence of menses and/or lack of 2° sexual characteristics by age 15 **or** absence of menses or 2° sexual characteristics by age 13. Associated with gonadal failure, congenital abnormalities, and constitutional symptoms (see Figure 15-2).
- **2° amenorrhea:** Absence of menses for 3 cycles or for 6 months with previously normal menses. Etiologies include pregnancy, anorexia nervosa, stress, strenuous exercise, intrauterine adhesions, chronic anovulation, hypothyroidism, hyperprolactinemia, and premature ovarian insufficiency (see Figure 15-3).

DIAGNOSIS

- **Check β-hCG** to make sure the patient is not pregnant.
- 1° amenorrhea: See Figure 15-2.
- 2° amenorrhea: See Figure 15-3.

TABLE 15-2. **Causes of Abnormal Uterine Bleeding**

STRUCTURAL CAUSES (PALM)	NONSTRUCTURAL CAUSES (COEIN)
Polyp	**C**oagulopathy
Adenomyosis	**O**vulatory dysfunction
Leiomyomas	**E**ndometrial
Malignancies	**I**atrogenic
	Not yet classified

KEY FACT

Always rule out pregnancy in a patient with amenorrhea.

KEY FACT

Amenorrhea is a symptom, not a diagnosis.

Q

A 46-year-old woman presents to her gynecologist with intermittent and painless noncyclic vaginal bleeding of 6 months' duration. She otherwise feels well and has a normal cervical exam. What is the next step?

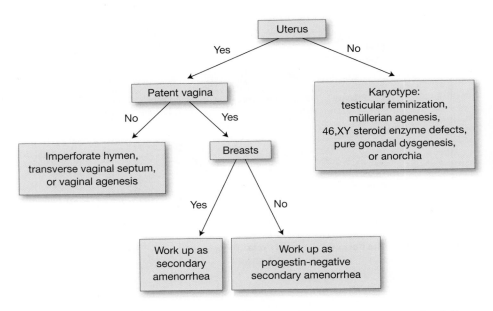

FIGURE 15-2. **Workup for patients with 1° amenorrhea.** (Adapted with permission from DeCherney AH, Nathan L. *Current Diagnosis & Treatment: Obstetrics & Gynecology,* 10th ed. New York: McGraw-Hill, 2007, Fig. 56-2.)

TREATMENT

Depends on the etiology; may include surgery or hormonal therapy +/− drug therapy.

Dysmenorrhea

Defined as pain with menstrual periods that requires medication and prevents normal activity. It is defined as either 1° or 2° dysmenorrhea.

- **1° dysmenorrhea:** No clinically detectable pelvic pathology. Most likely due to ↑ uterine prostaglandin production.

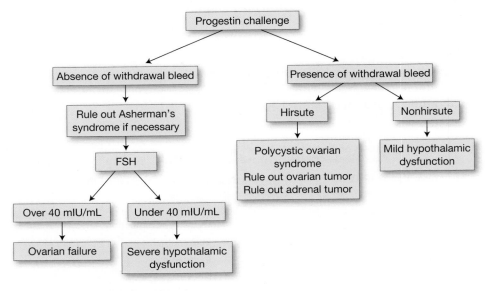

A

You must rule out endometrial cancer by performing an endometrial biopsy or a D&C (the gold standard).

FIGURE 15-3. **Workup for patients with 2° amenorrhea.** (Modified with permission from DeCherney AH, Nathan L. *Current Diagnosis & Treatment: Obstetrics & Gynecology,* 10th ed. New York: McGraw-Hill, 2007, Fig. 56-4.)

2° dysmenorrhea: Menstrual pain due to pelvic pathology, most commonly endometriosis, adenomyosis, or leiomyomas.

Endometriosis

Abnormal growth of endometrial tissue in locations other than the uterine lining, usually in the ovaries (called endometriomas or "chocolate cysts"), cul-de-sac, and uterosacral ligament. Associated with premenstrual pelvic pain due to stimulation from estrogen and progesterone during the menstrual cycle.

SYMPTOMS/EXAM

- Presents with pelvic pain, dysmenorrhea, dyspareunia, and infertility.
- On pelvic exam, patients may have tender nodularity along the uterosacral ligament +/– a fixed, retroflexed uterus or enlarged ovaries.

DIAGNOSIS

The history and physical can suggest the diagnosis, but the gold standard is direct visualization during laparoscopy with biopsy showing endometrial glands.

TREATMENT

- Treatment depends on the patient's symptoms, age, desire for future fertility, and disease stage. The extent of pelvic disease does not correlate with the patient's symptoms.
- If the patient's main complaint is **infertility,** operative laparoscopy should be performed to cauterize or excise the implants and resect ovarian endometriomas.
- If the patient's main complaint is **pain,** the objective is to induce a state of anovulation.
  - For mild pain, first-line treatment is NSAIDs and/or continuous OCPs.
  - For moderate to severe pain, options include medical treatment to induce anovulation (GnRH agonists) or **excision.**
- Hysterectomy with bilateral salpingo-oophorectomy is used as a final therapeutic option.

Polycystic Ovarian Syndrome (PCOS)

The most common cause of female hirsutism (male-pattern hair growth). Typically affects adolescent women. The cause is unknown.

SYMPTOMS

Look for an obese woman with hirsutism, oligo- or amenorrhea, infertility, acne, and diabetes or insulin resistance.

EXAM

- Patients may be obese.
- Exam may reveal hirsutism and/or acne; pelvic exam may show palpably enlarged ovaries.
- Patients may have acanthosis nigricans suggestive of insulin resistance.

 A 23-year-old woman with a history of irregular menses has been unable to conceive for 2 years. Her partner's infertility workup has been ⊖. The patient was diagnosed with diabetes at age 14 but is otherwise healthy. She is 5'2", weighs 165 lbs (74.8 kg), and has acne. What would you expect to find on exam and imaging?

DIAGNOSIS

- Two out of three of the following clinical signs must be present to diagnose PCOS:
  - Oligo- or anovulation.
  - Hyperandrogenism (acne, hirsutism, or elevated testosterone).
  - Polycystic ovaries on ultrasound.
  - An ↑ LH/FSH ratio (> 2) is also characteristic.
- Women with PCOS have an ↑ risk of **diabetes and cardiac disease.** Once PCOS has been diagnosed, order a glucose tolerance test and a lipid panel.

TREATMENT

Treat the specific symptoms:

- **Hyperglycemia/diabetes:** Weight loss; hypoglycemic agents.
- **Infertility:** May also improve with diet and exercise. Induce ovulation with clomiphene and/or metformin.
- **Hirsutism:** Start combination OCPs to suppress ovarian steroidogenesis. Combination OCPs also protect the uterine lining from unopposed estrogen.

Gestational Trophoblastic Disease

Can range from benign (eg, hydatidiform mole) to malignant (eg, choriocarcinoma). Hydatidiform mole accounts for approximately 80% of cases.

SYMPTOMS/EXAM

- Suspect in patients with first-trimester uterine bleeding and excessive nausea and vomiting.
- Look for **preeclampsia or eclampsia at < 24 weeks.**
- Other findings include uterine size greater than dates and hyperthyroidism.
- **No fetal heartbeat** is detected.
- Pelvic exam may show enlarged ovaries and possible expulsion of **grape-like molar clusters** into the vagina or blood in the cervical os.

DIAGNOSIS

- β-hCG levels are markedly ↑ (usually > 100,000 mIU/dL).
- Pelvic ultrasound shows a **"snowstorm" appearance** (see Figure 15-4) with no gestational sac and no fetus or heart tones present.
- Obtain a CXR to look for metastases.

TREATMENT

- D&C.
- Carefully monitor β-hCG levels after D&C for possible progression to malignant disease.
- Pregnancy prevention (contraception) is needed for 6 months to 1 year to ensure accurate monitoring of β-hCG levels.
- Treat malignant disease with chemotherapy and residual uterine disease with hysterectomy.

The patient probably has PCOS. You would expect to find enlarged ovaries on bimanual exam and many follicles in her ovaries on ultrasound/CT scan.

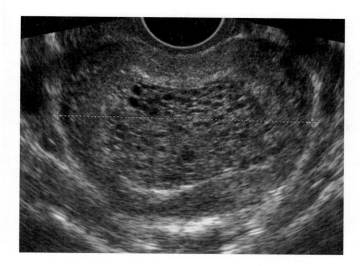

FIGURE 15-4.   Gestational trophoblastic disease. The classic "snowstorm" appearance is seen on transverse ultrasound of a patient with gestational trophoblastic disease. The patient has a complete hydatidiform mole that fills the uterine cavity. (Reproduced with permission from Hoffman BL et al. *Williams Gynecology*, 2nd ed. New York: McGraw-Hill, 2012, Fig. 37-5.)

Vulvovaginitis

Vulvovaginitis is most commonly caused by bacterial vaginosis (*Gardnerella vaginalis*), fungal infection (*Candida albicans*), or protozoal infection (*Trichomonas vaginalis*). It can also be caused by STDs such as gonorrhea or chlamydia. Figure 15-5 depicts the histologic appearance of bacterial vaginosis and yeast.

SYMPTOMS/EXAM

- May present with ↑ vaginal discharge, a change in discharge odor, and/or vulvovaginal pruritus.
- Perform a complete exam of the vulva, vagina, and cervix. Look for vulvar edema, erythema, and discharge.

KEY FACT

Sexual abuse must be considered in any child with vulvovaginitis.

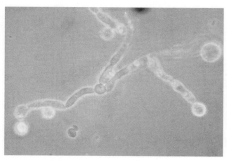

A

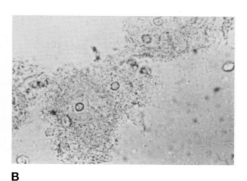

B

FIGURE 15-5.   Causes of vaginitis. (A) Candidal vaginitis. Note the pseudohyphae of *Candida albicans* organisms on KOH wet mount. **(B)** Bacterial vaginosis (*Gardnerella vaginalis*). Note the granular epithelial cells ("clue cells") and indistinct cell margins. (Image A reproduced with permission from Wolff K et al. *Fitzpatrick's Color Atlas & Synopsis of Clinical Dermatology*, 7th ed. New York: McGraw-Hill, 2013, Fig. 26-1. Image B reproduced with permission from Kasper DL et al. *Harrison's Principles of Internal Medicine*, 16th ed. New York: McGraw-Hill, 2005: 767.)

DIAGNOSIS/TREATMENT

Obtain swabs from the vagina to perform a wet mount and cultures for gonorrhea and chlamydia (see Table 15-3).

Pelvic Inflammatory Disease (PID)

The spectrum of PID ranges from endometritis to salpingitis, tubo-ovarian abscess, and pelvic peritonitis. Risk factors include age < 25, multiple sexual partners, lack of condom or barrier use, and a history of PID or STDs. The most common cause is gonorrhea or chlamydia infection.

SYMPTOMS/EXAM

Presents with abnormal bleeding, fevers, abdominal pain, abnormal discharge, and cervical motion tenderness.

DIAGNOSIS

- Diagnosed clinically.
- A finding of > 10 WBCs/low-power field on Gram stain and endocervical smear is consistent with a diagnosis of PID.
- Cervical and vaginal cultures should be obtained to rule out gonorrhea or chlamydia. However, do not delay treatment while awaiting results, as ⊖ results do not rule out PID.

TREATMENT

- **Inpatient management:**
    - **Indications:** Pregnancy, noncompliance with medications, severe illness, tubo-ovarian abscess.

> **KEY FACT**
>
> Additional tenderness in the RUQ can be a sign of Fitz-Hugh–Curtis syndrome, which is associated with gonorrhea infection.

TABLE 15-3.   Common Causes of Vulvovaginitis

	BACTERIAL VAGINOSIS	YEAST (USUALLY CANDIDA)	TRICHOMONAS VAGINALIS
Exam	Can be unremarkable except for discharge.	Erythema and irritation.	The vagina and cervix may be swollen and red.
Discharge	Grayish or white with a **fishy odor**; pronounced after intercourse.	White, curdlike.	Yellow-green, malodorous.
Wet mount	Reveals > 20% of epithelial cells with indistinct cell margins ("clue cells"; see Figure 15-5).	⊖.	Motile, flagellated protozoans.
KOH prep	⊕ **"whiff test"** (KOH placed on a slide leads to a fishy odor).	Pseudohyphae and spores (see Figure 15-5).	**Nothing.**
pH	Elevated (> 7).	Normal or < 7.	Elevated (> 7).
Treatment Nonpregnant	Metronidazole.	Topical antifungal × 3–7 days or oral fluconazole × 1 dose.	Metronidazole.
Pregnant	Metronidazole.	Use only topical antifungals × 7 days.	Metronidazole.

- **Tx:** Cefoxitin + doxycycline + metronidazole. Transition to PO doxycycline 24 hours after clinical improvement. Treatment duration is 14 days. If the patient does not improve, consider imaging (ultrasound) to evaluate for a tubo-ovarian abscess that requires drainage.
- **Outpatient management:**
  - **Indication:** Mild disease without the above findings.
  - **Tx:** Consider cefoxitin + doxycycline.

Ectopic Pregnancy

Defined as any pregnancy that is implanted outside the uterine cavity. The most common location is the fallopian tube (95%). Risk factors include a history of PID, prior ectopic pregnancy, tubal/pelvic surgery, and DES exposure in utero leading to abnormal tubal development.

SYMPTOMS/EXAM

- Patients may complain of lower abdominal or pelvic pain as well as abnormal vaginal spotting or bleeding and amenorrhea.
- The abdomen may be tender to palpation. Bimanual exam may also reveal cervical motion tenderness and an adnexal mass.
- A ruptured ectopic may present with unstable vital signs, diffuse abdominal pain, rebound tenderness, and shock.

DIFFERENTIAL

Spontaneous abortion, molar pregnancy, ruptured or hemorrhagic corpus luteum cyst, PID, ovarian torsion, appendicitis, pyelonephritis, diverticulitis, regional ileitis, ulcerative colitis.

DIAGNOSIS

- **An ↑ β-hCG in the absence of an intrauterine pregnancy on ultrasound is highly suspicious for an ectopic pregnancy.**
- Do an ultrasound to look for an intrauterine pregnancy, an adnexal mass, or free fluid (see Figure 15-6).
- The gestational sac may be visualized on transvaginal ultrasound when β-hCG is approximately 1500–3000 mIU/mL, or at approximately 4–5 weeks' gestational age (GA).

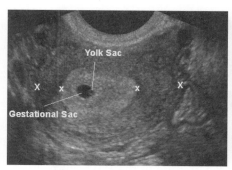

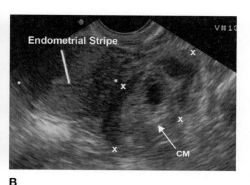

A   **B**

FIGURE 15-6. **Normal intrauterine pregnancy and ectopic pregnancy.** Transvaginal ultrasound showing (**A**) a normal intrauterine pregnancy with a gestational sac containing a yolk sac within the uterine cavity, and (**B**) a complex mass (CM)/ectopic pregnancy adjacent to an empty uterus. (Reproduced with permission from Tintinalli JE et al. *Tintinalli's Emergency Medicine: A Comprehensive Study Guide*, 6th ed. New York: McGraw-Hill, 2004, Figs. 113-15 and 113-22.)

KEY FACT

Any woman with abdominal pain needs a urine pregnancy test.

KEY FACT

A β-hCG of 3000 mIU/mL will not always show an intrauterine pregnancy. Therefore, it is important to repeat the β-hCG and ultrasound in 48 hours before treating the patient to confirm the abnormal pregnancy.

 Q — 1

A 19-year-old woman who is sexually active with multiple partners presents to your clinic with vaginal pruritus and ↑ discharge. A wet mount is ⊕ for protozoans, but KOH prep reveal no organisms. Which organism is likely contributing to her vulvovaginitis?

 Q — 2

A 28-year-old woman who found out that she was pregnant 1 week ago presents to the ED complaining of fevers and RLQ abdominal pain. Her exam is significant for RLQ tenderness and no cervical motion tenderness. What is the next step?

- Fetal heart motion of the embryo can be seen after 5–6 weeks' GA.
- Definitive diagnosis is made by laparoscopy, laparotomy, or ultrasound visualization of a pregnancy outside the uterus.

TREATMENT

- For **hemodynamically unstable** patients, immediate surgery is required.
- For **hemodynamically stable** patients:
  - Repeat the β-hCG in 24–48 hours.
  - Medical management with **methotrexate** is an option for:
    - No fetal cardiac motion
    - A β-hCG < 5000 mIU/mL
    - Pregnancy size < 3–4 cm
    - No baseline renal or hepatic dysfunction
    - No history of immune compromise or pulmonary disease
  - **Laparoscopy or laparotomy for removal of ectopic pregnancy.**
- Expectant management for stable, compliant patients with decreasing β-hCG levels or a β-hCG < 200 mIU/mL if the risk of rupture is low.
- Prevention of ectopic pregnancies includes prevention and thorough **treatment of STDs.**

> **KEY FACT**
>
> All women with ectopic pregnancies should be typed and screened and given RhoGAM if Rh is ⊖.

Contraception

ORAL CONTRACEPTIVES (OCPs)

There are 2 types of oral contraceptives: combined (estrogen and progesterone) and progesterone only. The long-term effects of combined OCP use include a ↓ in ovarian and endometrial cancers, a ↓ incidence of breast disease (but not breast cancer), ↓ menstrual flow, and ↓ dysmenorrhea. Contraindications to combined OCPs include:

- Pregnancy
- Migraines with aura
- Previous or active thromboembolic disease
- Smoking in patients > 35 years of age
- Undiagnosed genital bleeding
- Estrogen-dependent neoplasms
- Hepatocellular carcinoma
- Acute liver dysfunction

OTHER CONTRACEPTIVES

Table 15-4 contrasts hormonal contraceptives with nonhormonal methods.

INTRAUTERINE DEVICES (IUDs)

Two types of IUDs are approved for use in the United States. Both are highly effective, with > 99% efficacy during the first year of use.

- **Levonorgestrel IUD** (Mirena): The progesterone in the IUD causes thickening of the cervical mucus and thinning of the endometrium, which can ↓ menstrual blood loss or cause amenorrhea.
  - Lasts 5 years.

1 **A**

Trichomonas vaginalis.

2 **A**

Transvaginal ultrasound to look for an adnexal mass. It is too early to visualize an intrauterine gestational sac. Repeat the patient's β-hCG in 48 hours. If the value does not double in 48 hours, suspect ectopic pregnancy. It is also important to consider nongynecologic causes.

TABLE 15-4. **Hormonal vs Nonhormonal Methods**

METHOD	INDICATIONS/COMMENTS
HORMONAL	
Progesterone-only contraceptives	Indicated in woman for whom combined oral contraceptives are contraindicated. Less effective than combined OCPs and generally reserved for breast-feeding mothers who have lactational amenorrhea.
Injectable (Depo-Provera)	Administered intramuscularly every 3 months. Associated with irregular spotting and weight gain.
Subdermal progesterone implant	Approved for 3 years of use. Can be associated with irregular spotting.
Transdermal (Ortho Evra)	A patch that is changed weekly for 3 weeks followed by a 1-week holiday during which menses occur. Contains estrogen and must therefore be used in appropriate candidates.
Vaginal (NuvaRing)	A vaginal ring that is removed after 3 weeks followed by a 1-week holiday during which menses occur. Contains estrogen and must be used in appropriate candidates.
Intrauterine (Mirena)	See previous page.
NONHORMONAL	
Condoms, male or female	Provide protection against STDs.
Cervical diaphragm	Placed intravaginally over the cervix immediately before intercourse and removed within 3 hours afterward.
Spermicidal gel	Can be used in combination with condoms or diaphragm. When used alone, it is unreliable.
Copper IUD	See below.
Fertility awareness method	Relies on avoidance of intercourse during the ovulatory period.
Male or female sterilization	Either Fallopian tube interruption in females or ligation of the vas deferens in males.

- ↓ menstrual bleeding and dysmenorrhea; thus, a good choice for the treatment of heavy menstrual bleeding.
- **Side effects:** Irregular menstrual bleeding or amenorrhea.
- **Copper IUD (ParaGard):** Causes a sterile inflammatory response that prevents pregnancy implantation.
  - Lasts 10 years.
  - Nonhormonal; a good choice for women who have contraindications to hormone treatment.
  - **Side effects:** Dysmenorrhea and ↑ menstrual bleeding.

EMERGENCY CONTRACEPTION

- Should be taken immediately after intercourse; can be taken up to 5 days afterward, but with decreasing effectiveness.
- Options include oral levonorgestrel, oral ulipristal acetate, or placement of a copper IUD within 72 hours of unprotected intercourse.

 KEY FACT

The IUD itself does not ↑ the risk of ectopic pregnancy. However, it is so effective at preventing an intrauterine pregnancy that if a patient has a ⊕ pregnancy test with an IUD, suspect ectopic.

A 36-year-old G4P4004 presents to her gynecologist seeking a reliable, "hassle-free" birth control option. She has been in a long-term relationship with her husband. What method would you recommend?

KEY FACT

Endometriosis is the leading cause of female infertility, followed by PID.

Infertility

Defined as inability of a couple to conceive after 1 year of unprotected intercourse (or 6 months if > 35 years of age). Affects 10–15% of couples. Causes are listed in Table 15-5.

DIAGNOSIS

- Semen analysis to rule out male factors.
- Serum FSH/LH/TSH/prolactin to rule out endocrine dysfunction.
- Hysterosalpingography to rule out tubal and uterine cavity abnormalities.
- Basal body temperatures or ovulation kits to rule out ovulatory dysfunction.

TREATMENT

- Treat the underlying cause.
- Fertility rates in endometriosis can be improved through laparoscopic removal of implants outside the uterine cavity and resection of endometriomas.
- Ovulation can be induced with **clomiphene.** Caution should be exercised with this medication, as it can lead to ovarian hyperstimulation and multiple gestations.
- For refractory cases, assisted reproductive technologies such as in vitro fertilization can be used.

Menopause

Cessation of menstruation for 12 consecutive months. Average age of onset is 51. Surgical menopause occurs following removal or irradiation of the ovaries. Postmenopausal women are at ↑ risk for developing **osteoporosis** and **heart disease.**

SYMPTOMS/EXAM

- Patients may complain of menstrual irregularities, hot flashes, night sweats, sleep disturbances, mood changes, ↓ libido, and vaginal dryness.
- Exam may reveal vaginal dryness, ↓ breast size, and genital tract atrophy.

KEY FACT

Premature menopause occurs before age 40 and is often due to idiopathic premature ovarian insufficiency.

An IUD would be optimal for this patient.

TABLE 15-5. **Causes of Infertility**[a]

FEMALE (50%)	MALE (35%)
Uterine/tubal factors: Endometriosis or myomas that distort the endometrium or fallopian tubes; PID; congenital genital tract abnormalities.	**Congenital disorders:** Include Klinefelter's syndrome, androgen insensitivity, 5α-reductase deficiency, Kallmann syndrome, and Prader-Willi syndrome.
Ovulatory dysfunction: Ovarian failure, prolactinoma.	**Systemic disorders:** Obesity, chronic illness.
Endocrine dysfunction: Thyroid/adrenal disease, PCOS.	**Disorders of sperm production and transport:** Ejaculatory dysfunction, ↓ sperm count, abnormal morphology, or ↓ motility.

[a] The remaining 15% are attributable to unexplained fertility or rare problems.

DIAGNOSIS

- Requires **1 year** without menses with no other known cause.
- ↑↑ **serum FSH** (> **30 IU/L**) is suggestive.

TREATMENT

- Hormone therapy with estrogen or combined estrogen and progesterone can be used for short-term symptomatic relief.
- Absolute contraindications to hormone therapy include undiagnosed vaginal bleeding, active liver disease, recent MI, recent or active vascular thrombosis, and a history of endometrial or breast cancer.
- Alternatives to hormone therapy include:
  - **Vasomotor instability:** Venlafaxine and some SSRIs.
  - **Vaginal atrophy:** Vaginal lubricants or topical estrogens.
  - **Osteoporosis:** Calcium, vitamin D, calcitonin, bisphosphonates (eg, alendronate), selective estrogen receptor modulators (eg, raloxifene), denosumab.
- Unopposed estrogen (without progesterone therapy) can lead to endometrial hyperplasia and/or carcinoma.

KEY FACT

Use the lowest possible dose of hormone therapy for the shortest duration to treat menopausal symptoms.

Urinary Incontinence

Involuntary loss of urine that is a social or hygienic problem. See Table 15-6 for an outline of stress, urge, and mixed incontinence.

TABLE 15-6. Types of Urinary Incontinence

	STRESS INCONTINENCE	URGE INCONTINENCE (DETRUSOR INSTABILITY)	MIXED INCONTINENCE
History	Loss of urine with exertion (running) or straining (coughing, laughing).	Loss of urine with strong desire to void. Often associated with urinary frequency and urgency.	Stress and urge incontinence present simultaneously.
Mechanism	Poor support or poor function of the urethral sphincter.	Involuntary detrusor muscle contractions.	A combination of both mechanisms.
Etiology	Urethral hypermobility; weakened urethral closing mechanisms.	Idiopathic, neurologic (Alzheimer's, diabetes, MS).	As for both conditions.
Diagnosis	Patient history. Demonstrable leakage with stress (cough).	Patient history. Cystometry reveals involuntary detrusor muscle contraction associated with urinary leakage.	As for both conditions.
Treatment	Pelvic floor strengthening exercises (Kegel exercises) +/− biofeedback, pessaries, weight loss, surgery to restore bladder neck support.	Behavior modification (eg, limiting fluid intake; avoiding caffeinated or alcoholic beverages). Bladder training. Medical therapy (anticholinergic). Surgical therapy (sacral neurostimulators, intravesical Botox injections).	Based on the patient's worst symptom; some treatments overlap (eg, Kegel exercises).

EXAM/DIAGNOSIS

- Voiding diaries can help quantify the frequency and volume of urine lost, the circumstances of leakage (to diagnose stress or urge types of incontinence), voiding patterns, and the amount and type of fluid taken in.
- Patients with incontinence should have a screening neurologic exam to rule out neurologic causes.
- A standing cough stress test can be used to diagnose stress incontinence; cystometry can be used to diagnose urge incontinence.
- Urinary retention with overflow can be a cause of urinary incontinence and can be diagnosed with an elevated postvoid residual.

TREATMENT

Table 15-6 outlines treatment measures for urinary incontinence.

UTI must be ruled out in all women complaining of urinary incontinence.

Benign Breast Disorders

Include **fibrocystic change** (the most common), fibroadenoma, intraductal papilloma (a common cause of bloody nipple discharge), duct ectasia, fat necrosis, mastitis, and breast abscess. See Table 15-7 for a list of common examples.

TABLE 15-7. **Benign Breast Disease**

DISEASE TYPE	SYMPTOMS/EXAM	TREATMENT	ASSOCIATED WITH CARCINOMA
Fibrocystic changes	Mild to moderate pain in the breasts +/– lumps premenstrually; multifocal, bilateral nodularity. Most common in women 20–50 years of age.	OCPs.	Patients are at risk of breast cancer only in the presence of cellular atypia. Cancer must be excluded in high-risk groups.
Fibroadenoma	**The most common tumor in menstruating women** < 25 years of age. Presents as a small, firm, unilateral, nontender mass that is freely movable and slow growing. Ultrasound can be used to differentiate from a cyst.	Thirty percent will spontaneously disappear. Removal is not necessary, but surgical excision is both diagnostic and curative. Biopsy if the patient is in a high-risk group. Recurrence is common.	Risk is twice as high as that of control patients.
Intraductal papilloma	Clear, bloody, or discolored fluid from a single duct opening. Milking of the breast shows drainage from 1 duct opening.	Drainage and surgical exploration of the duct. **A malignant process must always be excluded.**	Risk is twice as high as that of control patients.
Mastitis	Seen in breast-feeding women; presents as a hard, red, tender, swollen area of breast accompanied by fever, myalgias, and general malaise.	Continued breast-feeding; NSAIDs and antibiotics to cover common etiologies (*Staphylococcus, Streptococcus, E coli*).	None.

TABLE 15-7. **Benign Breast Disease** *(continued)*

DISEASE TYPE	SYMPTOMS/EXAM	TREATMENT	ASSOCIATED WITH CARCINOMA
Abscess	Can develop if mastitis is inadequately treated. Exam reveals a fluctuant mass accompanied by systemic symptoms similar to those seen in mastitis.	Needle aspiration or surgical drainage in addition to antibiotics.	None.
Fat necrosis	Firm, tender, and ill defined with surrounding erythema; related to trauma/ischemia.	Analgesia. An excisional biopsy may be done to rule out malignancy.	None.

- **Nipple discharge:** Most commonly seen in women 20–40 years of age.
  - Discharge should raise concern if it is bloody, brown, black, unilateral, or persistent; appears spontaneously without manipulation; or is associated with systemic signs.
  - Unilateral discharge is most commonly from intraductal papilloma, which is rare and benign. Discharge is sticky and clear to straw-colored.
  - Bilateral discharge requires workup for prolactinoma (see Chapter 5 for a more detailed discussion).
  - The differential diagnosis includes malignancy and mastitis (presents with erythema, warmth, tenderness, pain, induration, and abscess).
- **Breast lumps:**
  - Evaluation includes assessing the general appearance of the breast (inverted nipple, change in size or symmetry) or any skin changes.
  - Determine if it is related to menses or was spontaneously discovered and has not gone away.
  - Exam should include evaluation of the lymph nodes.
  - For young women, it is reasonable to start with a breast ultrasound before mammography. For older women, start with mammography.

KEY FACT

Always rule out a breast malignancy with a biopsy in anyone who is high risk.

KEY FACT

Mammography should be performed for any new breast mass in an older woman even if the patient had a recent ⊖ study.

NOTES

CHAPTER 16

PEDIATRICS

Well-Child Care/Routine Health Screening

SCREENING BASICS

Routine health screening includes (1) monitoring of growth and development; (2) prevention of illness and promotion of safety; and (3) anticipatory guidance to help parents prepare for their child's next step. Routine screening should be conducted at the following intervals:

- **Metabolic/genetic diseases:** Start at 1 day of life with the newborn screen. The exact content of the screen varies by state but typically includes thyroid disease, cystic fibrosis (CF), and tyrosinemia, which, if identified early, can be treated to ↓ morbidity and mortality.
- **Growth parameters/development/behavior:** Screen at each visit—at 2–4 weeks, 2 months, 4 months, 6 months, 9 months, 12 months, 15 months, 18 months, 2 years, and annually thereafter.
- **Lead/anemia:** Begin screening during the developmental period in which children begin to explore their environment via hand-to-mouth interactions (ie, 9–15 months). Repeat at age 2, especially in high-risk communities (eg, those in which houses were built before 1950).
- **BP:** Screen with every medical exam starting at age 3. Norms are based on sex, age, and height percentile. Four-extremity blood pressures are performed in the newborn period to screen for coarctation of the aorta.
- **Vision and hearing screening:** Conduct subjective testing at each visit; red-reflex testing at all infant visits; and objective hearing and vision screening at birth and annually starting at age 3.
- **TB:** Conduct a risk assessment at each well-child check. PPD placement is appropriate for high-risk children.
- **High-risk behaviors/STD screening:** Screen at each adolescent visit beginning at approximately 10–11 years of age, and begin testing when appropriate.

GROWTH AND DEVELOPMENT

Nutrition

Guidelines for breast milk, formula, and the introduction of food are as follows:

- **Breast milk:**
  - Encouraged as an exclusive feeding source until 6 months of age. Confers immunogenic factors—including IgA, lymphocytes, and antibodies—that ↓ the risk of respiratory and GI tract infections. Also ↓ the risk of necrotizing enterocolitis.
  - Contraindications to breast-feeding/maternal breast milk include maternal HIV infection, TB infection, or an infant diagnosis of galactosemia. Maternal medications, including narcotic use, should be discussed with the mother's physician before breast-feeding is initiated.
- **Formula:**
  - All formulas are mixed to 20 kcal/oz unless concentrated to optimize growth. Types include cow's milk–protein-based, soy-protein-based, and hydrolyzed formulas. Infants with milk protein intolerance often demonstrate intolerance of soy-based formulas and need a semielemental or elemental formula.
  - Milk protein intolerance can be IgE mediated with anaphylaxis or non–IgE mediated; presentations include vomiting, diarrhea, constipation, GERD, and bloody stools 2° to proctocolitis.

KEY FACT

Neonate: Newborn to 28 days of life.
Infant: Neonatal period to 12 months of age.
Toddler: 1–3 years of age.

KEY FACT

Commonly tested disorders on newborn screens:
- Phenylketonuria
- Congenital hypothyroidism
- Galactosemia
- Sickle cell disease
- Biotinidase deficiency
- Congenital adrenal hyperplasia
- Maple syrup urine disease
- Tyrosinemia
- Cystic fibrosis
- Medium-chain acyl-CoA dehydrogenase deficiency
- Toxoplasmosis

- **Food introduction:** Recommended after 6 months of age with the introduction of a single food every 3–4 days followed by evaluation for evidence of food intolerance or allergy.

Failure to Thrive (FTT)

Although there is no consensus for the definition of FTT, criteria that are often used include:

- Weight less than the third to fifth percentile for gestation-corrected age and sex on growth charts on > 1 occasion.
- Pediatric growth chart comparison with a weight for length less than the 10th percentile.
- ↓ weight velocity with crossing of 2 major percentiles (90th, 75th, 50th, 25th, 10th, 5th) on the growth chart.
- Daily weight gain less than that expected for age.

Relevant definitions are as follows:

- **Failure to grow:** Growth that is significantly slower than that of children of the same age. Height and weight are both slow (eg, growth hormone deficiency, genetic disease).
- **Failure to gain weight:** The child is or was previously able to maintain normal height velocity, but weight is disproportionately low or has "fallen off" the growth curve. Height velocity will slow if the child is underweight for a prolonged period. Head circumference is the last to fall off the curve.
- **Short stature:**
    - Height less than the third percentile for age, with weight in the normal range.
    - ↓ height velocity with crossing of 2 major percentiles on the growth chart, with normal or ↑ weight gain for age.
    - Can have multiple underlying etiologies, including familial short stature, constitutional growth delay, genetic disorders, growth hormone deficiency, and hypothyroidism.

Symptoms/Exam

- Obtain a thorough feeding/nutrition history, and observe the parent or caretaker feeding the child.
- Ask about quality and frequency of stools to assess for malabsorption and/or systemic symptoms such as respiratory distress with feeding, vomiting, and excessive sweating with feeding.
- Obtain a detailed social history (eg, family stressors) and family history (eg, CF, genetic diseases, HIV).
- Conduct formal development and behavioral testing.
- Plot height, weight, and head circumference since birth.
- Conduct a complete physical exam.

Differential

- **Inadequate intake:**
    - The most common causes are overdilution of formula and infrequent feeding. Often 2° to psychosocial issues at home.
    - Can also result from mechanical problems such as cleft palate/nasal obstruction or sucking/swallowing dysfunction.
- **Inadequate absorption or ↑ losses:** Examples include malabsorption, infectious diarrhea, vomiting, biliary atresia, intestinal obstruction, necrotizing enterocolitis, and short gut.
- **↑ metabolic demand or ineffective utilization:** Examples include inborn errors of metabolism, CF/lung disease, HIV/infection, endocrine disorders, and congenital heart disease.

Q

An 11-month-old boy presents with his weight at the 10th percentile, length at the 25th percentile, and head circumference at the 20th percentile. His weight has trended between the 10th and 25th percentiles; length since birth has been at the 25th percentile and head circumference at the 20th percentile. His parents are concerned that he is smaller than his family members. What workup is needed?

TABLE 16-1. Developmental Milestones

Age	Gross Motor	Fine Motor	Language	Social/Cognitive
2 months	Lifts head/chest when prone.	Tracks past midline.	Alerts to sound; coos.	Recognizes parent; exhibits social smile.
4–5 months	**Rolls** front to back and back to front (5 months).	Grasps rattle.	Orients to voice; "ah-goo"; razzes.	Enjoys looking around; laughs.
6 months	**Sits unassisted** (7 months).	**Transfers objects;** exhibits raking grasp.	Babbles.	Exhibits **stranger anxiety.**
9–10 months	Crawls; pulls to stand.	Uses 3-finger pincer grasp.	Says **"mama/dada"** (nonspecific).	Waves "bye-bye"; plays pat-a-cake.
12 months	Cruises (11 months); **walks alone.**	Uses 2-finger pincer grasp.	Says **"mama/dada"** (specific).	Imitates actions.
15 months	Walks backward.	Uses cup.	Uses 4–6 words.	Has temper tantrums.
18 months	Runs; kicks a ball.	Builds tower of 2–4 cubes.	Names common objects.	Copies parent in tasks (eg, sweeping).
2 years	Walks up/down steps with help; jumps.	Builds tower of 6 cubes.	Uses **2-word** phrases.	Follows **2-step** commands; removes clothes.
3 years	Rides a **tricycle;** climbs stairs with alternating feet (3–4 years).	Copies a circle; uses utensils.	Uses **3-word** sentences.	Brushes teeth with help; washes/dries hands.
4 years	Hops.	Copies a cross.	Counts to 10.	Engages in cooperative play.

Adapted with permission from Le T et al. *First Aid for the USMLE Step 2 CK*, 7th ed. New York: McGraw-Hill, 2010: 402.

No further workup is indicated. The child's growth is appropriate, as demonstrated by consistency in growth since birth without the weight decreasing by > 2 growth percentile lines on the growth chart, length growing out of proportion to weight, or accelerated or decelerated head circumference growth.

DIAGNOSIS

- The history and physical (H&P) will dictate the extent of lab workup needed.
- First-line laboratory evaluation should include a CBC, electrolytes, BUN/creatinine, a lead level if appropriate, and a UA.
- If the child is severely malnourished, also check albumin (to assess protein status) as well as alkaline phosphatase, calcium, and phosphorus (to evaluate for rickets).

TREATMENT

- Treat the underlying cause.
- If the H&P does not suggest an organic cause, start a calorie count and consider nutritional supplementation.
- Hospitalization may be necessary for severe malnourishment or potential neglect.

Developmental Milestones

Table 16-1 highlights major developmental milestones. Red flags include:

Vaccine ▼ Age ▶	Birth	1 month	2 months	4 months	6 months	12 months	15 months	18 months	19–23 months	2–3 years	4–6 years
Hepatitis B	HepB	HepB			HepB						
Rotavirus			RV	RV	RV						
Diphtheria, Tetanus, Pertussis			DTaP	DTaP	DTaP		DTaP				DTaP
Haemophilus influenzae type b			Hib	Hib	Hib	Hib					
Pneumococcal			PCV	PCV	PCV	PCV				PPSV	
Inactivated Poliovirus			IPV	IPV	IPV						IPV
Influenza					Influenza (Yearly)						
Measles, Mumps, Rubella						MMR					MMR
Varicella						Varicella					Varicella
Hepatitis A						HepA (2 doses)				HepA Series	
Meningococcal										MCV	

Range of recommended ages for all children except certain high-risk groups

Range of recommended ages for certain high-risk groups

FIGURE 16-1. **Pediatric immunization timetable.** (Reproduced from the Centers for Disease Control and Prevention, Atlanta, GA.)

- Persistent primitive reflexes by 6 months.
- Handedness before 1 year.
- No pointing by 18 months.

IMMUNIZATIONS

Figure 16-1 summarizes the recommended timetable for childhood immunizations. Schedules may vary for children who are behind and require catch-up immunizations. Contraindications/considerations before immunization include:

- **Allergic reaction** to a vaccine or its components.
- **Live virus vaccines** (eg, varicella, MMR, combination vaccines, intranasal influenza): Contraindicated in patients who are immunocompromised, immunosuppressed, or pregnant. Consider administration of inactivated vaccines. Asthma patients should not receive intranasal influenza vaccine.
- **Egg allergy:** Consider the severity and type of reaction before influenza vaccination.
- **Mild acute illness is not a contraindication;** a delay in vaccination can be considered for moderate or severe acute intercurrent disease.

SAFETY

General Principles

- Anticipatory guidance should include guidance on the proper storage of chemicals, cleaners, and medications; use of plug covers on all electrical outlets; and counseling on helmet use.
- Car seats should be placed in the rear seat of the car, rear-facing, until the child is ≥ 2 years of age or until the height and weight determined by the car seat manufacturer is reached. Car seats should not be placed in seats with active air bags.
    - As children grow and develop, they progress to forward-facing car seats and booster seats.
    - Children should remain seated in the back seat until age 13.

KEY FACT

Immunocompromised and immunosuppressed patients should not be given live virus vaccines, including influenza, varicella, and MMR-containing vaccines.

KEY FACT

All infants should go **"back"** to sleep (ie, sleep on their **backs**) to ↓ the risk of sudden infant death syndrome (SIDS).

Q

You are seeing a formerly full-term female infant for a routine well-child checkup. The mother reports that the infant has started crawling, is saying "mama" and "dada" to everyone, and is waving "bye-bye." If the infant is developmentally on target, how old should she be?

KEY FACT

Consider nonaccidental trauma whenever the history of an injury is discordant with physical findings and developmental history.

Child Abuse

Workup must consider physical, sexual, and emotional abuse/neglect. Diagnosis is based on a history that is **discordant with physical findings.**

SYMPTOMS/EXAM

Presentation may include:

- Multiple injuries in varying stages of healing.
- Skeletal trauma in the absence of a developmentally plausible mechanism, especially spiral fracture of long bones, multiple/old/posterior rib fractures, or metaphyseal fractures (also known as corner or bucket-handle fractures).
- Pattern injuries (eg, cigarette/immersion burns).
- Oddly situated bruises (not over bony prominences) or bruises on a child who is not yet mobile.
- Irritability/lethargy.
- Retinal hemorrhage in infants.
- Intracranial hemorrhage, especially in the absence of a plausible mechanism.
- Growth failure.
- Signs/symptoms of STDs or genital trauma in prepubertal children.

DIAGNOSIS

- **Labs:** Evaluate for underlying disorders that would result in an acute presentation (eg, osteogenesis imperfecta, bleeding diathesis, acute infection).
  - **Bone metabolism:** Calcium, phosphorus, and alkaline phosphatase.
  - **Metabolic disorders:** LFTs, electrolytes.
  - **Coagulopathy:** CBC, PT/PTT, INR.
  - **Infection:** CBC, UA.
  - **General:** Consider toxicology and STD evaluation.
- **Imaging:** Skeletal survey to evaluate for fractures in various stages of healing; head CT for intracranial bleeding.
- **Consultation:** Consider an ophthalmology evaluation and consultation with a child abuse team.

MNEMONIC

Use the B-HEADSS interview for adolescents:

Body image
Home
Education and Employment
Activities
Drugs
Sexuality
Suicidality/depression

TREATMENT

- Physicians are mandated reporters of any suspected abuse or nonaccidental trauma and should immediately notify social services or Child Protective Services.
- Consider hospitalization to ensure the safety of the child. Be cognizant of other children in the home and their safety in the evaluation.
- The **B-HEADSS** interview (see mnemonic) can be used to gauge psychosocial risk in adolescents.

ANTICIPATORY GUIDANCE

Provide nutrition, dental hygiene, screen time, injury/violence prevention, and sleep counseling at each health maintenance visit.

A

Nine months.

Colic

- Defined as severe, paroxysmal crying for > 3 hours a day, > 3 days a week for > 3 weeks in a healthy, well-fed infant. Usually peaks at around 6 weeks of life, with spontaneous resolution by 3–4 months. A diagnosis of exclusion.

- **Tx:** Treatment consists of providing reassurance and teaching parents soothing techniques such as the **5 S's** (see mnemonic).

Neonatology

The specialty of pediatrics that concerns the care of infants from birth until they are ready to be discharged to home. A neonate is defined as an infant < 28 days old.

RESPIRATORY DISTRESS

- Common causes of neonatal respiratory distress are outlined in Table 16-2.
- Other causes include:
  - **Sepsis** (see below).
  - Congenital heart disease (if O_2 saturation fails to improve with supplemental O_2).
  - Anatomic airway anomalies (eg, choanal atresia, in which an NG tube cannot be passed through the nares at birth).
  - Pneumothorax (especially in an infant who suddenly decompensates), neurologic abnormalities, and pneumonia.
- **Dx/Tx:** The diagnosis and treatment of common neonatal respiratory disorders are outlined in Table 16-2.

NEONATAL SEPSIS

Serious bacterial infections are rare in the pediatric population but are relatively more common in infants < 2 months of age by virtue of their immature immune systems and waning maternal antibody protection. Risk factors in the immediate perinatal period include maternal group B streptococcal (GBS) infection or STD, rupture of membranes lasting > 18 hours, maternal fever, chorioamnionitis, premature labor, and limited or no maternal prenatal care.

- **Most frequent infections:** UTIs, followed by bacterial sepsis, meningitis, and pneumonia.
- **Most common pathogens:**
  - **Bacterial:** *E coli*; GBS and other gram-⊖ rods. *Listeria monocytogenes* is rare but is frequently tested on pediatric exams.
  - **Viral:** Mothers with active herpes lesions at the time of delivery or a first-time diagnosis of HSV in the peripartum period carry an ↑ risk of transmitting HSV to the infant. HSV should also be considered in any ill-appearing infant < 28 days of age.

Symptoms/Exam

Septic infants often present with nonspecific signs such as poor feeding, irritability, rapid breathing, vomiting, or ↓ activity.

Diagnosis

- All evaluations should include a CBC, a blood culture, a UA and urine culture, and an LP for CSF cell counts, glucose, protein, and culture.
- Workup for HSV should include HSV PCR from CSF/skin and LFTs for infants who appear toxic. Workup is also indicated if there is suspicion for first-time HSV infection in a mother during pregnancy.

MNEMONIC

The 5 S's for soothing crying babies:

Swaddling
Side/**S**tomach position (done under close supervision only)
Shushing sounds
Swinging
Sucking

KEY FACT

A fever in the first month of life is an indication for a full sepsis workup, admission, and IV antibiotics.

TABLE 16-2. **Common Neonatal Respiratory Disorders**

Disorder	Description	History	Exam/CXR Findings	Treatment	Complications
Respiratory distress syndrome/ hyaline membrane disease	**Surfactant deficiency** leads to poor lung compliance and respiratory failure.	Usually occurs in **premature infants.**	↓ air movement; CXR shows ↓ lung volumes and "ground-glass" appearance (see Figure 16-2A).	Maternal antenatal steroids for prevention; surfactant administration; respiratory support.	Chronic lung disease.
Transient tachypnea of the newborn	**Retained fetal lung fluid** leads to brief, **self-resolving,** mild respiratory distress. A diagnosis of exclusion.	Term or near-term infants; nonasphyxiated; born following short labor or via C-section without labor.	CXR shows perihilar streaking and fluid in interlobar fissures.	Usually only a mild to moderate O_2 requirement for support. Typically resolves over time.	None.
Meconium aspiration syndrome	Inhalation of meconium at or near the time of birth leads to **aspiration pneumonitis.**	**Term infants;** meconium is present at the time of delivery.	**Hypoxia;** coarse breath sounds; CXR shows coarse, irregular infiltrates, hyperexpansion, and lobar consolidation.	Nasopharyngeal suctioning at perineum if vigorous; tracheal suctioning at birth if not vigorous; ventilatory support and antibiotics. Nitric oxide if severe pulmonary hypertension.	Pulmonary hypertension. Suspect CF.
Persistent pulmonary hypertension of the newborn	Severe hypoxemia that results from ↑ pulmonary vascular resistance, leading to right-to-left fetal blood shunting.	Term infants; typically occurs concurrently with other respiratory pathologies (eg, pneumonia, meconium aspiration syndrome).	Hypoxemia, cyanosis and respiratory distress, prominent precordial impulse, and narrow S1/S2 with an accentuated S2.	Ventilatory support; investigation for concurrent etiologies of respiratory distress; circulatory support due to shunting and nitric oxide. Extracorporeal membrane oxygenation (ECMO) if unresponsive to other treatments.	Risk of developmental delay, hearing deficits, and motor disability.
Congenital diaphragmatic hernia	A defect in the diaphragm leads to herniation of abdominal contents into the chest cavity; limitation of lung growth leads to **pulmonary hypoplasia.**	Severe respiratory distress at birth; may be diagnosed by prenatal ultrasound.	Scaphoid abdomen; CXR may show bowel loops in the chest (see Figure 16-2B).	Immediate intubation, ventilatory support, and surgical correction after stabilization. Patients may require ECMO.	Severe pulmonary hypertension. Mortality is 25–40%.

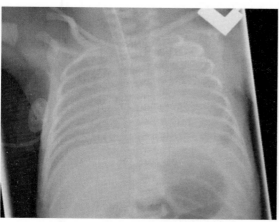
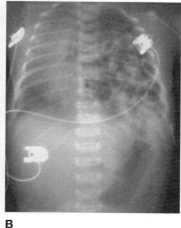

A   **B**

FIGURE 16-2. Neonatal respiratory distress. (A) Frontal CXR in a neonate with respiratory distress syndrome showing diffuse fine granular ("ground-glass") opacities and hypoaeration. (B) Frontal radiograph in a patient with congenital diaphragmatic hernia, demonstrating air-filled loops of bowel in the left chest and rightward displacement of mediastinal structures. (Image A reproduced with permission from USMLE-Rx.com. Image B reproduced with permission from Brunicardi FC et al. *Schwartz's Principles of Surgery*, 9th ed. New York: McGraw-Hill, 2010, Fig. 39-3.)

- Consider a CXR if a patient exhibits hypoxemia, respiratory distress, or clinical findings that raise concern for pneumonia.

TREATMENT

- **Initial treatment:** Begin IV ampicillin (to cover *Listeria*) plus either gentamicin or a third-generation cephalosporin such as cefotaxime. Consider acyclovir if there is a maternal history of HSV or if the infant appears ill.
- **Subsequent therapy:**
  - If the cause of sepsis is a UTI, a renal ultrasound and VCUG may be obtained to evaluate the infant for hydronephrosis and vesicoureteral reflux.
  - If the infant has meningitis, follow-up hearing and developmental tests may be recommended.

PREVENTION

Screen the mother for GBS at 36 weeks, and treat with prophylactic antibiotics during delivery.

CONGENITAL ToRCHeS INFECTIONS

Many congenital infections present with jaundice, hepatosplenomegaly, and thrombocytopenia. Table 16-3 outlines the diagnosis and treatment of each.

CONGENITAL ANOMALIES

Table 16-4 outlines the clinical presentation and treatment of common congenital anomalies and malformations.

KEY FACT

Ceftriaxone displaces bilirubin from albumin and should not be used in neonates < 28 days old.

Q 1

A 3-month-old infant presents to the pediatric ED with a broken left femur. Her parents explain that they had left her alone for only a minute when she "rolled off the living-room couch." In addition to obtaining leg x-rays, what other evaluations would you conduct?

Q 2

A father reports that his 2-week-old daughter has a rectal temperature of 38.5°C (101.3°F) but no other symptoms. She was born via an uncomplicated vaginal delivery and has been breast-feeding well with good wet diapers and stooling. Her 2-year-old sister has a cold, but the parents have taught her to wash her hands before going near the baby. What advice would you give?

TABLE 16-3. ToRCHeS Infections

Infection	Description	Treatment	Prevention
Toxoplasmosis	Hydrocephalus, seizures, chorioretinitis, intracranial calcifications, and ring-enhancing lesions on head CT.	Pyrimethamine, sulfadiazine, spiramycin.	Avoid exposure to cats and cat feces during pregnancy; avoid raw/undercooked meat; treat women with 1° infection.
Rubella	"Blueberry muffin" rash, cataracts, hearing loss, PDA and other cardiac defects, encephalitis.	None.	Immunize mothers prior to pregnancy.
Cytomegalovirus (CMV)	Petechial rash, periventricular calcifications, microcephaly, chorioretinitis.	Ganciclovir.	Avoid exposure.
Herpes simplex (HSV)	Skin, eye, and mouth vesicles; can progress to severe CNS/systemic infection.	Acyclovir.	Perform a C-section if the mother has active lesions at the time of delivery. The highest risk is from mothers with 1° infection.
Syphilis	Maculopapular skin rash on the palms and soles, lymphadenopathy, "snuffles," osteitis.	Penicillin.	Treat seropositive mothers with penicillin.

JAUNDICE

Physiologic Jaundice

Nearly all babies have some form of indirect (unconjugated) hyperbilirubinemia, commonly known as physiologic jaundice. Causes include:

- ↑ RBC breakdown.
- ↓ bilirubin breakdown due to ↓ conjugation in the immature liver and lack of appropriate bacterial components in the intestines.
- ↓ excretion due to less frequent stooling and urination.

SYMPTOMS/EXAM

- Physiologic jaundice usually presents in the first 36–48 hours of life and reaches peak total bilirubin levels of 10–15 mg/dL at 5–7 days of life.
- Visible jaundice starts at the head (or eyes) and travels down the body as bilirubin levels ↑.
- Initial evaluation should include both total and direct bilirubin to establish whether the hyperbilirubinemia is direct or indirect.
- Jaundice is less likely to be physiologic if it is severe or prolonged, occurs within the first 24 hours of life, or is associated with an ↑ direct (conjugated) component.

TREATMENT

- ↑ **feeding:** Most normal babies will be able to excrete bilirubin on their own with time, additional intake, and improved intestinal motility from the gastrocolic reflex.
- **UV phototherapy:** Phototherapy is more likely to be necessary if the mother's blood type is O negative or if the infant suffered birth trauma (bruising), is of Asian descent, was born preterm, or has a nonphysiologic form of jaundice. Phototherapy modifies the bilirubin molecule into a water-soluble form that can be more easily excreted.
- Exchange transfusion is indicated for severe jaundice.

1 A

Three-month-old infants rarely roll, and falls from couches should not cause a broken femur. Therefore, a full workup should be conducted for medical causes of unusual fractures (eg, osteogenesis imperfecta, nutritional deficiencies) as well as for injuries of abuse. Consider a skeletal survey, an ophthalmologic exam, and head imaging along with hematology labs, liver and pancreatic enzymes, bone labs, electrolytes, and a UA.

2 A

Infants < 28 days old with a temperature of ≥ 38°C require a full sepsis workup (CBC, blood culture, UA/urine culture, and CSF culture and cell counts). Admit for IV antibiotics with ampicillin and gentamicin or a third-generation cephalosporin until cultures return (usually in 48 hours). Strongly consider HSV workup and the addition of acyclovir.

TABLE 16-4.   Common Congenital Anomalies and Malformations

LESION	DESCRIPTION	AGE AT PRESENTATION	SYMPTOMS/SIGNS	TREATMENT
Cleft lip/palate	Abnormal ridge/division.	Presents at birth.	Poor feeding; aspiration; severe, recurrent otitis media. May be associated with other anomalies.	Surgical repair of the lip/palate.
Tracheoesophageal fistula	Four different types. A blind esophageal pouch with a fistula between the distal esophagus and trachea is most common.	Usually presents in the first few hours of life, but other types can present later in infancy.	Copious secretions, choking/coughing with feeds, cyanosis, respiratory distress/ aspiration.	Suctioning of the pouch with an NG tube; reflux precautions; supportive care; surgical repair.
Abdominal wall defects	Gastroschisis (extrusion of the intestine through the defect); omphalocele (a membrane-covered herniation of abdominal contents). (See Figure 16-3A and B.)	Present antenatally or at birth.	A visible defect. Associated anomalies are common with omphalocele but are rare in gastroschisis.	Coverage of abdominal contents with moist sterile dressing. NG decompressions, antibiotics, supportive care, and stabilization followed by 1° or staged closure.
Intestinal atresias	Intestinal obstruction.	Present antenatally or at birth.	Abdominal distention, bilious vomiting, obstipation/failure to pass meconium, polyhydramnios. With Down syndrome, look for the characteristic "double bubble" sign of duodenal atresia (see Figure 16-4).	Surgical resection.
Hirschsprung's disease	Absence of ganglion cells in the colon leads to narrowing of the aganglionic segment with dilation of the proximal normal colon. Can be a short (75%) or long segment.	Presents in infancy or usually within the first 2 years of life.	Failure to pass meconium, vomiting, abdominal distention, chronic constipation. Barium enema may show a region of marked dilation superior to the aganglionic segment.	Diagnosed by rectal suction biopsy at the anal verge to look for ganglion cells. Rectal irrigation for decompression. A staged procedure with an initial diverting colostomy followed by resection when the infant is > 6 months of age.
Neural tube defects	Include anencephaly (incompatible with life) and spina bifida (myelomeningocele, meningocele; see Figure 16-5).	Present at birth, but may be detected prenatally. Associated with ↑ maternal age and **amniotic fluid α-fetoprotein.**	Ranges from incompatibility with life to hydrocephalus, paralysis, and neurogenic bowel and bladder depending on the type of defect. Associated with an ↑ risk of latex allergy.	Risk ↓ with folate ingestion during the first trimester. Surgical repair.

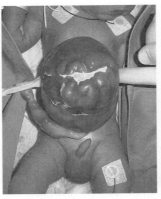
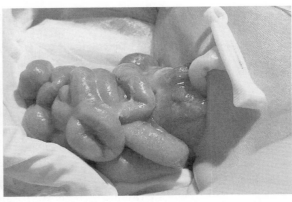

A   **B**

FIGURE 16-3. Omphalocele vs gastroschisis. (A) Giant omphalocele and **(B)** gastroschisis in a newborn. (Reproduced with permission from Brunicardi FC et al. *Schwartz's Principles of Surgery*, 9th ed. New York: McGraw-Hill, 2010, Figs. 39-30 and 39-31.)

KEY FACT

Both direct and indirect bilirubin should be checked in all neonates with hyperbilirubinemia to ensure that biliary atresia and other hepatobiliary diseases do not go undiagnosed.

■ Serum bilirubin levels should be trended during treatment for hyperbilirubinemia.

Breast Milk Jaundice

Breast milk contains an enzyme that further delays hepatic bilirubin conjugation and can prolong jaundice in newborns.

SYMPTOMS/EXAM

Affects exclusively breast-fed infants. Jaundice presents after the first 3–5 days of life and peaks at 2 weeks of age. Total bilirubin levels may reach 19–20 mg/dL and may persist for 1–2 months.

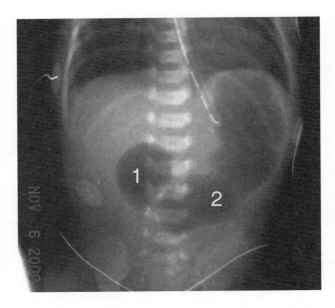

FIGURE 16-4. Duodenal atresia. Note the characteristic "double bubble" appearance of the duodenal bulb (1) and stomach (2) in a neonate with duodenal atresia presenting with bilious emesis. (Reproduced with permission from Brunicardi FC et al. *Schwartz's Principles of Surgery*, 9th ed. New York: McGraw-Hill, 2010, Fig. 39-13.)

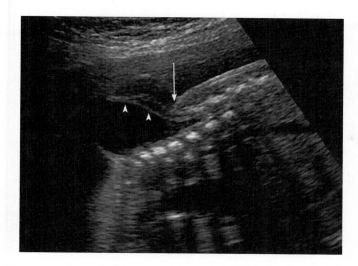

FIGURE 16-5. **Myelomeningocele.** Arrowheads indicate nerve roots within the anechoic herniated sac. The overlying skin is visible above the level of the spinal defect but abruptly stops at the defect (arrow). (Reproduced with permission from Cunningham FG et al. *Williams Obstetrics,* 24th ed. New York: McGraw-Hill, 2014, Fig. 10-7.)

DIAGNOSIS

A diagnosis of exclusion.

TREATMENT

Rarely requires phototherapy. Once the diagnosis is made, breast-feeding should be **encouraged** (not discouraged), as the problem will go away on its own.

Pathologic Jaundice

Jaundice is considered pathologic if it is severe or prolonged, occurs within the first 24 hours of life, or is associated with ↑ direct (conjugated) bilirubin. A direct bilirubin of > 10% or 2 mg/dL of the total suggests a hepatobiliary or general metabolic disorder. Very high levels of unconjugated bilirubin (> 30 mg/dL) can cross the blood-brain barrier and deposit in the basal ganglia, causing kernicterus, an irreversible, potentially fatal encephalopathy.

 KEY FACT

Remember that a direct bilirubin of > 10% or 2 mg/dL of total bilirubin points to a hepatobiliary or general metabolic disorder.

- Causes of pathologic **indirect hyperbilirubinemia** include:
  - ↑ **bilirubin production:** Hemolysis, sepsis, severe bruising/hematoma.
  - **Bilirubin conjugation abnormalities:** Hepatic enzyme deficiencies, hepatic dysfunction.
  - **Bilirubin excretion abnormalities:** Intestinal obstruction, poor motility.
- Causes of pathologic **direct hyperbilirubinemia** include:
  - **Intrahepatic:** Biliary obstruction/atresia (most common), choledochal cysts, neonatal hepatitis, Gilbert's syndrome, Crigler-Najjar syndrome, Dubin-Johnson syndrome, Rotor's syndrome, Alagille syndrome, α_1-antitrypsin deficiency, TPN cholestasis (affects premature infants on TPN). See also Table 16-5.
  - **Extrahepatic:** Sepsis, UTIs, hypothyroidism, CF, inborn errors of metabolism, RBC abnormalities such as sickle cell disease or hereditary spherocytosis.

SYMPTOMS/EXAM

- Look for hepatomegaly, acholic (white) stools, signs of anemia or plethora, evidence of sepsis, growth abnormalities, and congenital abnormalities.

TABLE 16-5.   Common Intrahepatic Causes of Hyperbilirubinemia

	CHARACTERISTICS	SIGNS/SYMPTOMS	TREATMENT
Gilbert's syndrome	The most common inherited disorder of bilirubin glucuronidation (see Figure 16-6). Due to a defect in UGT1A1. Presentation in adolescence is due to hormonal changes; rarely diagnosed before puberty.	Repeated episodes of jaundice with stressors such as illness, fever, dehydration, and fasting. Asymptomatic.	None.
Alagille syndrome	Chronic cholestasis due to paucity of bile ducts. Associated with the JAG1 or NOTCH2 mutation. Can be associated with dysmorphic facies and other congenital anomalies of the heart, eye, and vertebrae.	Pruritus due to cholestasis; growth failure due to malnutrition. Labs show ↑ bilirubin, ↑ GGT, and potentially ↑ AST/ALT. Diagnosed by liver biopsy showing a limited number of bile ducts.	Treat pruritus with ursodiol, rifampin, and bile acid–binding resins. Twenty percent of patients require liver transplantation. Optimize growth with nutrition.
Crigler-Najjar syndrome	Abnormal functioning of the bilirubin-UGT enzyme.	↑ unconjugated bilirubin; normal hepatic enzymes. Patients typically have persistent hyperbilirubinemia despite treatment with phototherapy and plasmapheresis.	Liver transplantation is the only curative therapy.

- **Kernicterus** (usually caused by extremely high levels of indirect hyperbilirubinemia) presents with jaundice, lethargy, poor feeding, a high-pitched cry, hypertonicity, and seizures.

DIAGNOSIS

- Order a CBC (to assess for anemia), a reticulocyte count, and a peripheral blood smear (to rule out hemolysis).

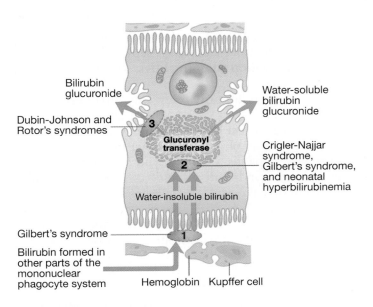

FIGURE 16-6.   Bilirubin metabolism. (Reproduced with permission from USMLE-Rx.com.)

- A Coombs' test can distinguish antibody-mediated disease (eg, ABO incompatibility) from non-immune-related disorders (eg, G6PD deficiency, hereditary spherocytosis).
- Additional testing should be guided by the patient's H&P with a focus on maternal pregnancy history, family history, and concerns for infection and feeding.

TREATMENT

- Phototherapy and, rarely, exchange transfusion.
- Treat associated conditions (eg, hemolysis, sepsis, hypothyroidism, biliary obstruction).

Dermatology

NEONATAL RASHES

The vast majority of skin findings in the neonatal period are benign. Nonetheless, they are often a cause for concern among new parents. Table 16-6 describes common neonatal rashes.

ECZEMA (ATOPIC DERMATITIS)

A chronic inflammatory skin condition that is driven by allergic sensitivities and affects nearly 20% of children in the United States. Onset generally occurs before age 5.

SYMPTOMS/EXAM

- Presents with dry, itchy, often erythematous skin. May be papular or excoriated in severe cases.
- In infants, it is usually found on the trunk, cheeks, and scalp. In older children, it is generally found on flexor surfaces and may include lichenified plaques.

TREATMENT

- **Avoid triggers** such as heat, perspiration, and dry climates. Allergic triggers may also include dust mites, molds, pet dander, and foods such as egg, milk, wheat, and peanuts.
- **Maintain hydration** by limiting bathing to every other day followed by the application of thick creams (eg, Eucerin, Cetaphil) or ointments (eg, petroleum jelly, Aquaphor) to lock in the skin's moisture.
- **Control itching** by using antihistamines such as diphenhydramine, hydroxyzine, and cyproheptadine. Cool baths and emollients covered with dry, loose cotton dressings may further reduce pruritus.
- **Treat inflammation** with topical corticosteroids (hydrocortisone for mild inflammation; triamcinolone or fluocinolone for more severe cases). Other treatment measures for severe disease include systemic corticosteroids, topical or oral calcineurin inhibitors, and phototherapy.
- **Aggressively treat superinfections** (impetigo or cellulitis), as patients with eczema are more susceptible to bacterial, viral (especially eczema herpeticum), and fungal skin infections.

TABLE 16-6.   **Presentation and Treatment of Common Neonatal Rashes**

Rash	Presentation	Treatment
Erythema toxicum neonatorum	Erythematous macules and papules that progress to pustules (see Figure 16-7A). Lesions usually appear within 24–48 hours after birth and resolve in 5–7 days.	None.
Transient neonatal pustular melanosis	There are 3 types of lesions: (1) pustules with a nonerythematous base; (2) erythematous macules with a surrounding scaly area; and (3) hyperpigmented macules. Lesions present at birth and resolve within weeks to months.	None.
Neonatal acne	Papules and pustules appearing on the face and/or scalp (see Figure 16-7B) at 3 weeks of age. Generally resolves by 4 months of age.	Gentle cleansing with soap and water; avoidance of oils and lotions.
Milia	White papules composed of retained keratin and sebaceous material. Present at birth; usually found on the cheeks and nose. Resolves within the first few weeks of life.	None.
Miliaria (crystallina, rubra, pustulosa, profunda)	Vesicles, papules, or pustules caused by the accumulation of sweat within sweat ducts blocked by keratin. More common in warm climates and among infants in incubators. Usually appears during the first week of life.	Provision of a cooler environment; loose clothing and cool baths.
Seborrheic dermatitis	Erythema and greasy scales, usually on the face and scalp (see Figure 16-7C). Resolves within weeks to months.	Application of emollient overnight followed by massage and shampooing with baby shampoo to loosen scales; use of a soft brush to remove scales. If gentle cleansing does not work, ketoconazole, selenium sulfide, or hydrocortisone may be tried.

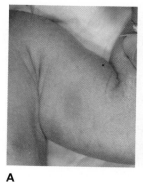
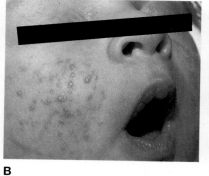
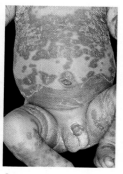

A   B   C

FIGURE 16-7.   **Common neonatal rashes.** (A) Erythema toxicum neonatorum. Erythematous macules are seen on the arm of a 1-day-old newborn. (B) Neonatal acne. Tiny papulopustules are seen on the face of a 3-week-old infant. (C) Seborrheic dermatitis. (Reproduced with permission from Goldsmith LA et al. *Fitzpatrick's Dermatology in General Medicine,* 8th ed. New York: McGraw-Hill, 2012, Figs. 107-3, 107-5, and 22-1.)

VIRAL EXANTHEMS

When considering pediatric viral exanthems, the history is as important as, if not more important than, the physical exam.

- **Timing:** Presence and timing of fever relative to exanthem eruption; seasonality/time of year.
- **Distribution:** The location of the first rash and subsequent spread.
- **Concurrent symptoms:** Rhinorrhea, congestion, oral sores, hematuria.
- **Exposures:** Recent travel, zoonotic exposures, sick contacts.

Table 16-7 describes several common viral exanthems, their infectious agents, and typical presentations and treatment.

TABLE 16-7.   Common Childhood Viral Exanthems

EXANTHEM	VIRAL AGENT	PRESENTATION	TREATMENT
Herpetic gingivostomatitis	HSV-1 and HSV-2	Vesicles on a red base that develop into shallow ulcers involving the gingivae, palate, and tongue. Fever, irritability, and pain with eating are common.	Supportive care; acyclovir if severe.
Varicella-zoster virus	VZV	Uncommon owing to vaccination; most often occurs in immunosuppressed and unvaccinated patients. Typically appear as pruritic vesicles on an erythematous base in multiple stages of eruption and healing (see Figure 16-8A). **Complications:** Systemic viremia or bacterial superinfection can occur. **Herpes zoster/"shingles":** Viral reactivation in sensory nerves, resulting in a painful vesicular rash in a dermatomal distribution.	Avoid aspirin in view of the risk of Reye's syndrome. Consider VZIG for immunocompromised patients who are exposed.
Rubeola (measles)	Measles virus	Fever with the **3 C's**—**C**ough, **C**oryza, and **C**onjunctivitis—and Koplik spots (see Figure 16-9A). Erythematous papules start 2–4 days later on the face and spread downward. **Complications:** Pneumonia, gastroenteritis, myocarditis, and encephalitis.	Consider vitamin A supplementation in patients with malnutrition or malabsorptive states.
Erythema infectiosum (fifth disease)	Parvovirus B19	Presents with fever, chills, and headache followed 2–3 days later by the development of a "slapped cheek" appearance with a flat, erythematous rash on the cheeks (see Figure 16-9B). Evolves to a lacy rash on the trunk and legs lasting 2–3 weeks.	Supportive care.
Roseola	HHV-6 or -7	High, spiking fevers lasting 3–5 days; rash develops as fever resolves. Begins as poorly defined erythematous macules and papules on the chest and spreads outward. **Complications:** The first febrile seizures may be associated with infection; encephalitis.	Supportive care.

TABLE 16-7.   **Common Childhood Viral Exanthems** *(continued)*

EXANTHEM	VIRAL AGENT	PRESENTATION	TREATMENT
Mumps	Mumps virus	Fever, malaise, headache, and anorexia. Affects glands and neural tissue. Commonly recognized by parotid swelling, but may also result in orchitis or meningoencephalitis.	Supportive care.
Hand-foot-and-mouth disease	Coxsackievirus	Begins with fever, malaise, and ↓ appetite followed 1–2 days later by painful oval vesicles on an erythematous base in the mouth and on the palms and soles of the feet.	Supportive care; resolves in 7–10 days.
Pityriasis rosea	Unclear	Often begins with a "herald patch"—a large, salmon-colored, scaly lesion followed 5–10 days later by lesions, especially on the trunk running along Blaschko's lines, in a "Christmas tree" distribution (see Figure 16-8B and C).	Supportive care; may improve more rapidly with UV light or erythromycin. Resolves in weeks to months.

DIAPER DERMATITIS ("DIAPER RASH")

The skin of the buttocks, groin, and mons pubis is in a moist, warm environment with frequent exposure to bacteria from stool and acidic urine, resulting in skin irritation and barrier disruption. Subtypes include:

- **Irritant diaper dermatitis:** Erythema and skin breakdown where the diaper contacts the skin. Results from allergy to diapers and/or prolonged contact with urine or stool. Treat with frequent diaper changes, cleansing with soap and water, and use of barrier creams or lubricants to protect the skin from contact exposure.
- **Staphylococcal diaper dermatitis:** Pustules rupture and dry, resulting in desquamation and skin breakdown. Treat with topical antibiotics or with oral antibiotics if severe.
- **Candidal diaper dermatitis:** Bright red, well-demarcated papules and pustules with satellite lesions, often in skin folds. Consider in the presence of antibiotic use, oral thrush, or diaper dermatitis that is unresponsive to symptomatic treatment. Treat with topical antifungals.

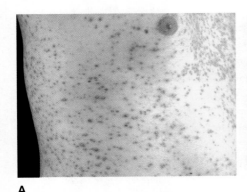
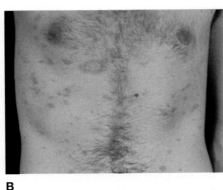
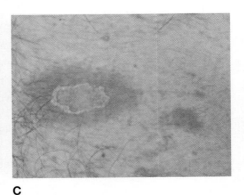

A   B   C

FIGURE 16-8.   **Varicella-zoster virus vs pityriasis rosea.** (**A**) Crusted pustules of VZV are shown in various stages of healing. (**B**) Classic presentation of pityriasis rosea showing a herald patch and scattered pink plaques. (**C**) The crusted, scaling herald patch of pityriasis rosea.
(Reproduced with permission from Wolff K et al. *Fitzpatrick's Color Atlas and Synopsis of Clinical Dermatology,* 7th ed. New York: McGraw-Hill, 2013, Figs. 27-57 and 3-20.)

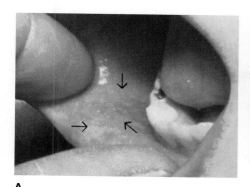
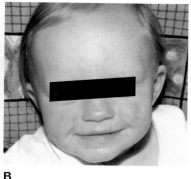

A **B**

FIGURE 16-9. **Measles vs fifth disease.** (**A**) Koplik spots of measles. (**B**) "Slapped-cheek" appearance of fifth disease. (Image A reproduced with permission from Goldsmith LA et al. *Fitzpatrick's Dermatology in General Medicine,* 8th ed. New York: McGraw-Hill, 2012, Fig. 192-1. Image B reproduced with permission from Longo DL et al. *Harrison's Principles of Internal Medicine,* 18th ed. New York: McGraw-Hill, 2012, Fig. 184-2.)

Endocrinology

CONGENITAL ADRENAL HYPERPLASIA (CAH)

A group of disorders caused by a defect in 1 or more of the enzymes required for cortisol synthesis. These defects lead to overproduction of the precursors in the pathway and to an excess of ACTH as the body attempts to stimulate the adrenal gland. The most common defect, which accounts for 90–95% of all cases, is in the 21-hydroxylase enzyme. Defects in 11β-hydroxylase and 17α-hydroxylase, as well as other enzymes in the pathway for adrenal steroid synthesis, are less common (see Figure 16-10).

SYMPTOMS/EXAM

- **Classic form:** Has 2 variants—**salt-losing** and **non-salt-losing** CAH.
    - **Girls with either variant:** Present as infants with ambiguous genitalia caused by excess androgen production in utero.
    - **Boys with the salt-losing variant:** Present in the first 1–2 weeks of life with hyponatremia, hyperkalemia, dehydration, and FTT.
    - **Boys with the non-salt-losing variant:** Present with early virilization, including the development of pubic hair, adult body odor, and a growth spurt at 2–4 years of age.
- **Nonclassic form:** Typically presents later with signs of excess androgen production such as hirsutism, acne, early pubarche, irregular menses, and premature closure of the physes.

TREATMENT

- **Glucocorticoid replacement** with hydrocortisone (in infants and younger children) or with dexamethasone or prednisone (in older adolescents) to replace cortisol and suppress androgen production.
- **Mineralocorticoid replacement** with fludrocortisone to normalize sodium and potassium concentrations. Infants should be given supplemental sodium chloride, which can be tapered as they begin to eat table food.
- **Monitoring:** Serum levels of 17-hydroxyprogesterone (17-OHP) and androstenedione, as well as plasma renin activity, should be measured every 3 months in infants and every 4–12 months in children. Bone-age films should be taken every 6 months.

KEY FACT

Children with CAH can have an adrenal crisis with any stressor, including illness or surgery. Immediate glucocorticoid administration at 2–3 times the maintenance dose is required.

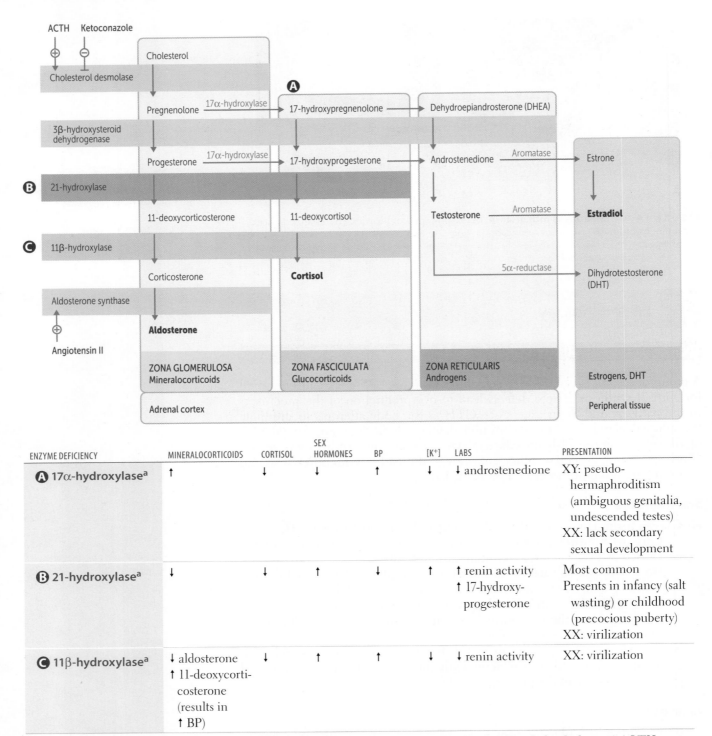

ENZYME DEFICIENCY	MINERALOCORTICOIDS	CORTISOL	SEX HORMONES	BP	[K⁺]	LABS	PRESENTATION
A 17α-hydroxylase[a]	↑	↓	↓	↑	↓	↓ androstenedione	XY: pseudo-hermaphroditism (ambiguous genitalia, undescended testes) XX: lack secondary sexual development
B 21-hydroxylase[a]	↓	↓	↑	↓	↑	↑ renin activity ↑ 17-hydroxy-progesterone	Most common Presents in infancy (salt wasting) or childhood (precocious puberty) XX: virilization
C 11β-hydroxylase[a]	↓ aldosterone ↑ 11-deoxycorti-costerone (results in ↑ BP)	↓	↑	↑	↓	↓ renin activity	XX: virilization

[a]All congenital adrenal enzyme deficiencies are characterized by an enlargement of both adrenal glands due to ↑ ACTH stimulation (due to ↓ cortisol).

FIGURE 16-10. **Adrenal steroids and CAH.** (Reproduced with permission from Le T, Bhushan V. *First Aid for the USMLE Step 1 2015.* New York: McGraw-Hill, 2015:318.)

PRECOCIOUS PUBERTY

Defined as the development of 2° sex characteristics before age 8 in girls and age 9 in boys. The lower limit of normal for girls is somewhat controversial; some use 7 years for Caucasian girls and 6 years for African American girls. Classified as follows:

- **Gonadotropin-dependent precocious puberty (GDPP):** Results from early activation of the hypothalamic-pituitary-gonadal (HPG) axis. Development occurs in the proper sequence and over a normal interval but begins early. Roughly 80% of cases are idiopathic. Other possible etiologies include CNS lesions; therefore, GDPP patients require brain imaging (CT or MRI).
- **Gonadotropin-independent precocious puberty (GIPP):** Not due to early activation of the HPG axis but rather to the secretion of sex hormones from the adrenals or the gonads. Possible causes include exogenous estrogen, ovarian tumors in girls, Leydig cell tumors, CAH, adrenal androgen-secreting tumors, pituitary gonadotropin-secreting tumors, and McCune-Albright syndrome (GIPP, café-au-lait spots, and fibrous dysplasia of bone).

DIAGNOSIS

- **Imaging:** X-rays of the hand and wrist to determine bone age.
- **Labs:** Serum estradiol or testosterone level; 17-OHP; basal and GnRH-stimulated LH; DHEA.
    - **GDPP:** Characterized by prepubertal LH and FSH levels. A GnRH stimulation test must demonstrate a pubertal response for this diagnosis to be made.
    - **GIPP:** Baseline FSH and LH levels are low because of feedback inhibition from exogenous steroid production. GnRH stimulation testing results in a suppressed LH response.
- **Ovarian tumors:** Estradiol levels are ↑ as a result of exogenous secretion.
- **CAH, adrenal androgen-secreting tumors, etc.:** Advanced bone age on x-ray with ↑ androgen levels and androgen metabolites.

TREATMENT

- **GDPP:** GnRH agonists are the therapy of choice if the projected height or rate of development results in a decision to treat.
- **GIPP:** Does not respond to GnRH agonists; treatment depends on the etiology.

Infectious Disease

FEVER WITHOUT A SOURCE (FWS)

Approximately 20% of children with fever do not have signs or symptoms of a bacterial or viral infection on history or exam. FWS is a concern because it may represent an occult serious bacterial infection (SBI). Risk factors include:

- **Girls:** Age < 1 year; fever for ≥ 2 days; temperature ≥ 39°C (102.2°F); Caucasian ethnicity; no other source of infection.
- **Boys:** Fever for > 24 hours; temperature ≥ 39°C; nonblack ethnicity; no other source of infection.

Q   **1**

A 10-day-old male infant is brought to the clinic because he is "acting funny." He is lethargic with poor skin turgor, a sunken fontanelle, and dry lips. His growth curve reveals that he is > 10% below his birth weight despite frequent breast-feeding with good latch. Labs show hyponatremia and hyperkalemia. Beyond evaluating for sepsis, which labs should you consider?

Q   **2**

An 11-month-old, fully immunized girl presents to urgent care with a fever of 39.2°C (102.6°F). She is non–toxic appearing and, although irritable, is consolable with an otherwise unremarkable exam. What workup, if any, should be performed for this child?

DIAGNOSIS

- The concern for SBI, and therefore the recommended workup for FWS, is age dependent.
    - **0–28 days:** See the discussion of neonatal sepsis.
    - **1–3 months:** Obtain a CBC; a blood culture; LP for CSF cell counts, glucose, and protein; and a UA and urine culture. Treat with empiric antibiotics (usually ceftriaxone) if the WBC count is > 15 or < 5.
    - **3–36 months:** If infants in this age group have been vaccinated and appear well, the risk of bacteremia and/or meningitis is low. Obtain a UA and urine culture if the infant is an uncircumcised boy < 1 year of age or a girl < 2 years of age, especially if the fever is > 39°C or has lasted > 48 hours. If unvaccinated, obtain a CBC and a blood culture. Obtain a blood culture and treat with ceftriaxone if the WBC count is > 15.
- **UTI** is the most common bacterial cause of FWS. In infants < 3 months of age, uncircumcised boys are at highest risk. Among infants > 3 months of age, Caucasian girls are at highest risk.
    - Children < 2 months of age with their first UTI require renal bladder ultrasound with VCUG (see Figure 16-11).
    - Significant debate exists in the literature and in practice regarding the utility of VCUG in the setting of a **first** febrile UTI in children > 2 months of age.

MENINGITIS

Inflammation of the meninges; may be bacterial, viral, or fungal. Most children are infected with viruses; however, it is estimated that > 75% of bacterial meningitis cases occur in children < 5 years of age. More than 90% of bacterial etiologies are 2° to *Streptococcus pneumoniae*, *Neisseria meningitidis*, and *Haemophilus influenzae*.

1   **A**

In this setting, congenital adrenal hyperplasia must be considered, and 17-hydroxyprogesterone and androstenedione levels must be sent. The newborn screen should also be reviewed to ensure that other metabolic disorders are not missed.

2   **A**

Aside from her fever and irritability, the child is asymptomatic—ie, she has a fever without an obvious source. In this age group, UTI must be considered. Labs include a UA with culture, a CBC with differential, and a blood culture. LP with CSF analysis should be considered if the patient appears ill or exhibits changes in mental status.

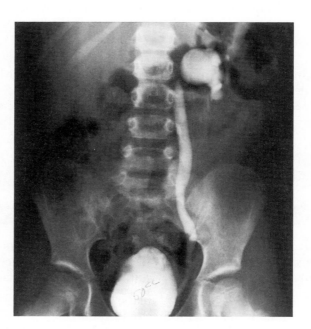

FIGURE 16-11.   Vesicoureteral reflux. Frontal radiograph from a voiding cystourethrogram shows reflux to the left ureter and intrarenal collecting system with hydronephrosis. Note the absence of reflux on the normal right side. (Reproduced with permission from Doherty GM. *Current Diagnosis & Treatment: Surgery,* 13th ed. New York: McGraw-Hill, 2010, Fig. 38-7.)

SYMPTOMS/EXAM

- Infants and children < 1 year of age may present with nondistinct symptoms such as irritability, vomiting, poor feeding, hypo- or hyperthermia, apnea, lethargy, and seizure activity.
- Older children may demonstrate similar symptoms but may also present with photosensitivity, headache, and neck stiffness, although these symptoms may be difficult to elicit depending on the child's age and cooperation with the examiner. Older children may also exhibit signs and symptoms commonly seen in adults, including $\oplus$ Kernig's and Brudzinski's signs.
- Children with Lyme and bacterial meningitis may demonstrate cranial nerve palsies.

DIAGNOSIS

- Depending on the clinical presentation and history, consider a CT scan if there is concern for intracranial bleeding, $\uparrow$ ICP, or trauma.
- Blood tests include a CBC, a chemistry panel that includes serum sodium and glucose levels, a blood culture, and a UA and urine culture. Serum sodium is important in view of risk of hyponatremia 2° to SIADH excretion. Serum glucose is used as a direct comparison to CSF glucose measurement. Consider full-panel sepsis labs.
- Additional tests include LP with CSF analysis to examine the color of the supernatant, cell counts with differential, protein, glucose, microscopic evaluation, and bacterial culture. Table 16-8 describes common characteristics of CSF findings in various infectious and inflammatory states.
- Consider viral PCR testing (including HSV and enteroviruses), encephalitis panels, and fungal cultures depending on clinical presentation and risk factors.

Immunology

IMMUNODEFICIENCY SYNDROMES

Present as recurrent or severe infections. In general, the frequency is roughly 1 in 10,000. Table 16-9 outlines the clinical presentation, diagnosis, and treatment of common pediatric immunodeficiency disorders.

KAWASAKI DISEASE (MUCOCUTANEOUS LYMPH NODE SYNDROME)

A relatively common medium-vessel vasculitis of childhood that predisposes to coronary artery aneurysms and to the subsequent development of myocardial ischemia. More common in children < 5 years of age and among those of Asian, particularly **Japanese**, ethnicity.

SYMPTOMS/EXAM

Presents as an acute illness characterized by the symptoms outlined in the **CRASH and BURN** mnemonic. Children tend to be highly irritable.

DIAGNOSIS

- A clinical diagnosis.
- Patients must have **fever** for **> 5 days** and meet 4–5 of the following criteria: conjunctivitis, rash, at least 1 cervical node > 1 cm, oropharyngeal mucosal changes, hand/foot swelling, and/or desquamation.

MNEMONIC

Kawasaki symptoms—

CRASH and BURN

Conjunctivitis (bilateral, limbic sparing, nonpurulent)
Rash
Adenopathy (at least 1 cervical node > 1 cm)
Strawberry tongue (or any change in oropharyngeal mucosa, including an injected pharynx or lip fissuring)
Hand/foot swelling and/or desquamation
BURN (fever for > 5 days)

TABLE 16-8.   CSF Findings in Normal, Infectious, and Inflammatory Conditions

CSF	INITIAL PRESSURE (mm H$_2$O)	APPEARANCE	CELLS/µL	PROTEIN (mg/dL)
Normal	< 160.	Clear.	0–5 lymphocytes; first 3 months, 1–3 PMNs; neonates, up to 30 lymphocytes, rare RBCs.	15–35 (lumbar), 5–15 (ventricular); up to 150 (lumbar) for a short time after birth; to 6 months up to 65.
Bloody tap	Normal or ↓.	Bloody (sometimes with clot).	One additional WBC/700 RBCs;[b] RBCs not crenated.	One additional milligram per 800 RBCs.[b]
Bacterial meningitis, acute	200–750+.	Opalescent to purulent.	Up to thousands, mostly PMNs; early, few cells.	Up to hundreds.
Bacterial meningitis, partially treated	Usually ↑.	Clear or opalescent.	Usually ↑; PMNs usually predominate.	↑.
Tuberculous meningitis	150–750+.	Opalescent; fibrin web or pellicle.	250–500, mostly lymphocytes; early, ↑ PMNs.	45–500; parallels cell count; ↑ over time.
Fungal meningitis	↑.	Variable; often clear.	10–500; early, ↑ PMNs; then mostly lymphocytes.	Elevated and increasing.
Aseptic meningoencephalitis	Normal or slightly ↑.	Clear unless cell count > 300/µL.	None to a few hundred, mostly lymphocytes; PMNs predominate early.	20–125.
Parainfectious encephalomyelitis	80–450, usually ↑.	Usually clear.	0–50+, mostly lymphocytes; lower numbers, even 0, in MS.	15–75.
Polyneuritis	Normal and occasionally ↑.	Early: normal; late: xanthochromic if protein ↑.	Normal; occasionally slight ↑.	Early: normal; late: 45–1500.

[a] CSF-IgG index = (CSF IgG/serum IgG)/(CSF albumin/serum albumin).

[b] Many studies document pitfalls in using these ratios due to WBC lysis. Clinical judgment and repeat LPs may be necessary to rule out meningitis in this situation.

[c] CSF WBC (predicated) = CSF RBC × (blood WBC/blood RBC). O:P ratio = (observed CSF WBC)/(predicted CSF WBC). Also do WBC:RBC ratio. If O:P ratio ≤ 0.01 and WBC:RBC ratio ≤ 1:100, meningitis is absent.

Adapted with permission from Stone CK, Humphries RL. *Current Diagnosis & Treatment: Emergency Medicine,* 7th ed. New York: McGraw-Hill, 2011, Table 50-14.

Glucose (mg/dL)	Other Tests	Comments
50–80 (two-thirds of blood glucose); may be ↑ after seizure.	CSF-IgG index < 0.7;[a] LDH 2–27 U/L.	CSF protein in the first month may be up to 170 mg/dL in small-for-date or premature infants; no ↑ in WBCs due to seizure.
Normal.	RBC number should ↓ between the first and third tubes; wait 5 minutes between tubes.	Spin down fluid, supernatant will be clear and colorless.[c]
↓; may be none.	Smear and culture are mandatory; LDH > 24 U/L; lactate, IL-8, TNF ↑, correlate with prognosis.	Very early, glucose may be normal; PCR meningococci and pneumococci in plasma; CSF may aid diagnosis.
Normal or ↓.	LDH usually > 24 U/L; PCR may still be ⊕.	Smear and culture may be ⊖ if antibiotics have been used.
↓; may be none.	Smear for acid-fast organisms; CSF culture and inoculation; PCR.	Consider AIDS, a common comorbidity of TB.
↓.	India ink preparations, cryptococcal antigen, PCR, culture, inoculations, immunofluorescence tests.	Often superimposed in patients who are debilitated or on immunosuppressive therapy.
Normal; may be ↓ in mumps, HSV, or other viral infections.	CSF, stool, blood, throat washings for viral cultures; LDH < 28 U/L; PCR for HSV, CMV, EBV, enterovirus, etc.	Acute and convalescent antibody titers for some viruses; in mumps, up to 1000 lymphocytes; serum amylase often ↑; up to 1000 cells present in enteroviral infection.
Normal.	CSF-IgG index, oligoclonal bands variable; in MS, moderate ↑.	No organisms; fulminant cases resemble bacterial meningitis.
Normal.	CSF-IgG index may be ↑; oligoclonal bands variable.	Try to find cause (eg, viral infections, toxins, lupus, diabetes).

TABLE 16-9.   Pediatric Immunodeficiency Disorders

DISORDER	DESCRIPTION	SYMPTOMS	DIAGNOSIS	TREATMENT
B-CELL DISORDERS				
	Most common.	Present with recurrent **URIs** and **bacteremia with encapsulated organisms** (pneumococci, *H influenzae*) and *Staphylococcus* after 6 months of age (when maternal antibodies taper).	**Quantitative Ig levels** (subclasses) and specific antibody responses.	Prophylactic antibiotics and IVIG.
X-linked (**B**ruton's) agammaglobulinemia	A profound **B**-cell deficiency found only in **B**oys.	Approximately 50% of patients are diagnosed by age 2; symptoms start after 3 months of age. Patients are at risk for pseudomonal infection.		
Common variable immunodeficiency (CVID)	Ig levels drop in the second and third decades of life.	Associated with an ↑ risk of lymphoma and autoimmune disease.		
IgA deficiency (most common)	Low IgA.	Usually asymptomatic. Recurrent infection or anaphylaxis to blood transfusion may be noted.		
T-CELL DISORDERS				
		Viral infection, fungal infection, intracellular bacteria (broader range of infections). Present at 1–3 months of age.	**Absolute lymphocyte count,** mitogen stimulation response, and delayed hypersensitivity skin testing.	
Thymic aplasia (DiGeorge syndrome)	Patients are unable to generate T cells because of the lack of a thymus.	**Tetany** (due to hypocalcemia) in the first few days of life.		Consider thymus transplant instead of bone marrow transplant (BMT).
Ataxia-telangiectasia	A DNA repair defect.	Oculocutaneous telangiectasias and progressive cerebellar ataxia.		**BMT** for severe disease; **IVIG** for antibody deficiency.
COMBINED DISORDERS				
			Absolute lymphocyte count and quantitative Ig levels.	
Severe combined immunodeficiency (SCID)	Severe lack of B and T cells.	Frequent and severe bacterial infections, chronic candidiasis, and opportunistic infections.		**BMT or stem-cell transplant;** IVIG for antibody deficiency; **PCP prophylaxis.**

TABLE 16-9. Pediatric Immunodeficiency Disorders *(continued)*

DISORDER	DESCRIPTION	SYMPTOMS	DIAGNOSIS	TREATMENT
COMBINED DISORDERS *(continued)*				
Wiskott-Aldrich syndrome	An X-linked disorder with less severe B- and T-cell dysfunction.	**Eczema,** ↑ IgE, ↑ IgA, ↓ IgM, and **thrombocytopenia.**		**Supportive treatment:** IVIG and aggressive antibiotics. Patients rarely survive to adulthood.
PHAGOCYTIC DISORDERS				
		Commonly caused by catalase-⊕ (*S aureus*) and enteric gram-⊖ organisms.	Absolute neutrophil count; adhesion, chemotactic, phagocytic, and bactericidal assays.	
Chronic granulomatous disease (CGD)	An X-linked or autosomal recessive disorder with deficient superoxide reduction by PMNs and macrophages.	Chronic GI and GU infections; osteomyelitis, hepatitis. Anemia, lymphadenopathy, and hypergammaglobulinemia.	A **nitroblue tetrazolium** test is diagnostic.	**Daily TMP-SMX,** judicious use of antibiotics, γ-interferon.
Chédiak-Higashi syndrome	An autosomal recessive defect in neutrophil chemotaxis.	**Recurrent pyogenic skin and respiratory infections.** Oculocutaneous albinism, neuropathy, neutropenia.	Blood smear shows PMNs with **giant cytoplasmic granules.**	Aggressive treatment of bacterial infections; corticosteroids, splenectomy.
COMPLEMENT DISORDERS				
		Recurrent **sinopulmonary infections,** bacteremia, and/or **meningitis** due to **encapsulated organisms** (*S pneumoniae, H influenzae* type b, *N meningitidis*).		
C1 esterase deficiency (hereditary angioneurotic edema)	An autosomal dominant disorder with recurrent angioedema lasting 21–72 hours.	Presents in late childhood or early **adolescence.** Provoked by stress, trauma, or puberty/menses. Can lead to **life-threatening airway edema.**	Measurement of complement components.	Daily prophylactic antifibrinolytic agents or **danazol.** Purified C1 esterase and FFP prior to surgery.
Terminal complement deficiency (C5–C9)	A deficiency of components of the membrane attack complex (C5–C9). Associated with meningococcal and gonococcal infection.	**Mild, recurrent** infection by *Neisseria* spp. **(meningococcal or gonococcal).** Rarely, SLE or glomerulonephritis.	**Total hemolytic complement (CH$_{50}$);** assess the quantity and function of complement pathway components.	Meningococcal vaccine and appropriate antibiotics.

Adapted with permission from Le T et al. *First Aid for the USMLE Step 2 CK,* 7th ed. New York: McGraw-Hill, 2010: 411–413.

- Occasional findings include arthritis, scrotal swelling, pericarditis, and gallbladder inflammation.
- Labs may reveal sterile pyuria on clean-catch urine (catheterization bypasses the urethral origin of pyuria), ↑ **ESR/CRP,** thrombocytosis, ↑ transaminases, hypoalbuminemia, and hyponatremia.
- Echocardiography may reveal coronary artery aneurysms.

TREATMENT

- Give **high-dose aspirin** during the acute phase for its anti-inflammatory properties and to ↓ the risk of thrombosis.
- Administer **IVIG** to prevent coronary artery aneurysms (given as a single infusion within the first 7–10 days of illness; repeat if the patient is still febrile 24 hours later).
- During the convalescent phase, switch to low-dose aspirin for its antiplatelet effect.
- Follow patients with repeated echocardiography and cardiology follow-up.

COMPLICATIONS

Myocarditis; pericarditis; coronary artery aneurysm predisposing to myocardial ischemia.

Rheumatology

JUVENILE IDIOPATHIC ARTHRITIS (JIA)

Diagnosed after > 6 weeks of arthritis symptoms after all other etiologies of childhood arthritides (eg, IBD) have been excluded. Classified on the basis of several factors:

- Age of symptom onset
- Number and type of joints involved
- The presence of other systemic symptoms
- Clinical course for 6 months after diagnosis

There are 3 main categories: systemic, pauciarticular, and polyarticular.

KEY FACT

Children with JIA are at risk for developing macrophage activation syndrome, which is similar to hemophagocytic lymphohistiocytosis and characterized by a proliferation of macrophages, T cells, and systemic involvement.

Systemic JIA

- **Sx/Exam:** Presents with intermittent fever, rash (macular and salmonpink), and arthritis (usually of the knees, wrists, and ankles, but can affect other joints as well). Diagnosed in patients < 16 years of age; after this age, it is considered adult-onset Still's disease. Affects boys and girls equally.
- **Dx:**
  - Patients are generally worked up for infectious processes and leukemia before a diagnosis is made.
  - WBC count, ESR, CRP, and platelets are ↑.
  - In order for the diagnosis of JIA to be made, the patient must have a daily fever for 2 weeks, typically > 38.5°C (101.3°F), and arthritis. Arthritis may develop after the initial fever and rash.
- **Tx:**
  - **First line:** NSAIDs.
  - **Second line:** Corticosteroids; nonbiologic disease-modifying antirheumatic drugs (DMARDs) such as methotrexate; biologic DMARDs, including IL-1 and IL-6 inhibitors.
  - **Other:** Agents such as thalidomide, IVIG, hydroxychloroquine, sul-

fasalazine, cyclosporine, and TNF inhibitors have been used with varying degrees of success.

- **Cx:** The initial episode of JIA may last 4–6 months. Some children will continue to have fever and rash for years. The long-term sequelae vary from none at all to severe destruction requiring joint replacement.

Pauciarticular JIA

- The most common form of JIA; affects girls more often than boys. Also called oligoarticular arthritis.
- **Sx/Exam:** Involves < 5 joints (generally large joints); usually presents at age 2–3.
- **Dx:** See above. Patients are ANA ⊕.
- **Tx:**
  - **First line:** NSAIDs and/or glucocorticoids injected into affected joints.
  - **Second line:** Methotrexate, TNF inhibitors (rarely used).
- **Cx:**
  - Usually resolves within 6 months.
  - More than 50% of patients will not have relapses; however, severe destructive arthritis may occur.
  - Children with pauciarticular JIA are at risk for uveitis, so routine screening by an ophthalmologist should be done every 3–12 months depending on age of onset and ANA status.

Polyarticular JIA

- Involves > 4 joints; affects girls more often than boys. Age of onset is 2–5 years and 10–14 years.
- **Dx:** See above. Patients may be ANA and/or RF ⊕; lab findings may include anemia, ↑ ESR, and hypergammaglobulinemia.
- **Tx:**
  - NSAIDs are first line but are unlikely to yield long-term control when used as a single agent.
  - **DMARDs** such as methotrexate, leflunomide, sulfasalazine, TNF inhibitors, cyclosporine, azathioprine, rituximab, corticosteroids (systemic and injected), and gold compounds should be added early in the course of treatment.
- **Cx:**
  - The prognosis is generally better for RF-seronegative patients than for those who are seropositive.
  - RF-seronegative patients often respond to NSAID therapy, whereas seropositive patients require treatment with DMARDs.
  - Patients are at risk for uveitis and require screening by an ophthalmologist.

HENOCH-SCHÖNLEIN PURPURA (HSP)

The most common small-vessel vasculitis of childhood. Usually affects children 3–15 years of age. Nearly one-half to two-thirds of cases are preceded by a URI a few weeks before symptom onset.

SYMPTOMS/EXAM

- Presents with palpable purpura (see Figure 16-12), arthritis/arthralgia, abdominal pain, and glomerulonephritis.
- Arthritis is usually oligoarthritis and migratory, affecting the large joints of the lower extremities more often than the upper extremities.

Q   **1**

A 2-year-old girl presents with fever and cough. She is found to have right lower lobe pneumonia both on exam and on CXR. She has been hospitalized twice—once with mastoiditis at 6 months and again with left-sided pneumonia with empyema and bacteremia at 15 months. Her weight is less than the third percentile for age. In addition to an acute workup, what tests would you consider?

Q   **2**

An 8-year-old boy comes to the ED for evaluation of abdominal pain and nausea. Three days ago he developed a fever and a purpuric rash on his lower extremities. Over the past few hours his abdominal pain has worsened. What is your concern, and which studies should be ordered for further evaluation?

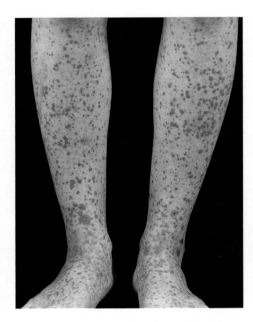

FIGURE 16-12. **Classic palpable purpura in Henoch-Schönlein purpura.** (Reproduced with permission from Wolff K, Johnson RA. *Fitzpatrick's Color Atlas & Synopsis of Clinical Dermatology*, 6th ed. New York: McGraw-Hill, 2009, Fig. 14-35.)

- If renal involvement occurs, it is usually seen within 4 weeks of presentation and is typically self-limited.
- Abdominal pain results from bowel wall edema and inflammation and may be treated with systemic corticosteroids if severe.

DIAGNOSIS

Diagnosis is clinical. If the clinical presentation is unclear, a skin or kidney biopsy with evidence of IgA deposits can confirm the diagnosis.

TREATMENT

Acetaminophen or NSAIDs for pain control +/− glucocorticoids.

COMPLICATIONS

- Intussusception due to bowel wall edema and inflammation can occur.
- Recurs in roughly one-third of cases, generally within 4 months of initial presentation. Recurrences are usually milder than the initial episode.

Cardiology

The incidence of congenital heart disease (CHD) is approximately 1%. The most common congenital heart lesion is VSD, followed by ASD. The most common cyanotic lesion is transposition of the great arteries (TGA).

VENTRICULAR SEPTAL DEFECT (VSD)

A hole in the ventricular septum. Can be membranous (least likely to close spontaneously), perimembranous, or muscular (most likely to close spontaneously).

---

1 **A**

A healthy child is unlikely to have multiple severe infections in different anatomic locations. Therefore, 1° immunodeficiency and other chronic diseases should be considered. Accordingly, a CBC, immunoglobulin levels, antibody titers to vaccinations, and a CH_{50} should be ordered. More specific tests (eg, HIV, CF) can be ordered if indicated.

2 **A**

The patient's history of Henoch-Schönlein purpura raises concern for intussusception. An abdominal ultrasound is the study of choice for initial evaluation.

SYMPTOMS/EXAM

- May be asymptomatic at birth if the lesion is small.
- Cardiac exam may reveal a **pansystolic, vibratory murmur** at the left lower sternal border **without radiation** to the axilla.
- May become symptomatic between 2 and 6 months of age. Symptoms result from flow across the defect, usually from the left to the right ventricle.
- If the lesion is large, it may present with symptoms of **CHF** (shortness of breath, pulmonary edema), frequent **respiratory infection**, FTT, and **exercise/feeding intolerance** (sweating with feeds).
- Look for cardiomegaly and crackles on exam (signs of right heart failure).

DIAGNOSIS

- ECG shows RVH and LVH.
- CXR may show pulmonary edema.
- Echocardiography is definitive.

TREATMENT

- Treat CHF if present.
- Follow small, asymptomatic VSDs.
- Surgically repair large or membranous VSDs to prevent subsequent development of heart failure and pulmonary hypertension.

COMPLICATIONS

If left untreated, VSD may lead to irreversible Eisenmenger's syndrome (pulmonary hypertension, RVH, and reversal of left-to-right shunt).

ATRIAL SEPTAL DEFECT (ASD)

A hole in the atrial septum.

SYMPTOMS/EXAM

- Typically asymptomatic until late childhood or early adulthood.
- Cardiac exam may reveal a **systolic murmur** at the **left upper sternal border.**
- A wide and fixed, split S2 and a heaving cardiac impulse at the left lower sternal border are characteristic signs.
- Progression to CHF and cyanosis may occur in the second or third decade of life and depends on the size of the lesion.

DIAGNOSIS

- ECG shows left-axis deviation.
- CXR reveals cardiomegaly and ↑ pulmonary vascularity (if the defect is large).
- Echocardiography is definitive.

TREATMENT

Treat CHF if present; follow small ASDs. Surgically repair large ASDs in patients with CHF, and repair before the third decade to prevent symptoms.

COMPLICATIONS

Eisenmenger's syndrome.

MNEMONIC

Causes of cyanotic congenital heart disease (right-to-left shunts):

The 5 T's

Truncus arteriosus (1 common artery off of both ventricles)

Transposition of the great arteries (2 vessels switched)

Tricuspid atresia (3 leaflets not well formed)

Tetralogy of Fallot (4 problems present)

Total anomalous pulmonary venous return (5 words)

KEY FACT

Patients with congenital heart disease no longer require prophylactic antibiotics before dental work. Antibiotic prophylaxis is required for:

- Unrepaired or incompletely repaired cyanotic CHD.
- Repaired CHD with a residual defect at or adjacent to the site of a prosthetic patch or device.
- Repaired CHD with prosthetic patches or devices within the first 6 months following the procedure.

PATENT DUCTUS ARTERIOSUS (PDA)

Failure of the ductus arteriosus (the connection between the pulmonary artery and aorta) to close in the first few days of life. Usually results in a **left-to-right shunt** (from the aorta to the pulmonary artery). Risk factors include **prematurity**, high altitude, and maternal first-trimester **rubella** infection.

Symptoms/Exam

- Presentation ranges from asymptomatic to CHF.
- Cardiac exam may reveal a **wide pulse pressure;** a continuous **"machinery" murmur** at the **left upper sternal border;** and bounding peripheral pulses.
- A loud S2 is characteristic.

Diagnosis

Echocardiography is definitive, showing shunt flow as well as left atrial and left ventricular enlargement.

Treatment

- If diagnosed within days of birth, use **indomethacin** to close the PDA.
- Surgical repair is indicated if indomethacin fails or the infant is > 6–8 months of age.

Complications

- In pulmonary hypertension of the newborn (eg, meconium aspiration syndrome), flow may be right to left across a PDA, resulting in persistent cyanosis/hypoxia. A reduction of pulmonary hypertension is required to reduce the right-to-left flow.
- Do not close the PDA in ductal-dependent cyanotic heart lesions (eg, TGA). To keep the ductus open, medications such as alprostadil (a form of prostaglandin E1) may be indicated until definitive repair can be performed.

TETRALOGY OF FALLOT

MNEMONIC

Anatomy of tetralogy of Fallot—

PROVe

Pulmonary stenosis (right ventricular outflow obstruction)
RVH
Overriding aorta
VSD

Consists of 4 lesions (see the mnemonic **PROVe**).

Symptoms/Exam

- Presentation ranges from acyanotic ("pink tet") to profound cyanosis. Most patients have some cyanosis depending on the severity of pulmonary stenosis and the relative right and left ventricular pressures (which determine the direction of flow across the VSD).
- Cyanotic "tet spells" may occur in a child who is crying or overheated. These children should be calmed and given O_2, and squatting or other measures can be used to ↑ systemic vascular resistance and restore left-to-right flow across the VSD.
- Cardiac exam may reveal a **systolic ejection murmur** at the left sternal border along with **right ventricular lift.**
- A single S2 is characteristic.

Diagnosis

- **Echocardiography** is definitive.
- CXR shows a **boot-shaped heart.**

TREATMENT

- If a newborn infant with this condition is cyanotic, administer **prostaglandin E** to maintain the PDA.
- Surgical repair is necessary.
- Treat spells with O_2, a **squatting position, fluids, morphine**, propranolol, and phenylephrine if severe.

TRANSPOSITION OF THE GREAT ARTERIES (TGA)

The aorta arises from the right ventricle and the pulmonary artery from the left ventricle.

SYMPTOMS/EXAM

- Presents with extreme cyanosis from birth.
- May have no murmur.
- **A single, loud S2** is characteristic.

DIAGNOSIS

- **Echocardiography** is definitive.
- CXR shows an **"egg on a string."**
- An O_2 saturation monitor on the right arm (measuring "preductal" saturation) will show a lower O_2 saturation than the one on the lower extremity ("postductal" saturation).

TREATMENT

- Administer **prostaglandin E** to maintain the PDA.
- If necessary, a "balloon septostomy" (Rashkind procedure) may be performed to rupture the atrial septum, thereby improving the mixing of venous and arterial blood and ensuring that adequately saturated blood enters the aorta.
- Surgical repair is necessary.

COARCTATION OF THE AORTA

Narrowing of the lumen of the aorta leads to ↓ blood flow below the obstruction and ↑ flow above it, resulting in upper extremity hypertension and cardiomegaly. Risk factors include **Turner's syndrome** and male gender; also associated with **bicuspid aortic valve.**

SYMPTOMS/EXAM

- Presents with dyspnea with exertion, systemic hypoperfusion/shock, and syncope.
- Cardiac exam may reveal **hypertension in the upper extremities** and a **lower BP in the lower extremities.**
- **↓ femoral and distal lower extremity pulses** are characteristic.

DIAGNOSIS

- **Echocardiography** or **catheterization** is definitive.
- CXR shows **rib notching** due to collateral circulation through the intercostal arteries.

Q

A 12-hour male infant in the nursery develops fussiness, ↑ work of breathing, diaphoresis, and pallor. Exam shows scattered crackles in the lungs and no evidence of murmur. However, his femoral pulses are difficult to appreciate with lower extremity mottling, and brachial-femoral pulse delay is noted. What simple test can you perform to confirm your suspected diagnosis?

TREATMENT

- Surgical repair or balloon angioplasty +/– stent placement.
- Patients require prophylactic antibiotics before dental work even after surgical repair.

COMPLICATIONS

Often recurs. Carries an ↑ risk of intracranial hemorrhage due to cerebral aneurysms.

Gastroenterology

PYLORIC STENOSIS

Hypertrophy of the pylorus leading to gastric outlet obstruction.

SYMPTOMS/EXAM

- Occurs at **3–4 weeks of life** (range 2 weeks to 4 months), predominantly in term, **firstborn** male infants.
- Presents with progressively **projectile, nonbilious emesis** that may lead to dehydration.
- Exam may reveal an **olive-shaped mass** in the epigastrium along with visible peristaltic waves.

DIAGNOSIS

- Electrolytes show **hypochloremic, hypokalemic metabolic alkalosis** 2° to emesis.
- Ultrasound is the gold standard, demonstrating a **hypertrophied pylorus** (see Figure 16-13).
- Barium studies show a **"string sign"** (a narrow pylorus) or a pyloric beak.

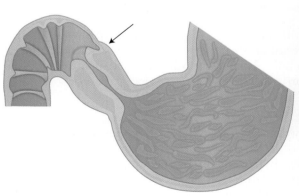
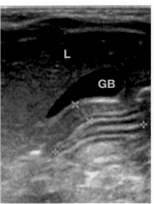

A   **B**

FIGURE 16-13. **Hypertrophic pyloric stenosis.** (A) Schematic representation of a hypertrophied pylorus. The arrow denotes protrusion of the pylorus into the duodenum. (B) Longitudinal ultrasound of the pylorus showing a thickened pyloric musculature (X's) over a long pyloric channel length (plus signs). L = liver; GB = gallbladder. (Image A adapted with permission from Doherty GM. *Current Diagnosis & Treatment: Surgery*, 13th ed. New York: McGraw-Hill, 2010, Fig. 43-9. Image B reproduced with permission from USMLE-Rx.com.)

You strongly suspect coarctation of the aorta, for which 4-extremity blood pressures are performed. A significant gradient is noted between upper and lower extremity blood pressures, and upper extremity hypertension is noted, confirming your diagnosis.

TREATMENT

- First **correct dehydration and electrolyte abnormalities.**
- Surgical repair consists of pyloromyotomy.

INTUSSUSCEPTION

Telescoping of a bowel segment into itself (see Figure 16-14). May lead to edema, arterial occlusion, gut necrosis, and death. Intussusception is the most common cause of bowel obstruction in the first 2 years of life. It is usually idiopathic in children < 2 years of age and often has an identifiable "lead point" (eg, a lymph node) in children > 5 years of age. Ileocecal intussusception is the most common type; ileoileal intussusception may have a pathologic cause.

SYMPTOMS/EXAM

- The classic presentation consists of bouts of **paroxysmal abdominal pain.** The child is often comfortable between paroxysms. Vomiting and heme-⊕ stools may be seen. "Currant jelly" stool (reddish-purple stool mixed with mucus and blood) is a late finding.
- May present with altered mental status (lethargy or even obtundation) and may be preceded by a viral illness.
- Abdominal exam may reveal a **palpable, sausage-shaped mass.**

DIAGNOSIS

- Abdominal ultrasound is the initial step for workup.
- An air-contrast enema or a water-soluble contrast enema is both **diagnostic and therapeutic for ileocecal intussusceptions.**

TREATMENT

- Following reduction via enema, treat with supportive care.
- If reduction fails or if perforation is suspected, surgical intervention may be required.

COMPLICATIONS

May be associated with HSP, CF, and ongoing viral infections.

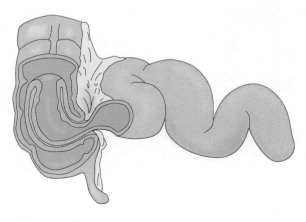

FIGURE 16-14. Intussusception.

MALROTATION/VOLVULUS

Distinguished as follows:

- **Malrotation:** Failure of gut rotation in the abdominal cavity during the tenth week of gestation. Results in abnormal location of intestinal contents as well as incomplete fixation to the posterior abdominal wall. May predispose to intestinal obstruction (by a tissue called "Ladd's bands" that abnormally lies over the proximal duodenum in malrotation) or volvulus.
- **Volvulus:** A complication of malrotation in which the malrotated gut twists on the axis of the superior mesenteric artery, resulting in intestinal obstruction and ischemia.

SYMPTOMS/EXAM

- **First 3 weeks of life:** Volvulus presents as acute onset of **bilious emesis,** small bowel obstruction, or bowel necrosis.
- **Later in infancy/early childhood:** Malrotation may present as acute or intermittent intestinal obstruction, malabsorption, protein-losing enteropathy, or diarrhea.

DIAGNOSIS

- **Malrotation:** An **upper GI series** shows the duodenojejunal junction on the right side of the spine (see Figure 16-15). Barium enema shows a mobile cecum that is not in the RLQ.
- **Volvulus:** Contrast studies show a **"bird's beak"** where the gut is twisted.

TREATMENT

Volvulus is a **surgical emergency requiring repair** because vascular occlusion may result in tissue ischemia and necrosis. Asymptomatic patients require surgical repair in view of the risk of volvulus and associated complications.

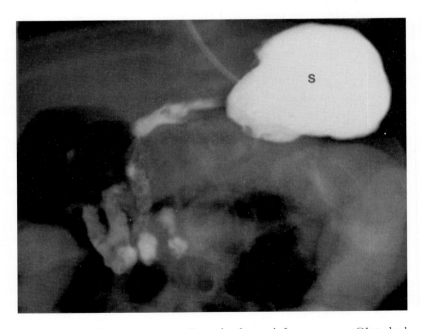

FIGURE 16-15.   **Midgut malrotation.** Frontal radiograph from an upper GI study shows a spiral pattern of duodenal and proximal jejunal loops in the right abdomen, consistent with midgut malrotation. The duodenal-jejunal junction should normally be to the left of the patient's spine. S = stomach. (Reproduced with permission from USMLE-Rx.com.)

COMPLICATIONS

- The 1° complication, "short bowel syndrome" following surgical bowel resection, occurs when < 30 cm of short bowel is left, resulting in poor intestinal absorption.
- If a large segment of bowel is lost as a result of bowel ischemia or surgery, the condition may also lead to malnutrition, TPN dependence, and liver failure.

MECKEL'S DIVERTICULUM

A remnant of the omphalomesenteric duct that persists as an outpouching of the distal ileum. Can contain ectopic (usually gastric or pancreatic) mucosa.

SYMPTOMS/EXAM

- Often asymptomatic.
- Patients may present with **painless rectal bleeding** or **intussusception** (with Meckel's as the lead point).

DIAGNOSIS

- Order a **technetium radionuclide scan** ("Meckel scan") to detect gastric mucosa.
- The gold standard is tissue obtained surgically.

TREATMENT

- Stabilize the patient with IV fluids; transfuse if needed.
- Surgical exploration is indicated if the patient is symptomatic.
- Bowel resection may be required with resection of diverticula depending on the location and complexity of the lesion.

NECROTIZING ENTEROCOLITIS

Intestinal necrosis occurring primarily in a watershed distribution. The most common GI emergency of newborns. Risk factors include prematurity and **CHD.**

SYMPTOMS/EXAM

- Presents with abdominal distention, retention of gastric contents and feeds, abdominal wall tenderness and discoloration, and bloody stools.
- **Nonspecific symptoms** include apnea, respiratory failure, lethargy, poor feeding, temperature instability, thrombocytopenia, hypoglycemia, and hypotension/shock.

DIAGNOSIS

AXR shows **pneumatosis intestinalis** and possibly portal venous gas and **free intraperitoneal air** (see Figure 16-16).

TREATMENT

- Medical management with IV fluids (no enteral feeds) and antibiotics if the patient is hemodynamically stable and/or too small or sick to go to the OR.
- **Surgical management (resection of necrotic bowel)** is necessary in the setting of extensive disease and/or hemodynamic instability.

MNEMONIC

Meckel's diverticulum rule of 2's:

2 feet proximal to the ileocecal valve
2 types of ectopic tissue (gastric, pancreatic)
2% of the population
2 times the number of males as females
Usually presents by age **2**
About **2** inches long
2 cm in diameter

A 3-week-old infant born at 28 weeks' gestation is at his goal feeds. This evening he developed emesis with heme-⊕ stools and an ↑ in abdominal girth. You obtain blood and stool cultures and AXRs. Pneumatosis is noted in the bowel wall and portal venous system. What are the next steps in management?

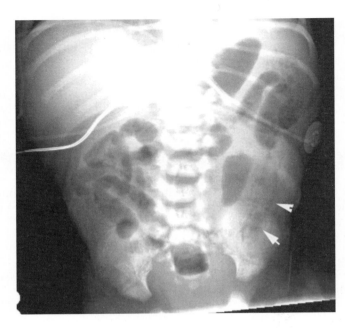

FIGURE 16-16. **Necrotizing enterocolitis.** Short arrows highlight pneumatosis intestinalis on an abdominal radiograph of a patient with NEC. (Reproduced with permission from Brunicardi FC et al. *Schwartz's Principles of Surgery,* 10th ed. New York: McGraw-Hill, 2015, Fig. 39-19.)

Pulmonology

CROUP (LARYNGOTRACHEOBRONCHITIS)

An acute viral inflammatory disease of the larynx/subglottic space (see Table 16-10). Most common in children 3 months to 3 years of age. Commonly caused by parainfluenza virus (PIV) type 1, but may also be caused by other PIVs as well as by RSV, influenza, rubeola, adenovirus, and *Mycoplasma pneumoniae.*

SYMPTOMS/EXAM

- Typically has a 1- to 2-day viral prodrome with URI symptoms.
- Also presents with low-grade fever, mild dyspnea, and inspiratory stridor that worsens with agitation and may improve with cool air or a warm shower.
- Listen for the characteristic **barking cough.**

DIAGNOSIS

- Based on clinical findings.
- A **"steeple sign"** formed by subglottic narrowing may be seen on frontal neck x-ray (see Figure 16-17A).

TREATMENT

- Mist therapy (for mild croup only); oral or IM/IV dexamethasone (for mild or moderate croup); nebulized racemic epinephrine if stridor is present at rest.

A

This patient has necrotizing enterocolitis, which is an emergency! The pediatric surgical team should be consulted and the patient made NPO. Intermittent NG suctioning should be started, IV antibiotics administered (piperacillin + tazobactam or ampicillin + gentamicin), electrolytes monitored, and TPN or IV fluids initiated.

TABLE 16-10. Characteristics of Croup, Epiglottitis, and Tracheitis

	TRACHEITIS	CROUP	EPIGLOTTITIS
Age group	3 months to 2 years	3 months to 3 years	3–7 years
Incidence in children presenting with stridor	2%	88%	8%
Pathogen	Often *S aureus*	PIV	Formerly *H influenzae;* now *S pneumoniae* and *S aureus.*
Onset	Prodrome (3 days) leads to acute decompensation (10 hours)	Prodrome (1–7 days)	Rapid (4–12 hours)
Fever severity	Intermediate grade	Low grade	High grade
Associated symptoms	Variable respiratory distress	Barking cough, hoarseness	Muffled voice, drooling
Position preference	None	None	Seated, neck extended
Response to racemic epinephrine	Slight improvement	Marked improvement	Slight improvement
Neck film findings	Subglottic narrowing may be seen on lateral film	"Steeple sign" on AP films	"Thumbprint sign" on lateral film

Adapted with permission from Le T et al. *First Aid for the USMLE Step 2 CK,* 7th ed. New York: McGraw-Hill, 2010: 417.

- Heliox and ICU admission for severe croup.
    - Heliox is typically administered at a ratio of 70% helium to 30% O_2 to ↓ the resistance of airflow through a narrowed airway by replacing nitrogen with helium.
    - This can act as an intermediary step before intubation for children who show evidence of airway compromise and risk progression to respiratory failure.
- Hospitalize patients with stridor at rest or those needing > 1 dose of racemic epinephrine.

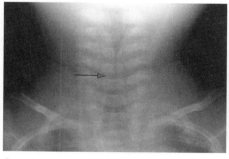
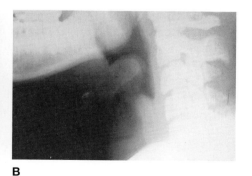

A   B

FIGURE 16-17. **Croup vs epiglottitis.** (A) Croup. X-ray shows marked subglottic narrowing of the airway (arrow). (B) Epiglottitis. The classic swollen epiglottis ("thumbprint sign") and obstructed airway are seen. (Reproduced with permission from Stone CK, Humphries RL. *Current Diagnosis & Treatment: Emergency Medicine,* 7th ed. New York: McGraw-Hill, 2011, Fig. 32-10A and 50-4.)

EPIGLOTTITIS

A serious and rapidly progressive infection of the epiglottis and contiguous structures that can lead to **life-threatening airway obstruction.** It is increasingly rare because of the Hib vaccine and is now most commonly caused by S *pneumoniae* or S *aureus.*

SYMPTOMS/EXAM

- Maintain a high index of suspicion in children with sudden-onset high fever, dysphagia, drooling, a muffled voice, inspiratory retractions, cyanosis, and soft stridor.
- Patients may be in the "sniffing" position, with the neck hyperextended and the chin protruding. These patients should be identified and stabilized rapidly, as the disease can quickly progress to complete airway obstruction and respiratory arrest.

DIAGNOSIS

- Diagnosis is based on the clinical picture.
- **Do not attempt to examine the throat unless the patient is in the OR** with an anesthesiologist present.
- Lateral neck films show the characteristic **"thumbprint sign"** of a swollen epiglottis obliterating the valleculae (see Figure 16-17B).

TREATMENT

- Keep the patient calm, call anesthesia and otolaryngology immediately, and transfer to the OR. If the patient is unstable, do not delay treatment by getting a neck film.
- Treat with endotracheal intubation and IV antibiotics.

KEY FACT

In epiglottitis, throat examination may cause laryngospasm and airway obstruction.

PERTUSSIS

Commonly known as "whooping cough." The causative agent is *Bordetella pertussis* or *Bordetella parapertussis.*

SYMPTOMS/EXAM

The disease has 3 stages:

- **Catarrhal:** Presents with nasal congestion, sneezing, and low-grade fever.
- **Paroxysmal:** Presents with intense coughing paroxysms followed by a "whoop" in young children. Neonates and infants may experience cyanosis and apnea after coughing fits.
- **Convalescent:** Characterized by a chronic cough that may last for weeks (also known as "hundred-day cough"). Patients are no longer shedding the organism during this phase.

DIAGNOSIS

Diagnosed by a nasopharyngeal swab that is ⊕ by PCR or culture for B *pertussis.*

TREATMENT

- Erythromycin or azithromycin is recommended if the diagnosis is made before the convalescent phase, when the patient is still contagious.
- Vaccination is key to preventing asymptomatic family members from spreading the infection to children.

BRONCHIOLITIS

The most common lower respiratory illness in childhood, and a leading cause of hospitalization in infants and young children. Peak incidence is at 2–8 months of age, from October to March. Symptoms are due to virally induced inflammation of the small airways, resulting in edema, mucous plugging, and sloughing of epithelial cells, causing bronchiolar obstruction.

SYMPTOMS/EXAM

- Infants present with fever, nasal congestion, and varying degrees of hypoxemia, tachypnea, retractions, and loud rhonchi on lung exam.
- Wheezing can occur, especially in children with no personal or family history of wheeze.

DIAGNOSIS

- Diagnosis is clinical and is based on the characteristic age, history, and exam findings.
- Can be caused by many viruses; RSV, influenza, human metapneumovirus, and rhinovirus are commonly tested for by nasopharyngeal swab.
- CXR shows nonspecific bilateral perihilar infiltrates as well as hyperinflation and peribronchial cuffing.

TREATMENT

- Supportive care with nasal suctioning, nebulized hypertonic saline, and O_2. Because infants and young children are obligate nose breathers, feeding difficulties may occur when they are in respiratory distress, necessitating close management of hydration and nutrition.
- Patients may or may not respond to albuterol, racemic epinephrine, and/or systemic corticosteroids. Use of these medications is not routinely recommended.
- Ribavirin can be used for immunocompromised patients and/or severe cases. Endotracheal intubation is indicated for respiratory failure.

CYSTIC FIBROSIS (CF)

A mutation of the CFTR gene in which an abnormal CFTR protein functions as a cAMP-regulated chloride channel and other ion channels, resulting in multisystem dysfunction.

- Frequently diagnosed in childhood; only ~ 5% of cases are diagnosed in adulthood.
- Most often affects the lungs, resulting in chronic bacterial infections and bronchiectasis, exocrine pancreatic dysfunction, abnormal sweat production, intestinal dysfunction, and urodynamics. See Chapter 18 for more detailed coverage.

Neurology

FEBRILE SEIZURES

Benign, self-limited seizures that occur in children 6 months to 6 years of age at the onset of a febrile illness. A ⊕ family history is common. Febrile seizures may be simple or complex:

- **Simple:** A generalized seizure characterized by a short duration (< 15 minutes), 1 seizure per 24-hour period, and a quick return to normal function with no residual focal neurologic deficit.
- **Complex:** A seizure associated with a febrile illness that does not meet the above criteria. The seizure may be focal; may have a longer duration (> 15 minutes); may recur in a 24-hour period; or may result in incomplete or slow return to normal neurologic status.

DIAGNOSIS/TREATMENT

- **Simple:** Treatment is focused on determining the source of the fever and providing supportive care, but no further neurologic evaluation is needed.
- **Complex:** Depending on the history, the severity of the seizure, and exam findings, consider performing laboratory or radiologic workup for other etiologies of seizure, such as electrolyte abnormalities, toxic ingestion, sepsis, CNS infection, or CNS trauma.
- **Strongly consider LP in patients < 12 months of age with complex febrile seizures** as well as in any child who has focal neurologic deficits before or after the seizure.
- EEG and MRI are not routinely recommended for children with febrile seizures. They may be considered on an outpatient basis in a child with a complex febrile seizure, especially a focal seizure or one resulting in prolonged neurologic defects.
- Family education and anticipatory guidance are essential. Although febrile seizures are benign, 30–50% of children with a febrile seizure will have another one before they outgrow the syndrome.
- Febrile seizures cannot be prevented with the use of antipyretics, and anticonvulsants are not routinely recommended. Complications from anticonvulsant use typically outweigh their utility.

EPILEPSY SYNDROMES

Table 16-11 outlines the presentation and treatment of common epilepsy syndromes affecting the pediatric population.

KEY FACT

Hypsarrhythmia on EEG is characterized by slow, high-amplitude waves with random spikes that originate in all cortical areas with no identified pattern or rhythm.

Oncology

Hematologic malignancies (leukemia and lymphoma) are the most common form of malignancy in children. Solid tumors in pediatrics most commonly occur in the CNS, bone, and kidneys. These topics are covered in Chapter 9.

WILMS' TUMOR

An embryonal tumor of renal origin. Wilms' tumor is the most common renal tumor in children and is usually seen in those 1–4 years of age. Risk factors include a ⊕ family history, neurofibromatosis, aniridia (WAGR syndrome), Beckwith-Wiedemann syndrome, and congenital GU anomalies (eg, Denys-Drash syndrome).

SYMPTOMS/EXAM

- Patients may have abdominal pain or may present with a painless abdominal or flank mass.
- Hematuria and hypertension are commonly seen.

TABLE 16-11. **Common Pediatric Epilepsy Syndromes**

Syndrome	Syndrome/Exam	Diagnosis	Treatment
Absence seizures	Multiple, brief staring episodes.	A generalized, **3-Hz, spike-and-wave** pattern on EEG.	Ethosuximide.
Infantile spasms (West syndrome)	Affects infants < 1 year of age, presenting with **"jackknife"** spasms and psychomotor arrest/**developmental regression.**	**Hypsarrhythmia** on EEG. Associated with tuberous sclerosis.	ACTH.
Lennox-Gastaut syndrome	The first seizure occurs between 1 and 7 years of age. Presents with multiple, progressive, difficult-to-treat seizure types, including generalized tonic-clonic seizures (GTCS) and drop attacks.	An atypical **spike-and-wave** pattern, primarily in the frontal region, on EEG. Progressive mental retardation. Associated with refractory infantile spasms and tuberous sclerosis.	No effective treatment.
Juvenile myoclonic epilepsy	Affects healthy adolescents, presenting with myoclonic jerks or GTCS in the **early-morning hours/upon awakening.**	May have a genetic basis; patients often have a ⊕ family history.	Easily treated with a variety of antiepileptic medications.
Benign partial epilepsy	Affects healthy children, presenting with partial seizures during wakefulness (oral, vocal, upper extremity symptoms). May spread to GTCS during sleep.	Classic **interictal** spikes from the centrotemporal (rolandic) region.	Seizures usually disappear by adolescence.
Landau-Kleffner syndrome	Those affected are developmentally normal children who **lose language ability** between 3 and 6 years of age. Often confused with autism.	A bilateral temporal spike and sharp waves on EEG.	Antiepileptic medications may improve the long-term prognosis but cannot reverse language loss.

Data from Hay WW et al. *Current Pediatric Diagnosis & Treatment,* 18th ed. New York: McGraw-Hill, 2007: 721–725.

- Systemic symptoms include weight loss, nausea, emesis, bone pain, dysuria, and polyuria.

DIAGNOSIS

- Initially, an abdominal CT or ultrasound should be obtained.
- CXR, chest CT, CBC, LFTs, and BUN/creatinine can be used to assess severity and spread.
- Excisional biopsy to confirm.

TREATMENT

- Transabdominal nephrectomy followed by postoperative chemotherapy (vincristine/dactinomycin).
- Flank irradiation is of benefit in some cases.
- The prognosis is usually good but depends on staging and tumor histology.

NEUROBLASTOMA

A tumor of neural crest cell origin that most commonly affects children < 5 years of age; the most common solid tumor during infancy. Risk factors include neurofibromatosis, tuberous sclerosis, pheochromocytoma, and Hirschsprung's disease.

SYMPTOMS/EXAM

- Lesions can appear anywhere in the body (eg, the skin or skull).
- Presentations include abdominal mass/distention/hepatomegaly, anorexia, weight loss, respiratory distress, fatigue, fever, diarrhea, irritability, or neuromuscular symptoms (if paraspinal).
- Other symptoms include leg edema, hypertension, and periorbital bruising ("raccoon eyes").

DIAGNOSIS

- Definitive diagnosis is based on a tumor tissue sample with or without ↑ urine catecholamines (VMA and HVA) or on metastases to bone marrow with ↑ urine catecholamines.
- The initial workup generally includes a CBC, electrolytes, LDH, ferritin, LFTs, a coagulation screen, urine catecholamines, and BUN/creatinine.
- To stage and assess severity, obtain bilateral iliac crest bone marrow biopsies, an abdominal CT or MRI, a CXR, bone radiographs, and a technetium radionuclide scan or ^{131}I-metaiodobenzylguanidine (MIBG) scan.

TREATMENT

- Localized tumors are usually cured with excision.
- Chemotherapy includes cyclophosphamide, carboplatin or cisplatin, etoposide or teniposide, vincristine, and doxorubicin.
- Radiation can be used as an adjunct.
- The prognosis is improved if the diagnosis is made before age 1. Staging is based on the International Neuroblastoma Staging System.

RETINOBLASTOMA

The most common intraocular malignancy in children; usually diagnosed before age 2. One-quarter of cases are bilateral.

SYMPTOMS/EXAM

- Usually presents with leukocoria and/or strabismus.
- Can be sporadic or inherited; the inherited form is associated with an ↑ risk of additional malignancies, including osteogenic sarcoma, soft tissue sarcomas, and malignant melanoma.
- Generally begins to metastasize within 6 months, so early diagnosis is critical.

DIAGNOSIS

Diagnosis is made by indirect ophthalmoscopic exam (with dilated pupils).

TREATMENT

- Determined by the size and location of the tumor.
- Treatment options include enucleation, external beam radiation therapy, radioactive plaque therapy (^{125}I brachytherapy), cryotherapy with laser photocoagulation, and chemotherapy.

- The chemotherapy regimen of vincristine, carboplatin, and etoposide is also used for chemoreduction of large tumors before the initiation of other therapies.
- Tumor cell lysis results in severe hyperkalemia, hyperphosphatemia, and large amounts of serum nucleic acids, leading to hyperuricemia. Hypocalcemia is also present 2° to calcium phosphate deposition.
- The condition can quickly lead to renal failure.
- Clinical manifestations may also include seizure, cardiac arrhythmia, or sudden death.

TREATMENT

The most effective approach is to prevent the syndrome from occurring by providing adequate IV hydration, urinary alkalinization using sodium bicarbonate and/or acetazolamide, and uric acid reduction using allopurinol or rasburicase (the drug of choice if uric acid levels are high before the initiation of chemotherapy).

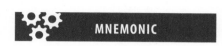
MNEMONIC

Mnemonic for trisomies:

Down syndrome: **D**rinking age/trisomy **21**.
Edwards' syndrome: **E**lection age/trisomy **18**.
Patau's syndrome: **P**uberty/trisomy **13**.

Genetics

COMMON GENETIC DISORDERS

Table 16-12 outlines the presentation and diagnosis of genetic syndromes.

TABLE 16-12. Common Genetic Syndromes

SYNDROME	SYMPTOMS	EXAM	DIAGNOSIS	PROGNOSIS
Trisomy 21 (incidence 1:600)	Hypotonia, brachycephalic head, slanted palpebral fissures, dysplasia of the midphalanx of the fifth finger, single transverse palmar crease.	Cognitive delay, cardiac defects, thyroid disease, GI atresias, atlantoaxial instability, leukemia.	Karyotype, baseline echocardiogram, TFTs, LFTs, CBC.	Fifty percent of those with congenital heart defects survive to 30 years; 80% of those without such defects survive to 30 years. Most who reach age 40 develop Alzheimer's disease.
Trisomy 18 (incidence 1:4000; 3:1 female predominance)	Clenched hand/overlapping fingers, intrauterine growth retardation, cardiac defects, rocker-bottom feet.	Profound cognitive delay.	Karyotype with fluorescence in situ hybridization (FISH) analysis.	Fifty percent die by 1 week and 90% by 1 year.
Trisomy 13 (incidence 1:12,000)	CNS malformations, polydactyly, seizures, deafness, sloping forehead, aplasia cutis, cleft lip/cleft palate, microphthalmia/eye defects, cardiac defects.	Profound cognitive delay.	Karyotype with FISH analysis.	Forty-four percent die within 1 month; > 70% die by 1 year.

TABLE 16-12. **Common Genetic Syndromes** *(continued)*

SYNDROME	SYMPTOMS	EXAM	DIAGNOSIS	PROGNOSIS
22q11 syndrome (DiGeorge syndrome, velocardiofacial syndrome) (incidence 1:4000)	Congenital heart disease, palatal abnormalities, prominent/ squared nose, thymic hypoplasia/immune deficiency, absent parathyroid glands/ hypocalcemia.	Mild to moderate cognitive delay. Most have speech and language delay, learning disabilities, and feeding difficulties. Psychotic symptoms are common.	FISH analysis for 22q11.2 deletion. Serum calcium, absolute lymphocyte count, renal ultrasound, baseline echocardiogram.	Parents should be tested for being carriers of the deletion.
Turner's syndrome (45,XO) (incidence 1:10,000)	Short female with shield chest, widely spaced nipples, a webbed neck, and congenital lymphedema.	Cognitive delay, gonadal dysgenesis, renal anomalies, cardiac defects (coarctation of the aorta), hearing loss.	Karyotype for diagnosis. Baseline echocardiogram, renal ultrasound, BP, hearing screen.	Infertility; normal life span.
Fragile X syndrome (incidence 1:1500 males)	Boys present with macrocephaly, large ears, macroorchidism, and tall stature. Girls may present only with learning disabilities.	Mild to profound cognitive delay, autism.	DNA analysis shows expansion of a CGG nucleotide repeat in the FMR1 gene. The size of the repeat correlates with disease severity.	Normal life span.
Marfan's syndrome (incidence 1:10,000)	Tall stature, low upper-to-lower-segment ratio, arachnodactyly, joint laxity, scoliosis, pectus excavatum or carinatum, lens dislocation, retinal detachment, dilation of the aortic root, mitral valve prolapse, lumbosacral dural ectasia, high-arched palate.	Normal intelligence.	Slit-lamp examination, echocardiography, genetic evaluation. Diagnosis is clinical.	With treatment/ corrective surgery of aortic root dilation, patients have a normal life span.

Data from Hay WW et al. *Current Diagnosis & Treatment: Pediatrics,* 18th ed. New York: McGraw-Hill, 2007: 721–725.

PSYCHIATRY

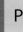

Pharmacotherapy

Benzodiazepines

- **Applications:** Used for anxiety, alcohol withdrawal, insomnia, anesthesia, seizures, and muscle spasms. Have **rapid onset of action; augment sedation and respiratory depression** from other CNS depressants (eg, alcohol). Where possible, use only on a short-term basis (eg, no more than 2–3 months) or occasionally PRN.
- **Interactions:** P-450 inhibitors (eg, cimetidine, fluoxetine) ↑ levels; carbamazepine and rifampin ↓ levels.
- **Relative contraindications:** Disadvantages include a risk of abuse, tolerance, dependence, and withdrawal. May also induce delirium in the elderly and/or critically ill patients. Avoid in patients who are at high risk for falling.

Zolpidem

A nonbenzodiazepine used for insomnia. ↓ sleep latency and ↑ total sleep time. Has rapid onset; withdrawal is rare.

Buspirone

- **Mechanism of action:** A 5-HT$_{1A}$ partial agonist.
- **Applications:** Used for GAD and chronic anxiety; for the augmentation of depression or OCD therapy; and for patients with a history of substance abuse. May also be used when sedation poses a potential risk. Unlike benzodiazepines, it has **no anticonvulsant or muscle relaxant properties.** Also has few side effects and no tolerance, dependence, or withdrawal.
- **Relative contraindications:** Has slow onset of action and lower efficacy than benzodiazepines. Should not be used with MAOIs. **Not effective as a PRN anxiolytic** (chronic increases in 5-HT are anxiolytic, but acute increases cause anxiety).

Antihistamines

Used for the short-term management of insomnia and for preoperative sedation.

Selective Serotonin Reuptake Inhibitors (SSRIs)

- Include **fluoxetine, sertraline, paroxetine, citalopram, escitalopram,** and **fluvoxamine.**
- **Applications:** First-line therapy for **depression** and many **anxiety disorders.** Well tolerated, effective, and relatively safe in overdose.
- **Interactions:** Can ↑ warfarin levels because of P-450 interactions.
- **Side effects: Sexual dysfunction,** nausea, diarrhea, anorexia, headache, anxiety, weight gain, tremor, sleep disturbance.

Atypical Antidepressants

- **Bupropion:**
  - **Mechanism of action:** Dopamine reuptake inhibition. Metabolite weakly blocks norepinephrine (NE) reuptake.

MNEMONIC

Benzodiazepines are metabolized—

Outside The Liver

Oxazepam
Temazepam
Lorazepam
(Metabolized via hepatic glucuronidation; safe to use in liver failure.)

KEY FACT

Diazepam is longer-acting than lorazepam.

KEY FACT

Antidepressant use during pregnancy carries the risk of abstinence syndrome and pulmonary hypertension in the neonate. However, untreated depression carries a risk of low birth weight.

- **Applications:** First-line therapy for depression and **smoking cessation.** Effective for patients who have had sexual side effects from other antidepressants.
- **Side effects:** Common side effects include anxiety, agitation, and insomnia. Can worsen tics. Also **lowers seizure threshold,** especially in the setting of rapid or large dose increases or immediate-release preparations. Not associated with weight gain.
- **Relative contraindications:** A history of seizure disorder, eating disorders, or head trauma.
- **Venlafaxine:**
  - **Mechanism of action:** The main action is 5-HT and NE reuptake inhibition.
  - **Applications:** Used for major depression and GAD.
  - **Side effects:** Adverse effects include **diastolic hypertension (monitor BP),** insomnia, nervousness, sedation, **sexual dysfunction,** anticholinergic effects, and nausea.
- **Mirtazapine:**
  - **Mechanism of action:** An α_2-antagonist that enhances NE and 5-HT. Does not affect the P-450 system. More effective as part of dual therapy.
  - **Side effects:** Sedation (worse in **lower** doses) and **weight gain.** Has little effect on sexual function.
- **Trazodone:**
  - **Mechanism of action:** Primarily inhibits 5-HT reuptake. At lower doses, may be **helpful in insomnia.**
  - **Side effects:** Sedation, **priapism.**

Tricyclic Antidepressants (TCAs)

- Include **nortriptyline, desipramine, imipramine, amitriptyline, clomipramine,** and **doxepin.** TCAs are considered to be **second-line agents** owing to their relatively poor side effect profile compared with the newer antidepressants, along with the risk of dysrhythmias, and even death, from an overdose.
- **Mechanism of action:** Block the reuptake of NE and serotonin.
- **Applications:** Useful for chronic pain and migraines. **OCD responds to clomipramine.**
- **Interactions:** Levels ↑ when used with SSRIs because of P-450 competition. Also interact with ranitidine and warfarin.
- **Side effects:**
  - **Anticholinergic:** Dry mouth, blurry vision, constipation, urinary retention.
  - **Cardiac:** Orthostatic hypotension; cardiac conduction delays with **prolonged PR and QRS intervals.** Contraindicated in patients with a history of heart block and in those at high risk of suicide. Obtain a baseline ECG before initiating therapy, and use with caution in the elderly.
  - **Other:** Sedation, weight gain.

Monoamine Oxidase Inhibitors (MAOIs)

- Include **phenelzine, selegiline,** and **tranylcypromine.** MAOIs are considered to be **second-line agents** owing to their relatively poor side effect profile compared to the newer antidepressants.
- **Side effects:**
  - Common side effects include orthostatic hypotension, insomnia, weight gain, edema, and sexual dysfunction.
  - May lead to **tyramine-induced hypertensive crisis.** Dietary restric-

KEY FACT

Antidepressants are the preferred long-term treatment for anxiety but can initially be anxiogenic. Bupropion in particular should not be used with anxiety disorders.

KEY FACT

Duloxetine has a profile similar to that of venlafaxine but has a less pronounced effect on BP.

KEY FACT

- **"Activating" antidepressants:** Bupropion, venlafaxine, SSRIs/MAOIs.
- **"Sedating" antidepressants:** Trazodone, mirtazapine, amitriptyline.

KEY FACT

TCAs may be lethal in an overdose.

MNEMONIC

TCA toxicity—

Trembling (convulsions)
Coma
Arrhythmias

MNEMONIC

Side effects of MAOIs—

The 6 H's

Hepatocellular jaundice/necrosis
Hypotension (postural)
Headache
Hyperreflexia
Hallucinations
Hypomania

KEY FACT

"Augmentation" strategies for antidepressants:
1. Lithium (with TCAs)
2. Triiodothyronine (with TCAs or SSRIs)
3. Mirtazapine
4. Aripiprazole (with SSRIs)
5. Buspirone
6. Bupropion

tions include aged cheeses, sour cream, yogurt, pickled herring, cured meats, and certain alcoholic beverages (eg, Chianti wine).

- Potentially fatal **serotonin syndrome** can occur if MAOIs are combined with SSRIs, TCAs, meperidine, fentanyl, or indirect sympathomimetics (eg, those found in some **OTC cold remedies**).

ANTIPSYCHOTICS

First-Generation ("Typical") Antipsychotics

- **Mechanism of action:** Act through dopamine receptor blockade.
- **Applications:** Used for psychotic disorders and acute agitation. Cheap and effective. Examples include:
  - **High-potency agents** (haloperidol, fluphenazine): ↓ only positive symptoms of psychosis. **Associated with more extrapyramidal symptoms (EPS).**
  - **Low-potency agents** (thioridazine, chlorpromazine): Associated with more sedation, anticholinergic effects, and hypotension.
- **Side effects:** Key side effects include:
  - **EPS:** Result from excessive cholinergic effect (see Table 17-1).
  - **Hyperprolactinemia:** Amenorrhea, gynecomastia, galactorrhea.
  - **Anticholinergic effects:** Dry mouth, blurry vision, constipation, urinary retention.
  - **Neuroleptic malignant syndrome.**
  - **Other:** Cardiac arrhythmias, weight gain, sedation.

Second-Generation ("Atypical") Antipsychotics

- **Risperidone, olanzapine, quetiapine, ziprasidone,** and **aripiprazole** are commonly used. **Lurasidone, iloperidone,** and **paliperidone** are newer agents.
- **Clozapine** is second-line therapy and is used for treatment-refractory patients.

TABLE 17-1. Extrapyramidal Symptoms and Treatment

SYMPTOM	DESCRIPTION	TREATMENT
Acute dystonia	Involuntary muscle contraction or spasm (eg, torticollis, oculogyric crisis). More common in young men.	Give an anticholinergic (benztropine) or diphenhydramine. To prevent, give prophylactic benztropine with an antipsychotic.
Dyskinesia	Pseudoparkinsonism (eg, shuffling gait, cogwheel rigidity).	Give an anticholinergic (benztropine) or a dopamine agonist (amantadine). ↓ the dose of neuroleptic or discontinue (if tolerated).
Akathisia	Subjective/objective restlessness.	↓ neuroleptic and try β-blockers (propranolol). Benzodiazepines or anticholinergics may help.
Tardive dyskinesia	Stereotypic oral-facial movements. Likely from dopamine receptor sensitization. Often irreversible (50%). More common in older women.	Discontinue or ↓ the dose of neuroleptic, attempt treatment with more appropriate drugs, and consider changing neuroleptic (eg, to clozapine or risperidone). Treat symptoms with β-blockers or benzodiazepines. Giving anticholinergics or decreasing neuroleptics may initially worsen tardive dyskinesia.

- **Mechanism of action:** Act through 5-HT_2 and dopamine antagonism.
- **Applications:** Currently first-line therapy for schizophrenia. Benefits are fewer EPS and anticholinergic effects than first-generation agents.
- **Side effects:**
    - ↑ risk of death in elderly patients with dementia-related psychosis.
    - May cause **sedation, weight gain, metabolic syndrome, anticholinergic effects,** and **QT prolongation.** Obtain baseline values, and monitor the patient's weight, lipid profile, and glucose levels.
    - Olanzapine and clozapine cause the most weight gain and carry the risk of **diabetogenesis.**
    - Common side effects of clozapine include sedation, constipation, weight gain, and sialorrhea (drooling). **Clozapine may also cause agranulocytosis and seizures** (requires weekly CBCs during the first 6 months followed by biweekly monitoring).

MOOD STABILIZERS

Lithium

- **Applications:** Used for long-term maintenance or prophylaxis of bipolar disorder. Effective in mania and in augmenting antidepressants in depression and OCD. ↓ suicidal behavior/risk in bipolar disorder. Has a **narrow therapeutic index** and requires monitoring of serum levels.
- **Side effects:**
    - Thirst, polyuria, fine tremor, weight gain, diarrhea, nausea, acne, and hypothyroidism.
    - Lithium toxicity presents with a **coarse tremor, ataxia,** vomiting, confusion, seizures, and arrhythmias.
    - Teratogenic.

Valproic Acid

- **Applications:** First-line agent for **acute mania** and bipolar disorder; effective in **rapid cyclers** (those with 4 or more episodes per year).
- **Side effects:**
    - Sedation, **weight gain,** hair loss, tremor, ataxia, GI distress.
    - Pancreatitis, thrombocytopenia, and fatal hepatotoxicity are uncommon. Do not use in patients with hepatitis or cirrhosis.
    - Monitor platelets, LFTs, and serum drug levels.
    - **Teratogenic.**

Carbamazepine

- **Applications:** Second-line agent for acute mania and bipolar disorder.
- **Side effects:**
    - Common side effects include nausea, sedation, rash, and ataxia.
    - Rare side effects include hepatic toxicity, SIADH (leading to hyponatremia), **bone marrow suppression** (leading to life-threatening dyscrasias such as aplastic anemia), and **Stevens-Johnson syndrome.**
    - Monitor blood counts, transaminases, and electrolytes. Drug interactions complicate its use (eg, cannot be used with MAOIs).
    - Teratogenic.

Other Anticonvulsants

- Include **oxcarbazepine, lamotrigine, gabapentin,** and **topiramate.**
- Efficacy is not well documented.
- Do not require blood level monitoring and do not cause weight gain.

MNEMONIC

Evolution of EPS—

4 hours: Acute dystonia
4 days: Akinesia
4 weeks: Akathisia
4 months: Tardive dyskinesia

KEY FACT

Metoclopramide is actually a more common cause of tardive dyskinesia than antipsychotics.

KEY FACT

When using lithium, monitor renal and thyroid function. Chronic use can lead to hypothyroidism and nephrotoxicity.

KEY FACT

Lithium toxicity treatment may include hemodialysis.

KEY FACT

Lamotrigine or lithium may be used as first-line agents for bipolar depression.

KEY FACT

The bioavailability of gabapentin actually ↓ with larger doses.

- Lamotrigine is associated with Stevens-Johnson syndrome and toxic epidermal necrolysis.

Diagnostic and Statistical Manual of Mental Disorders (DSM)

Psychiatric disorders affect (but do not always limit) a person's ability to handle daily living and/or social or occupational situations. The American Psychiatric Association's *Diagnostic and Statistical Manual of Mental Disorders* (DSM) provides diagnostic criteria useful for guiding treatment in psychiatric disorders. The fifth edition, DSM-5, was released in 2013.

Neurodevelopmental Disorders

AUTISM SPECTRUM DISORDERS

More common in males. Symptoms are usually recognized by age 2 and are characterized by lack of social interaction. Has a genetic component.

SYMPTOMS

- Characterized by **abnormal social interaction**; deficits in nonverbal communication (eg, eye contact, facial expressions); and restricted, repetitive, and **stereotyped patterns of behavior**, interests, and activities.
- Children **may or may not have intellectual and language impairment.**

DIFFERENTIAL

- **Fragile X syndrome:** A trinucleotide CGG repeat disorder. Children have long faces, a large body size, and macro-orchidism. **The most common inherited cause of mental retardation.**
- **Rett's disorder:** An X-linked genetic disorder that **affects only girls.** Characterized by **normal development until 6–18 months with arrest or deterioration of mental (especially language) and motor skills;** progressive microcephaly; and purposeless, stereotyped hand movements. Epilepsy is comorbid in 70–90% of cases.

TREATMENT

- **Early intervention** to treat speech delays and help with socialization.
- **Applied behavioral analysis** helps reinforce positive behaviors. Other forms of therapy, including occupational, speech, and sensory integration, may be helpful as well.
- **Irritability** can be treated with antipsychotics, including risperidone and aripiprazole.

ATTENTION-DEFICIT/HYPERACTIVITY DISORDER

The most common childhood psychiatric disorder.

SYMPTOMS

- Presents **before age 12.**
- Involves 6 or more symptoms for 6 months of either **inattention** (eg, easy distractibility, difficulty following instructions/finishing tasks, disorganiza-

---

KEY FACT

Fetal alcohol syndrome is the main preventable cause of mental retardation; fragile X is the most common inherited cause. Down syndrome is not inherited but is caused by a chromosome disorder (trisomy 21).

KEY FACT

Always do a hearing test in a child who shows poor language development or does not respond to his name.

tion) or **hyperactivity/impulsivity** (eg, fidgeting/interrupting others/difficulty waiting) in **2 or more settings** (school, work, home).

DIAGNOSIS

Although parents often think of this diagnosis immediately, first consider physical and social factors that may contribute to the problem (eg, poor vision that prevents the child from seeing the chalkboard).

TREATMENT

Initial treatment generally includes behavior modification. Pharmacologic approaches include psychostimulant (eg, amphetamines, **methylphenidate**) or nonstimulant medications (eg, **bupropion, atomoxetine,** SSRIs, α_2-agonists).

LEARNING DISORDERS

- Weaker academic performance than expected for age, intelligence, and education.
  - May involve specific deficits such as reading, writing, or mathematics disorder or more general problems with understanding and processing new information.
  - Tend to occur more frequently in males and in those of lower socioeconomic status (SES), and may have a familial pattern.
- **Dx:** As with ADHD, consider physical and social factors before making a diagnosis.

TIC DISORDERS

Distinguished as follows:

- **Tic:** A sudden, rapid, recurrent, nonrhythmic motor movement or vocalization. Common but often transient.
- **Tourette's syndrome:** Multiple **motor and vocal tics** such as blinking, grimacing, or grunting that occur many times a day for > 1 year and cause functional impairment. Associated with ADHD, learning disorders, and OCD. Treat with **dopamine receptor antagonists** (eg, haloperidol, pimozide), clonidine, behavioral therapy, and counseling. Stimulants can worsen or precipitate tics.

Psychotic Disorders

SCHIZOPHRENIA

Thought to be related to dysregulation of dopamine ($\uparrow$ in the limbic system and $\downarrow$ in the frontal cortex). Lifetime prevalence is 1%, with peak onset in the late teens to 30s. A $\oplus$ family history $\uparrow$ risk.

- Few patients have a complete recovery, and as with other psychiatric disorders, social/occupational dysfunction can be significant.
- Associated with an $\uparrow$ risk of substance abuse and suicide.

SYMPTOMS

- Two or more positive or negative symptoms must be present for at least 1 month and must result in impairment of functioning. Of these, delusions, hallucinations, or disorganized speech must be present. Continuous signs of the disturbance **must persist for at least 6 months.**

KEY FACT

Tourette's syndrome is often depicted in the media as including coprolalia (the repetition of obscene words), but this is found in only 10–30% of cases.

Q 1

A 29-year-old male attorney is being treated for depression. He blushingly admits that since starting SSRIs, he has had diminished interest in sex and difficulty maintaining an erection. What other antidepressant medications should be considered to prevent these sexual side effects?

Q 2

A mother brings her 18-month-old son to the pediatrician because he is nonverbal. He was born full term and met all milestones. He rarely gestures or points at things and always plays alone. On exam, he does not respond to his name or make eye contact. A hearing test was normal. What is the most likely diagnosis?

KEY FACT

A **bizarre delusion** is an absurd, implausible, fixed false belief that is not shared by other members of the society or culture—eg, the conviction that Martians have implanted electrodes into one's brain.

KEY FACT

Negative symptoms are harder to treat.

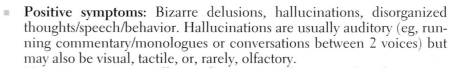

- **Positive symptoms:** Bizarre delusions, hallucinations, disorganized thoughts/speech/behavior. Hallucinations are usually auditory (eg, running commentary/monologues or conversations between 2 voices) but may also be visual, tactile, or, rarely, olfactory.
- **Negative symptoms:** Affective flattening, avolition, apathy, alogia.
- **Catatonic:** Involves a marked ↑ or ↓ in speech and motor function. Rare (affects only 10–15% of cases).

DIFFERENTIAL

- **Brief psychotic disorder:** Symptoms are of < 1 month's duration; onset often follows a psychosocial stressor. Associated with a better prognosis. (Postpartum psychosis can last up to 3 months.)
- **Schizophreniform disorder:** Diagnostic criteria are the same as those for schizophrenia, but symptoms have a duration of **1–6 months.**
- **Schizoaffective disorder:** Mood symptoms are present for a significant portion of the illness, but psychotic symptoms have been present without a mood episode.
- **Delusional disorder: Nonbizarre delusions for 1 month or more** in the absence of other psychotic symptoms; often chronic.
- **Other: Schizotypal personality disorder**; mood disorder with psychotic features (contrast with schizoaffective disorder); substance-induced psychosis (eg, amphetamines) or drug withdrawal (eg, alcoholic hallucinosis); psychosis due to a general medical condition (eg, brain tumor); delirium or dementia; shared psychotic disorder.

TREATMENT

- Antipsychotic medications (neuroleptics).
- Hospitalize when the patient is a danger to himself/herself or to others.
- Psychosocial treatments, individual supportive psychotherapy, and family therapy for relapse prevention.

Mood (Affective) Disorders

MAJOR DEPRESSIVE DISORDER (MDD)

The average age of onset is in the mid-20s. Often associated with a life stressor. Associated with a high (15%) incidence of suicide.

SYMPTOMS

Diagnosis requires depressed mood or **anhedonia** (loss of interest or pleasure) and at least 5 of the following symptoms during a 2-week period:

- Insomnia or hypersomnia
- Feelings of worthlessness or excessive guilt
- Fatigue or loss of energy
- ↓ ability to concentrate or indecisiveness
- Significant weight loss or weight gain/change in appetite
- Psychomotor agitation or retardation
- Recurrent thoughts of death or suicide

DIFFERENTIAL

- **Dysthymia:** A milder, chronic depressed state of 2 or more years' duration.
- **Bereavement:** Does not involve severe impairment or suicidality; usually improves within 2 months (but can last up to 1 year). Symptoms may vary

1   Bupropion or mirtazapine.

2   Autism spectrum disorder.

with cultural norms. For example, visual and auditory hallucinations (eg, thinking that a deceased person is still alive) are common and considered normal. Feelings of grief around anniversaries and other special events beyond the 1-year period are also common.

- **Adjustment disorder with depressed mood:** Has fewer symptoms; occurs within 3 months of a stressor and lasts < 6 months.
- **Bipolar disorder:** Patients can present with depression, so carefully screen for a history of a manic episode. **Use caution with SSRIs, as they can precipitate a manic episode.**
- **Other:** Substance-induced mood disorder (eg, illicit drugs, β-blockers, OCPs); mood disorder due to a medical condition (eg, hypothyroidism, ACA stroke); dementia.

DIAGNOSIS

Symptoms last 2 or more weeks and must lead to significant dysfunction or impairment.

TREATMENT

- **Pharmacotherapy:**
  - Most antidepressants have equal efficacy.
  - **SSRIs** (eg, fluoxetine, paroxetine), **SNRIs** (eg, venlafaxine), and **bupropion** are the main treatments; SSRIs are generally first line.
  - Take 4–6 weeks for full effect.
  - Generally safe, but common side effects include GI upset, akathisia, sexual side effects (most common with SSRIs; add or use bupropion instead), and ↑ thoughts of suicide **(black box warning).**
  - Abrupt discontinuation can lead to withdrawal.
  - Continue treatment for 6–12 months.
- **Electroconvulsive therapy (ECT):**
  - Safe and effective.
  - Best for refractory or catatonic depression, but may also be used for acute mania or acute psychosis as well as for patients who refuse to eat or drink (eg, severely depressed elderly) or are suicidally depressed.
  - Adverse effects include postictal confusion, arrhythmias, headache, and **retrograde amnesia** (inability to recall memories before the event).
  - Relative contraindications include intracranial mass, aneurysm, and recent MI/stroke. **Pregnancy is not a contraindication.**
- **Psychotherapy:** Psychotherapy combined with antidepressants is more effective than either modality alone.

BIPOLAR DISORDER

Prevalence is 1–2%. A family history of bipolar illness significantly ↑ risk. The male-to-female ratio is 1:1, but women more frequently seek treatment. Symptoms usually appear around age 20, and the number of cycles actually ↑ with age. About 10–15% of those affected die by suicide.

SYMPTOMS

- A **manic episode** is defined as follows:
  - **One week** of an abnormally and persistently **elevated ("euphoric"), expansive, or irritable mood.**
  - At least 3 of the symptoms (4 if the mood is irritable) in the mnemonic **DIGS FAR.**
- A **mixed episode** must meet the criteria for both manic and depressive episodes for 1 week or more.

MNEMONIC

Symptoms of depression—

SIG E CAPS

Sleep (↓/↑)
Interest (↓)
Guilt
Energy (↓)
Concentration
Appetite (↓/↑)
Psychomotor agitation or retardation
Suicidal ideation

KEY FACT

Cognitive decline is a common sign of major depressive disorder in the elderly ("pseudodementia").

KEY FACT

Severe MDD can present with psychotic symptoms, in which case an antipsychotic in addition to an antidepressant may be temporarily required.

KEY FACT

Seasonal affective disorder (SAD), which is typified by fall/winter depression, is treated with bright-light therapy (phototherapy).

KEY FACT

Catatonia may be observed in both schizophrenia and mood disorders. Of the latter, it is more often associated with mania than with depression.

MNEMONIC

Symptoms of a manic episode—

DIGS FAR

Distractibility
Insomnia (↓ need for sleep)
Grandiosity (inflated self-esteem)
Pressured **S**peech
Flight of ideas (racing thoughts)
Psychomotor **A**gitation/↑ goal-directed
  Activity
Recklessness/pursuit of pleasurable but
  Risky behaviors (eg, gambling, sexual
  indiscretions)

 KEY FACT

Screen for bipolar disorder before starting antidepressants, as they can induce acute mania or psychosis in bipolar patients.

- Mania and mixed episodes are considered **psychiatric emergencies** 2° to impaired judgment and the risk of hurting oneself or others.

DIFFERENTIAL

- **Hypomania:** Has no marked functional impairment or psychosis. Symptoms last for **4 days or less**. Does not require hospitalization.
- **Cyclothymic disorder:** Chronic cycles of mild depression (dysthymia) and hypomania for 2 or more years. Effectively a milder form of bipolar II disorder.
- **Other:** Substance-induced mood disorder, schizophrenia, schizoaffective disorder, personality disorders, medical conditions (eg, temporal lobe epilepsy, hyperthyroidism), ADHD.

DIAGNOSIS

- **Bipolar I disorder:** Diagnosis is made after just **1 mixed or manic episode**. Depressive episodes are common but are not required for diagnosis.
- **Bipolar II disorder:** Characterized by at least **1 hypomanic** (rather than manic) **episode** alternating with at least **1 major depressive episode**.

TREATMENT

- **Acute mania:** Lithium, anticonvulsants, antipsychotics, benzodiazepines, ECT.
- **Bipolar depression:** Mood stabilizers (lithium or lamotrigine are first line) +/− antidepressants. **Monotherapy with an antidepressant is not recommended.** If the patient does not respond to first-line treatment, the next step may include adding lamotrigine (if started with lithium), bupropion, or SSRIs. In severe cases, consider ECT.

Anxiety Disorders

PHOBIAS

The 3 categories of phobia are agoraphobia, social phobia, and specific phobia.

SYMPTOMS

- Defined as persistent, excessive, or unreasonable fear and/or avoidance of an object or situation that leads to significant distress or impairment.
- Exposure to the object or stimulus may precipitate **panic attacks**.

DIFFERENTIAL

Other anxiety disorders, depression, avoidant and schizoid personality disorders, schizophrenia, appropriate fear, normal shyness.

DIAGNOSIS

- **Social phobia** is characterized by unreasonable, marked, and persistent **fear of scrutiny and embarrassment in social or performance situations** (also referred to as social anxiety disorder). Usually begins in adolescence.
- **Specific phobia** is immediately **cued by an object or a situation** (eg, spiders, animals, heights). Usually begins in childhood.
- In adults, the **duration is 6 or more months**.
- As in OCD, symptoms interrupt the patient's life, and patients recognize that their fears are excessive.

TREATMENT

- Cognitive-behavioral therapy (CBT) and pharmacotherapy (eg, SSRIs, benzodiazepines, β-blockers) are effective for social phobias.
- **Behavioral therapy** that uses exposure and desensitization is best for specific phobia.

PANIC DISORDER

More common in women, with a mean age of onset of 25. Often accompanied by **agoraphobia,** a fear of being in places or situations from which escape is difficult; of being outside the home alone; or of being in public places.

SYMPTOMS

- Characterized by discrete periods of intense fear or discomfort.
- Attacks are not brought about by an identifiable trigger.
- There is excessive worry about having recurrent panic attacks.
- At least 4 of the symptoms in the **PANICS** mnemonic develop abruptly and peak within 10 minutes (may also include depersonalization).

DIFFERENTIAL

Medical conditions (eg, angina, hyperthyroidism, hypoglycemia), substance-induced anxiety disorder, other anxiety disorders.

DIAGNOSIS

- Characterized by recurrent, **unexpected** panic attacks.
- At least **1 month** of worry about and/or behavioral change to avoid subsequent attacks.

TREATMENT

- Behavioral therapy.
- Pharmacotherapy includes SSRIs, either alone or in combination with benzodiazepines.
- TCAs or MAOIs should be used only if SSRIs are not tolerated or are ineffective.
- Benzodiazepines (eg, alprazolam, clonazepam) are effective for immediate relief but have abuse potential.

GENERALIZED ANXIETY DISORDER (GAD)

Can be associated with panic attacks but are **expected and triggered by an identifiable stressor** (vs unexpected panic attacks in panic disorder). Clinical diagnosis is usually made in the early 20s.

SYMPTOMS

- Characterized by **excessive and pervasive worry** about a number of activities or events, leading to significant impairment or distress.
- Patients may seek medical care for somatic complaints.

DIFFERENTIAL

- Substance-induced anxiety disorder.
- Anxiety disorder due to a general medical condition (eg, hyperthyroidism).
- Other anxiety disorders (eg, panic disorder, social phobia).

MNEMONIC

Symptoms of panic disorder—

PANICS

Palpitations
Abdominal distress
Numbness, **N**ausea
Intense fear of death
Choking, **C**hills, **C**hest pain
Sweating, **S**haking, **S**hortness of breath

KEY FACT

CBT helps patients learn new ways to cope by:
- Identifying automatic thoughts, or "cognitive distortions."
- Testing the automatic thoughts.
- Identifying and testing the validity of maladaptive assumptions.
- Strategizing on alternative ways to deal with problems.

KEY FACT

In general, OCD is ego dystonic (causes distress), whereas OCPD is ego syntonic (does not cause distress).

DIAGNOSIS

Diagnostic criteria are as follows:

- **Anxiety/worry on most days for at least 6 months.**
- **Three or more somatic symptoms,** including restlessness, fatigue, difficulty concentrating, irritability, muscle tension, and sleep disturbance.

TREATMENT

- Pharmacologic therapy includes venlafaxine, SSRIs, benzodiazepines, and buspirone; second-line treatment with TCAs is appropriate if other antidepressants are ineffective or are not tolerated.
- Benzodiazepines offer acute relief, but tolerance and dependence may result from their use. Use them as a bridge to chronic treatment with SSRIs, as above.
- Psychotherapy (CBT) and relaxation training are important adjuncts.

Obsessive-Compulsive and Related Disorders

OBSESSIVE-COMPULSIVE DISORDER (OCD)

Typically presents in late adolescence or early adulthood; can lead to severe functional impairment.

SYMPTOMS

- Obsessions are **persistent, intrusive thoughts, impulses, or images** that lead to anxiety/distress and interfere with daily life. Common themes are contamination and fear of harm to oneself or to others.
- Compulsions are **conscious, repetitive behaviors** (eg, hand washing) or mental acts (eg, counting) that patients feel driven to perform to neutralize anxiety from obsessions.

DIFFERENTIAL

OCPD, other anxiety disorders, medical conditions (eg, brain tumor, temporal lobe epilepsy, group A β-hemolytic streptococcal infection).

DIAGNOSIS

Patients recognize that their obsessions and/or compulsions are excessive, unreasonable productions of their own minds (rather than thought insertion). Nonetheless, their behaviors cause marked distress and are time consuming (take > 1 hour/day).

TREATMENT

Pharmacotherapy (eg, SSRIs, clomipramine, fluvoxamine) and **CBT** (eg, exposure and response prevention).

BODY DYSMORPHIC DISORDER

- Preoccupation with an imagined defect in appearance. Multiple visits to surgeons and dermatologists are common. Associated with depression.
- **Tx:** Treat with SSRIs.

HOARDING

- Persistent difficulty discarding or parting with possessions, regardless of actual value, in order to save the items and avoid distress associated with discarding them. The items cause clogging and congestion in main areas of the home.
- Hoarding behavior causes **distress and impairment.**
- **Hoarding with excessive acquisition** affects 80% of cases.
- **Tx:** Treatment involves CBT and addressing comorbid diagnoses.

Trauma- and Stressor-Related Disorders

POSTTRAUMATIC STRESS DISORDER (PTSD)

Results from exposure to a traumatic event that involved **actual or threatened death or serious injury** and evoked **intense fear, helplessness, or horror.**

SYMPTOMS

- Examples of traumatic events include war, torture, natural disasters, assault, rape, and serious accidents.
- Patients may have experienced the trauma personally, or they may have witnessed the event in a way that leads them to feel personally threatened, helpless, and horrified (eg, a child witnessing a parent being assaulted).
- Nightmares and flashbacks are common.
- Watch for **survival guilt,** personality change, substance abuse, depression, and suicide.

DIFFERENTIAL

- **Acute stress disorder:** Symptoms are the same as or similar to those of PTSD but last < **1 month,** occur within 1 month of a trauma, and are primarily dissociative.
- **Adjustment disorder with anxiety:** Emotional or behavioral symptoms occurring within 3 months of a stressor and lasting < 6 months.
- **Other:** Depression, OCD, acute intoxication or withdrawal, factitious disorders, malingering, borderline personality disorder.

DIAGNOSIS

Symptoms persist for > **1 month** and include:

- **Reexperiencing** the event (eg, nightmares, flashbacks).
- Avoidance of trauma-related stimuli or **numbing** of general responsiveness.
- **Hyperarousal** (eg, hypervigilance, exaggerated startle, irritability, difficulty falling or staying asleep).

TREATMENT

- Pharmacotherapy includes first-line treatment with SSRIs; if SSRIs are not tolerated or are ineffective, use TCAs or MAOIs.
- Second-generation antipsychotics (eg, risperidone, olanzapine, quetiapine), anticonvulsants (eg, divalproex, topiramate), α_2-adrenergic agonists (clonidine), or β-blockers (propranolol) may be helpful for some patients.
- CBT, exposure therapy, and group therapy are also effective.

KEY FACT

Victims of human trafficking may present with symptoms similar to those of PTSD.

Q

A 30-year-old high school guidance counselor presents to her dermatologist for irritation of her hands. She states that she washes her hands under hot water about 20 times a day and uses a variety of alcohol-based hand sanitizer products to avoid picking up germs. What is the best treatment for her disorder?

ADJUSTMENT DISORDER

- The development of emotional or behavioral symptoms in response to an **identifiable stressor** occurring within **3 months** of the stressor.
- Sx/Dx:
  - Distress is out of proportion to the severity of the stressor, but symptoms **do not** meet the criteria for MDD or other disorders.
  - Once the stressor has passed, **symptoms do not persist for > 6 months.**
- Tx: Supportive therapy, CBT, or medication management of distinct symptoms (eg, sleep aids for insomnia); if symptoms become more severe or meet the criteria for another mood or anxiety disorder, antidepressants or anxiolytics may be indicated.

Dissociative Disorders

DISSOCIATIVE IDENTITY DISORDER

- Formerly known as multiple personality disorder.
- Sx/Dx:
  - Patients present with **2 or more distinct personalities** (aka "alters").
  - Each of these identities interprets and interacts with the world differently—eg, they may be of different ages, levels of intelligence, or even genders. Patients usually claim no memory when the other identities take over.
  - Often associated with severe and prolonged abuse and/or neglect in childhood. Comorbid PTSD is common.

DISSOCIATIVE FUGUE

- **Temporary amnesia for one's own identity.** Typically lasts hours to days.
- Sx/Dx:
  - **Usually precipitated by acute stressors.**
  - Classically, the affected individual is found after having traveled to a different city or state and having established a new identity. Upon recovery, he or she is amnestic for the fugue episode as well as for the original stressor that caused it.
  - Like other dissociative disorders, fugue cannot be attributed to the ingestion of illicit substances or to other psychiatric conditions (eg, delirium).

Somatic Symptoms and Related Disorders

All of the following disorders consist primarily of somatic symptoms without obvious medical diagnoses that cause significant impairment and distress. Because somatic symptom disorders often accompany medical diagnoses, **a medical cause of symptoms must be ruled out** before a diagnosis of somatic disorder is made.

SSRIs and CBT.

SOMATIC SYMPTOM DISORDER

- Defined as somatic symptoms that are highly distressing and/or result in significant disruption of function. Onset is before age 30, and women are affected more often than men.

- **Sx/Dx:**
  - Symptoms are accompanied by disproportionate thoughts, feelings, or behaviors regarding symptoms.
  - The patient's suffering is authentic even if no medical cause is identified.
- **Tx:**
  - Psychotherapy.
  - SSRIs for comorbid depression/anxiety.
  - Consistent follow-up with the primary care physician and/or psychiatric providers.

ILLNESS ANXIETY DISORDER

- Preoccupation for > 6 months with **fear of having a serious disease** based on **misinterpretation of symptoms** (rather than delusions). Formerly known as hypochondriasis.
  - Patients usually recognize that their concerns are excessive, but they are not reassured by negative medical evaluations.
  - **With predominant pain (formerly pain disorder):** Pain intensity or a pain profile that is inconsistent with physiologic processes. Affects women more often than men, with a peak onset at 40–50 years of age.
- **Sx:** Symptoms are exacerbated by or related to psychological factors, especially depression.
- **Tx:** Treat with physical therapy, psychotherapy, and antidepressants. Analgesics rarely provide relief.

KEY FACT

Medical students are prone to thinking they have the symptoms of whatever disease they are studying. This may be nosophobia, or fear of contracting disease, rather than true hypochondriasis.

CONVERSION DISORDER

- Characterized by **sensory symptoms, motor deficits (eg, paralysis), or "psychogenic seizures."**
- **Sx/Dx:**
  - Symptoms **are not volitionally produced** and are an attempt to avoid emotional distress following a stressful event (eg, a patient who presents with blindness after witnessing a fatal car accident).
  - **Relation to a stressful event** suggests association with psychological factors (eg, a mother who has paralysis of the right arm after hitting her child).
  - Symptoms cannot be explained by a known organic etiology, although neurologic causes have been speculated. Symptoms usually subside spontaneously.
  - **Hoover's sign** is used to separate organic from nonorganic leg paresis. The sign is ⊕ (ie, nonorganic) when weakness of hip extension returns to normal strength with contralateral hip flexion against resistance.
- **Tx:** Reassurance, psychotherapy, and close monitoring and follow-up.

FACTITIOUS DISORDER

- Falsification of physical or psychological symptoms, or inducing injury or illness (eg, a patient who injects himself with insulin), that is **associated with identified deception.** More common among health care workers than in the general population.
- **Sx:**
  - Symptoms are **consciously produced,** but the reason may be unconscious (eg, **wanting to assume the sick role or be taken care of**).

KEY FACT

Munchausen's syndrome refers to repeated episodes of factitious disorders (either the same or new complaints). The sufferer feels a deep psychological need to play the role of patient and feels comforted by assuming this role.

- Symptoms can be produced on oneself or on others (eg, a mother who gives her child nuts in order to induce anaphylactic shock).
- **Tx:** Therapy to resolve underlying issues; medication for comorbid diagnoses.

MALINGERING

Conscious feigning of symptoms for anticipated external rewards (eg, money, food, shelter).

Feeding and Eating Disorders

PICA

- Eating nonnutritive, nonfood substances (eg, ice, clay, sand, chalk, soil) over a period of at least a month.
- Possibly attributed to deficiencies in vitamins/minerals.
- More common with intellectual disability.

ANOREXIA NERVOSA

Females account for 90% of cases. Peak incidence is at age 14 and age 18.

- Risk factors include a ⊕ family history, higher SES, poor self-esteem, psychiatric comorbidities (eg, major depression, OCD, anxiety), and body-conscious careers/activities such as modeling, ballet, and wrestling.
- Mortality from suicide or medical complications is 10%.

SYMPTOMS

- Classified as **restricting type** (excessive dieting or exercising) or **binge-eating/purging type** (vomiting, laxatives, diuretics). Presents with the following:
    - **Refusal to maintain normal body weight** (ie, the patient is < 85% of ideal body weight)
    - Intense fear of weight gain
    - Distorted body image
- Amenorrhea is no longer required for a diagnosis of anorexia nervosa.

DIAGNOSIS

- Measure height and weight. Check CBC, electrolytes, TSH/FT_4, and an ECG.
- Look for **lanugo** (fine body hair), dry skin, lethargy, bradycardia, hypotension, and peripheral edema.

TREATMENT

- Patients often deny the health risks of their behavior. Monitor caloric intake and **focus on slow weight gain.** Individual, family, and group psychotherapy is crucial.
- Pharmacotherapy has not been successful, although some SSRIs (fluoxetine) and atypical antipsychotics (olanzapine) have been used with minimal success. Avoid bupropion in light of the risk of seizure.

KEY FACT

Amenorrhea is no longer required for the diagnosis of anorexia.

BULIMIA NERVOSA

Affects 1–3% of young adult females. The prognosis is more favorable than that of anorexia nervosa. Associated with an ↑ frequency of affective disorders, substance abuse, and borderline personality disorder.

SYMPTOMS

Patients have normal weight or are overweight but engage in the following behaviors at least once a week for 3 or more months:

- **Binge eating** with a sense of lack of self-control.
- **Compensatory behavior** to prevent weight gain (eg, self-induced vomiting, laxatives, diuretics, overexercise).

DIAGNOSIS

- The same as that for anorexia nervosa. Look for poor dentition, **enlarged parotid glands,** scars on the dorsal hand surfaces (from finger-induced vomiting), **electrolyte imbalances,** and **metabolic alkalosis.**
- In contrast to anorexia nervosa, **patients are typically distressed about their symptoms and behaviors** and are consequently easier to treat.

TREATMENT

- Restore the patient's nutritional status and electrolytes and then rebuild his/her weight.
- **CBT** is the most effective treatment. Antidepressants are useful even in nondepressed patients, but **avoid bupropion** in light of its seizure risk.

BINGE-EATING DISORDER

Occurs in normal-weight/overweight or obese individuals. Begins in adolescence or young adulthood; common in those who are college-age.

DIFFERENTIAL

- **Anorexia, binge-purge type:** Differentiated by weight; patients are underweight in anorexia but are of normal weight or overweight in binge eating.
- **Bulimia nervosa:** Patients with binge-eating disorder do not have compensatory behaviors such as purging, as seen in bulimia nervosa.
- Patients who seek treatment are usually older than those with anorexia or bulimia.

DIAGNOSIS

- **Recurrent episodes of binge eating:** Episodes are characterized by eating, in a discrete period of time, more than most people would eat in similar situation, with a sense of lack of control over eating.
- **Binge eating associated with 3 (or more) of the following:** Eating more rapidly than normal; eating until feeling uncomfortably full; eating large amounts of food when not feeling physically hungry; eating alone because of feeling embarrassed by how much one is eating; feeling disgusted with oneself, depressed, or guilty afterward.

TREATMENT

- Address the underlying psychopathology.
- **CBT** and interpersonal psychotherapy (IPT) can be helpful.
- May need to address obesity.

Q

A 15-year-old boy presents to the pediatrician. He states that he has been exercising more and eating less so that he can make the school wrestling team. His growth curve has dropped from the 50th to the 15th percentile for weight. Which psychiatric diagnoses should be considered?

- In general, binge-eating disorder has a better rate of remission than bulimia nervosa or anorexia nervosa.

Elimination Disorders

ENURESIS

- Enuresis (bed-wetting) is not a clinical disorder until a child is > 5 years of age (the child may not feel/understand neurologic impulses until then).
- **Tx: Treat initially with behavioral therapy** (eg, bed alarms); imipramine should be reserved for refractory cases.

Sleep-Wake Disorders

INSOMNIA DISORDER

- Significant **difficulty falling or staying asleep.**
- Can have early-morning awakening; associated with nonrestorative sleep.
- Sx/Dx:
  - The disorder cannot be attributed to physical or mental conditions but is often precipitated by anxiety.
  - Symptoms occur 3 or more times a week for at least 3 months.
- **Tx:** Sleep hygiene, hypnotics.

NARCOLEPSY

- Usually presents before age 30. May be familial. Often associated with mood disorders, substance abuse, and GAD.
- Sx:
  - Presents with excessive daytime sleepiness and daytime **sleep attacks** characterized by ↓ REM sleep latency. Symptoms occur at least 3 times per month for 3 or more months.
  - May involve hypnagogic (just before sleep) or hypnopompic (just before awakening) hallucinations.
  - Can involve **hypocretin deficiency,** as measured by CSF.
- **Tx:** Amphetamines (**methylphenidate**) or nonamphetamine stimulants (modafinil).

CIRCADIAN RHYTHM SLEEP-WAKE DISORDER

Discrepancy between when the patient would like to sleep and when he or she actually does so. **Often 2° to jet lag or shift work.**

PARASOMNIAS

Non-REM Sleep Arousal Disorders

- **Sleepwalking:** Repeated episodes of rising from bed during sleep and walking about. Not responsive to efforts of others to communicate.

KEY FACT

- Hypna**GO**gic hallucinations occur when you **GO** to sleep.
- Hypno**POMP**ic hallucinations occur when you awaken and **"PUMP"** yourself up for the day.

KEY FACT

Cataplexy is sudden loss of muscle tone leading to collapse, usually in the setting of strong emotions or excitement. It is treated with SSRIs.

Depression and anorexia nervosa. Eating disorders are much less common in males than in females, but the diagnosis should still be considered.

- **Sleep terrors:** Abrupt terror arousals from sleep, often starting with a panicky scream. The individual cannot be comforted by others.

REM Sleep Disorders

- **Nightmare disorder:** Repeated occurrence of extended, frightening, and **well-remembered dreams.** Individuals are at greater risk for suicide. **If comorbid with PTSD, treat with α-blockers.** Systematic desensitization and relaxation may be helpful.
- **REM sleep behavior disorder:** Arousal from sleep with vocalizations and complex motor behaviors, such as running, kicking, and punching. Can cause injury to the bed partner. Present in 30% of patients with narcolepsy. **Fifty percent of those affected will eventually develop a neurodegenerative disease such as Parkinson's disease.** Treat with **clonazepam** and **melatonin.**
- **Restless leg syndrome:** An urge to move legs that begins or worsens during periods of rest or inactivity, **particularly at night.** Partially relieved by movement. Can be associated with iron deficiency, so check serum ferritin level. Often comorbid with depression. **Treat with dopamine agonists** (eg, pramipexole, ropinirole).

Disruptive, Impulse Control, and Conduct Disorders

- **Oppositional defiant disorder: A negative, hostile, and defiant attitude toward authority figures** of 6 or more months' duration. Patients often lose their temper and are easily annoyed. May lead to conduct disorder. The most effective treatments are parent management training, family therapy, and CBT.
- **Conduct disorder:** A disorder in which a patient repeatedly and significantly **violates societal norms and the rights of others** (eg, bullies, tortures animals, steals/destroys property) for 1 or more years. Treatment usually involves behavioral therapy. Considered a precursor to antisocial personality disorder.

 KEY FACT

Conduct disorder is diagnosed in **C**hildren and can eventually lead to in**C**arceration. **A**dults suffer from **A**ntisocial personality disorder.

Substance-Related and Addictive Disorders

SUBSTANCE USE DISORDER

The lifetime prevalence of using 1 or more illicit substances in the United States is roughly 40%. Comorbid psychiatric disorders are common.

SYMPTOMS

The signs, symptoms, and physical findings of acute intoxication and withdrawal are outlined in Table 17-2.

DIAGNOSIS

- Check urine and serum toxicology. Offer HIV testing; check LFTs and consider hepatitis testing.
- Patients display loss of control over substance use, continued use despite knowledge of harm, and accumulating consequences from use (eg, arrest, job loss). These lead to clinically significant impairment and, in general, to an overall worsening of the situation.

KEY FACT

DSM-5 no longer distinguishes substance abuse from substance dependence. Rather, it now uses modifiers—low, moderate, or severe— to define severity of use.

TABLE 17-2. **Signs and Symptoms of Intoxication and Withdrawal**

DRUG	INTOXICATION	WITHDRAWAL
Alcohol	Disinhibition/impaired judgment, emotional lability, slurred speech, ataxia, aggression, hypoglycemia, blackouts (retrograde amnesia), coma.	Tremor, tachycardia, hypertension, malaise, nausea, seizures, DTs, agitation, hallucinations. **May be life threatening and require hospitalization.**
Opioids	Euphoria leading to apathy, CNS depression, nausea, vomiting, constipation, pupillary constriction, respiratory depression (life threatening in overdose). Naloxone/naltrexone will block opioid receptors and reverse effects (beware of the antagonist clearing before the opioid, particularly with long-acting opioids such as methadone).	Anxiety, insomnia, anorexia, diaphoresis, dilated pupils, fever, rhinorrhea, piloerection, nausea, stomach cramps, diarrhea, yawning, myalgias. Extremely uncomfortable, but rarely life threatening.
Amphetamines, cocaine	Psychomotor agitation, impaired judgment, tachycardia, pupillary dilation, fever, diaphoresis, hypertension, paranoia, angina, arrhythmias, seizures, hallucinations, sudden death. Treat with sedatives and benzodiazepines for severe agitation and with symptom-targeted medications.	Post-use "crash" with hypersomnolence, dysphoria/nightmares, depression, malaise, severe craving, suicidality.
Phencyclidine hydrochloride (PCP)	Belligerence, psychosis, **violence,** impulsiveness, psychomotor agitation, fever, tachycardia, vertical/horizontal nystagmus, ataxia, seizures, delirium. Give benzodiazepines or haloperidol for severe symptoms; otherwise reassure.	Recurrence of intoxication symptoms due to reabsorption in the GI tract; sudden onset of severe, random violence.
LSD	Marked anxiety or depression, delusions, visual hallucinations, pupillary dilation. Flashbacks are a possible long-term consequence. Treat by providing reassurance and a low-stimulation environment. Give benzodiazepines for severe symptoms.	—
Marijuana (THC)	Euphoria, slowed sense of time, impaired judgment, "heightened senses," social withdrawal, ↑ appetite, dry mouth, diaphoresis, conjunctival injection, hallucinations, anxiety, paranoia, tachycardia, hypertension, amotivation.	—
Barbiturates	Low safety margin; respiratory depression.	Anxiety, seizures, delirium, life-threatening cardiovascular collapse.
Benzodiazepines	Interactions with alcohol, amnesia, ataxia, somnolence, mild respiratory depression.	Rebound anxiety, seizures, tremor, insomnia, hypertension, tachycardia.
Caffeine	Restlessness, insomnia, diuresis, muscle twitching, arrhythmias, psychomotor agitation.	Headache, lethargy, depression, weight gain, irritability, craving.
Nicotine	Restlessness, insomnia, anxiety	Irritability, headache, anxiety, weight gain, craving.

TREATMENT

- Group therapy, Narcotics Anonymous, recovery housing. Hospitalization may be necessary for acute withdrawal. Consider methadone or buprenorphine maintenance for opiate use disorder.
- Treatment for tobacco use disorder includes counseling/physician advice, nicotine replacement, and bupropion or varenicline.

ALCOHOL USE DISORDER

More common in men than in women. Evidence of a problem usually begins to surface between 18 and 25 years of age. A ⊕ family history ↑ risk. Common causes of death include suicide, cancer, heart disease, and hepatic disease.

DIAGNOSIS

- Screen with the **CAGE** questionnaire (see mnemonic).
- Monitor vital signs for tachycardia and ↑ BP associated with withdrawal; look for stigmata of liver disease such as palmar erythema or spider angiomata.
- Labs may reveal macrocytosis and an ↑ **AST** and GGT.

TREATMENT

- Rule out medical complications; correct electrolyte abnormalities and hydrate.
- Start a **benzodiazepine taper** (eg, chlordiazepoxide, lorazepam) for withdrawal symptoms—ie, the CIWA protocol.
- Give multivitamins and folic acid; **administer thiamine before glucose** to prevent Wernicke's encephalopathy.
- Individual or group counseling, Alcoholics Anonymous, disulfiram, naltrexone, or acamprosate may be of benefit.

COMPLICATIONS

- **GI bleeding** (eg, gastritis, varices, Mallory-Weiss tears), **pancreatitis, liver disease,** delirium tremens (DTs), alcoholic hallucinosis, peripheral neuropathy, cerebellar degeneration.
- **Wernicke's encephalopathy:** Acute and usually reversible ataxia accompanied by confusion and ophthalmoplegia.
- **Korsakoff's syndrome:** A chronic and often irreversible condition marked by anterograde amnesia +/− confabulation.

Neurocognitive Disorders

DELIRIUM

Delirium is common in hospitalized medical or surgical patients and is a medical, not a psychiatric, disorder. May mimic psychosis or depression.

SYMPTOMS

Characterized by the following:

- **Disturbance of consciousness** and/or perception.
- Altered cognition (memory, orientation, language)—eg, diminished attention span, impaired short-term memory, or unclear speech.

KEY FACT

Alcoholism can to**AST** your liver.

MNEMONIC

CAGE questions:

1. Have you ever felt the need to **C**ut down on your drinking?
2. Have you ever felt **A**nnoyed by criticism of your drinking?
3. Have you ever felt **G**uilty about your drinking?
4. Have you ever had a morning **E**ye opener?

More than 1 "yes" answer on the CAGE questionnaire makes alcohol use disorder more likely.

KEY FACT

Alcohol use is related to 50% of all homicides and automobile fatalities.

KEY FACT

DTs are a medical emergency with an untreated mortality rate of 20%. Give IV lorazepam.

MNEMONIC

Causes of delirium—

I WATCH DEATH

Infectious (encephalitis, meningitis, UTI)
Withdrawal (alcohol, benzodiazepines)
Acute metabolic disorder (electrolyte imbalance)
Trauma (head injury, postoperative)
CNS pathology (stroke, hemorrhage, tumor)
Hypoxia (anemia, cardiac failure)
Deficiencies (vitamin B$_{12}$, folic acid, thiamine)
Endocrinopathies (thyroid, glucose)
Acute vascular (shock, vasculitis, hypertension)
Toxins, substance use, medications
Heavy metals (arsenic, lead, mercury)

- Acute onset.
- A history suggesting a probable medical cause of delirium.
- Symptoms that "wax and wane" during the day and feature lucid intervals.
- May be due to disruption in acetylcholine.

DIFFERENTIAL

In contrast to delirium, dementia usually has an insidious onset; includes chronic memory and executive function deficits; and is characterized by symptoms that tend not to fluctuate during the day (see Table 17-3).

DIAGNOSIS

- Evaluate for recent medication changes, hypoglycemia, hepatic encephalopathy, or UTI.
- Workup may include a CBC, electrolytes, BUN/creatinine, glucose, LFTs, UA, urine toxicology, vitamin B$_{12}$/folate, TSH, RPR, HIV, blood culture, serum calcium/phosphorus/magnesium, pulse oximetry, ABGs, CSF, or serum drug screening.
- The mnemonic **I WATCH DEATH** lists common etiologies of delirium.

TREATMENT

- **Treat the underlying medical condition.**
- Minimize or discontinue delirium-inducing drugs (eg, benzodiazepines, anticholinergics) and simplify medication regimens if possible.
- Recommend reorientation techniques (eg, clocks or wall calendars) and provide an environment that will facilitate healthy sleep/wake cycles.
- Pharmacotherapy may be beneficial and includes **low-dose antipsychotics** (haloperidol, risperidone, olanzapine, quetiapine), usually for short-term use. Physical restraints may be necessary to prevent physical harm to self/others.

DEMENTIA

- General deterioration of function 2° to **chronic, progressive cognitive decline** with intact attention and consciousness.

TABLE 17-3.   Delirium vs Dementia

	DELIRIUM	DEMENTIA
Course	**Acute** (abrupt onset) lasting hours to days; usually reversible.	**Chronic** (progressive degradation) lasting months to years; usually irreversible.
Functionality	Fluctuating ability to focus and shift attention. **Clouded consciousness.**	Alert; intact consciousness.
Cognition	Similar to dementia, but more likely to include perceptual disturbances (hallucinations) and paranoia.	Disrupted memory, orientation, and language. Hallucinations are present in ~ 30% of those with advanced disease.
Causes	Evidence of a general medical condition causing the problem (seizures, postictal state, infections, thyroid disorders, UTI, vitamin deficiencies); substances (eg, cocaine, opioids, PCP); head trauma, kidney disease, sleep deprivation.	Insidious processes such as Alzheimer's disease, Huntington's disease, vascular dementia, AIDS dementia, and MDD in the elderly.

- Most common among the elderly (those > 85 years of age), and most often caused by Alzheimer's disease (50%) or multi-infarct dementia (25%).
- Refer to the Dementia section of Chapter 13 for further details.

DEPRESSION AND ANXIETY DUE TO A GENERAL MEDICAL CONDITION

- Depression can be 2° to drug intoxication (alcohol or sedative-hypnotics; antihypertensives such as methyldopa, clonidine, and propranolol) or to stroke, hypothyroidism, MS, or SLE.
- Anxiety may be caused by drugs (caffeine, sympathomimetics, steroids), endocrinopathies (pheochromocytoma, hypercortisolism, hyperthyroidism, hyperparathyroidism), metabolic disorders (hypoxemia, hypercalcemia, hypoglycemia), or SLE.

Personality Disorders

Defined as enduring patterns of inner experience and behavior that deviate from cultural standards; are pervasive and inflexible; begin in adolescence or early adulthood; are stable and predictable over time; and lead to distress or impairment (see Table 17-4). In some cases, however (eg, OCPD), personality disorders are more annoying to others than to the person they affect. **Treat with psychotherapy;** pharmacotherapy is generally used only if psychiatric comorbidities exist.

Psychiatric Emergencies

SUICIDE RISK ASSESSMENT

The tenth leading cause of death in the United States. Protective factors include religious affiliation or civic groups, married status, and parenthood. Risk factors include the following:

- **Gender:** Men **complete** suicide 3 times more often than do women, whereas women **attempt** suicide 3 times more frequently. Men also prefer more violent methods (eg, hanging, **firearms,** jumping from high places) as opposed to overdose.
- **Age:** Those > 75 years of age account for 25% of completed suicides. Suicide is also the third leading cause of death in 15- to 24-year-olds, after homicides and accidents.
- **Ethnicity:** Two-thirds of completed suicides are Caucasian males.
- **Psychiatric illness:** MDD, bipolar disorder, psychotic disorder, substance abuse or dependence.
- **Other risk factors:** Include unemployment or job dissatisfaction; chronic, debilitating illness; a history of prior suicide attempts; and a family history of suicide. **Access to firearms should always be assessed and is a risk factor for completed suicide.**

NEUROLEPTIC MALIGNANT SYNDROME (NMS)

A life-threatening complication of antipsychotic treatment. May also be precipitated in patients with Parkinson's disease following the abrupt withdrawal of the dopamine precursor levodopa. Mortality is 10–20%.

MNEMONIC

Characteristics of personality disorders—

MEDIC

Maladaptive
Enduring
Deviate from cultural norms
Inflexible
Cause impairment in social or occupational functioning

KEY FACT

To differentiate between schizoid and schizotypal, remember that schiz**OID**s feel like "**O**h, **I D**on't care."

TABLE 17-4.   **Signs and Symptoms of Personality Disorders**

DISORDER	CHARACTERISTICS	CLINICAL DILEMMA/STRATEGIES
CLUSTER A: "WEIRD"		
Paranoid	Distrustful and suspicious; interpret others' motives as malevolent. Litigious.	Patients are suspicious and distrustful of doctors and rarely seek medical attention.
Schizoid	Isolated, detached "loners." Have restricted emotional expression.	Be clear, honest, noncontrolling, and nondefensive. Avoid humor. Maintain emotional distance.
Schizotypal	Odd behavior/appearance. Exhibit cognitive or perceptual distortions (eg, magical thinking, ideas of reference).	
CLUSTER B: "WILD"		
Borderline	Unstable mood/relationships and feelings of emptiness. Impulsive. Have a history of suicidal ideation or self-harm.	Patients change the rules, demand attention, and feel that they are special.
Histrionic	Excessively emotional and attention seeking. Sexually provocative.	Will manipulate staff and doctor ("splitting"). Be firm: Stick to the treatment plan.
Narcissistic	Grandiose; need admiration; have sense of entitlement. Lack empathy.	Be fair: Do not be punitive or derogatory. Be consistent: Do not change the rules.
Antisocial	Violate the rights of others, social norms, and laws. Impulsive; lack remorse. May have a criminal history. **Begins in childhood as conduct disorder.**	
CLUSTER C: "WORRIED AND WIMPY"		
Obsessive-compulsive	Preoccupied with perfectionism, order, and control. Miserly. Have inflexible morals and values.	Patients are controlling and may sabotage their treatment. Words may be inconsistent with actions.
Avoidant	Socially inhibited; sensitive to rejection. Have fear of being disliked or ridiculed.	Avoid power struggles. Give clear recommendations, but do not push patients into decisions.
Dependent	Submissive, clingy, need to be taken care of. Have difficulty making decisions. Feel helpless.	

SYMPTOMS

- **Can occur at any time** during the course of treatment.
- Presents with **muscular rigidity** and dystonia, akinesia, mutism, obtundation, and agitation.
- Autonomic symptoms include **high fever**, diaphoresis, hypertensive episodes, and tachycardia.
- Look for $\uparrow\uparrow$ **CK** and $\uparrow$ **liver enzymes.** May progress to **rhabdomyolysis** and/or renal dysfunction.

TREATMENT

Stop the offending medication; give **dantrolene**, bromocriptine, or amantadine.

SEROTONIN SYNDROME

Caused by the administration of **multiple serotonergic agents.** These can include **MAOIs with SSRIs or venlafaxine.** Less commonly, it may involve SSRIs with lithium, SSRIs with levodopa, or SSRIs with an atypical antipsychotic.

SYMPTOMS

- Presents with delirium, agitation, tachycardia, diaphoresis, and diarrhea.
- Exam reveals **myoclonus and hyperreflexia.** In severe cases, patients may present with hyperthermia, seizures, rhabdomyolysis, renal failure, cardiac arrhythmias, and DIC.

TREATMENT

Stop the offending medications; give supportive care. Administer a serotonin antagonist or cyproheptadine.

KEY FACT

NMS is characterized by rigidity, whereas serotonin syndrome is characterized by myoclonus and hyperreflexia. Both can result in fever but are due to different offending agents.

NOTES

CHAPTER 18

PULMONARY

Pulmonary Function Tests (PFTs)

The measurements most often used in PFTs are forced expiratory volume in 1 second (FEV₁), forced vital capacity (FVC), and total lung capacity (TLC) (see Figure 18-1). Two major patterns of pulmonary diseases are identified by PFTs: **obstructive** and **restrictive**.

- **Obstructive pattern** (COPD, chronic bronchitis, bronchiectasis, asthma):
    - A disproportionate ↓ in FEV₁ compared to FVC = **an FEV₁/FVC ratio of < 0.7.**
    - TLC is ↑ in some obstructive processes, such as COPD, but may be normal or ↑ in asthma.
    - As FEV₁ ↓, the severity of obstructive airway diseases ↑.
- **Restrictive pattern** (obesity, kyphosis, inflammatory/fibrosing lung disease, interstitial lung disease):
    - **TLC is ↓ in restrictive processes.**
    - Although FEV₁ and FVC are low, the FEV₁/FVC ratio is normal or ↑.
    - An FVC of < 80% is suggestive of restriction when the FEV₁/FVC ratio is normal.

Table 18-1 outlines PFT findings in the setting of common lung conditions.

KEY FACT

Although obstructive in nature, asthma is a reversible condition. It usually has a normal DL_{CO} because the alveoli are unaffected. By contrast, COPD is characterized by a ↓ DL_{CO} because some alveoli are destroyed and unavailable for gas diffusion.

Asthma

An obstructive disease characterized by intermittent airway inflammation and hyperreactivity.

SYMPTOMS

- Presents with **intermittent wheezing,** coughing, chest tightness, or shortness of breath.

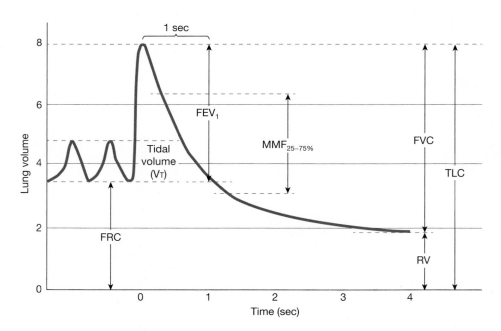

FIGURE 18-1. Normal forced exhalation curve. FRC = functional reserve capacity (volume of air in the lungs remaining after passive expiration); MMF₂₅₋₇₅% = maximum mid-expiratory flow rate; RV = residual volume (volume of air in the lungs remaining after maximum expiratory effort).

TABLE 18-1.   **PFTs in Common Settings**

	FEV$_1$/FVC	TLC	DL$_{CO}$[a]
Asthma	Normal/↓	Normal/↑	Normal/↑
COPD	↓	↑	↓
Fibrotic disease	Normal/↑	↓	↓
Extrathoracic restriction	Normal	↓	Normal

[a] DL$_{CO}$ (the diffusing capacity of carbon monoxide) measures the gas exchange capacity of the capillary-alveolar interface.

- Symptoms may be seasonal or may follow exposure to **triggers** (eg, URIs, dust, pet dander, cold air) or occur with exercise.

EXAM

- **Acute asthma exacerbations:**
  - During attacks, patients classically demonstrate a **prolonged expiratory phase** that is **sometimes accompanied by wheezing or cough.**
  - Determine severity by assessing **mental status, the ability to speak in full sentences,** use of accessory muscles, and vital signs. A normal or ↓ respiratory rate suggests respiratory fatigue.
  - Patients with severe exacerbations may have ↓ **wheezing** and will need prompt assessment of their gas exchange (with ABG analysis) along with aggressive treatment.
- **Chronic intermittent asthma:** Exam may be normal if the patient is not having an exacerbation.

DIFFERENTIAL

- **Not all that wheezes is asthma!** Rule out foreign body aspiration, endobronchial mass, laryngeal spasm or irritation, and CHF.
- In patients with chronic cough, think about asthma as well as allergic rhinitis, postnasal drip, or GERD.

DIAGNOSIS

- Definitive diagnosis is made with an **obstructive** pattern on PFTs supported by **reversibility** with bronchodilators, as demonstrated by an ↑ **in FEV$_1$ of 12% and at least 200 mL.**
- If PFTs are normal but suspicion for asthma remains high, a **methacholine challenge** can be used to provoke symptoms in a monitored setting, or an exhaled nitric oxide (Fe$_{NO}$) level can be measured. An ↑ Fe$_{NO}$ is suggestive of an asthma diagnosis.
- CXR is usually normal but can exclude other causes (eg, pneumonia, interstitial lung disease, sarcoid).

TREATMENT

- **Chronic asthma:** See Table 18-2.
- **Acute asthma exacerbations:**
  - **Short-acting β-agonist (albuterol) therapy** (nebulizer or MDI): β-agonists activate β$_2$ receptors, leading to smooth muscle relaxation of the bronchial passages and thus dilation of the airways.

KEY FACT

A ⊖ methacholine challenge generally excludes asthma.

Q

A patient with a history of asthma that was previously controlled with once-monthly albuterol states that he has been using his albuterol inhaler 4–5 times a week but denies any nighttime symptoms. How would you adjust his treatment regimen?

TABLE 18-2.   **Medications for the Treatment of Chronic Asthma**

TYPE	SYMPTOMS (DAY/NIGHT)	MEDICATIONS
Mild intermittent	≤ 2 days/week ≤ 2 nights/month	No daily medications. **PRN short-acting bronchodilator.**
Mild persistent	> 2/week but < 1/day > 2 nights/month	**Low-dose inhaled corticosteroids.** PRN short-acting bronchodilator.
Moderate persistent	Daily > 1 night/week	Low- to medium-dose inhaled corticosteroids + **long-acting inhaled β-agonists.** PRN short-acting bronchodilator.
Severe persistent	Continual frequent	**High-dose inhaled corticosteroids** + long-acting inhaled β-agonists. Possible PO steroids. PRN short-acting bronchodilator.

Reproduced with permission from Le T et al. *First Aid for the USMLE Step 2 CK,* 8th ed. New York: McGraw-Hill, 2012: 423.

KEY FACT

Inhaled corticosteroids are safe for use in pregnancy.

- **Systemic corticosteroids** such as methylprednisolone or prednisone + **inhaled corticosteroids.**
- A single 2-g dose of magnesium sulfate can be administered intravenously in severe exacerbations.
- Follow patients closely with **peak flows,** and tailor therapy to the response. A peak flow that is < 50% of baseline flow suggests a "medical alert." Consider noninvasive positive-pressure ventilation or intubation if necessary.
- Antibiotics (in the absence of infection), anticholinergics, cromolyn, and leukotriene antagonists are generally of no utility.

Chronic Obstructive Pulmonary Disease (COPD)

Defined as chronic airflow obstruction that is not fully reversible. It is often accompanied by chronic cough and sputum production. A combination of emphysema and chronic bronchitis, COPD generally involves the destruction of lung parenchyma. This results in ↓ elastic recoil, which leads to air trapping. **TLC** ↑ as a result of rising **residual volume** (RV). Chronic bronchitis is defined as a chronic productive cough for 3 or more months in each of 2 successive years.

SYMPTOMS

- Patients complain of cough, excessive sputum production, dyspnea, and wheezing. Dyspnea is usually progressive.
- Look for a **history of smoking** (or exposure to biomass fuels such as indoor wood fires in the developing world).

EXAM

Add a low-dose inhaled corticosteroid, as the patient now has mild persistent asthma.

- Exam may show ↓ breath sounds, cough (productive and nonproductive), pursed-lip breathing, barrel chest, rhonchi, or wheezing.
- Hypercarbia/hypoxia and weight loss are seen in later stages.
- Patients may show evidence of **cor pulmonale** (right heart failure from pulmonary hypertension caused by chronic hypoxia).

DIAGNOSIS

- **FEV$_1$/FVC is < 0.7** and FEV$_1$ < 80% of predicted. **TLC** is usually ↑.
- The condition is **not fully reversible** with bronchodilators.
- **DL$_{CO}$** tends to be ↓.
- CXR shows hyperlucent, **hyperinflated** lungs with **flat diaphragms** (see Figure 18-2).
- Disease severity, and hence stage, is determined by the ↓ in FEV$_1$ in relation to predicted, the patient's symptoms, and the number of annual COPD exacerbations.

TREATMENT

- **Chronic COPD:**
    - **Inhaled β-agonists** (albuterol) **and anticholinergics** (ipratropium): Short-acting agents for less severe symptoms; long-acting agents for more severe symptoms.
    - **O$_2$ therapy:** Indicated for patients with an O$_2$ saturation of < 88%, a **partial pressure of oxygen (Pao$_2$) of < 55 mm Hg**, or a Pao$_2$ of 55–60 mm Hg and evidence of cor pulmonale.
    - Inhaled corticosteroids do **not** play a critical role unless PFTs reveal significant reversible airway disease or the patient has frequent exacerbations.
    - Vaccinate patients against influenza (yearly) and pneumococcal pneumonia (at least once).
- **Acute COPD exacerbations:** Defined as ↑ **dyspnea** or a **change in cough or sputum production.**
    - Check a **CXR** to look for causes of the exacerbation (eg, pneumonia, CHF).
    - Administer O$_2$ to maintain a saturation of 90–95% (there is no need to go higher!).
    - Start patients on an inhaled β-agonist (albuterol) and an **anticholinergic** (ipratropium).
    - **Systemic corticosteroids** (prednisone) may ↓ the duration of hospital stay but should be tapered over 3–14 days.

> **KEY FACT**
>
> Think α$_1$-antitrypsin deficiency in young patients with COPD and bullae.

> **KEY FACT**
>
> Only O$_2$ therapy and smoking cessation have been unequivocally shown to improve survival in patients with COPD.

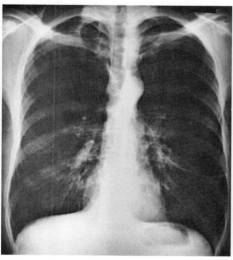

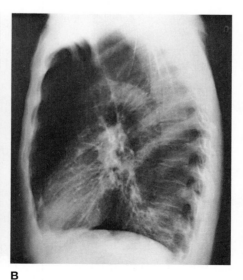

A   **B**

FIGURE 18-2. **Chronic obstructive pulmonary disease.** Note the hyperinflated and hyperlucent lungs, flat diaphragms, increased AP diameter, narrow mediastinum, and large upper lobe bullae on AP (**A**) and lateral (**B**) CXR. (Reproduced with permission from Stobo JD et al. *The Principles and Practice of Medicine*, 23rd ed. Stamford, CT: Appleton & Lange, 1996: 135.)

> **Q**
>
> You order PFTs for a patient with worsening shortness of breath. Which of the following values would be consistent with a diagnosis of COPD?
>
> (A) Low FEV$_1$, low FVC, low FEV$_1$/FVC, high TLC, low DL$_{CO}$.
> (B) Low FEV$_1$, low FVC, high FEV$_1$/FVC, low TLC, low DL$_{CO}$.

KEY FACT

Treat all hypoxic patients with O_2. CO_2 retention won't kill the patient, but hypoxia will.

KEY FACT

Think of methemoglobinemia, or an ↑ in methemoglobin (an altered state of hemoglobin that cannot bind to O_2), in patients with clinical cyanosis but a normal Pao_2. Treat with methylene blue, which reduces methemoglobin to hemoglobin.

The answer is A. Choice B describes a restrictive pattern.

- Hypoventilation leading to acute hypercarbia (an ↑ in Pco_2) may necessitate mechanical ventilation.
- **Empiric antibiotics** with coverage of *Streptococcus*, *H influenzae*, and *Moraxella* are indicated in an acute setting.
  - **Outpatient:** Amoxicillin/clavulanate, TMP-SMX, or doxycycline.
  - **Hospitalized:** Azithromycin, a respiratory fluoroquinolone, or a third-generation cephalosporin.

Hypoxia and Hypoxemia

Hypoxia is a state of deficient O_2 supply to the body or its organs. Hypoxemia is a ↓ Pao_2. Both conditions can be caused by a number of processes, outlined below.

DIAGNOSIS

1. **Determine if there is an alveolar-arterial (A-a) oxygen gradient.**
   a. **No gradient:** Consider a low Fio_2 state or high altitude. **Corrects with supplemental O_2.**
   b. **Positive gradient:**
      - **Shunt physiology: Does not correct with supplemental O_2.** Causes may be pulmonary or extrapulmonary.
        - **Pulmonary processes:** Alveolar collapse (atelectasis), lobar pneumonia, ARDS.
        - **Extrapulmonary processes:** PDA, patent foramen ovale.
      - **Ventilation-perfusion (V/Q) mismatch: Corrects with supplemental O_2.** Causes include asthma, COPD, pneumonia, interstitial lung disease, and pulmonary embolism (PE).
2. Hypoxia can also be accompanied by **hypercarbia** (↑ $Paco_2$). Causes include:
   - ↓ respiratory drive from CNS depression (opiates, stroke) or central sleep apnea.
   - Neuromuscular disease (normal A-a gradient).
   - COPD or obstructive lung disease. (generally ↓ A-a gradient).

TREATMENT

Always treat hypoxic patients with adequate amounts of O_2 to maintain saturations of > 90% or a Pao_2 of > 60 mm Hg.

Pleural Effusion

Effusions are characterized as either **transudative** or **exudative** on the basis of their composition.

SYMPTOMS/EXAM

- Presents with shortness of breath and occasionally with pleuritic chest pain.
- Patients may be asymptomatic or show symptoms of an underlying process (eg, CHF, pneumonia).
- Exam reveals ↓ **breath sounds, dullness** to percussion, and ↓ tactile fremitus on the side with the effusion.

DIAGNOSIS

- **CXR:**
    - Blunting of the costophrenic angle can be seen on a PA film if > 200–500 mL of fluid is present (see Figure 18-3).
    - A lateral decubitus film can reveal a 100-mL effusion.
- **Ultrasound:** Helps distinguish a free from a loculated effusion; can assist with thoracentesis.
- **CT:** Can better visualize fluid and characterize loculations.
- **Thoracentesis:**
    - To aid in management, obtain the following assays on pleural fluid: Gram stain and culture, AFB, glucose, triglycerides, cell count with differential, and pH. Serum total protein and LDH values will also be needed (see Table 18-3).
    - If the fluid is **transudative**, focus on treating the underlying cause (CHF, ascites, nephrotic syndrome, peritoneal dialysis, ventriculoperitoneal shunt, atelectasis, hypoalbuminemia).
    - If the fluid is **exudative**, refer to Table 18-4 to help determine the cause.

TREATMENT

- **Thoracentesis** for an effusion > 10 mm thick (or about 100 mL) may be both therapeutic (relieves dyspnea) and diagnostic.
- **Indications for a chest tube (any one of these)** are:
    - A pleural WBC count > 100,000/mm^3 or frank pus, or gram-$\oplus$ fluid.
    - Glucose < 40 mg/dL.
    - pH < 7.0.

COMPLICATIONS

- An untreated pleural effusion in the setting of pneumonia may become infected and turn into an empyema.
- Over time, exudative effusions may become loculated and require drainage by video-assisted thoracoscopy (VATS) or surgical decortication.
- Complications of thoracentesis include pneumothorax and bleeding (remember, the neurovascular bundle runs along the inferior side of the rib). Use ultrasound during the procedure to minimize the risk of pneumothorax, and obtain a CXR afterward.

> **KEY FACT**
>
> Consider a pleural biopsy if you suspect TB. Send the fluid for cytology if you suspect malignancy.

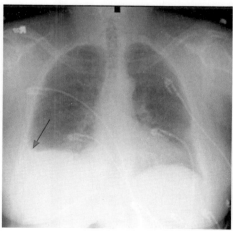
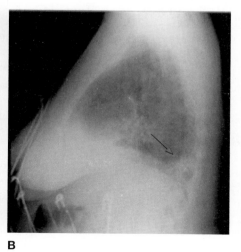

A

B

FIGURE 18-3. **Pleural effusion.** PA (A) and lateral (B) CXRs show blunting of the right costophrenic sulcus (arrows). (Reproduced with permission from USMLE-Rx.com.)

> **Q**
>
> A 33-year-old man presents with cough, night sweats, and pleuritic chest pain. CXR shows a left pleural effusion. PPD demonstrates 16 mm of induration. Thoracentesis reveals a glucose level of 50 mg/dL, LDH 340 U/L, pleural fluid protein 4.6 g/dL, and serum protein 3.0 mg/dL. A sputum culture for acid-fast bacilli (AFB) is $\ominus$. What is the next step?

TABLE 18-3. Thoracentesis Findings in Transudative vs Exudative Pleural Effusions

	PLEURAL/SERUM PROTEIN (RATIO)	PLEURAL/SERUM LDH (RATIO)	PLEURAL LDH
Transudative	< 0.5 **or**	< 0.6 **or**	< 200
Exudative	> 0.5 **or**	> 0.6 **or**	> 200

KEY FACT

Suspect pneumothorax with shortness of breath and chest pain plus underlying COPD, CF, chest procedures (eg, central lines), or trauma. A 1° pneumothorax may be seen in young adults with a tall, thin body habitus.

KEY FACT

The differential for shortness of breath/chest pain includes pneumothorax, MI, PE, pleuritis, and aortic dissection.

Pneumothorax

Defined as air that becomes trapped in the pleural space.

SYMPTOMS/EXAM

- Presents with acute shortness of breath and pleuritic chest pain.
- Exam reveals **tachypnea**, ↓ tactile fremitus, ↓ breath sounds, **tympany** on percussion on the side involved, and tracheal deviation toward the affected side.

DIAGNOSIS

- CXR shows a distinct lack of lung markings within the pneumothorax along with collapse of the lung on that side (see Figure 18-4).
- Tracheal deviation away from the side of the pneumothorax suggests tension pneumothorax (see below).

TREATMENT

- Chest tube insertion is required in patients with a pneumothorax of > 30%.
- Smaller pneumothoraces may be managed simply with supplemental O_2 and observation.
- For patients with recurrent pneumothorax, consider pleurodesis.

TABLE 18-4. Assays for Exudative Fluid and Their Differential Diagnosis

PLEURAL ASSAY	VALUE	DIFFERENTIAL
Glucose	< 60	Empyema or parapneumonia, TB, RA, malignancy.
WBCs	> 10,000	Empyema or parapneumonia, rheumatoid arthritis (RA), malignancy.
RBCs	> 100,000	Gross blood—think of trauma, PE.
Cellular differential		
Lymphocytes		TB, sarcoid, malignancy, chylothorax.
PMNs		Empyema, PE.
Eosinophils		Bleeding, pneumothorax.
pH	< 7.20	Complicated effusion or empyema.
Triglycerides	> 150	Diagnostic of chylothorax.

This patient has an exudative pleural effusion with suspected TB. A pleural biopsy is needed to confirm the diagnosis despite the fact that the patient's sputum smear was ⊖ for AFB.

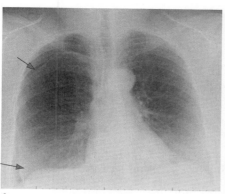
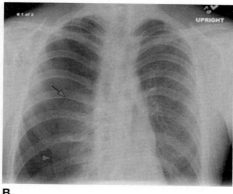

A   **B**

FIGURE 18-4. **Pneumothorax.** (A) Small right pneumothorax. (B) Right tension pneumothorax with collapse of the right lung and shifting of mediastinal structures to the left. Arrows
denote pleural reflections. (Reproduced with permission from USMLE-Rx.com.)

TENSION PNEUMOTHORAX

An emergent complication of pneumothorax in which a disruption in the
bronchial or alveolar wall acts as a 1-way valve, allowing air to be drawn
into the pleural space and become trapped. Airway wall injury can be due
to trauma (eg, penetrating chest trauma, iatrogenic injury) or to rupture of
an abnormal alveolar wall (seen in COPD). The result is **rapid decompensation**, hypotension, and circulatory collapse leading to **shock.**

DIAGNOSIS

Look for a **pneumothorax** along with **tachycardia, hypotension,** $\uparrow O_2$ requirements, and $\uparrow$ JVP. The trachea deviates **away** from the side with tension.

TREATMENT

If you suspect that the patient has a tension pneumothorax, **don't wait for
imaging!** Insert a large-bore needle with a syringe superior to the second or
third rib at the midclavicular line on the side of $\downarrow$ breath sounds to decom-
press the chest, and then insert a chest tube.

Pulmonary Embolism (PE)

The causes of PE can be remembered with **Virchow's triad:**

- **Stasis:** Immobility, CHF, obesity, $\uparrow$ JVP.
- **Endothelial injury:** Trauma, surgery, recent fracture, prior DVT.
- **Hypercoagulable state:** Pregnancy, OCP use, coagulation disorders,
  malignancy, burns.

SYMPTOMS

- Acute-onset chest pain (especially pleuritic) or shortness of breath.
- Syncope.
- Consider in patients who have risk factors for DVT/PE or leg pain and
  swelling.

Q   **1**

A 34-year-old man with COPD
comes to the ED with sudden-onset
shortness of breath that requires high
levels of supplemental O_2. Physical
exam reveals $\downarrow$ breath sounds on the
left side and tracheal deviation to the
right. What is your next step?

Q   **2**

A 72-year-old patient who was
admitted to the hospital for a
hemorrhagic stroke develops
shortness of breath. Imaging reveals a
pulmonary embolus and a left lower
extremity DVT. How do you proceed?

KEY FACT

Consider PE in any hospitalized patient who has dyspnea or unexplained tachycardia.

KEY FACT

Upper extremity DVTs and superficial thromboses are usually associated with IV catheters. About 6% of PEs are from upper extremity DVTs.

EXAM

- Exam shows **tachypnea, tachycardia,** cyanosis, a loud P2 or S2, ↑ JVP, and signs of right heart failure.
- Patients may occasionally have hemoptysis or a low-grade fever.

DIFFERENTIAL

Acute MI, pneumonia, pneumothorax, CHF, aortic dissection.

DIAGNOSIS

Initial assessment should include the following (see also Figures 18-5 and 18-6):

- **ABGs** may show a 1° respiratory alkalosis and an ↑ A-a gradient.
- **CXR** is usually **normal** but may show:
  - A wedge-shaped infarct (Hampton's hump).
  - Oligemia in the affected lobe (Westermark's sign).
  - Pleural effusion.
- **ECG** most commonly demonstrates **sinus tachycardia** but may also reveal an S wave in lead I, a Q wave in lead III, and T-wave inversion in lead III (neither sensitive nor specific).

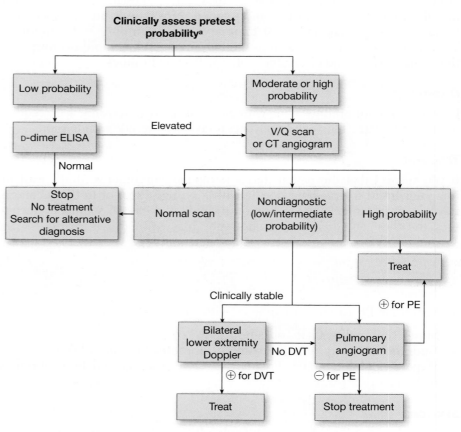

^a Clinical clues:
1. Sudden onset of dyspnea or worsening of chronic dyspnea
2. Pleuritic chest pain or pleural rub
3. Hypoxemia ($SaO_2 < 92\%$)
4. Hemoptysis
5. Recent surgery or immobilization
6. Prior history of DVT or PE

FIGURE 18-5. Diagnostic algorithm for pulmonary embolism. (Adapted with permission from Toy EC, Patlan JT. *Case Files: Internal Medicine,* 3rd ed. New York: McGraw-Hill, 2009, Fig. 82-1.)

1 **A**

Needle decompression for presumed left-sided tension pneumothorax.

2 **A**

Place an IVC filter.

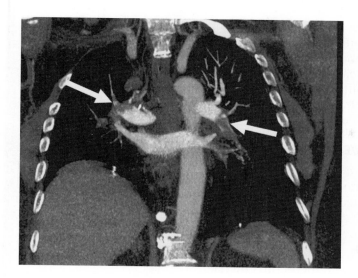

FIGURE 18-6. **Bilateral pulmonary emboli.** CT angiogram shows filling defects in the main and segmental pulmonary arteries (arrows) of a lung cancer patient who developed sudden shortness of breath and chest heaviness. (Reproduced with permission from Longo DL et al. *Harrison's Principles of Internal Medicine,* 18th ed. New York: McGraw-Hill, 2012, Fig. 262-3.)

- **Chest CT with contrast** has largely replaced V/Q scanning as the **1° diagnostic modality** unless it is contraindicated by renal insufficiency, pregnancy, or dye allergy.
- **Pulmonary angiography** can be considered for the diagnosis of PE and may be needed if other testing is intermediate. (Now rarely necessary.)

TREATMENT

- Treat venous thromboembolism (VTE) patients with anticoagulation to prevent recurrent VTE. Without anticoagulation, the risk of recurrent PE is 25%.
- Initially use **IV heparin or low-molecular-weight heparin.** Patients who are not adequately anticoagulated within 24 hours have a high rate of recurrence.
- Patients should then be transitioned to warfarin therapy with a goal INR of 2.0–3.0.
- In patients with documented large **central PEs** (saddle PEs) and hypotension or shock, consider administering **tPA** along with heparin. The duration of anticoagulation therapy will vary with risk factors.
- For patients with a **first event** and **reversible** or time-limited risk factors (eg, surgery, pregnancy), treat for at least **3–6 months.**
- Consider **lifelong anticoagulation** in patients with **chronic risk factors** (eg, malignancy, paraplegia, genes for hypercoagulable conditions, recurrent DVTs, PEs).
- In patients who cannot safely be anticoagulated, an IVC filter may be useful. Although these filters can ↓ the risk of PE, they are associated with a **higher risk** of recurrent DVT.

> **KEY FACT**
>
> Don't forget to order DVT prophylaxis for all your high-risk hospitalized patients!

Acute Respiratory Distress Syndrome (ARDS)

Acute lung injury characterized by noncardiogenic pulmonary edema, resulting in bilateral, diffuse alveolar damage and hypoxia. It can be caused by a range of pulmonary and nonpulmonary conditions, including:

- Sepsis
- Aspiration (usually massive aspiration of gastric contents)
- Pneumonia
- Trauma (particularly trauma to the chest or massive tissue injury)
- Transfusion-related lung injury (TRALI)
- Lung transplant
- Stem cell transplant

SYMPTOMS/EXAM

Look for a patient with risk factors, usually in an **ICU setting.** Patients will have **acute** onset of hypoxia along with diffuse rales on exam and will be difficult to oxygenate. Intubation is usually required to maintain an acceptable Pao_2.

DIAGNOSIS

Diagnose with the Berlin criteria:

- Lung injury that develops within 1 week of clinical insult or respiratory decompensation.
- Imaging that shows diffuse **bilateral pulmonary opacities** (see Figure 18-7).
- ↓ **oxygenation** as defined by the **Pao_2/Fio_2 ratio** (ratio of the arterial O_2 level on ABG divided by the fraction of inhaled O_2 the patient is on).
  - **Mild:** 200–300.
  - **Moderate:** 100–200.
  - **Severe:** < 100.

TREATMENT

- Patients typically require intubation and mechanical ventilation for the management of hypoxia.
- **Low tidal volumes** (6 mL/kg) and associated permissive hypercapnia (ie, letting Pco_2 rise) lead to a ↓↓ risk of barotrauma.
- **Positive end-expiratory pressure (PEEP)** improves oxygenation and thus ↓ the Fio_2 requirement and associated O_2 toxicity.
- Look for the **underlying cause** and focus treatment on that as you stabilize the patient and treat hypoxia.

KEY FACT

Remember—use low tidal volumes and PEEP for the treatment of ARDS.

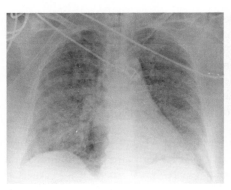 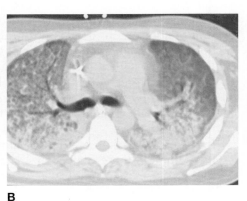

A   B

FIGURE 18-7. Acute respiratory distress syndrome. (A) Frontal CXR showing patchy areas of airspace consolidation in a patient with ARDS. **(B)** Transaxial CT showing ground-glass opacity anteriorly and consolidations dependently in a patient with exudative-phase ARDS. (Reproduced with permission from Longo DL et al. *Harrison's Principles of Internal Medicine,* 18th ed. New York: McGraw-Hill, 2012, Figs. 262-2 and 268-4.)

Solitary Pulmonary Nodule (SPN)

Defined as a radiodense lesion seen on chest imaging that is **< 3 cm in diameter** and is not associated with infiltrates, adenopathy, or atelectasis.

SYMPTOMS/EXAM

Most SPNs are detected on routine CXR in patients who are otherwise **asymptomatic**. Benign and malignant lesions can be distinguished as follows:

- **Benign lesions** (eg, histoplasmosis, coccidioidomycosis, TB, hamartoma):
  - **No growth** on serial imaging 2 years apart.
  - **A diffuse, dense and central, popcorn-like, or concentric "target" calcification pattern.**
  - Occurrence in patients who are **lifelong nonsmokers**, are **< 30 years of age**, and have **no history of malignancy.**
- **Malignant lesions** (ie, lung cancer or metastases):
  - **Size > 2 cm.**
  - **Spiculation** (ie, ragged edges).
  - Sunburst pattern.
  - Upper lobe location.
  - Occurrence in patients who are **smokers**, are **> 40 years of age**, or have a **prior diagnosis of cancer.**

DIAGNOSIS/TREATMENT

- Start by examining old radiographs to determine age and change in size. Lesions with > 1 malignant feature should be further evaluated with CT imaging.
- If imaging points to a malignancy, biopsy tissue via bronchoscopy, needle aspiration, or VATS. If the probability of malignancy is low, evaluate with serial CXRs or CTs every 3 months for 1 year and then every 6 months for 1 year.
- For patients who lack previous imaging, follow the Fleischner Society guidelines (see Table 18-5).

KEY FACT

The appearance of "popcorn" calcification within an SPN likely represents a benign hamartoma.

Sarcoidosis

An idiopathic illness characterized by the formation of **noncaseating granulomas** in various organs. Most patients have pulmonary involvement.

TABLE 18-5. Guidelines for the Diagnosis of Solitary Pulmonary Nodules

| | FOLLOW-UP | |
NODULE SIZE	LOW RISK	HIGH RISK
< 4 mm	None.	CT at 12 months.
4–6 mm	CT at 12 months.	CT at 6–12 and 18–24 months.
6–8 mm	CT at 6–12 and 18–24 months.	CT at 3–6, 9–12, and 24 months.
> 8 mm	Serial CT, PET scan, or excision based on radiographic characteristics.	

Q

A chest CT of a 61-year-old patient with no smoking history reveals a noncalcified 1.7-cm nodule. What is your next step?

MNEMONIC

Features of sarcoidosis—

GRUELING

Granulomas
Rheumatoid arthritis
Uveitis
Erythema nodosum
Lymphadenitis
Interstitial fibrosis
Negative PPD
Gammaglobulinemia

SYMPTOMS/EXAM

Typical features include **fever, cough, malaise, weight loss, dyspnea,** and **arthritis,** particularly of the knees and ankles.

DIFFERENTIAL

Sarcoidosis is a **diagnosis of exclusion,** so be sure to rule out other diseases that present similarly, such as **TB, lymphoma,** fungal infection, idiopathic pulmonary fibrosis, HIV, and berylliosis.

DIAGNOSIS

- Look for **bilateral hilar lymphadenopathy** on CXR and/or infiltrates (see Figure 18-8).
- PFTs show a **restrictive or mixed restrictive-obstructive** pattern. Patients may also have **hypercalcemia caused by the production of calcitriol by activated macrophages.**
- Tissue biopsy shows **noncaseating granulomas without organisms.**

TREATMENT

Therapy includes systemic **corticosteroids** such as prednisone. Gear other medications toward the control of symptoms such as coughing or wheezing.

Sleep Apnea

Intermittent episodes of hypoxia and recurrent arousal during sleep, resulting in daytime sleepiness. May be obstructive or central.

- **Obstructive sleep apnea (OSA):** Upper airway collapse during sleep (↓ airflow but normal effort).
- **Central sleep apnea (CSA):** Diminished central ventilator drive (↓ airflow and effort). May be 1° (idiopathic) or 2° (stroke, heart failure, CNS depressants).

Compare the CT scan with an old CXR.

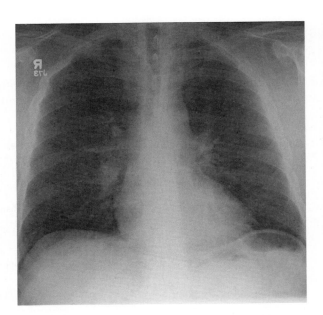

FIGURE 18-8. **Bilateral hilar lymphadenopathy in a patient with sarcoidosis.** (Reproduced with permission from Imboden JB et al. *Current Diagnosis & Treatment: Rheumatology,* 3rd ed. New York, McGraw-Hill, 2013, Fig. 54-1B.)

Symptoms

- Presents with neurocognitive impairment, morning headache, poor sleep, or impotence.
- With OSA, the patient may report snoring, choking, or gasping during sleep.

Exam

Patients with OSA are typically **obese** and **hypertensive**. They may also have a **large neck circumference.** Look for **micrognathia/retrognathia,** a **large tongue,** or large tonsils.

Differential

Rule out other causes of excessive daytime sleepiness, including **obesity hypoventilation syndrome,** narcolepsy, and restless leg syndrome.

Diagnosis

- **Overnight polysomnography (sleep study)** is the gold standard for diagnosis. Severity is measured by the apnea-hypopnea index (AHI), defined as the number of apneas and/or hypopneas (shallow breathing) per hour of sleep. An **AHI of > 5** is diagnostic of sleep apnea.
- OSA is associated with observed physical attempts to breathe.

Treatment

- The most effective treatment for both central and obstructive sleep apnea is **continuous positive airway pressure (CPAP)** or bilevel positive airway pressure (BiPAP) ventilation to keep the airways open during sleep.
- For OSA, other treatment options include weight loss, oral appliances to relieve the obstruction, and surgery such as uvulopalatopharyngoplasty (effective in 40–50% of cases).
- For CSA, treat the underlying condition whenever possible (eg, CHF, excessive opiates).

Complications

Patients with OSA are at ↑ risk of **hypertension, left ventricular dysfunction, cardiac dysrhythmias, pulmonary hypertension,** and insulin resistance.

> **KEY FACT**
>
> Central sleep apnea with Cheyne-Stokes breathing—which is characterized by deep, rapid breathing followed by ↓ ventilation and apnea—is often caused by stroke or heart failure.

Cystic Fibrosis (CF)

An **autosomal recessive** disorder with mutations located in the CFTR gene, leading to **abnormal transfer of sodium and chloride.** Multiple exocrine glands and cilia in various organs become dysfunctional. The **most common genetic disease in the United States and among Caucasians, affecting 1 in 3200.**

Symptoms

- Patients typically present in childhood or adolescence.
- Look for **recurrent pulmonary infections,** sinusitis, or **bronchiectasis.**
- Infants may present with **meconium ileus** or **intussusception.**
- Also presents with pancreatic insufficiency characterized by steatorrhea and poor weight gain due to malabsorption.
- Adult males may present with infertility.

> **Q**
>
> A 46-year-old African American woman presents with chronic dyspnea and a mild cough with clear sputum. Exam reveals raised, painful lesions on her legs. Labs show a serum calcium level of 9.6 mg/dL, and CXR demonstrates hilar adenopathy. What will confirm the diagnosis of sarcoidosis?

EXAM

- Patients may have short stature and nasal polyps.
- Lung exam often reveals **wheezing, crackles,** or **squeaks. Clubbing** may be present.
- Hyperinflation is seen early and is followed by peribronchial cuffing, mucous plugging, and bronchiectasis (see Figure 18-9).

DIAGNOSIS

- Diagnosis is made with a sweat chloride test of **> 60 mEq/L** (must be confirmed on 2 different days).
- Genetic testing can confirm the presence of many of the genetic mutations (ΔF508 is the most common genetic mutation).

TREATMENT

- Pulmonary symptoms are treated with **chest physiotherapy, bronchodilators, and mucolytics** (DNase).
- Patients need supplemental pancreatic enzymes, **fat-soluble vitamins (A, D, E, K)** to address fat malabsorption, and stool softeners (fiber).
- **Chronic** and **chronic intermittent oral antibiotics (azithromycin)** or **inhaled antibiotics (tobramycin)** may also be beneficial. *Pseudomonas aeruginosa* is common; therapies are tailored to treat the infecting organism.
- In severe end-stage pulmonary disease, bilateral **lung transplantation** is the **only definitive treatment.**

KEY FACT

In CF patients with signs of pulmonary infection, think *Pseudomonas* and/or *Staphylococcus.*

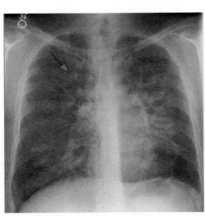
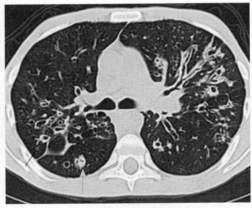

A   B

FIGURE 18-9. **Cystic fibrosis.** (A) Frontal CXR showing central cystic bronchiectasis (arrow) in a patient with CF. (B) Transaxial CT image showing cystic bronchiectasis (red arrow), with some bronchi containing impacted mucus (yellow arrow). (Reproduced with permission from USMLE-Rx.com.)

An endobronchial biopsy revealing a noncaseating granuloma is confirmatory. A biopsy specimen of erythema nodosum will not show granulomatous involvement and is not diagnostically helpful.

CHAPTER 19

HIGH-YIELD CCS CASES

How to Use This Section

In this section are 100 **minicases** reflecting the types of clinical situations encountered on the actual CCS. Each case consists of **columns** that start on the left-hand page and end on the right-hand page with the **Final Diagnosis.** As you read each column, ask yourself what you should do and/or think next (see Table 19-1). If no results are given for a test, assume that it is **normal.** To get the most out of these minicases, we **strongly** recommend that you do at least a few of the CCS cases on the USMLE CD-ROM (or from the USMLE Web site) to get a feel for the case flow and key decision points. This will allow you to place the minicases in context. Happy studying!

TABLE 19-1. Approaching the CCS Minicases

WHEN READING . . .	ASK YOURSELF . . .
History	What should I be looking for on VS and PE?
	Do I need to stabilize the patient or perform an emergency procedure before conducting a PE?
Physical exam	What are the most likely diagnoses that explain the patient's presentation?
Differential	What are the initial diagnostic tests and treatment that should be done?
	Does the patient need to be transferred to another location (eg, from the ER to the ICU)?
	Does the clock need to be advanced?
Initial management	What additional workup and management should occur?
	Can the patient be discharged or transferred to another setting?
Continuing management	What should be done in follow-up, including long-term disease management, health maintenance, and patient counseling?
	Should any treatment or monitoring be stopped?
Follow-up	What is the final diagnosis?

HEADACHE

CASE 1

HX	PE	DDX
21 yo F presents with a severe headache. She has a history of throbbing left temporal pain that lasts for 2–3 hours. Before these episodes start, she sees flashes of light in her right visual field and feels weakness and numbness on the right side of her body for a few minutes. The headaches are often associated with nausea and vomiting. She has a family history of migraine.	VS: T 37°C (99.2°F), P 70, BP 120/80, RR 15, O_2 sat 100% room air Gen: NAD Lungs: WNL CV: WNL Abd: WNL Ext: WNL Neuro: WNL	▪ Cluster headache ▪ Intracranial neoplasm ▪ Migraine (complicated) ▪ Partial seizure ▪ Pseudotumor cerebri ▪ Tension headache ▪ Trigeminal neuralgia

CASE 2

HX	PE	DDX
29 yo F presents with daily episodes of bilateral bandlike throbbing pain in her frontal-occipital region that last between 30 minutes and a few hours. She usually experiences these episodes when she is either tired or under stress. She denies any associated nausea, vomiting, phonophobia, photophobia, or aura. She also feels pain and stiffness in her neck and shoulder.	VS: Afebrile, P 70, BP 120/80, RR 15 Gen: NAD Lungs: WNL CV: WNL Abd: WNL Ext: WNL Neuro: WNL	▪ Cluster headache ▪ Intracranial neoplasm ▪ Meningitis ▪ Migraine headache ▪ Pseudotumor cerebri ▪ Sinusitis ▪ Tension headache

CASE 3

HX	PE	DDX
65 yo F presents with a severe intermittent headache in the right temporal lobe together with blurred vision in her right eye and pain in her jaw during mastication.	VS: T 37°C (99°F), P 85, BP 140/85, RR 18, O_2 sat 100% room air Gen: NAD HEENT: Tenderness on temporal artery palpation Neck: No rigidity Lungs: WNL CV: WNL Abd: WNL Ext: WNL Neuro: WNL	▪ Cluster headache ▪ Glaucoma ▪ Intracranial neoplasm ▪ Meningitis ▪ Migraine ▪ Temporal arteritis (giant cell arteritis) ▪ Tension headache ▪ Trigeminal neuralgia

INITIAL MGMT	CONTINUING MGMT	F/U
Emergency room W/U ■ CT–head ■ CBC ■ Chem 8 ■ ESR **Rx** ■ IV normal saline ■ IV promethazine, prochlorperazine, or metoclopramide ■ Aspirin, NSAIDs, or acetaminophen ■ Caffeine ■ IM sumatriptan (if the patient does not improve)		■ Follow up in 1 month ■ Prophylactic therapy if the migraine recurs—eg, β-blockers, antidepressants (SSRIs, TCAs), anticonvulsants (valproic acid, gabapentin), calcium channel blockers

Final Dx: Migraine (complicated)

INITIAL MGMT	CONTINUING MGMT	F/U
Office W/U ■ CBC with differential ■ Chem 8 ■ ESR **Rx** ■ Cold compresses ■ Acetaminophen ■ NSAIDs		■ Follow up in 1 month ■ Relaxation exercises

Final Dx: Tension headache

INITIAL MGMT	CONTINUING MGMT	F/U
Emergency room STAT ■ IV normal saline ■ Prednisone **Emergency room W/U** ■ CBC ■ Chem 8 ■ MRI/MRA—brain: ⊖ ■ CXR: ⊖ ■ ESR: ↑↑ ■ CRP: ↑↑	**Ward W/U** ■ Ophthalmology consult ■ Temporal artery biopsy: ⊕ for temporal arteritis ■ ESR every morning ■ Screen for polymyalgia rheumatica **Rx** ■ Continue high-dose prednisone for at least 2 weeks; then taper	■ Discharge home ■ Continue low-dose maintenance prednisone with slow taper ■ ESR in 2 weeks ■ Adequate dietary calcium and vitamin D if steroids are to be used chronically

Final Dx: Temporal arteritis (giant cell arteritis)

CASE 4

HX	PE	DDX
25 yo M presents with a high fever, severe headache, and photophobia.	VS: T 39°C (103°F), P 95, BP 150/85, RR 18, O$_2$ sat 100% room air Gen: Moderate distress Neck: Nuchal rigidity Lungs: WNL CV: WNL Abd: WNL Ext: WNL Neuro: ⊕ Kernig's and Brudzinski's signs	• Encephalitis • Intracranial or epidural abscess • Meningitis • Migraine • Sinusitis • Subarachnoid hemorrhage

CASE 5

HX	PE	DDX
60 yo M with a past medical history of hypertension presents with severe headache, nausea, and vomiting. The patient states that he stopped taking his metoprolol because he thought that he did not need it anymore.	VS: T 37°C (99.3°F), P 100, BP 220/120, RR 20, O$_2$ sat 95% room air Gen: Severe distress HEENT: Funduscopy reveals papilledema Lungs: WNL CV: WNL Abd: WNL Ext: WNL Neuro: WNL	• Cluster headache • Intracranial hemorrhage • Intracranial neoplasm • Malignant hypertension • Migraine • Partial seizure

INITIAL MGMT	CONTINUING MGMT	F/U
Emergency room STAT	**Ward W/U**	■ Improved within 48 hours
■ IV normal saline	■ CSF culture: ⊕ for *S pneumoniae*	■ Discharge home
■ Blood culture	■ Blood culture: ⊖	■ Follow up in 1 month
■ CT—head	**Rx**	
■ Ceftriaxone and vancomycin	■ Continue ceftriaxone + vancomycin +	
■ LP-CSF: ↑ WBCs, ↑ protein, ↓ CSF/blood	steroids	
glucose ratio, gram-⊕ cocci, ↑ opening		
pressure		
■ IV dexamethasone		
Emergency room W/U		
■ CBC: ↑ WBC count		
■ Chem 8		
■ CT—head: ⊖		
■ CXR: ⊖		
Rx		
■ Acetaminophen		

Final Dx: Bacterial meningitis

INITIAL MGMT	CONTINUING MGMT	F/U
Emergency room STAT	**ICU W/U**	■ Transfer to the floor
■ O_2	■ Continuous cardiac monitoring	■ Counsel patient re medication compliance
■ IV labetalol	■ Lipid profile	■ Discharge home
■ BP in both arms	■ Echocardiography: EF < 45%	■ Follow up in 1 week
■ CT—head: White matter changes	**Rx**	
consistent with hypertension	■ Switch to oral agents after first 24 hours;	
■ ECG: LVH	labetalol or metoprolol if good control	
■ CXR	previously	
Emergency room W/U	■ ACEIs (low EF)	
■ Cardiac/BP monitoring	■ HCTZ	
■ CPK-MB, troponin × 3: ⊖		
■ CBC		
■ Chem 8		
■ UA		

Final Dx: Hypertensive emergency

ALTERED MENTAL STATUS/LOSS OF CONSCIOUSNESS

CASE 6

HX	PE	DDX
84 yo F brought in by her son complains of forgetfulness (eg, forgets phone numbers, loses her way home) along with difficulty performing some of her daily activities (eg, bathing, dressing, managing money, answering the phone). The problem has gradually progressed over the past few years.	VS: P 90, BP 120/60, RR 12 Gen: NAD Lungs: WNL CV: WNL Abd: WNL Ext: WNL Neuro: On mini-mental status exam, patient cannot recall objects, follow 3-step commands, or spell "world" backward; cranial nerves intact; strength and sensation intact	▪ Alzheimer's disease ▪ B_{12} deficiency ▪ Chronic subdural hematoma ▪ Depression ▪ Hypothyroidism ▪ Intracranial tumor ▪ Neurosyphilis ▪ Pressure hydrocephalus ▪ Vascular dementia

CASE 7

HX	PE	DDX
79 yo M is brought in by his family complaining of a 7-week history of difficulty walking accompanied by memory loss and urinary incontinence. Since then he has had ↑ difficulty with memory and more frequent episodes of incontinence.	VS: P 92, BP 144/86, RR 14 Gen: NAD Lungs: WNL CV: WNL Abd: WNL Ext: WNL Neuro: Difficulty with both recent and immediate recall on mini-mental status exam; spasticity and hyperreflexia in upper and lower extremities; problem initiating gait (gait is shuffling, broad-based, and slow)	▪ Alzheimer's disease ▪ B_{12} deficiency ▪ Chronic subdural hematoma ▪ Frontal lobe syndromes ▪ Huntington's disease ▪ Intracranial tumor ▪ Meningitis ▪ Normal pressure hydrocephalus ▪ Parkinson's disease ▪ Vascular dementia

INITIAL MGMT	CONTINUING MGMT	F/U
Office W/U • CBC • Chem 14 • TSH • Serum B$_{12}$ • Serum folic acid • VDRL/RPR • CT—head **Rx** • Donepezil		• Patient counseling • Support group • Advance directives • Family counseling

Final Dx: Alzheimer's disease

INITIAL MGMT	CONTINUING MGMT	F/U
Emergency room W/U • CBC • Chem 8 • LFTs • TSH • CT—head: Enlarged lateral ventricles with no prominence of cortical sulci • LP • Serum B$_{12}$ • Serum folic acid	**Ward W/U** • Neurosurgery consult • Neurology consult • Ventriculoperitoneal shunt	• Advance directives • Family counseling • Supportive care

Final Dx: Normal pressure hydrocephalus

CASE 8

HX	PE	DDX
The on-call physician is called to see a 46 yo M patient because of seizures. The patient was admitted to the surgical ward 2 days ago, after emergency trauma surgery. The nurse reports that the patient was anxious, agitated, irritable, and tachycardic last night. Later on, the nurse noted nausea, diarrhea, sweating, and insomnia. The patient had tremors, startle response, and hallucinations earlier tonight.	VS: T 37°C (99°F), P 133, BP 146/89, RR 22, O₂ sat 92% room air Gen: Sweating; cigarette burns on hands; multiple tattoos and rings Chest: WNL Abd: Hepatomegaly Ext: Evidence of recent surgery Neuro: Tremor, confusion, delirium, clouded sensorium, and evidence of peripheral neuropathy	▪ Alcohol withdrawal ▪ Amphetamine psychosis ▪ Delirium ▪ Sedative withdrawal ▪ SLE

CASE 9

HX	PE	DDX
24 yo M is brought to the ER in a drowsy state. His wife reports that he was working at home when he suddenly stiffened, fell backward, and lost consciousness. While he was lying on the ground, he was noted to have no respiration for about 1 minute, followed by jerking of all 4 limbs for about 5 minutes. He was unconscious for another 5 minutes.	VS: T 37°C (98.2°F), P 90, BP 120/80, RR 12 Gen: NAD Lungs: WNL CV: WNL Abd: WNL Ext: WNL Neuro: In a state of confusion and lethargy but oriented; no focal neurologic deficits	▪ Alcohol withdrawal ▪ Cardioembolic stroke ▪ Frontal lobe epilepsy ▪ Migraine headache ▪ Psychiatric conditions ▪ Seizures ▪ Syncope ▪ Vascular conditions

INITIAL MGMT	CONTINUING MGMT	F/U
Ward W/U ▪ CBC: MCV 110 fL ▪ Chem 8: Hypokalemia, hypomagnesemia ▪ Urine toxicology: WNL ▪ LFTs: GGT 40 U/L ▪ ECG: Sinus tachycardia ▪ CT—head: Cerebral atrophy, no subdural hematoma **Rx** ▪ Thiamine before IV D_5W NS ▪ Pyridoxine ▪ Folic acid ▪ IV diazepam ▪ Replete K and Mg	**Ward W/U** ▪ Chem 8: Corrected hypokalemia, hypomagnesemia **Rx** ▪ IV normal saline ▪ IV diazepam ▪ Naltrexone (for maintenance therapy if indicated)	▪ Follow up in 4 weeks ▪ Patient counseling ▪ Smoking cessation ▪ Dietary supplements ▪ Addiction unit consult ▪ Social work consult

Final Dx: Alcohol withdrawal

INITIAL MGMT	CONTINUING MGMT	F/U
Emergency room W/U ▪ CBC ▪ Chem 8 ▪ LFTs ▪ ABG ▪ Serum prolactin ▪ Serum calcium, magnesium, phosphate ▪ ECG ▪ EEG ▪ CT—head ▪ MRI—brain ▪ UA ▪ Urine toxicology	**Ward W/U** ▪ Continue IV **Rx** ▪ Neurology consult	▪ Follow up in 3–4 weeks ▪ Patient counseling ▪ Family counseling ▪ Advise patient to use seat belts ▪ Advise patient not to drive

Final Dx: Grand mal seizure (complex tonic-clonic seizure)

CASE 10

HX	PE	DDX
72 yo M is brought to the ER complaining of syncope. He underwent a coronary artery bypass graft (CABG) 3 years ago. He reports fatigue and dizziness over the past 5 days. The patient's fall was broken by his wife, and as a result he has no head trauma. His wife reports loss of consciousness of about 3 minutes' duration. Before the syncopal episode, the patient recalls a prodrome of lightheadedness. His medications include propranolol, digoxin, and diltiazem.	VS: T 37°C (98.1°F), P 35, BP 114/54, RR 15 Gen: NAD Lungs: WNL CV: Irregular S1 and S2, bradycardia Abd: WNL Ext: WNL Neuro: Alert and oriented; CN II–XII intact; 5/5 motor strength in all extremities	▪ Aortic stenosis ▪ Asystole ▪ Atrial fibrillation ▪ Dilated cardiomyopathy ▪ Heart block ▪ MI ▪ Myocarditis ▪ Myopathies ▪ Restrictive cardiomyopathy ▪ Vasodepressor/vasovagal response ▪ VT/VF

CASE 11

HX	PE	DDX
25 yo F with no significant past medical history is brought to the ER after having been found unresponsive with an empty bottle lying next to her.	VS: T 38°C (99.8°F), P 50, BP 110/50, RR 9, O_2 sat 92% room air Gen: Drowsy HEENT: Pinpoint pupils Lungs: WNL CV: Bradycardia Abd: WNL Ext: WNL Neuro: Opens eyes to painful stimuli Limited PE with ABCs	▪ Acetaminophen overdose ▪ Benzodiazepine overdose ▪ Hypoglycemia ▪ Narcotic overdose ▪ TCA overdose

INITIAL MGMT	CONTINUING MGMT	F/U
Emergency room W/U	**ICU W/U**	▪ Cardiac rehabilitation program
▪ IV normal saline	▪ Continuous cardiac monitoring	▪ Smoking cessation
▪ CBC	▪ ECG	▪ Counsel patient to limit alcohol intake
▪ Chem 8	▪ Lipid profile	▪ Counsel patient not to drive
▪ LFTs	▪ Echocardiography	▪ Low-fat, low-sodium diet
▪ ECG: Third-degree AV block	**Rx**	
▪ Cardiac enzymes	▪ Lipid-lowering agents	
▪ Serum troponin I	▪ Cardiology consult	
▪ Serum calcium, magnesium, phosphate	▪ Cardiac catheterization, angiocardiography	
▪ CXR	▪ Permanent cardiac pacemaker	
▪ UA		
▪ O_2		
▪ Continuous cardiac monitoring		
Rx		
▪ Temporary transvenous cardiac pacemaker		
▪ Withhold AV nodal agents		

Final Dx: Complete heart block

INITIAL MGMT	CONTINUING MGMT	F/U
Emergency room STAT	**ICU W/U**	▪ Monitor for at least 24 hours
▪ Suction airway	▪ Gastric lavage: Pill fragments	
▪ Fingerstick blood glucose	▪ Continuous monitoring: Patient started to become drowsy again (monitor events)	
▪ IV normal saline	**Rx**	
▪ IV naloxone: Patient responded	▪ IV naloxone: Patient responded	
▪ Dextrose 50%	▪ Psychiatry consult	
▪ IV thiamine	▪ Suicide precautions	
▪ ABG		
Emergency room W/U		
▪ CBC		
▪ ECG		
▪ Urine pregnancy		
▪ Urine toxicology		
▪ UA		
▪ Serum acetaminophen, salicylate		
▪ INR		
▪ Serum lactate		
▪ CXR, PA		

Final Dx: Narcotic overdose

CASE 12

HX	PE	DDX
60 yo M was found unconscious by his wife, who called the paramedics. She left him in bed at 7 A.M. to go to her volunteer job. When she returned for lunch at 1 P.M., she found an empty bottle of amitriptyline next to him. When paramedics arrived, he was noted to be in respiratory distress and was transferred to the ER.	VS: T 38°C (101°F), P 110, BP 95/45, RR 35, O_2 sat 89% on 100% face mask Gen: Acute distress; shallow, rapid breathing HEENT: Dilated pupils Lungs: WNL CV: Tachycardia Abd: WNL Neuro: Opens eyes to painful stimuli **Limited PE**	▪ Anticholinergic toxicity ▪ TCA intoxication

---

FATIGUE/WEAKNESS

CASE 13

HX	PE	DDX
68 yo M presents following a 20-minute episode of slurred speech, right facial drooping and numbness, and weakness of the right hand. His symptoms had totally resolved by the time he got to the ER. He has a history of hypertension, diabetes mellitus, and heavy smoking.	VS: T 37°C (98°F), P 75, BP 150/90, RR 16, O_2 sat 100% room air Gen: NAD Neck: Right carotid bruit Lungs: WNL CV: WNL Abd: WNL Ext: WNL Neuro: WNL	▪ Intracranial tumor ▪ Seizure ▪ Stroke ▪ Subdural or epidural hematoma ▪ TIA

INITIAL MGMT	CONTINUING MGMT	F/U
Emergency room STAT - Intubate **Emergency room W/U** - Cardiac/BP monitoring - Chem 14 - Fingerstick blood glucose - CBC - ABG - Serum lactate - Serum osmolality - Blood ketones - Urine toxicology: $\oplus$ for TCAs - ECG: Widened QRS - Serum magnesium - CXR, PA - Cardiac enzymes - CT—head **Rx** - IV D_5W 0.9 NS - Thiamine - Central line placement - NG tube gastric lavage - Activated charcoal - IV bicarbonate	**ICU W/U** - Continuous monitoring of urine output q 1 h - Continuous BP monitoring - Continuous cardiac monitoring - Neuro check **Rx** - Cardiology consult - Lidocaine for TCA-induced ventricular arrhythmias - IV magnesium sulfate, 1 time	- Psychiatry consult

Final Dx: Tricyclic antidepressant (TCA) intoxication

INITIAL MGMT	CONTINUING MGMT	F/U
Emergency room STAT - Assess ABCs - O_2 - Blood glucose - IV normal saline - CT—head **Emergency room W/U** - Continuous cardiac monitoring - BP monitoring - ECG - CBC - Chem 8 - PT/PTT, INR - Neurology consult **Rx** - Aspirin	**Ward W/U** - Repeat neurologic exam - Continuous cardiac monitoring - BP monitoring - Telemetry - Lipid profile, HbA_{1c} - Echocardiography: EF 60% - Carotid duplex: > 75% stenosis in right carotid artery **Rx** - Vascular surgery consult - Patient is scheduled for elective carotid endarterectomy - Aspirin	- Counsel patient re smoking cessation, exercise - Treat hypertension - Treat diabetes - Diabetic diet - Diabetic teaching - Treat cholesterol - Low-fat, low-sodium diet

Final Dx: Transient ischemic attack (TIA)

CASE 14

HX	PE	DDX
40 yo F presents with numbness, lower extremity weakness, and difficulty walking. She reports having had a URI approximately 2 weeks ago. She says that her weakness spread from her lower limbs to her hip and then progressed to her upper limbs. She also complains of lightheadedness on standing and shortness of breath.	VS: Afebrile, P 115, BP 130/80 with orthostatic changes, RR 16 Gen: NAD Lungs: WNL CV: WNL Ext: WNL Neuro: Loss of motor strength in lower limbs; absent DTRs in patella and Achilles tendon; sensation intact	▪ Conversion disorder ▪ Guillain-Barré syndrome ▪ Myasthenia gravis ▪ Paraneoplastic neuropathy ▪ Poliomyelitis ▪ Polymyositis

CASE 15

HX	PE	DDX
40 yo F presents with fatigue, weight gain, sleepiness, cold intolerance, constipation, and dry skin.	VS: T 36°C (97°F), BP 100/60, HR 60 Gen: Obese Skin: Dry HEENT: Scar on neck from previous thyroidectomy Lungs: WNL CV: WNL Neuro: Delayed relaxation of DTRs	▪ Anemia ▪ Depression ▪ Diabetes ▪ Hypothyroidism

CASE 16

HX	PE	DDX
16 yo M complains of myalgia, fatigue, and sore throat. He also reports loss of appetite and nausea but no vomiting. He reports that his girlfriend recently had similar symptoms that lasted a few weeks.	VS: T 38°C (101°F), P 85, BP 125/80, RR 18 Gen: Maculopapular rash HEENT: Posterior and auricular lymphadenopathy and pharyngitis with diffuse exudates and petechiae at junction of hard and soft palates Lungs: WNL CV: WNL Abd: Soft, nontender; mild hepatosplenomegaly Ext: WNL Neuro: WNL	▪ CMV ▪ Hepatitis ▪ Infectious mononucleosis ▪ 1° HIV infection ▪ Streptococcal pharyngitis ▪ Toxoplasmosis

INITIAL MGMT	CONTINUING MGMT	F/U
Emergency room W/U	**Ward Rx**	■ Follow up in 3–4 weeks
■ CBC	■ Immunoglobulins	■ Patient counseling
■ Chem 8	■ Plasmapheresis	■ Family counseling
■ TSH	■ Rehabilitative medicine consult	■ Advise patient to use seat belts
■ ESR	■ Neurology consult	
■ CRP	■ Immunology consult	
■ RF	■ Measure forced vital capacity or inspiratory and expiratory pressure	
■ VDRL		
■ Serum B_{12}		
■ Serum folic acid		
■ ECG		
■ Serum CPK		
■ CXR		
■ LP: ↑ CSF protein		
■ HIV testing, ELISA		

Final Dx: Guillain-Barré syndrome

INITIAL MGMT	CONTINUING MGMT	F/U
Office W/U		■ Check TSH after 1 month
■ CBC		
■ Chem 14		
■ TSH: ↑		
■ FT_4: ↓		
■ ECG		
■ Lipid profile		
■ Depression index		
Rx		
■ Levothyroxine		

Final Dx: Hypothyroidism

INITIAL MGMT	CONTINUING MGMT	F/U
Office W/U		■ Follow up in 2 weeks with CBC
■ CBC: ↑ WBC count		■ Advise patient to rest at home
■ Peripheral smear: Atypical lymphocytes		■ Advise patient to avoid sports
■ Chem 14: ↑ SGOT and SGPT		
■ ESR		
■ CRP		
■ Mono test: ⊕		
■ Serum EBV titer: ↑, rapid strep		
Rx		
■ Acetaminophen or NSAIDs		
■ Hydrate; patient counseling		

Final Dx: Infectious mononucleosis

CASE 17

HX	PE	DDX
40 yo F complains of feeling tired, hopeless, and worthless. She also reports depressed mood, inability to sleep, and impaired concentration. She has been missing work. She denies any suicidal thoughts or attempts and denies having hallucinations. She has no history of alcohol or drug abuse and has not lost a loved one within the last 12 months. She is married and has 1 child and a supportive husband.	VS: P 70, BP 120/60, RR 12 Gen: NAD Lungs: WNL CV: WNL Abd: WNL Ext: WNL Neuro: WNL	▪ Adjustment disorder ▪ Anemia ▪ Anxiety ▪ Cancer ▪ Chronic fatigue syndrome ▪ Dementia ▪ Depression ▪ Fibromyalgia ▪ Hypothyroidism

COUGH/SHORTNESS OF BREATH

CASE 18

HX	PE	DDX
2 yo M is brought in by his mother because of sudden-onset shortness of breath and cough. He had a URI 4 days ago. Earlier in the day he was playing with peanuts with his brother. His immunizations are up to date.	VS: T 37°C (98°F), P 110, BP 80/50, RR 38, O$_2$ sat 99% room air Gen: Respiratory distress; using accessory muscles HEENT: WNL Neck: WNL Lungs: Inspiratory stridor; ↓ breath sounds in right lower base CV: Tachycardia Abd: WNL	▪ Angioedema ▪ Asthma ▪ Croup ▪ Epiglottitis ▪ Foreign-body aspiration ▪ Laryngitis ▪ Peritonsillar abscess ▪ Pneumonia ▪ Retropharyngeal abscess

CASE 19

HX	PE	DDX
75 yo F presents with chest pain and shortness of breath. She reports having fallen 5 days ago and has a long cast for her femoral fracture.	VS: Afebrile, BP 120/75, HR 100, RR 24 Gen: Respiratory distress HEENT: WNL Lungs: Rales, wheezing, ↓ breath sounds in left lower lung CV: Loud P2 and splitting of S2 Abd: WNL	▪ CHF ▪ Lung cancer ▪ MI ▪ Pericarditis ▪ Pneumothorax ▪ Pulmonary embolism ▪ Syncope

INITIAL MGMT	CONTINUING MGMT	F/U
Office W/U - CBC - Chem 14 - TSH - Urine/serum toxicology **Rx** - Suicide contract - SSRI (eg, sertraline) or - SNRI (eg, venlafaxine) - Psychiatry consult		- Follow up in 1 week - Supportive psychotherapy - Exercise program - Patient counseling

Final Dx: Major depression

INITIAL MGMT	CONTINUING MGMT	F/U
Emergency room STAT - CXR, PA and lateral - XR—neck - Bronchoscopy: Foreign body is removed and patient improves **Rx** - Consider IV methylprednisolone before removal of the foreign body		- Follow up in 2 weeks

Final Dx: Foreign-body aspiration

INITIAL MGMT	CONTINUING MGMT	F/U
Emergency room W/U - IV normal saline - NPO - CBC - Chem 14 - ABG: Hypoxia and hypocapnia - CXR: Left lower lobe atelectasis, Hampton's humps - CT—chest: Pulmonary embolism - ECG - DVT U/S: Venous DVT - Heparin IV and warfarin	**Ward W/U** - Continuous cardiac and BP monitoring - Pulmonary medicine consult - PT/PTT, INR **Rx** - Discontinue heparin 2 days after INR is therapeutic - Warfarin	- Follow up in 2 weeks with PT/INR - Chest physical therapy - Warfarin - Rehabilitative medicine consult

Final Dx: Pulmonary embolism

CASE 20

HX	PE	DDX
5 yo M is brought to the ER with a harsh barking cough. He has a history of URIs with coryza, nasal congestion, and sore throat. His symptoms have been present for about a week.	VS: T 38°C (101°F), BP 110/65, HR 100, RR 22, O_2 sat 100% room air Gen: Pallor and mild respiratory distress with intercostal retraction and nasal flaring HEENT: WNL Lungs: Stridor, hoarseness, barking cough CV: WNL Abd: WNL	▪ Bacterial tracheitis ▪ Croup ▪ Diphtheria ▪ Epiglottitis ▪ Measles ▪ Peritonsillar abscess ▪ Retropharyngeal abscess

CASE 21

HX	PE	DDX
75 yo M presents with shortness of breath on exertion along with cough and blood-streaked sputum. He reports progressive malaise and weight loss together with loss of appetite over the past 6 months. He smokes 40 packs of cigarettes per year.	VS: Afebrile, BP 130/85, HR 90, RR 15 Gen: WNL Chest: Barrel-shaped chest, gynecomastia Lungs: Rales, wheezing, ↓ breath sounds, dullness on percussion in left upper lung CV: WNL Abd: Mild tenderness in RUQ with mild hepatomegaly Ext: Finger clubbing; dark-colored, pruritic rash on both forearms	▪ Lung cancer ▪ Lymphoma ▪ Sarcoidosis ▪ Tuberculosis

INITIAL MGMT	CONTINUING MGMT	F/U
Emergency room W/U ▪ O$_2$ ▪ CBC ▪ Chem 8 ▪ Throat culture ▪ XR—neck: Subglottic narrowing	**Ward Rx** ▪ Humidified air ▪ Epinephrine ▪ Dexamethasone	▪ Follow up in 1 month ▪ Family counseling

Final Dx: Croup

INITIAL MGMT	CONTINUING MGMT	F/U
Office W/U ▪ CBC: ↓ hemoglobin ▪ Chem 8 ▪ LFTs: ↑ transaminases ▪ ABG ▪ ESR: ↑ ▪ CXR: Infiltrate and nodules in upper left lobe ▪ Sputum cytology: Adenocarcinoma ▪ Sputum culture ▪ PPD: ⊖ ▪ CT—chest: Left upper lobe mass	**Office W/U** ▪ PFTs ▪ Oncology consult ▪ Surgery consult ▪ Dietary consult ▪ Bronchoscopy with biopsy ▪ CT—abdomen and pelvis ▪ CT—head ▪ Antiemetic medication	▪ Smoking cessation ▪ Patient counseling ▪ Family counseling ▪ Follow up in 3–4 weeks with CXR and CBC ▪ Counsel patient to limit alcohol intake

Final Dx: Lung cancer

CASE 22

HX	PE	DDX
60 yo M presents with ↑ dyspnea, sputum production, and a change in the color of his sputum to yellow over the past 3 days. He is a smoker with a history of COPD.	VS: T 38°C (100.6°F), P 90, BP 130/70, RR 28, O₂ sat 92% on 2-L NC Gen: Moderate respiratory distress Lungs: Rhonchi at left lower base; diffuse wheezing CV: WNL Abd: WNL Ext: WNL	▪ Bronchitis ▪ CHF ▪ COPD exacerbation ▪ Lung cancer ▪ Pneumonia ▪ URI

CASE 23

HX	PE	DDX
50 yo Mexican immigrant M presents with cough productive of bloody sputum accompanied by night sweats, weight loss, and fatigue of 3 months' duration.	VS: T 38°C (100°F), BP 130/85, HR 90, RR 22, O₂ sat 99% room air Gen: Pallor Lungs: ↓ breath sounds in upper lobes of both lungs CV: WNL Abd: WNL	▪ Bronchiectasis ▪ Fungal lung infection ▪ Lung cancer ▪ Lymphoma ▪ Sarcoidosis ▪ TB ▪ Vasculitis

INITIAL MGMT	CONTINUING MGMT	F/U
Emergency room STAT - O$_2$ - IV normal saline - IV steroids - Albuterol by nebulizer - Ipratropium by nebulizer - Sputum culture - Blood culture **Emergency room W/U** - CBC: ↑ WBC count - CXR: Left lower lobe infiltrate - ECG - ABG - Peak flow: < 200 L/min - Sputum Gram stain: Gram-⊕ cocci - Chem 8 **Rx** - Third-generation cephalosporin + azithromycin vs levofloxacin or gatifloxacin IV	**Ward W/U** - Peak flow: 300 L/min - FEV$_1$: 2 L - Sputum culture: ⊕ for *S pneumoniae* sensitive to levofloxacin - Blood culture: ⊖ **Rx** - Change to PO levofloxacin - Change to PO prednisone	- PO prednisone - Smoking cessation - Consider pneumococcal vaccine and flu shot

Final Dx: Chronic obstructive pulmonary disease (COPD) exacerbation/pneumonia

INITIAL MGMT	CONTINUING MGMT	F/U
Emergency room W/U - CXR: Infiltrate/nodules in upper lobes - AFB sputum/culture × 3 days: ⊕ stain - Sputum Gram stain and culture - PPD: 16 mm - CBC - Chem 14 - HIV testing - CT—chest: Infiltrates and cavity consistent with TB **Rx** - Respiratory isolation - Transfer to the ward	**Ward W/U** - Social worker consult **Rx** - INH + rifampin + pyrazinamide + ethambutol - Vitamin B$_6$	- Sputum culture and smear at 3 months - LFTs - Ophthalmology consult - Family education - Family PPD placement - Report case to the local public health department

Final Dx: Tuberculosis (TB)

CASE 24

HX	PE	DDX
55 yo M presents with cough that is exacerbated when he lies down at night and improves when he props his head up on 3 pillows. He also reports worsening exertional dyspnea for the past 2 months (he now has dyspnea at rest). He has had a 25-pound weight gain since his symptoms began. His past medical history is significant for hypertension, an MI 5 years ago, hyperlipidemia, and smoking.	VS: P 70, BP 120/70, RR 28, O_2 sat 86% room air Gen: Moderate respiratory distress Neck: JVD Lungs: Bibasilar crackles CV: S1/S2/S3 RRR, 3/6 systolic murmur at apex Abd: WNL Ext: +2 bilateral pitting edema	▪ CHF ▪ COPD exacerbation ▪ MI ▪ Pericardial tamponade ▪ Pulmonary embolism ▪ Pulmonary fibrosis ▪ Renal failure

CASE 25

HX	PE	DDX
5 yo F presents with shortness of breath. She has a history of recurrent pulmonary infection and fatty, foul-smelling stool. She has also shown failure to thrive and has a history of meconium ileus.	VS: T 38°C (101°F), BP 110/65, HR 110, RR 24 Gen: Pallor, mild respiratory distress, low weight and height for age, dry skin HEENT: Nasal polyps Lungs: Barrel-shaped chest, rales, dullness and ↓ breath sounds over lower lung fields CV: WNL Abd: Abdominal distention, hepatosplenomegaly	▪ Asthma ▪ Cystic fibrosis ▪ Failure to thrive ▪ Malabsorption syndrome ▪ Sinusitis

INITIAL MGMT	CONTINUING MGMT	F/U
Emergency room STAT • O_2 • IV furosemide • CXR: Pulmonary edema • ECG: Old Q wave in anterior leads **Emergency room W/U** • Cardiac/BP monitoring • CPK-MB, troponin q 8 h • CBC • Chem 8: K 3.4 • Serum calcium, magnesium, phosphate **Rx** • IV KCl • Daily weight • SQ heparin • Low-fat, low-sodium diet	**Ward W/U** • TSH • Lipid profile • HbA_{1c} • Echocardiography: Hypokinesia in anterior wall; EF 20% • Chem 8: K 3.7 **Rx** • Fluid restriction • Lisinopril • Atorvastatin • Aspirin • Digoxin • Spironolactone • Change IV furosemide • β-blockers (when euvolemic)	• Cardiac rehabilitation • Counsel patient re smoking cessation, hypertension, exercise, relaxation, and lipids • Follow up in 1 week • Repeat echocardiogram at 3–6 months • Refer to cardiology; with ischemic cardiomyopathy and EF < 30%, patients may benefit from an automatic implantable cardiac defibrillator (AICD)

Final Dx: Congestive heart failure (CHF) exacerbation

INITIAL MGMT	CONTINUING MGMT	F/U
Emergency room W/U • CBC: ↓ hemoglobin • Chem 8: ↑ glucose, ↓ albumin • ABG: Hypoxia • CXR: Hyperinflation • Sputum Gram stain and culture • O_2	**Ward W/U** • PFTs • Sweat chloride test: ⊕ • Pancreatic enzymes • 24-hour fecal fat • Dietary consult • Genetics consult • Cystic fibrosis specialist • Pulmonary medicine, pediatrics consults **Rx** • IV normal saline • O_2 • IV piperacillin • Albuterol, inhalation	• Follow up in 2 months • Chest physical therapy • Regular multiple vitamins • Influenza vaccine • Pneumococcal vaccine • Family counseling

Final Dx: Cystic fibrosis (CF)

CASE 26

HX	PE	DDX
65 yo F with a history of hypertension and diabetes mellitus presents with LUQ pain accompanied by fever and a productive cough with purulent yellow sputum.	VS: T 38°C (101°F), P 105, BP 130/75, RR 22, O₂ sat 95% room air Gen: NAD Neck: WNL Lungs: ↓ breath sounds and rhonchi on left side CV: Tachycardia Abd: Tenderness in LUQ	▪ Bronchitis ▪ Infectious mononucleosis ▪ Lung abscess ▪ Lung cancer ▪ Pneumonia ▪ Pyelonephritis ▪ Spleen abscess

CASE 27

HX	PE	DDX
25 yo HIV-⊕ M presents with shortness of breath, malaise, dry cough, fatigue, and fever.	VS: T 38°C (101°F), BP 110/65, HR 110, RR 24 Gen: Pallor, mild respiratory distress, generalized lymphadenopathy HEENT: Oral thrush Lungs: Intercostal reaction; rales and ↓ breath sounds over both lung fields CV: WNL Abd: Soft, nontender; hepatosplenomegaly Ext: Reddish maculopapular rash	▪ CMV ▪ Interstitial pneumonia ▪ Kaposi's sarcoma ▪ Legionellosis ▪ *Mycobacterium avium–intracellulare* ▪ *Pneumocystis jiroveci* pneumonia ▪ TB

INITIAL MGMT	CONTINUING MGMT	F/U
Office W/U - CBC: ↑ WBC count - Chem 8 - UA - Sputum Gram stain: Gram-⊕ cocci - Sputum culture: Pending - CXR: Left lower lobe infiltrate - U/S—abdomen	**Ward W/U** - Sputum culture: ⊕ for *S pneumoniae* **Rx** - IV normal saline - PO levofloxacin - Chest physiotherapy - SQ heparin	- Discharge home - Continue PO levofloxacin × 14 days

Final Dx: Pneumonia

INITIAL MGMT	CONTINUING MGMT	F/U
Office W/U - CBC - CD4: 200 - Chem 8 - ABG: Hypoxia - Sputum Gram stain and culture - Sputum AFB smear - Bronchial washings—*Pneumocystis* stain (bronchoscopy is a prerequisite along with thoracic surgery consult): ⊕ - CXR: Bilateral interstitial infiltrate - PPD: ⊖	**Office W/U** - LFTs - VDRL - Anti-HCV - HBsAg - Anti-HBc - Serum *Toxoplasma* serology - HIV viral load **Rx** - TMP-SMX or pentamidine (if patient cannot tolerate TMP-SMX) - Prednisone - Begin antiretroviral therapy within 2 weeks	- Regular follow-up visits - LFTs - Influenza vaccine - Pneumococcal vaccine after acute event - Counsel patient re safe sex practices - HIV support group - Patient counseling - Family counseling

Final Dx: *Pneumocystis jiroveci* pneumonia (PCP)

CHEST PAIN

CASE 28

HX	PE	DDX
40 yo F presents with sudden onset of 8/10 substernal chest pain that began at rest, has lasted for 20 minutes, and radiates to the jaw. The pain is accompanied by nausea. The patient has a prior history of hypertension, hyperlipidemia, and smoking.	VS: P 80, BP 130/60, RR 14, O_2 sat 99% room air Gen: Moderate distress Lungs: WNL CV: WNL Abd: WNL Ext: WNL	▪ Angina ▪ Aortic dissection ▪ Costochondritis ▪ GERD ▪ MI ▪ Pericarditis ▪ Pneumothorax ▪ Pulmonary embolism

CASE 29

HX	PE	DDX
58 yo M was working in his office 30 minutes ago when he suddenly developed right-sided chest discomfort and shortness of breath. He has a prior history of asthma and emphysema.	VS: P 123, BP 101/64, RR 28, O_2 sat 91% room air Gen: Cyanosis, severe respiratory distress Trachea: Deviated to left Lungs: No breath sounds on right side with hyperresonance on percussion CV: Tachycardia; apical impulse displaced to the left Abd: WNL	▪ Angina ▪ Aortic dissection ▪ Asthma exacerbation ▪ Pneumothorax ▪ Pulmonary embolism ▪ Tension pneumothorax

INITIAL MGMT	CONTINUING MGMT	F/U
Emergency room STAT	**ICU W/U**	▪ Cardiac rehabilitation
▪ O_2	▪ ECG	▪ Counsel patient re smoking cessation,
▪ Chewable aspirin	▪ Lipid profile	hypertension, exercise, relaxation, and
▪ SL nitroglycerin	▪ TSH	lipids
▪ IV normal saline	▪ Echocardiography: 60%	▪ Advise patient to rest at home
▪ IV morphine	▪ Cardiac catheterization	▪ Low-fat, low-sodium diet
▪ ECG: T-wave inversions	▪ Stress test (if cardiac catheterization is	
Emergency room W/U	unavailable)	
▪ Cardiac/BP monitoring	**Rx**	
▪ CPK-MB, troponin q 8 h: ⊖	▪ Enoxaparin	
▪ CBC	▪ Aspirin	
▪ Chem 14	▪ Clopidogrel	
▪ PT/PTT	▪ β-blocker	
▪ CXR	▪ ACEI (enalapril)	
▪ Cardiac catheterization	▪ Atorvastatin	
	▪ Cardiology consult	

Final Dx: Unstable angina

INITIAL MGMT	CONTINUING MGMT	F/U
Emergency room STAT	**Ward W/U**	▪ Pleurodesis if indicated
▪ IV normal saline	▪ Thoracic surgery consult	
▪ O_2	▪ CXR: Inflated right lung	
▪ Needle thoracostomy	**Rx**	
▪ Chest tube	▪ Morphine	
▪ CXR: Collapsed right lung, mediastinal shift to left	▪ Chest tube to water seal and vacuum device	
▪ IV morphine		
Emergency room W/U		
▪ Cardiac/BP monitoring		
▪ ECG: Sinus tachycardia		
▪ CBC		
▪ Chem 14		
▪ PT/PTT		

Final Dx: Tension pneumothorax

CASE 30

HX	PE	DDX
34 yo F presents with stabbing retrosternal chest pain that radiates to the back. The pain improves when she leans forward and worsens with deep inspiration. She had a URI 1 week ago.	VS: T 37°C (99.2°F), P 80, BP 130/70, RR 16, O₂ sat 98% room air Gen: NAD Neck: WNL Lungs: WNL CV: S1/S2, pericardial friction rub Abd: WNL Ext: WNL	▪ Angina/MI ▪ Aortic dissection ▪ Costochondritis ▪ Esophageal rupture ▪ GERD ▪ Pericarditis ▪ Pneumothorax ▪ Pulmonary embolism

CASE 31

HX	PE	DDX
48 yo F presents with palpitations and anxiety. She reports that she feels hot and has to run the air conditioner all the time. She also reports hand tremors. She has lost 10 pounds over the past few months despite her good appetite.	VS: P 113, BP 145/85, RR 20 Gen: Mild respiratory distress, dehydration, sweaty palms and face, warm skin, hand tremor HEENT: Exophthalmos with lid lag, generalized thyromegaly, thyroid bruit Lungs: WNL CV: Tachycardia Abd: WNL Ext: Edema over the tibia bilaterally	▪ Anxiety ▪ Atrial fibrillation ▪ Early menopause ▪ Hyperthyroidism ▪ Mitral valve prolapse ▪ Panic attack ▪ Withdrawal syndrome

INITIAL MGMT	CONTINUING MGMT	F/U
Emergency room W/U	**Ward W/U**	▪ Discharge home
▪ Continuous cardiac and BP monitoring	▪ Discontinue continuous monitoring	▪ Follow up in 2 weeks
▪ Stat ECG: Diffuse ST elevation, PR depression	▪ Echocardiography: Minimal pericardial effusion	
▪ CPK-MB, troponin × 3	**Rx**	
▪ CBC	▪ Reassure patient	
▪ Chem 8	▪ NSAIDs, colchicine	
▪ CXR: No cardiomegaly		
▪ ESR		
Rx		
▪ NSAIDs		
▪ Start IV		
▪ O_2		

Final Dx: Pericarditis

INITIAL MGMT	CONTINUING MGMT	F/U
Office W/U	**Office W/U**	▪ Check thyroid studies in 1 month
▪ CBC	▪ Endocrinology consult	▪ Patient counseling
▪ BMP		
▪ Thyroid studies (T_4, T_3RU, T_3, TSH): ↑ T_3/T_4, ↓ TSH		
▪ Serum thyroid autoantibodies: ⊕		
▪ ECG		
▪ CXR		
▪ Nuclear scan—thyroid: ↑ uptake		
Rx		
▪ Propranolol		
▪ Methimazole or PTU (if pregnant)		

Final Dx: Hyperthyroidism

CASE 32

HX	PE	DDX
65 yo M presents with sudden onset of severe tearing anterior chest pain that radiates to the back. He is anxious and diaphoretic. He has a history of long-standing hypertension.	VS: T 36°C (97°F), BP 195/110 right arm, 160/80 left arm, HR 100, RR 30, O_2 sat 98% room air Gen: Acute distress Lungs: WNL CV: Tachycardia, S4, diastolic decrescendo heard best at left sternal border Abd: WNL Ext: Unequal pulse in both arms **Limited PE**	▪ Aortic dissection ▪ MI ▪ Pericarditis ▪ Pulmonary embolism

CASE 33

HX	PE	DDX
34 yo F is brought to the ER after a car accident. She is gasping for air and complains of weakness, chest pain, and dizziness.	VS: Afebrile, BP 100/50, HR 115, RR 22, pulsus paradoxus Gen: Confusion, cyanosis, respiratory distress Neck: ↑ JVP, engorged neck veins, Kussmaul's sign Lungs: WNL CV: Muffled heart sounds, ↓ PMI Abd: WNL Ext: WNL	▪ Aortic dissection ▪ Cardiogenic shock ▪ MI ▪ Pericardial tamponade ▪ Pericarditis ▪ Pneumothorax ▪ Pulmonary embolism

INITIAL MGMT	CONTINUING MGMT	F/U
Emergency room STAT • O_2 • IV normal saline • CXR: Widened mediastinum • IV β-blockers • ECG: LVH • IV morphine **Emergency room W/U** • Cardiac/BP monitoring • CPK-MB, troponin × 3: ⊖ • CBC • Chem 8 • TEE: Aortic dissection type A or • CT—chest with IV contrast: Aortic dissection **Rx** • Thoracic surgery consult	**ICU W/U** • Continuous cardiac and BP monitoring • Blood type and cross-match • PT/PTT, INR **Rx** • Continuing IV β-blockers • Emergent surgery	• Diet and lifestyle modifications • Lipid/BP management

Final Dx: Aortic dissection

INITIAL MGMT	CONTINUING MGMT	F/U
Emergency room W/U • O_2 • IV normal saline • NPO • Pulse oximetry • ECG: Tachycardia, low voltage, nonspecific ST- and T-wave changes • CPK-MB • CBC • Chem 8 • ABG • Coagulation profile • Blood type and cross-match • CXR: Cardiomegaly • Echocardiography: Tamponade • Pericardiocentesis	**ICU W/U** • Continuous cardiac and BP monitoring • ECG • Echocardiography • CXR • Cardiac surgery consult • ABG **Rx** • NPO to liquid • O_2 • Follow up in 2 weeks	• CXR • Echocardiography • Patient counseling

Final Dx: Pericardial tamponade

CASE 34

HX	PE	DDX
28 yo F presents with palpitations, chest pain, nausea, and dizziness that last for almost 5–6 minutes. She has had several attacks over the past few weeks. During these episodes, she becomes diaphoretic and occasionally has diarrhea. In the course of some of her attacks, she describes feeling as if she might die.	VS: P 90, BP 125/75, RR 20 Gen: Mild respiratory distress, dehydration, sweating, cold hands HEENT: WNL Lungs: WNL CV: WNL Abd: WNL Ext: WNL	■ Anxiety ■ Asthma attack ■ Atrial fibrillation ■ Early menopause ■ Hyperthyroidism ■ Hyperventilation ■ Hypoglycemia ■ Mitral valve prolapse ■ Panic attack ■ Pheochromocytoma ■ Pulmonary embolus ■ Substance abuse

CASE 35

HX	PE	DDX
32 yo F presents with new-onset palpitations, chest pain, and dizziness. Her symptoms are intermittent and occur 3–4 times a day. She also reports shortness of breath and chest tightness during her attacks.	VS: P 90–200 (variable), BP 125/75, RR 20 Gen: Mild cyanosis HEENT: WNL Lungs: Bibasilar crackles CV: Irregularly irregular, tachycardia Abd: WNL Ext: WNL	■ Anxiety ■ Atrial fibrillation ■ Hyperthyroidism ■ Hyperventilation ■ Mitral valve prolapse ■ Panic attack

INITIAL MGMT	CONTINUING MGMT	F/U
Office W/U		■ Outpatient follow-up in 4 weeks
■ CBC		■ Psychiatry consult
■ Chem 8		■ Patient counseling
■ UA		■ Behavioral modification program
■ Urine toxicology: ⊖		■ Relaxation exercises
■ TFTs		
■ ECG		
■ CXR		
Rx		
■ Reassure patient		
■ Benzodiazepines (eg, alprazolam, lorazepam, clonazepam) or		
■ SSRIs		

Final Dx: Panic attack

INITIAL MGMT	CONTINUING MGMT	F/U
Emergency room W/U	**ICU W/U**	■ Follow up in 2 weeks
■ IV normal saline	■ ECG	■ Patient counseling
■ O$_2$	■ Continuous cardiac monitoring	
■ CBC	■ Continuous BP monitoring	
■ Chem 8	■ Warfarin	
■ TFTs	■ Aspirin	
■ ECG: Atrial fibrillation		
■ CXR: Pulmonary vascular congestion		
■ Echocardiography: Enlarged left atrium		
Rx		
■ Synchronous cardioversion		
■ Propranolol		
■ Heparin		

Final Dx: Atrial fibrillation

ABDOMINAL PAIN

CASE 36

HX	PE	DDX
38 yo M presents with RUQ abdominal pain of 48 hours' duration. The pain radiates to his right groin and scrotal area and comes in waves of severe intensity that prevent him from finding a comfortable resting position.	VS: T 36°C (96°F), BP 130/85, HR 110, RR 22 Gen: In pain Lungs: WNL CV: Tachycardia Abd: Soft, nontender, no distention, tenderness in right flank, no peritoneal signs, normal BS Rectal exam: WNL, guaiac ⊖	▪ Gastroenteritis ▪ Nephrolithiasis ▪ Pancreatitis ▪ Perforated duodenal ulcer ▪ Retrocecal appendicitis

CASE 37

HX	PE	DDX
60 yo M presents with generalized weakness, left flank discomfort, nausea, and constipation of 2 weeks' duration. He has lost 20 pounds over the past 4 months.	VS: T 37°C (99.2°F), P 90, BP 120/60, RR 18 Gen: NAD Lungs: WNL CV: WNL Abd: ↓ BS, left flank tenderness with deep palpation Rectal exam: WNL Ext: WNL Neuro: WNL	▪ Colorectal cancer ▪ Renal abscess ▪ Renal cell carcinoma

CASE 38

HX	PE	DDX
32 yo F presents with 2 days of progressive flank pain, urinary frequency, and a burning sensation during urination. She also reports associated fever and shaking chills.	VS: T 39.1°C (102°F), BP 130/85, HR 86, RR 18 Gen: Mild discomfort with exam Lungs: WNL CV: Tachycardia Abd: ⊕ BS, mild suprapubic tenderness, no peritoneal signs Back: Mild CVA tenderness on the left Pelvic: WNL Rectal exam: WNL, guaiac ⊖	▪ Acute cervicitis ▪ Acute cystitis ▪ Acute PID ▪ Acute pyelonephritis ▪ Acute urethritis ▪ Ectopic pregnancy ▪ Nephrolithiasis

INITIAL MGMT	CONTINUING MGMT	F/U
Emergency room W/U ▪ CBC: Normal WBC count ▪ Chem 8 ▪ Serum amylase, lipase ▪ UA: Microscopic hematuria ▪ Urine culture ▪ KUB: Radiopaque 3-mm stone ▪ CT—kidney: Stone visualized in distal ureter **Rx** ▪ Analgesia: Narcotics and NSAIDs ▪ Counsel patient re oral hydration	▪ Serum calcium, magnesium, phosphate ▪ Serum uric acid ▪ Urine strain ▪ Stone analysis: Calcium oxalate	▪ ↑ fluid intake ▪ Follow up in 4 weeks ▪ Patient counseling ▪ Counsel patient to limit alcohol intake ▪ Counsel patient to limit caffeine intake ▪ Smoking cessation

Final Dx: Nephrolithiasis

INITIAL MGMT	CONTINUING MGMT	F/U
Office W/U ▪ CBC: Hemoglobin 9.0 ▪ Chem 14: Ca 15, BUN 40, creatinine 2.0 ▪ UA: ⊕ for RBCs ▪ CXR ▪ U/S—complete abdominal: Left renal mass ▪ Admit to ward **Rx** ▪ IV normal saline ▪ Bisphosphonate (pamidronate)	**Ward W/U** ▪ Intact PTH: ↓ ▪ Chem 7: Ca 10, BUN 20, creatinine 1.5 ▪ CT—abdomen and chest: Left renal mass ▪ Renal mass biopsy ▪ Bone scan ▪ CT—head ▪ Ferritin, TIBC, serum iron **Rx** ▪ Oncology consult ▪ Surgery consult	

Final Dx: Renal cell carcinoma

INITIAL MGMT	CONTINUING MGMT	F/U
Office W/U ▪ CBC: ↑ WBC count ▪ Chem 8 ▪ UA: WBC, bacteria, nitrite ⊕ ▪ Urine culture: Pending ▪ Urinary β-hCG: ⊖ ▪ U/S—renal **Rx** ▪ Ciprofloxacin (fluoroquinolone)	**Office W/U** ▪ Urine culture: ⊕ for *E coli*	▪ Follow up in 3–5 days ▪ Patient counseling ▪ Counsel patient re medication compliance ▪ Counsel patient to limit alcohol intake

Final Dx: Pyelonephritis

CASE 39

HX	PE	DDX
10 yo African American M presents with sudden onset of jaundice, dark-colored urine, back pain, and fatigue. He was started on TMP-SMX for an ear infection a few days ago. He has a family history of blood disorders.	VS: T 38°C (99.8°F), P 90, BP 110/50, RR 14 Gen: NAD Skin: Jaundice HEENT: Icterus, pallor Lungs: WNL CV: WNL Abd: WNL Ext: WNL	▪ Autoimmune hemolytic anemia ▪ DIC ▪ G6PD deficiency ▪ Sickle cell anemia ▪ Spherocytosis ▪ Thalassemias ▪ TTP

CASE 40

HX	PE	DDX
58 yo alcoholic M presents with a 1-day history of sharp epigastric pain that radiates to his back. He is nauseated and has vomited several times. He also complains of anorexia. The patient reports heavy alcohol use over the past 2–3 days. He has no previous history of peptic ulcer disease.	VS: T 38.2°C (101°F), BP 138/68, HR 110, RR 22 Gen: WD/WN but agitated, lying on bed with knees drawn up Lungs: ↓ breath sounds over left lower lung CV: Tachycardia Abd: Tender and distended with ↓ BS	▪ Acute cholecystitis ▪ Acute gastritis ▪ Acute pancreatitis ▪ Aortic dissection ▪ Cholelithiasis ▪ Intestinal perforation ▪ MI ▪ Perforated duodenal ulcers ▪ Pneumonia

INITIAL MGMT	CONTINUING MGMT	F/U
Office W/U	**Ward W/U**	▪ Discharge home
▪ CBC stat and q 12 h: ↓↓ hemoglobin, ↓↓ hematocrit	▪ Reticulocyte count: Elevated	▪ Follow up in 2 months
▪ Peripheral smear: Bite cells, fragment cells	▪ LDH: ↑	▪ Educate patient/family
▪ Chem 14: ↑ indirect bilirubin	▪ Haptoglobin: ↓	
▪ PT/PTT, INR	▪ UA: Hemoglobinuria	
Rx	▪ G6PD assay: Consistent with G6PD deficiency	
▪ Discontinue TMP-SMX	▪ Type and cross 2 units of packed RBCs	
	Rx	
	▪ Start IV	
	▪ IV normal saline	
	▪ Transfuse 2 units of packed RBCs	

Final Dx: G6PD deficiency

INITIAL MGMT	CONTINUING MGMT	F/U
Emergency room W/U	**Ward W/U**	▪ Follow up in 7 days
▪ IV normal saline	▪ Monitor, continue BP cuff	▪ Patient counseling
▪ NPO	▪ Continue NPO	▪ Counsel patient to cease alcohol intake
▪ Monitor, continue BP cuff	▪ U/S—liver, gallbladder and bile duct, pancreas	▪ Smoking cessation
▪ NG tube suction	▪ PT/PTT	
▪ ECG: No evidence of ischemia	▪ CT—abdomen	
▪ CBC	▪ Surgery consult	
▪ Chem 14	▪ GI consult	
▪ Serum amylase, lipase: ↑	▪ Advance diet as tolerated	
▪ ABG		
▪ O_2		
▪ Pulse oximetry		
▪ LFTs		
▪ Serum calcium		
▪ AXR, upright		
▪ CXR		
Rx		
▪ NG tube		
▪ IV meperidine		

Final Dx: Acute pancreatitis

CASE 41

HX	PE	DDX
1-day-old M born at home is brought to the ER because of bilious vomiting, irritability, poor feeding, lethargy, and an acute episode of rectal bleeding.	VS: T 38°C (100°F), P 170, BP 69/44, RR 43, O₂ sat 89% room air Skin: Evidence of poor perfusion Chest: WNL CV: WNL Abd: Distention; evidence of intestinal obstruction **Limited PE**	▪ Duodenal web ▪ Intestinal atresia ▪ Malrotation with volvulus ▪ Meconium plug/ileus ▪ Necrotizing enterocolitis

CASE 42

HX	PE	DDX
21-month-old M is brought to the ER because of intermittent abdominal pain that causes him to become still while drawing up his legs. He also presents with irritability and vomiting that initially was clear but then became bilious. The child seemed lethargic between the pain episodes. In the ER, the child passes some dark red stool.	VS: T 38.5°C (101°F), P 157, BP 81/59, RR 35, O₂ sat 93% room air Skin: No evidence of purpura Chest: WNL CV: WNL Abd: Soft and mildly tender; examination of RUQ fails to identify presence of bowel; ill-defined mass in the RUQ **Limited PE**	▪ Intoxication ▪ Intussusception ▪ Metabolic disease ▪ Neurologic disease ▪ Small bowel obstruction ▪ Volvulus

INITIAL MGMT	CONTINUING MGMT	F/U
Emergency room STAT	**Ward W/U**	▪ Follow up in 48 hours
▪ IV normal saline	▪ Upper GI series: Bird's beak, corkscrew appearance of proximal jejunum	▪ Family counseling
▪ O_2	▪ Barium enema: Cecum in RUQ	
▪ ABG: Metabolic acidosis	**Rx**	
Emergency room W/U	▪ NG tube suction	
▪ CBC: ↑ WBC count, mildly ↓ hemoglobin	▪ IV normal saline	
▪ Chem 8		
▪ AXR: Airless rectum; large gastric bubble		
▪ CXR: No evidence of diaphragmatic hernia		
Rx		
▪ NG tube suction		
▪ IV bicarbonate (to correct acidosis if pH < 7.0)		
▪ Pediatric surgery consult		

Final Dx: Malrotation with volvulus

INITIAL MGMT	CONTINUING MGMT	F/U
Emergency room STAT	**Ward W/U**	▪ Follow up in 48 hours
▪ IV normal saline	▪ AXR: Gastric bubble; no air-fluid levels	▪ Family counseling
▪ O_2	▪ ABG: Derangements being resolved	
Emergency room W/U	**Rx**	
▪ CBC: ↑ WBC count	▪ D/C NG tube suction	
▪ Chem 14	▪ IV normal saline	
▪ ABG: Metabolic acidosis	▪ Advance diet	
▪ AXR: Distended bowel with air-fluid levels; mass in right abdomen		
▪ U/S—abdomen: Compatible with intussusception		
Rx		
▪ NG tube suction		
▪ Barium enema: Coiled-spring appearance; disorder is relieved by air insufflation		
▪ Pediatric surgery consult		

Final Dx: Intussusception

CASE 43

HX	PE	DDX
27-month-old M presents to the ER with seizures, irritability, anorexia, altered sleep patterns, emotional lability, and vomiting. His mother states that the family has been living for about a year in an old, poorly maintained building that has only recently begun to undergo renovation. Since she was laid off at the battery plant, the family has been considering moving out of town.	VS: T 37°C (99°F), P 129, BP 89/61, RR 20, O_2 sat 92% room air Neuro: Lethargy, ataxia, seizures. Remainder of physical examination is noncontributory (except for some conjunctival pallor)	▪ Lead toxicity ▪ Metabolic disease ▪ Neurologic disease ▪ Nonmetal intoxication ▪ Other heavy metal toxicity

CASE 44

HX	PE	DDX
7-day-old alert M presents to a clinic with jaundice that started 2 days ago. The baby was born at term via an uneventful vaginal delivery and started breast-feeding after some delay. The mother states that she took the baby to the doctor's office at that time and that the baby's bilirubin was 14 mg/dL. The mother does not take any drugs. She is very concerned that the baby's jaundice is not improving and asks if the baby has kernicterus.	VS: T 37°C (99°F), P 129, BP 80/51, RR 29, O_2 sat 94% room air PE: WNL except for jaundice Neuro: WNL	▪ Breast-feeding jaundice ▪ Hereditary spherocytosis ▪ Physiologic hyperbilirubinemia ▪ Unconjugated hyperbilirubinemia (Gilbert's/Crigler-Najjar)

CASE 45

HX	PE	DDX
31 yo M comes to the office complaining of midepigastric pain that usually begins 1–2 hours after eating and sometimes awakens him at night. He also has occasional indigestion. He is taking an antacid for his problem. He denies melena or hematemesis.	VS: T 37.1°C (99°F), BP 130/75, HR 100, RR 16 Gen: Pallor, no distress Lungs: WNL CV: WNL Abd: Epigastric tenderness Rectal exam: WNL	▪ Acute gastritis ▪ Diverticulitis ▪ GERD ▪ Mesenteric ischemia ▪ Pancreatic disease ▪ Peptic ulcer disease

INITIAL MGMT	CONTINUING MGMT	F/U
Emergency room W/U	**Ward Rx**	▪ Follow up in 7 days
▪ CBC: Hemoglobin 9 g/dL, MCV 75, blood smear reveals coarse basophilic stippling in RBCs	▪ IV normal saline	▪ Family counseling
	▪ Serum lead	▪ Lead paint assay in home
	▪ IM EDTA (if necessary)	
▪ Chem 8	▪ Family counseling	
▪ Serum lead: 80 µg/dL		
▪ UA: Glycosuria		
▪ Free erythrocyte protoporphyrin: ↑		
▪ Serum toxicology: ↑ lead levels		
Rx		
▪ IV normal saline		
▪ IM EDTA		

Final Dx: Lead intoxication with encephalopathy

INITIAL MGMT	CONTINUING MGMT	F/U
Office W/U	**Office W/U**	▪ Follow up in 7 days
▪ CBC: WNL, smear WNL	▪ Breast-feeding suppression test: Bilirubin levels ↓ on cessation of breast-feeding; levels ↑ again when breast-feeding restarted	▪ Family counseling
▪ Direct Coombs' test: Noncontributory		
▪ Serum bilirubin: ↑ indirect bilirubin		
▪ TSH: WNL	**Rx**	
	▪ Continue breast feedings	
	▪ Consider phototherapy (if bilirubin levels do not ↓)	

Final Dx: Breast-feeding neonatal jaundice

INITIAL MGMT	CONTINUING MGMT	F/U
Office W/U		▪ Follow up in 4 weeks; patient reports that he is feeling better (if symptoms persist or if *H pylori* is still present, may proceed to endoscopy)
▪ CBC		
▪ Chem 8		▪ Patient counseling
▪ Serum amylase, lipase		▪ Counsel patient to limit alcohol intake
▪ Serum *H pylori* antibody: ⊕		▪ Smoking cessation
▪ Stool *H pylori* antibody: ⊕		
Rx		
▪ Proton pump inhibitor		
▪ Clarithromycin (Biaxin)		
▪ Metronidazole		

Final Dx: Gastritis (*H pylori* infection)

CASE 46

HX	PE	DDX
45 yo M presents with a 6-week history of jaundice, pale stools, tea-colored urine, and epigastric pain that radiates to the back. He also reports that he has bilateral lower extremity swelling.	VS: T 37°C (98°F), BP 130/70, HR 90, RR 16 Gen: Jaundice Lungs: WNL CV: WNL Abd: Palpable epigastric mass Ext: Lower extremity swelling with pain on dorsiflexion of ankle	▪ Cholangiocarcinoma ▪ Colon/stomach cancer with metastases in the porta hepatis region causing biliary obstruction ▪ Pancreatic cancer

CASE 47

HX	PE	DDX
60 yo F G0 presents with a 2-month history of ↑ abdominal girth, ↓ appetite, and early satiety. She also has mild shortness of breath.	VS: T 36°C (97°F), BP 140/60, HR 90, RR 23 Gen: Pallor Breast: WNL Lungs: WNL CV: WNL Abd: Distended, nontender, normal BS, no palpable hepatosplenomegaly Pelvic: Solid right adnexal mass Rectal exam: Solid right adnexal mass; no involvement of rectovaginal septum	▪ CHF ▪ Liver cirrhosis ▪ Ovarian cancer

CASE 48

HX	PE	DDX
32 yo F presents with sudden onset of left lower abdominal pain that radiates to the scapula and back and is associated with vaginal bleeding. Her last menstrual period was 5 weeks ago. She has a history of pelvic inflammatory disease and unprotected intercourse.	VS: T 37°C (99°F), P 90, BP 120/50, RR 14 Gen: Moderate distress 2° to pain Lungs: WNL CV: WNL Abd: RLQ tenderness, rebound, and guarding Pelvic: Slightly enlarged uterus with small amount of dark bloody discharge from cervix; right adnexal tenderness	▪ Ectopic pregnancy ▪ Ovarian torsion ▪ PID ▪ Ruptured ovarian cyst

INITIAL MGMT	CONTINUING MGMT	F/U
Office W/U - CBC - Chem 14 - Bilirubin, ALT, AST, alkaline phosphatase - CT—abdomen: Large necrotic pancreatic mass in head - ERCP/EUS: Biopsy to obtain histology	**Ward Rx** - Medical oncology consult; palliative care - Surgery is not an option owing to advanced disease	

Final Dx: Pancreatic cancer

INITIAL MGMT	CONTINUING MGMT	F/U
Office W/U - CBC - Chem 14 - CA-125: 900 - CT—abdomen and pelvis: 10- × 12-cm right complex ovarian cyst; severe ascites - CXR: Right moderate pleural effusion - ECG - Pap smear - Mammogram - Colonoscopy - Gynecology consult	**Ward W/U** - Blood type and cross-match - PT/PTT, INR **Rx** - Exploratory laparotomy - TAH-BSO, laparotomy - Staging, laparotomy	- Carboplatin - CA-125 - CBC - Chem 14

Final Dx: Ovarian cancer

INITIAL MGMT	CONTINUING MGMT	F/U
Emergency room W/U - Urinary β-hCG: ⊕ - Quantitative serum β-hCG: 2500 - CBC - Chem 8 - Cervical Gram stain and G&C culture - U/S—transvaginal: 2-cm right adnexal mass, no intrauterine pregnancy, free fluid in cul-de-sac **Rx** - IV normal saline	- Blood type and cross-match - PT/PTT, INR - Gynecology consult - Laparoscopy - Rh IgG (RhoGAM) if Rh-⊖	- Counsel patient on contraception - Counsel patient re safe sex practices

Final Dx: Ectopic pregnancy

CASE 49

HX	PE	DDX
74 yo M presents with LLQ abdominal pain, fever, and chills for the past 3 days. He also reports recent-onset episodes of alternating diarrhea and constipation. He consumes a low-fiber, high-fat diet.	VS: T 38°C (101°F), BP 130/85, HR 100, RR 22 Gen: Pallor, diaphoresis Lungs: WNL CV: Tachycardia Abd: LLQ tenderness, no peritoneal signs, sluggish BS Rectal exam: Guaiac ⊖	▪ Crohn's disease ▪ Diverticular abscess ▪ Diverticulitis ▪ Gastroenteritis ▪ Ulcerative colitis

CASE 50

HX	PE	DDX
41 yo F presents with sudden-onset RUQ abdominal pain of 6 hours' duration. She also reports nausea and emesis. The pain started after lunch and has become more severe and constant. She reports that the pain is exacerbated by deep breathing and that it radiates to her shoulder. She had a similar attack almost 1 year ago. She is taking OCPs and has 3 children.	VS: T 39.0°C (102°F), BP 130/82, HR 80, RR 16 Gen: WD, slightly obese, moderate distress Lungs: WNL CV: WNL Abd: Obesity, tenderness and guarding to palpation on RUQ, ⊕ Murphy's sign, ↓ BS Rectal exam: WNL, guaiac ⊖	▪ Acute appendicitis ▪ Acute cholangitis ▪ Acute cholecystitis ▪ Acute hepatitis ▪ Acute pancreatitis ▪ Acute peptic ulcer disease with or without perforation ▪ Biliary atresia ▪ Cardiac ischemia ▪ Cholelithiasis ▪ Fitz-Hugh–Curtis syndrome (gonococcal perihepatitis) ▪ Gastritis ▪ Renal colic ▪ Right-sided pneumonia ▪ Small bowel obstruction

INITIAL MGMT	CONTINUING MGMT	F/U
Emergency room W/U ▪ CBC: ↑ WBC count ▪ Chem 14 ▪ Serum amylase, lipase ▪ UA ▪ Urine culture: Pending ▪ Blood culture: Pending ▪ Stool culture and sensitivity ▪ Stool for ova and parasites ▪ CXR ▪ KUB ▪ CT—abdomen: Diverticulitis **Rx** ▪ NPO ▪ IV normal saline ▪ IV metronidazole + ciprofloxacin	**Ward W/U** ▪ Urine culture: Pending ▪ Blood culture: Pending **Rx** ▪ NPO or clear liquid diet ▪ Surgery consult ▪ Metronidazole + ciprofloxacin × 7–10 days ▪ Discharge home in 3–4 days	▪ High-fiber diet ▪ Colonoscopy 4 weeks after recovery

Final Dx: Diverticulitis

INITIAL MGMT	CONTINUING MGMT	F/U
Emergency room W/U ▪ IV normal saline ▪ NPO ▪ Monitor, continue BP cuff ▪ ECG ▪ CBC ▪ Chem 14 ▪ Serum amylase, lipase ▪ LFTs ▪ Blood/urine cultures ▪ AXR/CXR ▪ Pregnancy test—urine ▪ U/S—abdomen: Gallstones with gallbladder edema **Rx** ▪ IM prochlorperazine ▪ IV hydromorphone ▪ IV cefuroxime	**Ward W/U** ▪ Blood type and cross-match ▪ PT/PTT, INR ▪ Surgery consult for cholecystectomy ▪ Vitals q 4 h ▪ CBC next day ▪ Chem 8 next day **Rx** ▪ NPO → advance diet as tolerated ▪ Continue antibiotic therapy	▪ Follow up in 2 weeks ▪ Patient counseling ▪ Counsel patient to limit alcohol intake

Final Dx: Acute cholecystitis

CASE 51

HX	PE	DDX
24 yo F presents with bilateral lower abdominal pain that started with the first day of her menstrual period. The pain is associated with fever and a thick, greenish-yellow vaginal discharge. She has had unprotected sex with multiple sexual partners.	VS: T 38°C (100.4°F), P 90, BP 110/50, RR 14 Gen: Moderate distress 2° to pain Lungs: WNL CV: WNL Abd: Diffuse tenderness (greatest in the lower quadrants), no rebound, no distention, ↓ BS Pelvic: Purulent, bloody discharge from cervix; cervical motion and bilateral adnexal tenderness Rectal exam: WNL Ext: WNL	▪ Dysmenorrhea ▪ Endometriosis ▪ PID ▪ Pyelonephritis ▪ Vaginitis

CASE 52

HX	PE	DDX
25 yo M is brought to the ER because of abdominal pain and ↓ appetite for 4 days. This episode was preceded by ↑ urinary frequency, nausea, and vomiting.	VS: T 37°C (98°F), P 120, BP 100/60, RR 25 Gen: Moderate distress Skin: Poor skin turgor HEENT: Dry mucous membranes, sweet-smelling breath Lungs: WNL CV: Tachycardia Abd: Generalized tenderness Ext: WNL Neuro: WNL **Limited PE**	▪ Acute intestinal obstruction ▪ Alcoholic ketoacidosis ▪ Appendicitis ▪ DKA ▪ Drug intoxication ▪ Gastroenteritis ▪ Pancreatitis ▪ Pyelonephritis

INITIAL MGMT	CONTINUING MGMT	F/U
Emergency room W/U	**Ward W/U**	▪ Counsel patient re safe sex practices
▪ Urinary β-hCG: ⊖	▪ Cervical culture: *N gonorrhoeae*	▪ Treat partners
▪ CBC: ↑ WBC count	**Rx**	
▪ Chem 14	▪ Discontinue **IV** ceftriaxone when	
▪ Cervical Gram stain and G&C culture	symptoms improve (usually in 24–48	
▪ U/S—pelvis	hours)	
▪ UA and urine culture	▪ Switch to PO doxycycline or clindamycin	
Rx		
▪ IV normal saline		
▪ IV ceftriaxone + PO doxycycline or PO azithromycin		
▪ Acetaminophen		

Final Dx: Pelvic inflammatory disease (PID)

INITIAL MGMT	CONTINUING MGMT	F/U
Emergency room STAT	**ICU W/U**	▪ Diabetic diet
▪ Glucometer: 480 mg/dL	▪ Continuous monitoring	▪ Diabetic teaching
▪ IV normal saline	▪ Random glucose q 1 h	▪ HbA_{1c} q 3 months
Emergency room W/U	▪ Chem 8 q 4 h: ↓ K, glucose < 250	▪ Follow up in 2 weeks in the office
▪ Continuous monitoring	**Rx**	▪ Diabetic foot care
▪ Chem 14: Normal K, normal Na, ↑ anion gap	▪ Switch IV fluid to D_5W	▪ Ophthalmology consult
▪ CBC: ↑ WBC count	▪ IV potassium	▪ Lipid profile
▪ Serum amylase, lipase	▪ SQ insulin NPH	▪ Instruct patient in home glucose monitoring
▪ UA and urine culture: ⊕ glucose, ⊕ ketones	▪ SQ insulin regular	▪ Home glucose monitoring, glucometer
▪ Urine/serum toxicology	▪ Discontinue IV insulin 2 hours after starting long-acting insulin (NPH or Lantus)	
▪ Phosphate: ↓		
▪ ECG		
▪ ABG: Metabolic acidosis (pH = 7.1)		
▪ Quantitative serum ketones: ↑		
▪ Serum osmolality: Normal		
▪ CXR/AXR		
Rx		
▪ IV regular insulin, continue		
▪ Phosphate therapy		

Final Dx: Diabetic ketoacidosis (DKA)

CONSTIPATION/DIARRHEA

CASE 53

HX	PE	DDX
67 yo M presents with constipation, ↓ stool caliber, and blood in his stool for the past 8 months. He also reports unintentional weight loss. He is on a low-fiber diet and has a family history of colon cancer.	VS: P 85, BP 140/85, RR 14, O_2 sat 98% room air Gen: NAD HEENT: Pale conjunctivae Lungs: WNL CV: WNL Abd: WNL Pelvic: WNL Rectal exam: Guaiac ⊕	▪ Angiodysplasia ▪ Colorectal cancer ▪ Diverticulosis ▪ GI parasitic infection (ascariasis, giardiasis) ▪ Hemorrhoids ▪ Hypothyroidism ▪ Inflammatory bowel disease ▪ Irritable bowel syndrome

CASE 54

HX	PE	DDX
28 yo M presents with diffuse abdominal pain, loose stools, perianal pain, mild fever, and weight loss over the past 4 weeks. He denies any history of travel or recent use of antibiotics.	VS: T 37°C (99°F), BP 130/65, HR 70, RR 14 Gen: NAD Lungs: WNL CV: WNL Abd: WNL Rectal exam: Perianal skin tags, guaiac ⊕	▪ Crohn's disease ▪ Diverticulitis ▪ Gastroenteritis ▪ Infectious colitis ▪ Irritable bowel syndrome ▪ Ischemic colitis ▪ Lactose intolerance ▪ Pseudomembranous colitis ▪ Small bowel lymphoma ▪ Ulcerative colitis

CASE 55

HX	PE	DDX
30 yo F presents with periumbilical crampy pain of 6 months' duration. The pain never awakens her from sleep. It is relieved by defecation and worsens when she is upset. She has alternating constipation and diarrhea but no nausea, vomiting, weight loss, or anorexia.	VS: Afebrile, P 85, BP 130/65, RR 14 Gen: NAD Lungs: WNL CV: WNL Abd: WNL Pelvic: WNL Rectal exam: Guaiac ⊖	▪ Celiac disease ▪ Chronic pancreatitis ▪ Colorectal cancer ▪ Crohn's disease ▪ Diverticulosis ▪ Endometriosis ▪ GI parasitic infection (ascariasis, giardiasis) ▪ Hypothyroidism ▪ Inflammatory bowel disease ▪ Irritable bowel syndrome

INITIAL MGMT	CONTINUING MGMT	F/U
Office W/U ■ CBC: ↓ hematocrit, ↓ MCV ■ Chem 8: Normal ■ Ferritin: ↓ ■ Serum iron: ↓ ■ TIBC: ↑ ■ TSH: Normal ■ Stool for ova and parasites ■ ESR: Normal ■ Stool guaiac: ⊕	**Office W/U** ■ GI consult ■ Colonoscopy: Polyp with adenocarcinoma ■ CT—abdomen and pelvis with contrast ■ CEA **Rx** ■ Iron sulfate ■ General surgery consult ■ Plan partial colectomy	

Final Dx: Colorectal cancer

INITIAL MGMT	CONTINUING MGMT	F/U
Office W/U ■ CBC ■ Chem 14 ■ Serum amylase, lipase ■ Stool for ova and parasites ■ Stool *C difficile* ■ AXR ■ Colonoscopy: Crohn's disease **Rx** ■ 5-ASA ■ Metronidazole (for perianal abscess or fistula)		■ Follow up in 2 weeks ■ Counsel patient re medication compliance and adherence

Final Dx: Crohn's disease

INITIAL MGMT	CONTINUING MGMT	F/U
Office W/U ■ CBC ■ Chem 14 ■ TSH ■ Stool for ova and parasites ■ Stool for WBCs ■ Stool culture and sensitivity ■ Transglutaminase antibody **Rx** ■ Educate patient ■ Reassurance ■ High-fiber diet ■ Lactose-free diet		■ Follow up in 4 weeks ■ Call with questions

Final Dx: Irritable bowel syndrome

CASE 56

HX	PE	DDX
8 yo M is brought to the clinic by his mother for intermittent diarrhea alternating with constipation together with vomiting and cramping abdominal pain. His mother also reports that he has had progressive anorexia.	VS: T 37°C (98°F), BP 110/65, HR 90, RR 16 Gen: Pale and dry mucosal membranes; lack of growth Lungs: WNL CV: WNL Abd: WNL Ext: Muscle wasting, especially in gluteal area	▪ Bacterial gastroenteritis ▪ Celiac disease ▪ Food allergy ▪ Giardiasis ▪ Protein intolerance ▪ Viral gastroenteritis

CASE 57

HX	PE	DDX
28 yo M reports intermittent episodes of vomiting and diarrhea along with cramping abdominal pain for the past 2 days. He describes his stool as watery. He returned from Mexico 3 days ago.	VS: T 39°C (101.9°F), BP 135/85, HR 100, RR 22 Gen: Mild dehydration Lungs: WNL CV: WNL Abd: Mild tenderness, no peritoneal signs, hyperactive BS Rectal exam: WNL, guaiac ⊖	▪ *Campylobacter* infection ▪ Cholera ▪ *C difficile* colitis ▪ Crohn's disease ▪ Gastroenteritis ▪ Giardiasis ▪ Salmonellosis ▪ Shigellosis

CASE 58

HX	PE	DDX
40 yo F presents with fever, anorexia, nausea, profuse and watery diarrhea, and diffuse abdominal pain. Last week she was on antibiotics for a UTI.	VS: T 38°C (100.4°F), BP 100/50, HR 100, RR 22, orthostatic hypotension Gen: WNL Lungs: WNL CV: Tachycardia Abd: Diffuse tenderness, no peritoneal signs, ⊕ BS Rectal exam: Guaiac ⊕	▪ Amebiasis ▪ Food poisoning ▪ Gastroenteritis ▪ Giardiasis ▪ Hepatitis A ▪ Infectious diarrhea (bacterial, viral, parasitic, protozoal) ▪ Inflammatory bowel disease ▪ Pseudomembranous (*C difficile*) colitis ▪ Traveler's diarrhea

INITIAL MGMT	CONTINUING MGMT	F/U
Office W/U	**Ward W/U**	▪ Follow up in 1 week
▪ CBC	▪ CXR: Normal	▪ Patient counseling
▪ Chem 14	▪ KUB: Normal	▪ Pneumococcal vaccine
▪ UA	▪ D-xylose tolerance test: Carbohydrate malabsorption	
▪ Stool for ova and parasites	▪ Peroral duodenal biopsy: Villi are atrophic or absent	
▪ Stool occult blood	▪ Dietary consult	
▪ Stool Gram stain	**Rx**	
▪ Stool fat stain	▪ Gluten-free diet	
▪ Barium enema	▪ Prednisone	
▪ CT—abdomen	▪ Vitamin D	
▪ Ferritin	▪ Calcium	
▪ Serum folate		
▪ Serum B$_{12}$		
▪ Serum endomysial antibody: ⊕ titers		
▪ Serum transglutaminase antibody: ⊕ titers		

Final Dx: Celiac disease

INITIAL MGMT	CONTINUING MGMT	F/U
Emergency room W/U	**Emergency room W/U**	▪ Follow up in 1 week
▪ CBC	▪ Stool culture: ⊕ for *E coli*	▪ Patient counseling
▪ Chem 14	▪ Stool Gram stain: ⊕ for gram-⊖ rods and ↑ leukocytes	▪ Counsel patient to limit alcohol intake
▪ Stool culture	**Rx**	▪ Smoking cessation
▪ Fecal leukocyte stain	▪ Oral hydration	
▪ Stool for *C difficile*	▪ Ciprofloxacin	
▪ Stool Gram stain		
▪ Stool for ova and parasites		
▪ Stool occult blood		
▪ Stool fat stain		
▪ UA and urine culture		

Final Dx: Gastroenteritis

INITIAL MGMT	CONTINUING MGMT	F/U
Emergency room W/U	**Ward W/U**	▪ Counsel patient re oral hydration
▪ Stool culture	▪ No orthostatic hypotension	
▪ Stool *Giardia* antigen	**Rx**	
▪ Stool for ova and parasites	▪ Send home on metronidazole (when diarrhea improves); no Lomotil/Imodium	
▪ Stool WBCs: ⊕		
▪ Stool for *C difficile:* ⊕		
▪ CBC: ↑ WBC count		
▪ Chem 14		
Rx		
▪ IV normal saline		
▪ Metronidazole		

Final Dx: Pseudomembranous (*C difficile*) colitis

CASE 59

HX	PE	DDX
33 yo M presents with foul-smelling, watery diarrhea together with diffuse abdominal cramps and bloating that began yesterday. He also vomited once. He was recently in Mexico.	VS: T 37°C (98°F), BP 110/50, HR 85, RR 22, no orthostatic hypotension Gen: WNL Lungs: WNL CV: WNL Abd: No tenderness, no peritoneal signs, active BS Rectal exam: Guaiac ⊖	▪ Amebiasis ▪ Food poisoning ▪ Gastroenteritis ▪ Giardiasis ▪ Hepatitis A ▪ Infectious diarrhea (bacterial, viral, parasitic, protozoal) ▪ Inflammatory bowel disease ▪ Pseudomembranous (*C difficile*) colitis ▪ Traveler's diarrhea

GI BLEEDING

CASE 60

HX	PE	DDX
38 yo M presents with intermittent hematemesis of 2 weeks' duration. He has a history of epigastric pain for almost 2 years that occasionally worsens when he eats food or drinks milk. He also reports melena of 3 weeks' duration. His social history is significant for alcohol and tobacco use.	VS: T 37°C (98.9°F), BP 90/65, HR 110, RR 24 Gen: Pallor Lungs: WNL CV: WNL Abd: No tenderness, no peritoneal signs, normal BS Rectal exam: WNL, guaiac ⊕ **Limited PE**	▪ Duodenal ulcers ▪ Esophageal tear ▪ Gastric carcinoma ▪ Gastric ulcer ▪ Portal hypertension

INITIAL MGMT	CONTINUING MGMT	F/U
Office W/U		▪ Counsel patient re oral hydration
▪ Stool culture		
▪ Stool *Giardia* antigen: $\oplus$		
▪ Stool for ova and parasites		
▪ Stool WBCs		
▪ Stool for *C difficile*		
▪ CBC		
▪ Chem 8		
Rx		
▪ Metronidazole		

Final Dx: Giardiasis

INITIAL MGMT	CONTINUING MGMT	F/U
Emergency room STAT	**ICU W/U**	▪ Follow up in 1 week
▪ IV normal saline	▪ CBC q 4 h until hematocrit is stable; then frequency can be ↓	▪ Patient counseling
▪ O_2	**Rx**	▪ Counsel patient to cease alcohol intake
▪ Orthostatic vitals: Drop on standing	▪ GI consult	▪ Smoking cessation
▪ Type and cross-match	▪ Combination therapy with epinephrine injection followed by thermal coagulation	▪ Dietary consult
Emergency room W/U	▪ Octreotide for varices	
▪ CBC: Hematocrit 24	▪ Advance diet	
▪ Chem 14	▪ Ranitidine	
▪ Upper GI series or STAT GI consult/ endoscopy: Gastric antral lesion with adherent clot	▪ Pantoprazole	
▪ PT/PTT, INR	▪ Transfer to wards if patient remains stable	
▪ CXR	▪ *H pylori* serology and eradication if $\oplus$	
▪ ECG		
Rx		
▪ NPO		
▪ Blood transfusion if hemoglobin < 7 or active ongoing bleeding		
▪ NG tube, iced saline lavage: Clears with 1 L of normal saline		
▪ IV pantoprazole		
▪ IV cimetidine		

Final Dx: Bleeding gastric ulcer

CASE 61

HX	PE	DDX
67 yo F presents with acute crampy abdominal pain, weakness, and black stool. She reports diffuse abdominal pain of 3 months' duration. Eating worsens the pain. She has had a 5-lb weight loss over the last 3 months.	VS: T 37°C (98.9°F), BP 90/65, HR 100, RR 24 Gen: Mild dehydration Lungs: WNL CV: WNL Abd: Tender and mildly distended; no rigidity or rebound tenderness Rectal exam: WNL, guaiac ⊕ **Limited PE**	▪ Adenocarcinoma of the colon ▪ Crohn's disease ▪ Diverticular bleed ▪ Infectious colitis ▪ Ischemic colitis ▪ Peptic ulcer disease ▪ Ulcerative colitis

CASE 62

HX	PE	DDX
30 yo M presents with loose, watery stools that are streaked with blood and mucus. He has also had colicky abdominal pain and weight loss over the past 3 weeks. He denies any history of travel, radiation, or recent medication use (antibiotics, NSAIDs).	VS: T 37°C (99°F), BP 130/65, HR 70, RR 14 Gen: NAD Lungs: WNL CV: WNL Abd: WNL Rectal exam: Blood-stained stool	▪ Crohn's disease ▪ Diverticulitis ▪ Gastroenteritis ▪ Infectious colitis ▪ Internal hemorrhoid ▪ Ischemic colitis ▪ Pseudomembranous colitis ▪ Radiation colitis ▪ Ulcerative colitis

INITIAL MGMT	CONTINUING MGMT	F/U
Emergency room STAT - IV normal saline - O$_2$ **Emergency room W/U** - CBC - Chem 14 - Serum amylase: Normal - LDH: ↑ - PT/PTT - CXR - ECG - AXR - CT—abdomen: Pneumatosis coli - Blood type and cross-match **Rx** - NPO - Surgery consult (for bowel resection) - Broad-spectrum antibiotics - NG tube suction if ileus	**Ward W/U** - Hemoglobin and hematocrit q 4 h **Rx** - Advance diet - Monitor carefully for persistent fever, leukocytosis, peritoneal irritation, diarrhea, and/or bleeding	- Follow up in 4 weeks - Patient counseling - Counsel patient to cease alcohol intake - Smoking cessation - Dietary consult

Final Dx: Ischemic colitis

INITIAL MGMT	CONTINUING MGMT	F/U
Office W/U - CBC: Mild anemia - Chem 14 - Serum amylase, lipase - Stool culture and sensitivity - Stool for ova and parasites - Stool WBCs - PT/PTT - Flexible sigmoidoscopy and rectal biopsy: Consistent with ulcerative colitis involving rectum and distal sigmoid colon **Rx** - IV steroids (for attack) or - 5-ASA enema/suppositories - Sulfasalazine		- Follow up in 2 weeks - Counsel patient re medication compliance and adherence

Final Dx: Ulcerative colitis

CASE 63

HX	PE	DDX
58 yo M presents with painless bright red blood in his stool. He reports that his diet is low in fiber.	VS: T 37°C (98°F), BP 130/85, HR 90, RR 20 Gen: Pallor, diaphoresis Lungs: WNL CV: WNL Abd: Soft, nontender, no peritoneal signs, ⊕ BS Rectal exam: Bloody stool	▪ Colon cancer ▪ Crohn's disease ▪ Diverticulitis ▪ Diverticulosis ▪ Ulcerative colitis

HEMATURIA

CASE 64

HX	PE	DDX
71 yo Asian M presents with a 3-month history of low back pain that is 3/6 in severity and steady with no radiation. He has BPH and denies any history of trauma.	VS: T 37°C (98.5°F), P 76, BP 140/75, RR 14 Gen: NAD Neck: WNL Back: Tenderness along lumbar spine (L4, L5) Lungs: WNL CV: WNL Abd: WNL Rectal exam: Irregular, enlarged prostate; guaiac ⊖ Ext: WNL Neuro: WNL	▪ Disk herniation ▪ Lumbar muscle strain ▪ Muscular spasm ▪ Osteoporosis ▪ Prostate cancer ▪ Sciatic irritation ▪ Spinal stenosis ▪ Tumor in the vertebral canal

CASE 65

HX	PE	DDX
40 yo M complains of a slow-onset dull pain in his left flank and blood in his urine. His father died of a stroke.	VS: T 37°C (98°F), P 98, BP 150/95, RR 18 Gen: WD/WN HEENT: WNL Lungs: WNL CV: WNL (no pericardial rub) Abd: Palpable, nontender mass on both flanks Ext: WNL	▪ Polycystic kidney disease ▪ Renal cell carcinoma ▪ Renal dysplasia ▪ Simple renal cysts ▪ Tuberous sclerosis ▪ Wilms' tumor

INITIAL MGMT	CONTINUING MGMT	F/U
Emergency room W/U - NPO - IV normal saline - CBC: ↓ hemoglobin - Chem 14 - PT/PTT - Serum amylase, lipase - UA - CXR - CT—abdomen: Diverticulosis	**Ward W/U** - Colonoscopy: Diverticulosis, no other source **Rx** - NPO → clear liquid diet - Surgery consult - GI consult	- Follow up in 4 weeks - Patient counseling - Counsel patient to cease alcohol intake - Smoking cessation - Dietary consult - High-fiber diet

Final Dx: Diverticulosis

INITIAL MGMT	CONTINUING MGMT	F/U
Office W/U - CBC - Chem 14 - UA: Hematuria - ESR: ↑ - PSA: ↑↑ - XR—back: Metastatic lesions in L4 and L5 - CT—lumbar spine: Mets to L4 and L5 - Echo—rectal: Multinodular enlarged prostate - Prostate biopsy: Pending **Rx** - Acetaminophen - Morphine or codeine if pain persists	**Office W/U** - Bone scan: Diffuse metastases - Prostate biopsy: Adenocarcinoma - CT—abdomen and pelvis: ⊕ for lymphatic involvement above aortic bifurcation **Rx** - Flutamide (antiandrogen therapy) or - Urology consult - Radiation oncology consult	- Patient counseling

Final Dx: Prostate cancer

INITIAL MGMT	CONTINUING MGMT	F/U
Office W/U - CBC - Chem 8 - UA: Hematuria - U/S—renal or CT—abdomen: Bilateral renal cysts, enlarged kidneys, no liver cysts - MRA—brain: No berry aneurysms **Rx** - ACEIs (eg, captopril, enalapril, lisinopril)	**Office W/U** - Nephrology consult (to look for evidence of renal insufficiency)—creatinine > 2 mg/dL - Urology consult (for nephrectomy, cyst decompression, or unroofing)	- Follow up in 8 weeks with blood testing and ultrasound - Patient counseling - Counsel patient to cease alcohol intake - Smoking cessation - Dietary consult - Low-sodium diet - Counsel patient to avoid sports

Final Dx: Polycystic kidney disease

CASE 66

HX	PE	DDX
10 yo M presents with tea-colored urine and periorbital edema. He had a fever and sore throat 1 week ago. He also complains of malaise, weakness, and anorexia.	VS: T 36°C (97.5°F), BP 140/85, HR 88, RR 18 Gen: Periorbital edema, pallor Lungs: WNL CV: WNL Abd: WNL Ext: Edema around ankles	▪ Cryoglobulinemia ▪ IgA nephropathy ▪ Membranoproliferative glomerulonephritis ▪ Poststreptococcal glomerulonephritis (PSGN)

OTHER URINARY SYMPTOMS

CASE 67

HX	PE	DDX
70 yo M complains of waking up 4–5 times a night to urinate. He also has urgency, a weak stream, and dribbling, and he needs to strain to initiate urination. He denies any weight loss, fatigue, or bone pain. He also has a sensation of incomplete evacuation of urine from the bladder.	VS: T 37°C (98.5°F), P 78, BP 140/85, RR 14 Gen: NAD Neck: WNL Lungs: WNL CV: WNL Abd: WNL Rectal exam: Enlarged, nodular, nontender, rubbery prostate gland Ext: WNL	▪ Benign prostatic hypertrophy ▪ Bladder cancer ▪ Bladder stones ▪ Bladder trauma ▪ Chronic pelvic pain ▪ Cystitis ▪ Neurogenic bladder ▪ Prostate cancer ▪ Prostatitis ▪ Urethral strictures ▪ UTI

CASE 68

HX	PE	DDX
39 yo M complains of sudden-onset fever and chills, urgency and burning on urination, and perineal pain. His symptoms started after he underwent urethral dilation for stricture.	VS: T 37.3°C (99°F), P 65, BP 101/64, RR 16 Gen: No acute distress Lungs: WNL CV: WNL Abd: Suprapubic tenderness GU: Genitalia WNL Rectal exam: Asymmetrically swollen, firm, markedly tender, hot prostate	▪ Acute cystitis ▪ Anal fistulas and fissures ▪ Epididymitis ▪ Obstructive calculus ▪ Orchitis ▪ Prostatitis ▪ Pyelonephritis ▪ Reiter's syndrome ▪ Urethritis

INITIAL MGMT	CONTINUING MGMT	F/U
Emergency room W/U ▪ CBC ▪ Chem 8 ▪ UA: Hematuria, proteinuria, RBC casts ▪ 24-hour urine protein: Proteinuria ▪ ASO titer: Normal ▪ Throat culture: Pending ▪ Total serum complement: ↓ **Rx** ▪ Furosemide ▪ Captopril ▪ Penicillin	**Office W/U** ▪ U/S—renal ▪ Throat culture: ⊕ **Rx** ▪ Furosemide ▪ Captopril ▪ Nephrology consult	▪ Follow up in 3 weeks with UA and periodic BP and BUN/Cr monitoring ▪ Family counseling ▪ Dietary consult ▪ Low-sodium diet ▪ Restrict fluid intake

Final Dx: Acute glomerulonephritis (PSGN)

INITIAL MGMT	CONTINUING MGMT	F/U
Office W/U ▪ CBC ▪ BMP: Creatinine ▪ UA ▪ Urine culture ▪ U/S—prostate ▪ ESR ▪ Total serum PSA ▪ Residual urinary volume **Rx** ▪ Finasteride ▪ Prazosin (selective short-acting α-blockers)	**Office W/U** ▪ Urology consult if refractory to treatment ▪ Urodynamic studies	▪ Follow up in 6 months with digital rectal examination and PSA ▪ Patient counseling ▪ Dietary consult

Final Dx: Benign prostatic hypertrophy (BPH)

INITIAL MGMT	CONTINUING MGMT	F/U
Office W/U ▪ UA ▪ Urine Gram stain and culture ▪ CBC ▪ Chem 8 ▪ VDRL, gonorrhea and chlamydia testing **Rx** ▪ TMP-SMX or fluoroquinolone	**Office W/U** ▪ Urology consult ▪ Cystoscopy	▪ Follow up in 4 weeks ▪ Patient counseling ▪ Counsel patient to cease alcohol intake ▪ Smoking cessation ▪ Counsel patient re safe sex practices ▪ Treat sexual partner

Final Dx: Prostatitis

CASE 69

HX	PE	DDX
21 yo M complains of a burning sensation during urination and urethral discharge. He recently began having unprotected sex with a new partner. He denies urinary frequency, urgency, fever, chills, sweats, or nausea.	VS: T 37.3°C (98.9°F), P 65, BP 101/64, RR 14 Gen: NAD Lungs: WNL CV: WNL Abd: Mild suprapubic tenderness GU: Erythema of urethral meatus, no penile lesions, pus expressed from urethra	▪ Acute cystitis ▪ Epididymitis ▪ Foreign body ▪ Nephrolithiasis ▪ Orchitis ▪ Prostatitis ▪ Pyelonephritis ▪ Reiter's syndrome ▪ Urethritis

CASE 70

HX	PE	DDX
20 yo F presents with a 2-day history of dysuria, ↑ urinary frequency, and suprapubic pain. She is sexually active only with her husband. She has no flank pain, fever, or nausea.	VS: P 65, BP 101/64, RR 16 Gen: NAD Lungs: WNL CV: WNL Abd: Mild suprapubic tenderness Pelvic: WNL	▪ Acute cystitis ▪ Nephrolithiasis ▪ PID ▪ Pyelonephritis ▪ Urethritis ▪ Vaginitis

INITIAL MGMT	CONTINUING MGMT	F/U
Office W/U • UA and urine culture • Urethral Gram stain: Many WBCs/hpf without bacteria • Urethral G&C culture (for *Neisseria gonorrhoeae* and *Chlamydia trachomatis*) • CBC • VDRL **Rx** • Azithromycin (single dose) • Ceftriaxone (single dose)		• Follow up in 4 weeks • Patient counseling • Treat partner • Counsel patient re safe sex practices

Final Dx: Urethritis

INITIAL MGMT	CONTINUING MGMT	F/U
Office W/U • UA: ↑↑ WBCs, +4 bacteria, ⊕ nitrites, ⊕ esterase • Urine culture • CBC • Chem 8 • Pregnancy test—urinary **Rx** • TMP-SMX × 3 days	**Office W/U** • Urine culture: ⊕ for *E coli* sensitive to TMP-SMX **Rx** • TMP-SMX	

Final Dx: Acute cystitis

AMENORRHEA

CASE 71

HX	PE	DDX
21 yo F complains of irregular menstrual periods every 3–5 months since menarche at age 15. She also complains of facial hair, weight gain, acne, and darkening of the skin in her axillae.	VS: T 36°C (97°F), P 80, BP 120/80, RR 14 Gen: Obese Skin: Thick hair on face, chest, and buttocks; thickened skin in axillae Lungs: WNL CV: WNL Abd: WNL Pelvic: WNL	▪ Adrenal tumor ▪ Cushing's syndrome ▪ Idiopathic hirsutism ▪ Late-onset congenital adrenal hyperplasia ▪ Ovarian neoplasm ▪ Polycystic ovarian syndrome

CASE 72

HX	PE	DDX
50 yo F presents with hot flashes and dyspareunia. Her last menstrual period was 6 months ago.	VS: T 36°C (97°F), BP 120/60, HR 70, RR 13 Gen: NAD HEENT: WNL Breast: WNL Lungs: WNL CV: WNL Abd: WNL Pelvic: Atrophy of vaginal mucosa	▪ Hyperthyroidism ▪ Hypothyroidism ▪ Menopause ▪ Pregnancy ▪ Prolactinoma

INITIAL MGMT	CONTINUING MGMT	F/U
Office W/U		▪ Follow up in 6 months
▪ DHEAS		
▪ Testosterone: ↑		
▪ Serum 17-hydroxyprogesterone		
▪ LH/FSH: ↑		
▪ Prolactin		
▪ TSH/free T$_4$		
▪ Insulin/fasting glucose		
Rx		
▪ Weight loss		
▪ Exercise program		
▪ OCPs		
▪ Spironolactone		
▪ Smoking cessation		

Final Dx: Polycystic ovarian syndrome (PCOS)

INITIAL MGMT	CONTINUING MGMT	F/U
Office W/U		▪ Follow up in 12 months
▪ Urine pregnancy test		▪ Counsel patient re HRT—not recommended unless only short-term treatment is planned and if the patient has no CAD, breast cancer, or thromboembolic risk factors
▪ Prolactin		
▪ TSH		
▪ FSH: ↑		
▪ Wet mount		
▪ Pap smear		
▪ Mammogram		
▪ DEXA scan		
Rx		
▪ Calcium		
▪ Vitamin D		
▪ SSRI for hot flashes		
▪ Premarin (vaginal estrogen)		
▪ Vaginal jelly for lubrication		

Final Dx: Menopause

CASE 73

HX	PE	DDX
14 yo F is brought into the office by her mother. The mother is concerned because her daughter is considerably shorter than her classmates and has not yet had her menses. The girl's parents are of normal height, and her sisters had their menses at age 13.	VS: Afebrile, BP 110/70, HR 70, RR 12 Gen: Short stature HEENT: Low posterior hairline, high-arched palate Neck: Short and wide Lungs: Widely spaced nipples CV: Tachycardia, irregular	▪ Constitutional growth delay ▪ Familial short stature ▪ Hypopituitarism ▪ Hypothyroidism ▪ Turner's syndrome

VAGINAL BLEEDING

CASE 74

HX	PE	DDX
21 yo F complains of prolonged and excessive menstrual bleeding and menstrual frequency for the past 6 months.	VS: T 36°C (97°F), P 65, BP 120/60, RR 14 Gen: NAD HEENT: WNL Lungs: WNL CV: WNL Abd: WNL GU: WNL	▪ Bleeding disorder ▪ Dysfunctional uterine bleeding ▪ Fibroids ▪ Hyperthyroidism ▪ Hypothyroidism ▪ Pregnancy

INITIAL MGMT	CONTINUING MGMT	F/U
Office W/U	**Office W/U**	■ Stop growth hormone when bone age > 15 years
■ TSH	■ 2D echocardiography	■ Audiogram every 3–5 years
■ FSH: ↑	■ U/S—renal	■ Check yearly for hypertension
■ LH: ↑	■ U/S—pelvis: Streaked ovaries	■ Monitor aortic root diameter every 3–5 years
■ Karyotyping: Consistent with Turner's syndrome	■ Skeletal survey: Short fourth metacarpal	
■ Lipid panel	■ Chem 13	
■ Fasting glucose	■ CBC	
Rx	■ UA	
■ Growth hormone therapy	■ Lipid profile	
■ Estrogen + progestin	■ Hearing test	
■ Psychiatry consult for IQ estimation	**Rx**	
■ Vitamin D	■ Continue growth hormone therapy until epiphysis is closed	
■ Calcium	■ Combination estrogen and progestin	
	■ Encourage weight-bearing exercises	

Final Dx: Turner's syndrome

INITIAL MGMT	CONTINUING MGMT	F/U
Office W/U		■ Follow up in 6 months
■ Qualitative urine pregnancy test		■ Counsel patient re safe sex practices
■ TSH		
■ CBC: Hypochromic microcytic anemia		
■ Bleeding time		
■ PT/aPTT, INR		
■ U/S—pelvis		
■ Pap smear		
Rx		
■ Iron sulfate		
■ NSAIDs		
■ OCPs		

Final Dx: Dysfunctional uterine bleeding

CASE 75

HX	PE	DDX
27 yo F whose last menstrual period was 7 weeks ago presents with lower abdominal cramping and heavy vaginal bleeding.	VS: T 36°C (97°F), BP 120/60, HR 80, RR 12 Gen: NAD Lungs: WNL CV: WNL Abd: Suprapubic tenderness with no rebound or guarding Pelvic: Active bleeding from cervix, cervical os open, 7-week-size uterus, mildly tender, no cervical motion tenderness, no adnexal masses or tenderness	▪ Cervical or vaginal pathology (polyp, infection, neoplasia) ▪ Cervical polyp ▪ Ectopic pregnancy ▪ Menstrual period with dysmenorrhea ▪ Spontaneous abortion

CASE 76

HX	PE	DDX
60 yo F G0 who had her last menstrual period 10 years ago presents with mild vaginal bleeding for the last 2 days. Her medical history is significant for type 2 diabetes, hypertension, and infertility.	VS: T 36°C (97°F), BP 120/60, HR 80, RR 14 Gen: NAD HEENT: WNL Lungs: WNL CV: WNL Abd: WNL Pelvic: WNL	▪ Atrophic endometritis ▪ Cervical cancer ▪ Endometrial cancer ▪ Endometrial polyp

CASE 77

HX	PE	DDX
32 yo F G2P1011 presents with vaginal bleeding after intercourse for the last month. She has no history of abnormal Pap smears or STDs and has had the same partner for the last 8 years. She uses OCPs.	VS: WNL Gen: NAD Abd: WNL Pelvic: Visible cervical lesion Rectal exam: ⊖, guaiac ⊖	▪ Cervical cancer ▪ Cervical polyp ▪ Cervicitis ▪ Ectropion ▪ Vaginal cancer ▪ Vaginitis

INITIAL MGMT	CONTINUING MGMT	F/U
Emergency room W/U - Qualitative urine pregnancy test: ⊕ - Quantitative serum β-hCG: 3000 - CBC: Hemoglobin 9 - Blood type and cross-match - Rh factor - U/S—pelvis: Intrauterine pregnancy sac, fetal pole, no fetal heart tones - Gynecology consult **Rx** - Fluids, IV normal saline - D&C	**Ward W/U** - CBC **Rx** - Methylergonovine - Doxycycline - Counsel patient re birth control - Grief counseling - Pelvic rest for 2 weeks	- Follow up in 3 weeks

Final Dx: Spontaneous abortion

INITIAL MGMT	CONTINUING MGMT	F/U
Office W/U - CBC - Chem 14 - PT/PTT, INR - Bleeding time - Pap smear - Endometrial biopsy: Poorly differentiated endometrioid adenocarcinoma - U/S—pelvis: 10-mm endometrial stripe - Gynecology consult	**Ward W/U** - CXR - ECG - CA-125 **Rx** - Exploratory laparotomy - TAH-BSO - Depending on staging, patient may benefit from adjuvant therapy (radiation vs chemo vs hormonal therapy)	

Final Dx: Endometrial cancer

INITIAL MGMT	CONTINUING MGMT	F/U
Office W/U - UA - Pap smear: HGSIL - Pelvic: Visible cervical lesion - G&C culture or PCR - Wet mount - Gynecology consult	**Office W/U** - Colposcopy - Cervical biopsy: Invasive squamous cell carcinoma of the cervix	- Radical hysterectomy vs radiation therapy - +/− adjuvant chemoradiotherapy

Final Dx: Cervical cancer

MUSCULOSKELETAL PAIN

CASE 78

HX	PE	DDX
28 yo F complains of multiple facial and bodily injuries. She claims that she fell on the stairs. She was hospitalized for some physical injuries 7 months ago. She denies any abuse.	VS: P 90, BP 120/64, RR 22, O_2 sat 95% room air Gen: Moderate distress with shallow breathing HEENT: 2.5-cm bruise on forehead; 2-cm bruise on left cheek Chest/lungs: Severe tenderness on left fifth and sixth ribs; CTA bilaterally CV: WNL Abd: WNL Ext: WNL Neuro: WNL	▪ Accident proneness ▪ Domestic violence ▪ Substance abuse

CASE 79

HX	PE	DDX
28 yo F presents with joint pain and swelling along with a butterfly-like rash over her nasal bridge and cheeks that worsens after exposure to the sun. She also reports pleuritic chest pain, shortness of breath, myalgia, and fatigue over the past few months. She says that her joint pain tends to move from joint to joint and primarily involves her hands, wrists, knees, and ankles. She also has weight loss, loss of appetite, and night sweats.	VS: T 38°C (101°F), BP 140/95, HR 80, RR 18 Gen: Pallor, fatigue HEENT: Oral ulcers, malar rash Lungs: CTA, pleural friction rub CV: WNL Abd: WNL Ext: Maculopapular rash over arms and chest; effusion in knees, wrists, and ankles	▪ Dermatomyositis ▪ Drug reaction ▪ Photosensitivity ▪ Polymyositis ▪ SLE

INITIAL MGMT	CONTINUING MGMT	F/U
Emergency room W/U ▪ XR—ribs: Fracture of left fifth and sixth ribs ▪ Urine toxicology ▪ CT—head ▪ Skeletal survey: Old fracture in forearm **Rx** ▪ Ibuprofen ▪ Oxycodone PRN ▪ Splint ▪ Assess for children at home ▪ Counsel patient re domestic abuse ▪ Counsel patient re safety plan		▪ Support group referral ▪ Social work referral

Final Dx: Domestic abuse

INITIAL MGMT	CONTINUING MGMT	F/U
Office W/U ▪ CBC: ↓ hemoglobin ▪ BMP ▪ PT/PTT ▪ ESR: ↑ ▪ Serum ANA: ⊕ ▪ UA: Proteinuria ▪ CXR ▪ Total complement: ↓ C3 and C4 **Rx** ▪ NSAIDs	**Office W/U** ▪ Anti-dsDNA or SLE prep: ⊕ ▪ Bone densitometry **Rx** ▪ Prednisone ▪ NSAIDs ▪ Rheumatology consult ▪ Nephrology consult ▪ Antimalarials ▪ Ophthalmology consult if using antimalarials	▪ Follow up in 4 weeks with UA ▪ Patient counseling ▪ Counsel patient to cease alcohol intake ▪ Smoking cessation ▪ Sunblock

Final Dx: Systemic lupus erythematosus (SLE)

CASE 80

HX	PE	DDX
35 yo M with a history of hypertension presents with pain and swelling in his left knee for the last 3 days. He was recently started on HCTZ for his hypertension. He is sexually active only with his wife and denies any history of trauma or IV drug abuse.	VS: T 38°C (100.7°F), P 80, BP 130/60, RR 12 Gen: In pain Skin: WNL HEENT: WNL Lungs: WNL CV: WNL Abd: WNL Ext: Left knee is swollen, erythematous, and tender with limited range of motion and effusion	▪ Bacterial arthritis ▪ Gout ▪ Infective endocarditis ▪ Lyme disease ▪ Pseudogout ▪ Psoriatic arthritis ▪ Reiter's arthritis

CASE 81

HX	PE	DDX
40 yo M with a history of diabetes mellitus presents with pain, swelling, and discoloration of his right leg for the last week. He denies any trauma.	VS: T 38°C (100.5°F), P 70, BP 120/60, RR 12 Gen: NAD Lungs: WNL CV: WNL Abd: WNL Ext: +2 edema in right lower extremity; warmth, erythematous discoloration of skin, 20-cm ulcer	▪ Calf tear or pull ▪ Cellulitis ▪ Deep venous thrombosis ▪ Lymphedema ▪ Osteomyelitis ▪ Popliteal (Baker's) cyst ▪ Venous insufficiency

CASE 82

HX	PE	DDX
50 yo M complains of a single episode of steady, diffuse, aching pain that affected his skeletal muscles and made it difficult for him to climb stairs. He states that he has never experienced anything like this before and that no one in his family has had a disease similar to his. Because of his ↑ LDL cholesterol, ↓ HDL cholesterol, and ↑ triglycerides, he was started on simvastatin and gemfibrozil about 1 year ago.	VS: T 37°C (99°F), P 85, BP 127/85, RR 20, O_2 sat 94% room air HEENT and neck: No dysarthria, dysphagia, diplopia, or ptosis; exam WNL Chest: WNL CV: WNL Abd: WNL Ext: Proximal muscle weakness that is more obvious in lower limbs; no evidence of myotonia	▪ Cocaine abuse ▪ Inclusion body myositis ▪ Myopathy due to drugs/toxins ▪ Myotonic dystrophy ▪ Polymyositis

INITIAL MGMT	CONTINUING MGMT	F/U
Office W/U ▪ CBC: ↑ WBC count ▪ Chem 14 ▪ ESR: ↑ ▪ PT/PTT, INR ▪ XR—left knee ▪ Joint aspiration fluid analysis: Gram stain ⊖, culture ⊖, ⊖ birefringent and needle-shaped crystals, WBC 8000 ▪ Urethral Gram stain: ⊖ **Rx** ▪ NSAIDs or corticosteroids ▪ Discontinue HCTZ and start losartan	**Ward W/U** ▪ Blood culture: ⊖ ▪ Urethral culture: ⊖ ▪ Lyme serology: ⊖ ▪ CBC: WBC is trending down **Rx** ▪ Continue NSAIDs and corticosteroids until patient improves ▪ Low-purine diet	▪ Follow up in 2 weeks in the clinic ▪ Uric acid ↑ ▪ Low-purine diet ▪ Start allopurinol or colchicine (to prevent an attack if serum uric acid > 12 or if the patient has tophaceous gout)

Final Dx: Gout

INITIAL MGMT	CONTINUING MGMT	F/U
Emergency room W/U ▪ CBC: ↑ WBC count ▪ Chem 14 ▪ PT/PTT ▪ U/S—left lower extremity: ⊖ for deep venous thrombosis ▪ ESR ▪ X-ray ▪ Blood culture: Pending **Rx** ▪ IV ampicillin-sulbactam ▪ Surgical consult: Debridement of ulcers	**Ward W/U** ▪ Blood culture: ⊖ ▪ Blood glucose: Controlled on insulin regimen ▪ CBC: WBC is trending down **Rx** ▪ Elevate the leg ▪ Switch to amoxicillin when patient is afebrile and symptoms improve (usually in 3–5 days) ▪ Discharge home	▪ Two weeks later his leg is back to normal ▪ Amoxicillin is discontinued after a course of 14 days

Final Dx: Cellulitis

INITIAL MGMT	CONTINUING MGMT	F/U
Emergency room W/U ▪ IV normal saline ▪ CBC ▪ BMP ▪ Serum CPK: ↑ ▪ LDH: ↑ ▪ EMG: Muscle injury ▪ UA: Myoglobinuria **Rx** ▪ Counsel patient re medication side effects ▪ NSAIDs	**Ward W/U** ▪ CPK, LDH: ↑ ▪ UA: ⊕ for myoglobin **Rx** ▪ Stop the offending simvastatin and gemfibrozil	▪ Follow up in 4 weeks ▪ Patient counseling ▪ Rest at home ▪ Counsel patient re medication side effects

Final Dx: Myopathy due to simvastatin and gemfibrozil

CASE 83

HX	PE	DDX
21 yo F stripper complains of hot, swollen, painful knee joints following an asymptomatic dermatitis that progressed from macules to vesicles and pustules. She admits using IV drugs, binge drinking, and having sex with multiple partners. She states that about 3 weeks ago, during a trip to Mexico, she had dysuria, frequency, and urgency during her menses, followed a few days later by bilateral conjunctivitis.	VS: T 39°C (102°F), P 122, BP 138/82, RR 28, O₂ sat 96% room air HEENT and neck: WNL Chest: Four vesicles on thoracic skin CV: WNL Abd: Three vesicles and 1 pustule on abdominal skin Ext: Knee joints are hot, swollen, and tender; ↓ ROM due to severe pain	▪ *Chlamydia trachomatis* infection ▪ *Neisseria gonorrhoeae* infection ▪ Reactive arthritis ▪ *S aureus* infection ▪ *Streptococcus* infection

CASE 84

HX	PE	DDX
25-month-old M is brought to the ER because of sudden respiratory distress. His mother does not remember the boy's immunization, developmental, or nutritional history. She calmly states that her son fell from a sofa a few days ago, and that this accident explains the boy's reluctance to walk. She adds that her son has been exposed to sick children lately and that she has used coin rubbing and cupping as folk medicine practices.	VS: T 37°C (99°F), P 129, BP 82/59, RR 40, O₂ sat 89% room air Gen: Undernourished HEENT: Circumferential cord marks around neck Lungs: Clear; pain with exam CV: Tachycardia; I/VI systolic murmur Abd: Bruising over nipples Ext: Circumferential burns of both feet and ankles with a smooth, clear-cut border; light brown bruises; pain on palpation of right lower limb Neuro/psych: Withdrawn, apprehensive	▪ Accidental trauma ▪ Child abuse ▪ Deliberate criminal violence (home invasion)

INITIAL MGMT	CONTINUING MGMT	F/U
Emergency room W/U	**Ward W/U**	■ Follow up in 1 week
■ CBC: ↑ WBC count	■ Joint fluid analysis and culture: 60,000 leukocytes/mL, ⊕ for *N gonorrhoeae*	■ Patient counseling
■ GC culture assay: ⊕	■ Throat culture	■ Counsel patient re safe sex practices
■ Blood culture: ⊖	■ Anorectal culture	■ Treat sexual partner
■ Arthrocentesis	**Rx**	■ Counsel patient to cease illegal drug use
■ Joint fluid analysis	■ Azithromycin (for *C trachomatis*), penicillin (if susceptible), ceftriaxone (if not resistant), or fluoroquinolones (if not resistant)	■ Counsel patient to cease alcohol intake
■ Joint fluid culture: Pending		■ Smoking cessation
■ Throat culture: Pending		■ Rest at home
■ Anorectal culture: Pending	■ Joint drainage and irrigation (if indicated)	
■ Urine β-hCG: ⊖	■ Arthroscopy (if indicated)	
Rx		
■ NSAIDs		
■ Antibiotics: Azithromycin (for *C trachomatis*), penicillin (if susceptible), ceftriaxone (if not resistant), or fluoroquinolones (if not resistant)		

Final Dx: Septic arthritis due to *N gonorrhoeae* infection

INITIAL MGMT	CONTINUING MGMT	F/U
Emergency room W/U	**Ward W/U**	■ Child Protective Services
■ CBC	■ Child abuse report	
■ PT/aPTT	■ Social work/Child Protective Services evaluation in hospital	
■ Electrolyte panel, BUN, creatinine	■ Ventilator (if necessary)	
■ CXR: Posterior rib fractures	■ IV fluids	
■ Skeletal survey: Posterior rib fractures; obliquely oriented callus formation in right femur		
■ CT—head: Short-length skull fractures; small subdural hemorrhages		
■ Ophthalmologic exam: Bilateral retinal hemorrhages		
Rx		
■ Admission to hospital		
■ IV fluids		
■ Neurosurgery consult		
■ Ventilator (if necessary)		

Final Dx: Nonaccidental trauma (child abuse)

CASE 85

HX	PE	DDX
36 yo F complains of malaise, anorexia, unintended weight loss, and morning stiffness together with swollen and painful wrist, knee, and ankle joints of 2 years' duration. Initially, she disregarded her symptoms, as they were insidious. However, over time they persisted and ↑ in severity. An acute disabling episode prompted her to visit the office.	VS: T 38°C (100°F), P 95, BP 132/86, RR 20, O$_2$ sat 95% room air HEENT and neck: Cervical lymphadenopathy Chest: WNL CV: WNL Ext: Symmetric wrist, knee, and ankle joint swelling with tenderness and warmth; subcutaneous nodules over both olecranon prominences; no ulnar deviation of fingers, boutonnière deformity, or swan-neck deformity; no evidence of carpal tunnel syndrome; knee valgus is observed	▪ Gout ▪ Lyme disease ▪ Osteoarthritis ▪ Paraneoplastic syndrome ▪ Rheumatoid arthritis ▪ Sarcoidosis

CASE 86

HX	PE	DDX
45 yo F bus driver comes to the clinic complaining of pain radiating down the leg that followed back pain. The pain is aggravated by coughing, sneezing, straining, or prolonged sitting.	VS: T 37°C (99°F), P 86, BP 128/86, RR 20, O$_2$ sat 93% room air Trunk: Lumbar spine mobility ↓ due to pain Ext: ⊕ straight leg raising (Lasègue) sign; ⊕ crossed straight leg sign Neuro: Weak plantar flexion of foot; loss of Achilles tendon reflex	▪ Cauda equina syndrome ▪ Compression fracture ▪ Facet joint degenerative disease ▪ Lumbar disk herniation ▪ Spinal stenosis ▪ Tumor involving the spine causing radiculopathy

INITIAL MGMT	CONTINUING MGMT	F/U
Office W/U ■ CBC: Hypochromic normocytic anemia, thrombocytosis ■ ESR: ↑ ■ XR—joints: Soft tissue swelling, juxta-articular demineralization, joint space narrowing, erosions in juxta-articular margin ■ RF: High titer **Rx** ■ Ibuprofen or celecoxib ■ Intra-articular triamcinolone (for acute disabling episodes)	**Office W/U** ■ RF: High titer ■ Joint fluid analysis: Abnormalities suggesting inflammation **Rx** ■ Methotrexate (if unresponsive to NSAIDs) ■ Etanercept (if unresponsive to methotrexate); place PPD; review vaccination history; check hepatitis titers ■ Hydroxychloroquine for mild disease	■ Follow up in 4 weeks ■ Patient counseling ■ Physical therapy ■ Occupational therapy ■ Rest at home ■ Exercise program ■ Splint extremity ■ Ophthalmologic consult if using hydrochloroquine

Final Dx: Rheumatoid arthritis

INITIAL MGMT	CONTINUING MGMT	F/U
Office W/U ■ None initially **Rx** ■ Conservative treatment ■ Pain control (NSAIDs)	**Office W/U** ■ MRI—lumbar spine: Disk herniation at L5–S1 level (MRI is not routinely ordered for a disk herniation; it is ordered if conservative treatment fails) **Rx** ■ Conservative treatment ■ Orthopedic surgery consult (if conservative treatment fails)	■ Follow up in 2 weeks ■ Patient counseling ■ Rest at home

Final Dx: Lumbar disk herniation

CHILD WITH FEVER

CASE 87

HX	PE	DDX
40-day-old M is brought to the ER because of irritability and lethargy, vomiting, and ↓ oral intake of 3 days' duration. Today his parents noted that he had a fever of 101.5°F, and he subsequently had a seizure. The baby's weight at delivery was 2500 grams, and he has been well.	VS: T 39°C (102°F), P 160, BP 77/50, RR 40, O$_2$ sat 92% room air Gen: Irritable infant Lungs: Clear CV: Tachycardia; I/VI systolic murmur Abd: WNL Neuro/psych: Bulging fontanelle, ↓ responsiveness	▪ CNS fungal infection (in immunocompromised patients) ▪ HIV infection (in immunocompromised patients) ▪ Meningitis (viral or bacterial) ▪ Osteomyelitis ▪ Pneumonia ▪ Sepsis ▪ UTI

CASE 88

HX	PE	DDX
4-month-old M is brought to the ER because of apneic episodes following a runny nose, cough, labored breathing, wheezing, and fever of 2 days' duration. His asthmatic mother was diagnosed with rubella infection during her pregnancy. The baby was delivered prematurely at 28 weeks. The boy has a history of respiratory difficulty and tachycardia, and he has missed several of his health maintenance appointments.	VS: T 39°C (102°F), P 160, BP 77/50, RR 40, O$_2$ sat 88% room air Gen: Irritable infant Lungs: Tachypnea, intercostal retractions, nasal flaring, expiratory wheezing, bilateral crackles CV: Tachycardia; continuous II/VI murmur Abd: WNL Neuro/psych: Fontanelle is soft and flat; infant is irritable	▪ Asthma ▪ CHF ▪ Cystic fibrosis ▪ Pneumonia ▪ RSV bronchiolitis

INITIAL MGMT	CONTINUING MGMT	F/U
Emergency room W/U ▪ CBC ▪ Blood cultures ▪ Electrolyte panel, BUN, creatinine, glucose ▪ CXR ▪ UA and urine culture ▪ LP: Cell count, differential, bacterial culture, viral PCR pending ▪ ABG: Metabolic acidosis, hyponatremia **Rx** ▪ Empiric IV antibiotics (ampicillin and cefotaxime) ▪ Admission to the hospital ▪ IV fluid bolus ▪ IV fluids with dextrose	**Ward W/U** ▪ Serum glucose: 75 mg/dL ▪ Urine culture: ⊖ ▪ Blood culture: ⊕ for *S pneumoniae* ▪ Ventilator (if necessary) **Rx** ▪ IV fluids, (D$_{5\frac{1}{2}}$NS) ▪ IV antibiotics × 10–14 days	▪ Follow up in 48 hours of discharge from hospital ▪ Family counseling

Final Dx: Meningitis

INITIAL MGMT	CONTINUING MGMT	F/U
Emergency room W/U ▪ CBC: WBC 14,000 ▪ Blood culture ▪ Electrolyte panel, BUN, creatinine, glucose ▪ CXR: Hyperinflation, bilateral patchy interstitial infiltrates, ↑ pulmonary blood flow, prominent left atrium and ventricle ▪ UA and urine culture ▪ ABG: Hypoxemia ▪ RSV PCR: Pending **Rx** ▪ Empiric IV antibiotics ▪ Admission to the ICU ▪ IV fluid bolus ▪ Supplemental O$_2$ ▪ Nebulized albuterol trial	**ICU W/U** ▪ Serum glucose: 70 mg/dL ▪ Urine culture: ⊖ ▪ CXR: No change ▪ Blood culture: ⊖ ▪ RSV PCR ⊕ ▪ Ventilator (if necessary) ▪ Echocardiogram: Patent ductus arteriosus **Rx** ▪ IV fluids (D$_{5\frac{1}{2}}$NS) ▪ Supplemental O$_2$ ▪ Nebulized albuterol (if effective) ▪ Cardiology consult	▪ Follow up in 48 hours of discharge from hospital ▪ Family counseling

Final Dx: Bronchiolitis with patent ductus arteriosus (PDA)

CASE 89

HX	PE	DDX
8-month-old F is brought to the urgent care clinic because of abrupt onset of fever that lasted a couple of days with 1 seizure episode (the girl and her parents were camping in a remote area). The fever resolved after a rash appeared on the girl's chest and abdomen. Her parents did not notice any lethargy, poor feeding, or vomiting. She has no history of seizures.	VS: T 37°C (100°F); other vital signs WNL HEENT and neck: Bilateral cervical lymphadenopathy, ears WNL, ophthalmologic exam WNL Trunk: Macular rash Neuro: Alert and active; no abnormalities	▪ Fifth disease ▪ Measles ▪ Meningitis ▪ Roseola infantum ▪ Rubella

CASE 90

HX	PE	DDX
3-day-old M presents to the ER with ↑ temperature, lethargy, respiratory distress, and poor feeding for the past 24 hours. His Apgar scores at birth were 6 and 8. His mother had a prolonged rupture of membranes (30 hours).	VS: T 39°C (102°F), P 170, BP 74/51, RR 70, O_2 sat 90% room air Lungs: Grunting respiration, chest indrawing with breathing, ↓ air entry CV: No murmurs or rubs Abd: Distended; ⊖ BS Neuro: Lethargy	▪ *Bordetella* lung infection ▪ *Chlamydia* lung infection ▪ Complicated congenital lung abnormalities (eg, sequestration) ▪ Foreign body causing obstruction ▪ Group B streptococcus bacterial pneumonia

INITIAL MGMT	CONTINUING MGMT	F/U
Office W/U • CBC: WNL **Rx** • Hydrate • Acetaminophen		• Follow up in 7 days or as needed • Family counseling

Final Dx: Roseola infantum (exanthem subitum)

INITIAL MGMT	CONTINUING MGMT	F/U
Emergency room W/U • CBC: ↑ WBC count • Random serum glucose: 60 mg/dL • CXR: Patchy infiltrates, pleural effusion, gastric dilation • Blood cultures: Pending • Viral culture ABG: Po_2 50 mm Hg, Pco_2 55 mm Hg **Rx** • O_2 • Fluids, $D_{5¼}NS$ • Empiric IV antibiotics • Respiratory and hemodynamic support (if necessary)	**Ward W/U** • Random serum glucose: 65 mg/dL • Blood cultures: Group B streptococcus • ABG: Po_2 60 mm Hg, Pco_2 50 mm Hg **Rx** • Antibiotics • Ventilatory and hemodynamic support (if necessary) • Antiviral drugs (if appropriate) • Bronchoscopy (if indicated)	• Follow up in 48 hours • Family counseling

Final Dx: Pneumonia

FEVER

CASE 91

HX	PE	DDX
49 yo F presents to the ER with fever of 3 days' duration. Since she turned 49 (about 7 months ago), she has had recurrent infections that have been treated with antibiotics. She has also been treated with anthracyclines and alkylating agents for another disease for the past 18 months. However, she has not seen a doctor lately. She works in a manufacturing plant that produces cosmetics.	VS: T 39°C (102°F), P 132, BP 108/77, RR 29, O_2 sat 88% room air Lungs: No evidence of consolidation CV: WNL Abd: WNL Ext: WNL Neuro: WNL	▪ Deep abscess (unknown location) ▪ Pneumonia ▪ Pyelonephritis ▪ Sepsis ▪ Severe infection (unknown location)

CASE 92

HX	PE	DDX
43 yo F presents to the ER with fever, fatigue, malaise, and diffuse musculoskeletal pain of 2 days' duration. She complains of difficulty moving her right eye. The patient has a history of diabetes mellitus and mitral valve prolapse with regurgitation.	VS: T 40°C (104°F), P 134, BP 113/83, RR 31, O_2 sat 93% room air Ophthalmology: Visual field defects, conjunctival hemorrhage Funduscopy: Abnormal spots Lungs: WNL CV: Regurgitant murmur Abd: WNL Ext: Petechiae on feet Neuro: CN III palsy	▪ Complicated pyelonephritis ▪ Infective endocarditis ▪ Infective process (undetermined location) ▪ Intracranial infection ▪ Sepsis

INITIAL MGMT	CONTINUING MGMT	F/U
Emergency room W/U ▪ CT—abdomen: WNL ▪ CBC: Neutropenia ▪ CXR: Bilateral infiltrates in both lungs ▪ Sputum cultures: ⊕ for several bacterial species, including *Klebsiella* ▪ Blood cultures: ⊕ for *Klebsiella* ▪ UA: WNL ▪ Urine cultures: ⊖ **Rx** ▪ IV antibiotics (empiric cefepime or quinolone) ▪ Acetaminophen ▪ IV normal saline	**Ward W/U** ▪ Bone marrow biopsy, needle: Low myelogenous progenitor cell lines ▪ CT—chest, spiral: Widespread bilateral infiltrates in both lungs **Rx** ▪ IV antibiotics (appropriate for *Klebsiella*); tailor antibiotics to sensitivities ▪ IV normal saline ▪ G-CSF (for neutropenia)	▪ Follow up in 4 weeks ▪ Patient counseling ▪ Counsel patient to cease alcohol intake ▪ Smoking cessation ▪ Chest physical therapy

Final Dx: Multilobar pneumonia in a neutropenic patient

INITIAL MGMT	CONTINUING MGMT	F/U
Emergency room W/U ▪ ESR: 59 mm/hr ▪ CBC : ↑WBC ▪ CXR: Some areas of patchy consolidation ▪ Blood cultures: Pending ▪ Echocardiography: Mobile mass attached to a valve ▪ ECG: RBBB ▪ UA: Microscopic hematuria **Rx** ▪ IV normal saline ▪ O_2 ▪ Empiric IV antibiotics (vancomycin, oxacillin/gentamicin) ▪ Acetaminophen	**Ward W/U** ▪ Blood cultures: ⊕ for viridans streptococci **Rx** ▪ IV antibiotics ▪ Acetaminophen ▪ IV normal saline	▪ Follow up in 4 weeks ▪ Patient counseling ▪ Counsel patient to cease alcohol intake ▪ Smoking cessation

Final Dx: Infective endocarditis

CASE 93

HX	PE	DDX
60 yo M presents with fever and altered mental status 8 hours after undergoing a diverticular abscess drainage.	VS: T 39°C (102°F), P 110, BP 60/35, RR 22, O$_2$ sat 92% on 2-L NC Gen: Acute distress HEENT: WNL Lungs: WNL CV: Tachycardia Abd: Lower abdominal tenderness Neuro: WNL	• Cardiogenic shock • Hypovolemic shock • Septic shock

CASE 94

HX	PE	DDX
17 yo F G0 whose last menstrual period was 2 days ago presents with fever, vomiting, myalgia, and a generalized skin rash.	VS: T 39°C (102°F), BP 75/30, HR 120 Gen: NAD Skin: Diffuse macular erythema; hyperemic mucous membranes Lungs: WNL CV: WNL Pelvic: Menstrual flow; foul-smelling tampon **Limited PE**	• Meningococcemia • Rocky Mountain spotted fever • Streptococcal toxic shock syndrome • Toxic shock syndrome • Typhoid fever

INITIAL MGMT	CONTINUING MGMT	F/U

Emergency room STAT

- O$_2$
- IV normal saline/central line
- Blood culture: Pending
- Wound culture
- UA and urine culture

Emergency room W/U

- CBC: ↑ WBC count
- Chem 14
- ABG: Metabolic acidosis
- ECG
- Serum amylase, lipase
- Serum lactate: 6
- Cardiac enzymes
- CXR
- CT—abdomen: Persistent diverticular abscess

Rx

- Ampicillin-gentamicin-metronidazole or piperacillin-tazobactam or ticarcillin-clavulanate

ICU W/U

- Urine output q 1 h
- 2D echocardiography
- Blood culture: ⊕ for *E coli* sensitive to gentamicin and ceftriaxone
- Wound culture: ⊕ for *E coli* sensitive to gentamicin and ceftriaxone

Rx

- Tailor antibiotics to sensitivities
- Surgery consult

Final Dx: Septic shock

INITIAL MGMT	CONTINUING MGMT	F/U

Emergency room STAT

- O$_2$ inhalation
- IV normal saline
- Tampon removal

Emergency room W/U

- CBC with differential
- Chem 14
- UA
- Blood culture: Pending
- Urine culture: Pending

Rx

- IV clindamycin + vancomycin
- Methylprednisolone

ICU W/U

- Blood culture: ⊖
- Urine culture: ⊖

Rx

- Continue IV clindamycin and vancomycin
- Wound care

Final Dx: Toxic shock syndrome

OUTPATIENT POTPOURRI

CASE 95

HX	PE	DDX
50 yo F presents with a painless lump in her right breast. She first noted this mass 1 month ago. There is no nipple discharge.	VS: Afebrile, P 70, BP 110/50, RR 12 Gen: NAD Skin: WNL HEENT: WNL Lymph nodes: ⊖ Breast: 3-cm, hard, immobile, nontender mass with irregular borders; no nipple discharge Lungs: WNL CV: WNL Abd: WNL	▪ Breast cancer ▪ Fibroadenoma ▪ Fibrocystic disease ▪ Mastitis ▪ Papillomas

CASE 96

HX	PE	DDX
62 yo F complains of vaginal itching, painful intercourse, and a clear discharge.	VS: WNL Gen: NAD Lungs: WNL CV: WNL Pelvic: Vulvar erythema, thin and pale mucosa with areas of erythema, clear discharge, mucosa bleeds easily during exam	▪ Atrophic vaginitis ▪ Bacterial vaginosis ▪ Candidal vaginitis ▪ Cervicitis (chlamydia, gonorrhea) ▪ Trichomonal vaginitis

CASE 97

HX	PE	DDX
33 yo Rh-negative F who currently lives in a battered-women's shelter calls the on-call physician because she noticed ↓ fetal movements. She is a G1P0 pregnant F at 36 weeks' gestational age. She states that fetal growth has been normal and that her obstetric ultrasound at 18 weeks showed a single normal fetus. The patient has no known preexisting diseases and does not smoke, drink alcohol, or take medications or illicit drugs. She received a dose of anti-D at 28 weeks.	VS: T 37°C (99°F), P 96, BP 141/91, RR 26, O_2 sat 93% room air Gen: No jaundice Eyes: Normal vision Lungs: No rales CV: No gallops or murmurs Pelvic: Fundal height in centimeters is appropriate for gestational age; cephalic presentation; speculum exam reveals unripe cervix, no ferning, Nitrazine ⊖ Ext: Slight pedal edema	▪ Preeclampsia ▪ Pregnancy-induced hypertension

INITIAL MGMT	CONTINUING MGMT	F/U

Office W/U
- Mammography: Suspicious of tumor
- FNA biopsy: Malignancy

Rx
- Surgery consult

Final Dx: Breast cancer

INITIAL MGMT	CONTINUING MGMT	F/U

Office W/U
- Vaginal pH: 6
- Chlamydia PCR
- Gonorrhea PCR
- Wet mount
- Pap smear

Rx
- Vaginal jelly for lubrication
- Counsel patient re local HRT
- Premarin (vaginal estrogen)

F/U:
- Follow up as needed

Final Dx: Atrophic vaginitis

INITIAL MGMT	CONTINUING MGMT	F/U

Office W/U
- BUN, creatinine, ALT, AST
- CBC
- Chem 8
- UA: ⊕ protein
- Random serum glucose
- Serum uric acid

Rx
- Complete bed rest
- Monitor, continue BP cuff
- Fetal monitoring

Ward W/U
- UA: Protein 0.3 g/L/24 hrs; normal sediment
- LFTs: WNL

Rx
- Complete bed rest
- Monitor, continue BP cuff
- Fetal monitoring

F/U:
- Patient counseling
- Admit to labor and delivery for induction of labor
- Obstetric consult

Final Dx: Antenatal disorder: Pregnancy-induced hypertension

CASE 98

HX	PE	DDX
30 yo F presents for her regular checkup. She denies any complaints but is concerned about her BP, as it has been high on both of her previous visits over the past 2 months.	VS: P 75, BP 160/90 (no difference in BP between both arms), RR 12 Gen: WNL HEENT: WNL Breast: WNL Lungs: WNL CV: WNL Abd: WNL Pelvic: WNL Ext: WNL Neuro: WNL	▪ Cushing's disease ▪ Essential hypertension ▪ Hyperaldosteronism ▪ Hyperthyroidism ▪ Pheochromocytoma ▪ Renal artery stenosis ▪ White coat hypertension/anxiety

CASE 99

HX	PE	DDX
6 yo M is brought by his mother with continuous oozing of blood from the site of a tooth extraction he underwent 2 days ago. The bleeding initially stopped but restarted spontaneously a few hours later. His mother denies any history of epistaxis, easy bruising, petechiae, or bleeding per rectum. The patient's mother has a brother with hemophilia.	VS: Afebrile, P 80, BP 80/50, RR 14 Gen: NAD Skin: WNL HEENT: Blood oozing from site of extracted tooth Lungs: WNL CV: WNL Abd: WNL Ext: WNL	▪ DIC ▪ Hemophilia ▪ ITP ▪ Liver disease ▪ TTP ▪ Vitamin K deficiency ▪ von Willebrand's disease

CASE 100

HX	PE	DDX
27 yo F complains of pain during intercourse. She has a long history of painful periods.	VS: WNL Gen: NAD Lungs: WNL CV: WNL Pelvic: Normal vaginal walls, normal cervix, mild cervical motion tenderness; uterus tender, retroverted, and fixed; right adnexa slightly enlarged and tender	▪ Endometriosis ▪ PID ▪ Vaginismus ▪ Vaginitis

INITIAL MGMT	CONTINUING MGMT	F/U
Office W/U - Lipid profile - Chem 14 - CBC - UA: +1 protein - ECG: LVH - Echocardiography: LVH - TSH **Rx** - Lisinopril - Exercise program - Low-sodium diet	**Office W/U** - Consider workup for 2° hypertension given the patient's young age (MRI/MRA renal arteries, urine catecholamines, urine cortisol)	- Follow up in 1 month

Final Dx: Essential hypertension

INITIAL MGMT	CONTINUING MGMT	F/U
Office W/U - CBC - Peripheral smear - Bleeding time - PTT: Prolonged - PT, INR - Plasma factor VIII: 3% - Plasma factor IX **Rx** - Factor VIII therapy - Genetics consult - Counsel parents		- Console and reassure patient - Patient counseling - Family counseling

Final Dx: Hemophilia

INITIAL MGMT	CONTINUING MGMT	F/U
Office W/U - Wet mount - Chlamydia DNA probe - Gonorrhea DNA probe - U/S—pelvis: Retroverted uterus of normal size; 2- × 3-cm cyst on the right adnexa that may represent a hemorrhagic corpus luteum or endometrioma **Rx** - NSAIDs - OCPs		- If initial treatment with OCPs and NSAIDs does not relieve pain, refer to a gynecologist for a trial of GnRH analogs, progestins, or danazol. - Follow up as needed

Final Dx: Endometriosis

NOTES

APPENDIX

ACRONYMS AND ABBREVIATIONS

Abbreviation	Meaning
A-a	alveolar-arterial (oxygen gradient)
AAA	abdominal aortic aneurysm
ABC	airway, breathing, circulation
ABG	arterial blood gas
AC	alternating current
ACA	anterior cerebral artery
ACE	angiotensin-converting enzyme
ACEI	angiotensin-converting enzyme inhibitor
ACh	acetylcholine
ACL	anterior cruciate ligament
ACLS	advanced cardiac life support (protocol)
ACM	Advanced Clinical Medicine
ACTH	adrenocorticotropic hormone
ADA	American Diabetes Association
ADH	antidiuretic hormone
ADHD	attention-deficit hyperactivity disorder
AF	atrial fibrillation
AFB	acid-fast bacillus
AFI	amniotic fluid index
AFP	α-fetoprotein
AG	anion gap
AHI	apnea-hypopnea index
AICD	automatic implantable cardiac defibrillator
AIDS	acquired immunodeficiency syndrome
AKI	acute kidney injury
ALL	acute lymphocytic leukemia
ALS	amyotrophic lateral sclerosis
ALT	alanine aminotransferase
AMA	antimitochondrial antibody
AML	acute myelogenous leukemia
ANA	antinuclear antibody
ANC	absolute neutrophil count
ANCA	antineutrophil cytoplasmic antibody
AP	anteroposterior
APC	activated protein C
APL	acute promyelocytic leukemia
ARB	angiotensin receptor blocker
ARDS	acute respiratory distress syndrome
ARR	absolute risk reduction
ART	antiretroviral therapy
5-ASA	5-aminosalicylic acid
ASCA	anti–*Saccharomyces cerevisiae* antibody
ASD	atrial septal defect
ASMA	anti–smooth muscle antibody

Abbreviation	Meaning
AST	aspartate aminotransferase
ATN	acute tubular necrosis
ATRA	*all*-transretinoic acid
AV	arteriovenous, atrioventricular
AVM	arteriovenous malformation
AVNRT	atrioventricular nodal reentrant tachycardia
AXR	abdominal x-ray
AZT	zidovudine
BCG	bacille Calmette-Guérin
BiPAP	bilateral positive airway pressure
BMI	body mass index
BMP	basic metabolic panel
BMT	bone marrow transplantation
BP	blood pressure
BPH	benign prostatic hyperplasia
BPP	biophysical profile
BSA	body surface area
BSO	bilateral salpingo-oophorectomy
BUN	blood urea nitrogen
CABG	coronary artery bypass graft
CAD	coronary artery disease
CAH	congenital adrenal hyperplasia
CBC	complete blood count
CBT	cognitive-behavioral therapy
CCB	calcium channel blocker
CCP	cyclic citrullinated peptide
CCS	Computer-based Case Simulations
CD	cluster of differentiation
CEA	carcinoembryonic antigen
CF	cystic fibrosis
CGD	chronic granulomatous disease
CH_{50}	total hemolytic complement
CHF	congestive heart failure
CI	confidence interval
CIN	Candidate Identification Number, cervical intraepithelial neoplasia
CK	creatine kinase
CKD	chronic kidney disease
CK-MB	creatine kinase, MB fraction
CLL	chronic lymphocytic leukemia
CML	chronic myelogenous leukemia
CMV	cytomegalovirus
CN	cranial nerve
CNS	central nervous system

Abbreviation	Meaning
COBI	cobicistat
COMT	catechol-O-methyltransferase
COPD	chronic obstructive pulmonary disease
CPAP	continuous positive airway pressure
CPR	cardiopulmonary resuscitation
CrCl	creatinine clearance
CRP	C-reactive protein
CRT	cardiac resynchronization therapy
CSA	central sleep apnea
CSF	cerebrospinal fluid
CST	contraction stress test
CT	computed tomography
CVA	costovertebral angle
CVID	common variable immunodeficiency
CXR	chest x-ray
D&C	dilation and curettage
DBP	diastolic blood pressure
DC	direct current
DCIS	ductal carcinoma in situ
DDAVP	desmopressin acetate
ddI	didanosine
DES	diethylstilbestrol
DEXA	dual-energy x-ray absorptiometry
DFA	direct fluorescent antibody
DHEA	dehydroepiandrosterone
DI	diabetes insipidus
DIC	disseminated intravascular coagulation
DIP	distal interphalangeal (joint)
DKA	diabetic ketoacidosis
DL_{CO}	diffusing capacity of carbon monoxide
DM	diabetes mellitus
DMARD	disease-modifying antirheumatic drug
DNA	deoxyribonucleic acid
DNR	do not resuscitate
DPoA	durable power of attorney
DPP	dipeptidyl peptidase
DRE	digital rectal examination
dsDNA	double-stranded DNA
DSM	Diagnostic and Statistical Manual of Mental Disorders
DTG	dolutegravir
DTRs	deep tendon reflexes
DTs	delirium tremens
DVT	deep venous thrombosis
EBV	Epstein-Barr virus
ECFMG	Educational Commission for Foreign Medical Graduates
ECG	electrocardiography
ECMO	extracorporeal membrane oxygenation
ECT	electroconvulsive therapy
ED	emergency department, erectile dysfunction
EEG	electroencephalography
EF	ejection fraction
EGD	esophagogastroduodenoscopy
EHEC	enterohemorrhagic *E coli*

Abbreviation	Meaning
ELISA	enzyme-linked immunosorbent assay
EM	erythema multiforme
ENT	ear, nose, and throat
EPS	extrapyramidal symptoms
ER	estrogen receptor
ERCP	endoscopic retrograde cholangiopancreatography
ESR	erythrocyte sedimentation rate
ESWL	extracorporeal shock-wave lithotripsy
EtOH	ethanol
EUS	endoscopic ultrasound
EVG	elvitegravir
FAP	familial adenomatous polyposis
FAST	focused abdominal sonography for trauma
Fe_{Na}	fractional excretion of sodium
Fe_{urea}	fractional excretion of urea
FEV_1	forced expiratory volume in one second
FFP	fresh frozen plasma
FIP	Foundations of Independent Practice
FISH	fluorescence in situ hybridization
FNA	fine-needle aspiration
FOBT	fecal occult blood test
FSH	follicle-stimulating hormone
FSMB	Federation of State Medical Boards
FTA-ABS	fluorescent treponemal antibody absorption (test)
FTC	emtricitabine
FTT	failure to thrive
5-FU	5-fluorouracil
FVC	forced vital capacity
FWS	fever without a source
G&C	gonorrhea and chlamydia (culture)
G6PD	gluciose-6-phosphate dehydrogenase
GA	gestational age
GAD	generalized anxiety disorder
GBM	glomerular basement membrane
GBS	group B streptococcus, Guillain-Barré syndrome
GCS	Glasgow Coma Scale
G-CSF	granulocyte colony-stimulating factor
GDPP	gonadotropin-dependent precocious puberty
GERD	gastroesophageal reflux disease
GFR	glomerular filtration rate
GGT	gamma-glutamyl transferase
GI	gastrointestinal
GIPP	gonadotropin-independent precocious puberty
GLP	glucagon-like peptide
GNR	gram-negative rod
GnRH	gonadotropin-releasing hormone
GTCS	generalized tonic-clonic seizure
GTD	gestational trophoblastic disease
GU	genitourinary
H&P	history and physical
HAV	hepatitis A virus
HbA_{1c}	hemoglobin A_{1c}

Abbreviation	Meaning
HBcAb	hepatitis B core antibody
HBeAg	hepatitis B early antigen
HBIG	hepatitis B immune globulin
HBsAb	hepatitis B surface antibody
HBsAg	hepatitis B surface antigen
HBV	hepatitis B virus
HCC	hepatocellular cancer
hCG	human chorionic gonadotropin
HCTZ	hydrochlorothiazide
HCV	hepatitis C virus
HD	Huntington's disease
HDL	high-density lipoprotein
HDV	hepatitis D virus
HEENT	head, eyes, ears, nose, and throat
HEV	hepatitis E virus
HFpEF	heart failure with preserved ejection fraction
HGSIL	high-grade squamous intraepithelial lesion
HHS	hyperglycemic hyperosmolar state
HHV	human herpesvirus
5-HIAA	5-hydroxyindoleacetic acid
HIDA	hepato-iminodiacetic acid (scan)
HIPAA	Health Insurance Portability and Accountability Act
HIT	heparin-induced thrombocytopenia
HIV	human immunodeficiency virus
HLA	human leukocyte antigen
HMG-CoA	hydroxymethylglutaryl coenzyme A
HNPCC	hereditary nonpolyposis colorectal cancer
HPA	hypothalamic-pituitary-adrenal (axis)
hpf	high-power field
HPV	human papillomavirus
HR	heart rate
HRIG	human rabies immune globulin
HRT	hormone replacement therapy
HSP	Henoch-Schönlein purpura
HSV	herpes simplex virus
5-HT	5-hydroxytryptamine
HTLV	human T-cell lymphotropic virus
HUS	hemolytic-uremic syndrome
HVA	homovanillic acid
IBD	inflammatory bowel disease
IBS	irritable bowel syndrome
ICH	intracerebral hemorrhage
ICP	intracranial pressure
ICU	intensive care unit
IE	infective endocarditis
Ig	immunoglobulin
IM	intramuscular
IMG	international medical graduate
INH	isoniazid
INR	International Normalized Ratio
INSTI	integrase strand transfer inhibitor
IPT	interpersonal psychotherapy
ITP	idiopathic thrombocytopenic purpura
IUD	intrauterine device

Abbreviation	Meaning
IUGR	intrauterine growth restriction
IV	intravenous
IVC	inferior vena cava
IVIG	intravenous immunoglobulin
IVP	intravenous pyelography
IVS	interventricular septum
JIA	juvenile idiopathic arthritis
JVD	jugular venous distention
JVP	jugular venous pressure
KOH	potassium hydroxide
KUB	kidney, ureter, bladder (study)
LAD	left anterior descending (artery)
LBBB	left bundle branch block
LBP	low back pain
LCIS	lobular carcinoma in situ
LDH	lactate dehydrogenase
LDL	low-density lipoprotein
LEEP	loop electrosurgical excision procedure
LES	lower esophageal sphincter
LFT	liver function test
LGSIL	low-grade squamous intraepithelial lesion
LH	luteinizing hormone
LKMA	liver/kidney microsomal antibody
LLQ	left lower quadrant
LMN	lower motor neuron
LMP	last menstrual period
LMWH	low-molecular-weight heparin
LP	lumbar puncture
LTBI	latent tuberculosis infection
LUQ	left upper quadrant
LV	left ventricle
LVEF	left ventricular ejection fraction
LVH	left ventricular hypertrophy
MAC	*Mycobacterium avium* complex
MAOI	monoamine oxidase inhibitor
MAT	multifocal atrial tachycardia
MCA	middle cerebral artery
MCHC	mean corpuscular hemoglobin concentration
MCI	mild cognitive impairment
MCP	metacarpophalangeal (joint)
MCV	mean corpuscular volume
MDD	major depressive disorder
MDI	metered-dose inhaler, multiple daily injection
MDRD	Modification of Diet in Renal Disease (equation)
MDRO	multi-drug-resistant organism
MEN	multiple endocrine neoplasia
MG	myasthenia gravis
MGUS	monoclonal gammopathy of undetermined significance
MHA-TP	microhemagglutination assay for *Treponema pallidum*
MI	myocardial infarction
MIBG	^{131}I-metaiodobenzylguanidine (scan)
MLF	medial longitudinal fasciculus

Abbreviation	Meaning
MMA	methylmalonic acid
MMR	measles, mumps, rubella (vaccine)
MoM	multiple of the mean
MPGN	membranoproliferative glomerulonephritis
MRA	magnetic resonance angiography
MRI	magnetic resonance imaging
MRSA	methicillin-resistant *S aureus*
MS	multiple sclerosis
MSAFP	maternal serum α-fetoprotein
MTP	metatarsophalangeal (joint)
MuSK	muscle-specific kinase
MVA	motor vehicle accident
NAD	no acute distress
NBME	National Board of Medical Examiners
NBTE	nonbacterial thrombotic endocarditis
NCS	nerve conduction study
NE	norepinephrine
NEC	necrotizing enterocolitis
NG	nasogastric
NK	natural killer (cells)
NMDA	N-methyl-D-aspartate
NNRTI	non-nucleoside reverse transcriptase inhibitor
NNT	number needed to treat
NPO	nil per os (nothing by mouth)
NPV	negative predictive value
NRTI	nucleoside reverse transcriptase inhibitor
NS	normal saline
NSAID	nonsteroidal anti-inflammatory drug
NSCLC	non–small cell lung cancer
NST	nonstress test
NSTEMI	non-ST-segment-elevation MI
NTD	neural tube defect
O&P	ova and parasites
OA	osteoarthritis
OCD	obsessive-compulsive disorder
OCP	oral contraceptive pill
17-OHP	17-hydroxyprogesterone
OR	odds ratio, operating room
OSA	obstructive sleep apnea
OTC	over the counter
PA	posteroanterior
PAC	plasma aldosterone concentration, premature atrial contraction
PAN	polyarteritis nodosa
p-ANCA	perinuclear antineutrophil cytoplasmic antibody
Pao_2	partial pressure of oxygen in arterial blood
$Paco_2$	partial pressure of carbon dioxide in arterial blood
PAPP-A	pregnancy-associated plasma protein A
PCA	posterior cerebral artery
PCL	posterior cruciate ligament
Pco_2	partial pressure of carbon dioxide
PCOS	polycystic ovarian syndrome
PCP	phencyclidine hydrochloride, *Pneumocystis carinii* (now *jiroveci*) pneumonia
P_{Cr}	plasma creatinine
PCR	polymerase chain reaction
PCV	polycythemia vera
PCWP	pulmonary capillary wedge pressure
PD	Parkinson's disease
PDA	patent ductus arteriosus, posterior descending artery
PDE-5a	phosphodiesterase type 5a
PE	pulmonary embolism
PEA	pulseless electrical activity
PEEP	positive end-expiratory pressure
PEG	polyethylene glycol
PET	positron emission tomography (scan)
PF	platelet factor
PFT	pulmonary function test
$PGF_{2\alpha}$	prostaglandin F2-α
PI	protease inhibitor
PID	pelvic inflammatory disease
PIP	proximal interphalangeal (joint)
PIV	parainfluenza virus
PMI	point of maximal impulse
PMN	polymorphonuclear (leukocyte)
PMR	polymyalgia rheumatica
P_{Na}	plasma sodium
PNH	paroxysmal nocturnal hemoglobinuria
PNS	peripheral nervous system
PO	per os (by mouth)
POC	product of conception
P_{osm}	plasma osmolarity
PPD	purified protein derivative (of tuberculin)
PPI	proton pump inhibitor
PPROM	preterm premature rupture of membranes
PPV	positive predictive value
PR	progesterone receptor
PRA	plasma renin activity
PRN	pro re nata (as needed)
PROM	premature rupture of membranes
PSA	prostate-specific antigen
PSGN	poststreptococcal glomerulonephritis
PT	prothrombin time
PTH	parathyroid hormone
PTHrP	parathyroid hormone–related peptide
PTSD	posttraumatic stress disorder
PTT	partial thromboplastin time
PTU	propylthiouracil
PUD	peptic ulcer disease
PUVA	psoralen and ultraviolet A
PVC	premature ventricular contraction
PVS	persistent vegetative state
RA	rheumatoid arthritis
RAA	renin-angiotensin-aldosterone (system)
RAI	radioactive iodine
RAL	raltegravir
RAST	radioallergosorbent testing
RBBB	right bundle branch block

Abbreviation	Meaning
RBC	red blood cell
RC	reticulocyte count
RCA	right coronary artery
RCT	randomized controlled trial
RDS	respiratory distress syndrome
RDW	red cell distribution width
REM	rapid eye movement
RF	rheumatoid factor
RLQ	right lower quadrant
ROM	rupture of membranes
RPR	rapid plasma reagin
RR	relative risk
RRR	regular rate and rhythm, relative risk reduction
RSV	respiratory syncytial virus
RTA	renal tubular acidosis
RUQ	right upper quadrant
RV	residual volume, right ventricle
RVH	right ventricular hypertrophy
SA	sinoatrial
SAAG	serum-ascites albumin gradient
SAB	spontaneous abortion
SAD	seasonal affective disorder
SAH	subarachnoid hemorrhage
SBFT	small bowel follow-through
SBI	serious bacterial infection
SBP	spontaneous bacterial peritonitis, systolic blood pressure
SCID	severe combined immunodeficiency
SCLC	small cell lung cancer
SERM	selective estrogen receptor modulator
SES	socioeconomic status
SIADH	syndrome of inappropriate secretion of antidiuretic hormone
SIDS	sudden infant death syndrome
SIFE	serum immunofixation electrophoresis
SIRS	systemic inflammatory response syndrome
SLE	systemic lupus erythematosus
SMA	superior mesenteric artery
SNRI	serotonin-norepinephrine reuptake inhibitor
SPEP	serum protein electrophoresis
SPN	solitary pulmonary nodule
SQ	subcutaneous
SSRI	selective serotonin reuptake inhibitor
STD	sexually transmitted disease
STEMI	ST-segment-elevation MI
SVO_2	mixed venous oxygen saturation
SVR	systemic vascular resistance
SVT	supraventricular tachycardia
T_3	triiodothyronine
T_4	thyroxine
TAH	total abdominal hysterectomy
TB	tuberculosis
3TC	lamivudine
Tc	technetium

Abbreviation	Meaning
TCA	tricyclic antidepressant
Td	tetanus and diphtheria toxoid
TD	traveler's diarrhea
TdT	terminal deoxynucleotidyl transferase
TEE	transesophageal echocardiography
TENS	transcutaneous electrical nerve stimulation
TGA	transposition of the great arteries
TIA	transient ischemic attack
TIBC	total iron-binding capacity
TIG	tetanus immune globulin
TIPS	transjugular intrahepatic portosystemic shunt
TLC	total lung capacity
TMP-SMX	trimethoprim-sulfamethoxazole
TNF	tumor necrosis factor
TNV	tenofovir
tPA	tissue plasminogen activator
TPN	total parenteral nutrition
TPO	thyroperoxidase
TRALI	transfusion-related acute lung injury
TSH	thyroid-stimulating hormone
TSS	toxic shock syndrome
TSS-T	toxic shock syndrome toxin
TTE	transthoracic echocardiography
TTP	thrombotic thrombocytopenic purpura
TURP	transurethral resection of the prostate
UA	urinalysis
U_{Cr}	urine creatinine
UIFE	urine immunofixation electrophoresis
UMN	upper motor neuron
U_{Na}	urine sodium
U_{osm}	urine osmolarity
UPEP	urine protein electrophoresis
URI	upper respiratory infection
USMLE	United States Medical Licensing Examination
USPSTF	United States Preventive Services Task Force
UTI	urinary tract infection
UV	ultraviolet
VCUG	voiding cystourethrography
VDRL	Venereal Disease Research Laboratory
VF	ventricular fibrillation
VIP	vasoactive intestinal peptide
VMA	vanillylmandelic acid
V/Q	ventilation-perfusion (ratio)
VRE	vancomycin-resistant enterococcus
VS	vital signs
VSD	ventricular septal defect
VT	ventricular tachycardia
VTE	venous thromboembolism
vWD	von Willebrand's disease
vWF	von Willebrand's factor
VZV	varicella-zoster virus
WBC	white blood cell
WD/WN	well developed, well nourished
WNL	within normal limits

NOTES

Index

NOTES

NOTES

NOTES